ANESTHESIA AND ORTHOPAEDIC SURGERY

ANESTHESIA AND ORTHOPAEDIC SURGERY

Editor

André P. Boezaart, MB ChB, MPraxMed, DA(CMSA), FFA(CMSA), MMed(Anaesth), PhD
Professor of Anesthesia and Orthopaedic Surgery
Director, Orthopaedic Anesthesia
Director, Regional Anesthesia Study Center of Iowa (RASCI)
University of Iowa
Iowa City, Iowa

Artwork by
Mary K. Bryson

McGraw-Hill
Medical Publishing Division

New York   Chicago   San Francisco   Lisbon   London   Madrid   Mexico City   Milan
New Delhi   San Juan   Seoul   Singapore   Sydney   Toronto

Anesthesia and Orthopaedic Surgery

1 2 3 4 5 6 7 8 9 0   CTP/CTP   0 9 8 7 6

ISBN: 0-07-144686-9

This book was set in Garamond by International Typesetting and Composition.
The editors were Joe Rusko, Robert Pancotti, and Lester A. Sheinis.
The production supervisor was Catherine H. Saggese.
The artwork was prepared by Mary K. Bryson, copyright © Bryson Biomedical Illustrations.
The cover designer was Mary McKeon.
The indexer was Alexandra Nickerson.
China Translation & Printing Services, Ltd., was printer and binder.

This book is printed on acid-free paper.

Library of Congress Cataloging-in-Publication Data

Anesthesia and orthopaedic surgery / editor, André P. Boezaart; artwork by Mary K. Bryson.
    p. cm.
    Includes bibliographical references and index.
    ISBN 0-07-144686-9 (alk. paper)
    1. Anesthesia in orthopedics. I. Boezaart, André P.

RD751.A52 2006
617.9'6747—dc22

                                                          2005054500

This work is dedicated to the loving memory of Anneli,
who was taken from us far too soon.

CONTENTS

PART IV Miscellaneous Topics

CONTRIBUTORS

Brian D. Adams, MD *(Chapters 8, 9)*
Professor of Orthopaedics
Department of Orthopaedics and Rehabilitation
University of Iowa
Iowa City, Iowa

Annunziato (Ned) Amendola, MD, FRCS(C)
(Chapter 17)
Professor of Orthopaedic Surgery
Department of Orthopaedic Surgery and
   Rehabilitation
Director, Sports Medicine
University of Iowa
Iowa City, Iowa

**Anthony G. Beeton, MB ChB, DA(CMSA),
FFA(CMSA)** *(Chapter 4)*
Anesthesiologist in Private Practice
Auckland Park
South Africa

G. Michael Blanchard, Jr., MD *(Chapter 17)*
Baton Rouge Orthopaedic Clinic
Baton Rouge, Louisiana

André P. Boezaart *(Chapters 4, 7, 8, 9, 10, 11, 12,
14, 15, 16, 17, 20, 23, 28)*
Professor of Anesthesia and Orthopaedic Surgery
Director, Orthopaedic Anesthesia
Director, Regional Anesthesia Study Center of
   Iowa (RASCI)
Department of Anesthesia and Orthopaedic Surgery
University of Iowa
Iowa City, Iowa

Steven C. Borene, MD *(Chapters 27, 33)*
Anesthesiologist
North Iowa Anesthesia Associates
Mason City, Iowa
Faculty, Regional Anesthesiology Study Center
   of Iowa (RASCI)
Iowa City, Iowa

Adrian T. Bösenberg, MB ChB, DA(SA), FFA(CMSA)
(Chapters 6, 31)
Professor and Second Chair
Department of Anesthesia
Faculty of Health Sciences
University of Cape Town
Cape Town, South Africa
Red Cross War Memorial Children's Hospital
Rondebosch, South Africa

Chester C. Buckenmaier III, MD *(Chapter 34)*
Lieutenant Colonel, United States Marine Corps
Chief, Army Regional Anesthesia and Pain
   Management Initiative
Assistant Professor of University Uniformed
   Services
Walter Reed Army Medical Center
Washington, DC

John J. Callaghan, MD *(Chapters 10, 11)*
Professor of Orthopaedics and Biomedical
   Engineering
Department of Orthopaedic Surgery and
   Rehabilitation
University of Iowa
Iowa City, Iowa

Xavier Capdevila, MD, PhD *(Chapter 29)*
Professor and Head
Chu de Montpellier
Hôpital Lapeyronie
Département d'Anesthesie et Réanimation A
Montpellier, France

Vincent W. S. Chan, MD, FRCPC *(Chapter 22)*
Professor of Anesthesia
The Toronto Hospital
Anesthesia Western Division
Toronto, Ontario, Canada

Jacques E. Chelly, MD, PhD, MBA *(Chapter 1)*
Professor of Anesthesia and Orthopedic Surgery
Vice-Chair of Clinical Research
Department of Anesthesiology
University of Pittsburgh Medical Center
Director of Orthopedic Anesthesia and Acute
  Interventional Pain Service
Department of Anesthesiology
University of Pittsburgh Medical Center
  Presbyterian-Shadyside Hospital
Pittsburgh, Pennsylania

**André R. Coetzee, MB ChB, PhD, MMed(Anes),
FFA(SA), FFARCS(Ireland), MD, PhD**
(Chapter 5)
Professor and Chairman
Department of Anesthesiology and Critical Care
School of Medicine
Faculty of Health Sciences
University of Stellenbosch
Tygerberg, South Africa

Carlo D. Franco, MD *(Chapters 23, 27)*
Chairman, Orthopedic Anesthesiology
Department of Anesthesiology
John H. Stroger Jr. Hospital of Cook County
Chicago, Illinois

Vijaya Gottumukkala, MB BS, MD(Anes), FRCA
(Chapter 12)
Associate Professor and Associate Clinical Director
University of Texas
M.D. Anderson Cancer Center
Houston, Texas

Basem Hamid, MD *(Chapter 32)*
Assistant Professor of Anesthesia
Assistant Professor of Neurology
Department of Anesthesia
University of Iowa
Iowa City, Iowa

William Harrop-Griffiths, MB BS, FRCA *(Chapter 25)*
Department of Anesthesia and Perioperative
  Medicine
Royal Brisbane and Women's Hospital
Herston, Queensland, Australia

Daniel G. Hoernschemeyer, MD *(Chapter 13)*
Assistant Professor of Orthopaedic Surgery
Department of Orthopaedic Surgery
  (Pediatric Orthopaedics)
University of Missouri
Columbia, Missouri

**Dominique Hopkins, DUES(France),
BSc(Hons), PhD, MB ChB, FFA(CMSA), FANZCA**
(Chapter 19)
Department of Anesthesia and Perioperative
  Medicine
Royal Brisbane and Women's Hospital
Herston, Queensland, Australia

Morgan H. Jones, MD *(Chapter 17)*
Associate Staff Orthopaedic Surgeon
Department of Orthopaedic Surgery
Cleveland Clinic Foundation
Cleveland, Ohio

R. Kumar Kadiyala, MD, PhD *(Chapter 7)*
Director of Upper Extremity Surgery
Department of Orthopaedic Surgery
Mount Sinai Medical Center
Miami Beach, Florida

Todd McKinley, MD *(Chapter 16)*
Assistant Professor
Department of Orthopaedic Surgery and Rehabilitation
University of Iowa
Iowa City, Iowa

Sergio Mendoza-Lattes, MD *(Chapter 14)*
Assistant Professor of Orthopaedic Surgery
Department of Orthopaedic Surgery and
  Rehabilitation
University of Iowa Hospitals and Clinics
Iowa City, Iowa

**John A. Myburgh, MB BCh, PhD, DA(SA), FANZCA,
FJFICM** *(Chapter 2)*
Director of Research
Senior Consultant in Intensive Care Medicine
Associate Professor, Faculty of Medicine
University of New South Wales
Department of Intensive Care Medicine
St. George Hospital
Sydney, New South Wales, Australia

Marie-Josée Nadeau, MD, FRCPC *(Chapter 29)*
Chu de Montpellier
Hôpital Lapeyronie
Département d'Anesthesie et Réanimation A
Montpellier, France

Michael R. O'Rourke, MD *(Chapters 10, 11)*
Assistant Professor
Department of Orthopaedic Surgery and
  Rehabilitation
University of Iowa Hospitals and Clinics
Iowa City, Iowa

Milton Raff, BSc, MB ChB, FCA(SA)
(Chapter 30)
Director, Pain Clinic
Christian Barnard Memorial Hospital
Consultant, Pain Clinic
Groote Schuur Hospital
Cape Town, South Africa

Robert M. Raw, MB ChB, MPraxMed, DA(CMSA), FFA(CMSA) *(Chapter 24)*
Associate Professor of Anesthesia
Department of Anesthesia
University of Iowa
Iowa City, Iowa

Theresa Rickelman, DO *(Chapter 28)*
Regional Anesthesia Fellow
Department of Anesthesia
University of Iowa
Iowa City, Iowa

Michael L. Salamon, MD *(Chapter 12)*
Orthopaedic Surgeon
Louisville, Kentucky

Francis V. Salinas, MD *(Chapter 26)*
Staff Anesthesiologist
Department of Anesthesia
Virginia Mason Medical Center
Clinical Assistant Professor of Anesthesiology
Department of Anesthesiology
University of Washington
Seattle, Washington

Charles L. Saltzman, MD *(Chapter 12)*
Professor of Orthopaedic Surgery and
  Biomedical Engineering and Heart
Department of Orthopaedic Surgery,
  Bioengineering and Physical Therapy
University of Utah
Salt Lake City, Utah

Hala H. Shamsuddin, MD *(Chapter 3)*
Assistant Professor
Department of Internal Medicine
University of Iowa
Iowa City, Iowa

Andrew C. Steel, BSc, MB BS, MRCP, FRCA
(Chapter 25)
Specialist Registrar in Anesthesia
St. Mary's Hospital–NHS Trust
London, United Kingdom

Curtis Steyers, MD *(Chapter 15)*
Professor of Orthopaedic Surgery
Division of Hand and Microsurgery
Department of Orthopaedics and Rehabilitation
University of Iowa
Iowa City, Iowa

Santhanam Suresh, MD, FAAP *(Chapter 31)*
Co-Director, Pain Treatment Services
Children's Memorial Hospital
Associate Professor of Anesthesiology and
  Pediatrics
Feinberg School of Medicine
Northwestern University
Chicago, Illinois

Joseph D. Tobias, MD *(Chapter 13)*
Vice-Chairman, Department of Anesthesiology
Chief, Division of Pediatric
  Anesthesiology/Pediatric Critical Care
Russell and Mary Shelden Chair of Pediatric
  Intensive Care Medicine
Professor of Anesthesiology and Pediatrics
Department of Anesthesiology
University of Missouri
Columbia, Missouri

Ban Chi-Ho Tsui, MSc, MD, FRCP(C) *(Chapter 19)*
Director of Clinical Research/Associate Professor
Department of Anesthesia and Pain Medicine
University of Alberta
Edmonton, Alberta, Canada

Peter Van de Putte, MD *(Chapters 18, 21)*
Anesthesiologist
Department of Anesthesia
Ziekenhuis O.L.V. Middelares
Deurne, Belgium

Martial van der Vorst, MD *(Chapters 18, 21)*
Anesthesiologist
Department of Anesthesiology
A.Z. St.-Elisabeth Herentals
Mortsel, Belgium

Brian R. Wolf, MD *(Chapter 17)*
Assistant Professor
Department of Orthopaedic Surgery and
  Rehabilitation
University of Iowa, Sports Medicine
Iowa City, Iowa

Lisa Zuccherelli, MB BCh, FCA(SA) *(Chapter 32)*
Dunkeld Anaesthetic Practice
Sandton, Gauteng, South Africa

FOREWORD

In recent years, orthopaedic anesthesia has generated growing interest as an anesthesia subspecialty of its own. This development has been driven by multiple factors, including an aging population, improved joint replacement hardware, improved surgical techniques, and a growing expectation that life need not be inevitably limited by joint degeneration. Interest in this specialty is not an entirely new phenomenon. A search for textbooks about orthopaedic anesthesia reveals eight textbooks published between 1980 and the present: one each in 1980, 1992, and 1993, two in 1994, one in 1995, and two in 2005. Each of these texts has addressed some of the unique characteristics of orthopaedic surgical procedures and the resulting anesthetic considerations.

However, little has been written about the way in which a real understanding of the surgical procedure affects anesthetic choice. Furthermore, contemporary anesthetic practice does not end in the recovery room. The formulation of a perioperative anesthetic plan should incorporate the patient's preexisting medical condition, the planned surgical procedure, postoperative surgical evaluation and monitoring, postoperative analgesia, rehabilitation plan, and reduction of postoperative complications. As an example, in a healthy patient scheduled for bilateral acetabular osteotomies, the use of combined epidural/general anesthesia with pharmacologic manipulation of the physiologic response to surgery produces both decreased blood loss and improved surgical conditions. Maintenance of the epidural provides excellent postoperative analgesia while minimizing the need for additional opioid analgesics. However, the epidural may be used for only a short period of time because postoperative anticoagulation is recommended to minimize the risk of thromboembolic complications. In other postoperative settings, the use of early and aggressive rehabilitation has been associated with shortened times to recovery and restoration of range of motion. Judicious use of regional analgesia has been demonstrated to facilitate this process.

In this text, the editor has assembled an extremely talented and knowledgeable group of chapter authors from a variety of specialties and seeks to address four specific areas of orthopaedic anesthesia. The first part of the book discusses basic principles. The second part addresses orthopaedic surgical procedures by region or joint and provides insight into the surgical technique, the type of anesthetic required, postoperative evaluation, rehabilitation, and complications associated with a given surgical procedure. The third part covers regional anesthesia, continuous nerve and neuraxial blocks, and ambulatory treatment of postoperative pain. The fourth part deals with a range of orthopaedic anesthesia topics: nerve injury, bone cement, and battlefield injuries.

Textbooks are written for a variety of purposes: to fill educational gaps, to record the learning of a lifetime, to promote one's academic institution or oneself, or in some cases to express passion for a topic or practice that other outlets are insufficient to express. This textbook has been written for the last-named purpose. The editor of this text is innovative, thoughtful, progressive, and passionate about the application of sound anesthetic practices to this unique subset of patients and surgical procedures. In addition, he is passionate about the education of orthopaedic anesthesia providers and he understands that success in this area will produce a wide-ranging impact on patient care in the United States and abroad. In his pursuit of excellence in education, he has developed a variety of new teaching tools, regional anesthetic approaches, and educational courses and is widely recognized—locally, nationally, and internationally—as an expert in regional and orthopaedic anesthesia.

On a personal note, it has been a unique pleasure to watch the editor assemble this text. He has invested countless hours in this project but has done so without complaint and frequently with unbridled excitement about the latest contribution of a chapter author. I have no doubt that this text will become a foundation for continuing orthopaedic anesthesia education and practice. I expect that this text will find its way onto the bookshelf of every serious regional and orthopaedic anesthesiologist. I know that it will grace my own shelf and will have well-worn corners from frequent use.

Richard W. Rosenquist, MD
President, American Society of Regional Anesthesia and Pain Medicine
Professor, Department of Anesthesia
University of Iowa
Iowa City, Iowa
Director, Center for Pain Medicine and Regional Anesthesia

PREFACE

Orthopaedic anesthesia as a fully fledged subspecialty of anesthesiology has acquired an extensive literature of its own. This book is an attempt to bring under one cover a survey of the most important topics that directly or indirectly affect the practice of this subspecialty. Although the subject matter covers a wide range, we do not claim exhaustiveness or final authority. Nevertheless, the editor and the contributing authors hope that readers will find this book useful as a guide to, and reminder of, the many problems that confront the orthopaedic anesthesiologist.

The importance of orthopaedic anesthesiology cannot be overstated. With the massive increase in the number of procedures for joint replacements, spinal surgery, and trauma, orthopaedic surgery now constitutes approximately 30 percent of all major surgical procedures performed in the United States.

Although this book is aimed mainly at anesthesiologists-in-training and practicing anesthesiologists, an attempt has also been made to highlight orthopaedic surgical problems. The aim has been to promote an increased mutual understanding between anesthesiologists and surgeons. It has been said that anesthesia without surgeons would be a pleasure. Surgeons, no doubt, have voiced similar feelings. Of course, the fact is that neither can function without the other. The welfare of our patients depends to a large extent on teamwork. If this book helps to promote better mutual understanding and more efficient teamwork between anesthesiologists and surgeons, the editor and the authors will have been well rewarded.

The editor was privileged to obtain contributions by experienced authors as well as by several first-time authors. In all cases, the choice of contributors was based on their acknowledged expertise and international recognition. Younger authors were usually paired with more established writers as the second author. This collaboration resulted in a blend of fresh (even exuberant) youthful approaches with the wisdom of more experienced practitioners. Although this was not a time-proven recipe, I believe that it has been successful for this book. I tried my best to avoid unnecessary repetition of work from other texts. To my knowledge, this is the first comprehensive textbook on orthopaedic anesthesia as a subspecialty.

All of the drawings of anatomy and surgical procedures were done from specially prepared cadaver dissections, photographs, or other primary illustrative material.

The book is divided into four parts. The first part deals with basic principles. Although they are applicable to anesthesia in general, these principles must be thoroughly understood by practitioners who provide anesthesia for orthopaedic surgery. The topics included here involve antimicrobial and thromboprophylaxis, homeostasis in trauma, fat embolism, and a special chapter on dysmorphic children. A selection of Adrian Bösenberg's unique collection of photographs, taken during his humanitarian work all over the world, is published here for the first time.

The second part has been written by orthopaedic surgeons paired with anesthesiologists and deals with orthopaedic surgical procedures organized by region or joint. Authors were asked to address basic anatomical and surgical aspects and to emphasize comorbidities, anesthetic management, intra- and postoperative pain management, and rehabilitation. These chapters also explain how surgeons, anesthesiologists, physical therapists, and nurses can work as a team to provide the best care for patients by understanding issues from the perspective of the different specialties. Todd McKinley wrote a unique chapter on fractures and crush injuries, which, among other things, makes the poorly understood compartment syndrome clearer. In addition to the major joints, there are chapters on hand and foot surgery and on spinal surgery in adults and children. Ned Amendola, Brian Wolf, and their team cover sports injuries in detail. In this second part, the authors' experience and a list of suggested readings are used instead of formal lists of references to primary literature.

The third part covers regional anesthesia, more specifically continuous nerve and neuraxial blocks and ambulatory treatment of postoperative pain. All of the nerve blocks required for routine orthopaedic anesthesia are discussed in detail. Basic principles on topics such as the physics of electrical nerve stimulation and the use of ultrasound are also discussed in detail. Also included are chapters on local anesthetic infusion strategies, home care of patients with continuous nerve blocks, and nerve blocks in children. This part of the book should provide the basic information that practitioners will need for regional anesthesia in orthopaedic surgery.

The final part deals with miscellaneous special topics of which the orthopaedic anesthesiologist should have a thorough knowledge. These topics include nerve injuries, their prevention and management, and problems associated with the use of bone cement. The final chapter covers battlefield orthopaedic anesthesia by Trip Buckenmaier, who recently served in the Iraq war theater.

ACKNOWLEDGMENTS

The idea for this book arose from a suggestion by my good friend and colleague Dr. Admir Hadzic, while we were teaching regional anesthesia (and fly-fishing) in Chile. I acknowledge with thanks all his behind-the-scenes help and sincerely thank him for always being there when I needed sound advice.

I acknowledge with gratitude the enormous contribution of Dr. Chris Theron (Oranjezicht, Cape Town, South Africa) in editing the text. I am also deeply indebted to Dr. Michael Todd and my other colleagues and partners in the Department of Anesthesia of the University of Iowa for their continuous encouragement, support, and advice. I am especially indebted to them for allowing me time away from the operating room to complete this work. A special word of thanks goes to Dr. Richard Rosenquist, a special friend, partner, and colleague, for his advice and continued encouragement and support. Of course, I am deeply indebted to the contributing authors of this book for their unstinting cooperation.

The orthopaedic surgeons and faculty members of the Department of Orthopaedic Surgery of the University of Iowa deserve special thanks. I appreciate their generosity of spirit in writing for a textbook not primarily intended for their fellow surgeons. I also offer my sincere thanks to my secretaries Teresa Schmidt and Judith Carney, who always placed this work at the top of their long and overburdened priority lists.

Sincere thanks go to Chris Spofford, MD, and her extremely competent team of fellow residents from the University of Iowa: Drs. Thom Cannon, Rebecca de Long, Bill Esham, Clint Rozycki, Wendy Wallskog, and Andrew Wilkey for final proofreading of the manuscript.

Mary Bryson stepped up to the challenge and I thank her for the tremendous value that she added to this work by her clear and beautiful artwork. I also thank the production team at McGraw-Hill for their guidance and professional support.

Last, but not least, are my heartfelt thanks to Karin Boezaart, my wife, and our children Dirk, Kim, Ted, and Johke, and grandchild, Dihan, for all their tolerance and patience with me over the years of my career. I also cannot neglect to thank my physician brothers, Drs. Louis and François Boezaart, for always being there for me. Finally, I thank my mother, Elma Boezaart, for all her love and support and for introducing me to the massive legacy of a great physician, Dr. Jan D. G. du Preez—her late father.

PART I

General Principles

CHAPTER 1

Orthopaedic Anesthesia as a Subspecialty of Anesthesia

JACQUES E. CHELLY

In the Preface to this book, the editor has pointed out that approximately 30 percent of all major surgical procedures in the United States now involve orthopaedic surgery. If any quantitative justification for the importance of orthopaedic anesthesia is still needed, this should suffice. The comprehensive survey presented in the following pages is, therefore, timely and appropriate.

Orthopaedic anesthesia has developed into a full fledged subspecialty of anesthesia and is now widely accepted. The writing of a detailed account of this development must be left to those colleagues who busy themselves with medical history. In this chapter, I can only indicate briefly and in general, a few factors which, to a large extent have contributed to this development.

There can be little doubt that the growth of orthopaedic anesthesia into a subspecialty has to a large extent been promoted by developments in orthopaedic surgery. Over the past 50 years, the focus of orthopaedic surgery has shifted from trauma to joint replacement, sports medicine, and spinal surgery with several subspecializations in between. Today increasing numbers of orthopaedic surgeons restrict themselves to highly specialized fields. Surgeons who initially specialized in joint replacements now specialize, more specifically, in knee, hip or ankle replacement. Other orthopaedic subspecializations include orthopaedic oncology and pediatric orthopaedic surgery, while spinal surgery has become a subspecialty shared with neurosurgeons.

Among the factors that have led to these changes are advances in endoscopic techniques as well as the development of biocompatible materials, imaging equipment, and computer-guided techniques. The increasing numbers of the elderly and the resultant greater demand for joint replacements has also had a major impact on the practice of orthopaedic surgery.

Meanwhile, it has become increasingly clear that a successful outcome with many of the new operative procedures depends to a significant extent on the use of specific and specialized anesthetic techniques during surgery and in postoperative pain management. In this respect, regional anesthesia and continuous nerve blocks have been preeminent. These techniques are, for example, especially important when surgery is done on an outpatient basis. Orthopaedic surgeons and hospital administrators now increasingly acknowledge the fact that orthopaedic anesthesiologists play a key role in promoting the speedy functional recovery of patients, thus decreasing the length of their hospitalization.

The use of neuraxial and peripheral nerve blocks is obviously not restricted to orthopaedic surgery. However, it often requires specialized knowledge and skills in the orthopaedic setting. For example, patients who undergo minimally invasive knee or hip surgery on an outpatient basis must be able to tolerate weight bearing during physical therapy within hours of surgery. This is made possible by using specific regional anesthetic techniques that differ from those used in, for example, cesarean sections or hysterectomies. Immediate or speedy postoperative functional recovery without any residual motor block is required in such instances. This is achieved with spinal or epidural anesthesia that utilize minidoses of local anesthetic.

The complexity and unique features of many modern orthopaedic operations also require specialized knowledge

▶ **TABLE 1-1.** ORTHOPAEDIC MARKET OVERVIEW

Orthopaedic procedures (U.S.)*	1996	1997	1998	1999	2000	2001	2002	2003	2004	2005	2006	2007	2008
Inpatient	3,795,000	3,719,100	3,644,718	3,571,824	3,500,387	3,430,379	3,361,772	3,294,536	3,228,646	3,164,073	3,100,791	3,038,775	2,978,000
Outpatient	4,200,000	4,284,000	4,369,680	4,457,074	4,546,215	4,637,139	4,729,882	4,824,480	4,920,969	5,019,389	5,119,777	5,222,172	5,326,616
Total procedures (U.S.)	7,995,000	8,003,100	8,014,398	8,028,898	8,046,602	8,067,518	8,091,654	8,119,016	8,149,615	8,183,462	8,220,568	8,260,947	8,304,616
Estimated number of procedures indicated for PNB (U.S.)†					**5,138,544**	**5,271,252**	**5,416,762**	**5,597,237**	**5,798,172**	**6,012,683**	**6,241,959**	**6,487,302**	**6,750,138**
Shoulder procedures (U.S.)	229,810	244,479	249,468	257,184	267,900	282,000	300,000	325,000	357,500	393,250	432,575	475,833	523,416
Hip arthroplasty (U.S.)	249,000	256,470	266,729	280,065	296,869	314,681	340,000	365,000	390,550	417,889	447,141	478,441	511,931
Knee replacement (U.S.)	265,000	272,950	283,868	298,061	315,945	334,902	350,000	385,000	423,500	465,850	512,435	563,679	620,046
Other fracture treatments	603,000	603,000	603,000	603,000	603,000	603,000	603,000	603,000	603,000	603,000	603,000	603,000	603,000

PNB = peripheral nerve blocks.
*Estimates and projections based on MDI 1998 RP611117, American Academy of Orthopedic Surgeons (1996–2000), National Center for Health Statistics (1996–2000).
†Estimates generated by Medtech Insight (1/03–5/03).

from the anesthesiologist. The anesthesiologist must, for example, be fully aware of and conversant with the possible complications associated with different specific orthopaedic surgical procedures, such as rimming of the bone and the use of bone cement. In addition, the difficulty involved in bone hemostasis requires special vigilance in estimating blood loss.

An optimal outcome in orthopaedic surgery is very difficult to achieve if the anesthesiologist does not have a thorough understanding of the technical aspects of an operation. Knowledge of the specific positioning of the patient, the duration of the operation, and the specific complications that a given procedures may entail is therefore essential in orthopaedic anesthesia. The surgeon's choice of anticoagulant may, for instance, determine the regional anesthetic technique used for a particular operation and for postoperative pain management. Serious complications have occurred when epidural anesthesia was used without considering the pharmacokinetics of the drug used prophylactically to prevent deep venous thrombosis and pulmonary emboli. Although, there are guidelines to help the anesthesiologist. The catastrophic consequences of epidural hematomas have led many practitioners to view the use of antithrombotic drugs as an absolute contraindication to the use of epidural analgesia.

In orthopaedic surgery, it is now not unusual to perform operations for hip fractures in the elderly population (85 to 90 years of age) or joint replacements in the obese population (130 kg or more). The orthopaedic anesthesiologist should be aware of the fact that, in younger patients, the use of 27-gauge needles reduces the incidence of postpuncture headache. In the very elderly, this complication occurs less frequently, so that lower-gauge needles (25 or even 22 gauge) can be used. Many elderly patients with arthritis of the hip or knee also suffer from arthritis of the spine. In these cases it is better to use sharp spinal needles.

A final example of the problems that have promoted orthopaedic anesthesia as a subspecialty is the fact that given surgical protocols must consider not only the operations but also the postoperative requirements, especially those related to pain management at rest and during mobilization. Thus, in traditional hip replacement, the patient undergoes minimal physical therapy on the first postoperative day, so that speedy motor recovery is not necessary. In these cases pain is mainly managed while the patient is resting in bed.

In contrast, patients who undergo minimally invasive hip replacement have to be able to tolerate extensive physical therapy within hours of surgery. Here, complete recovery of motor function is essential. This may be best achieved with a multimodal approach to pain management that commences before surgery. Because of this, it is important that anesthesiologists and acute pain specialists work closely together. Anesthesiologist groups who specialize in both orthopaedic anesthesia and acute pain management achieve this best. In our institution, one anesthesiologist is responsible for the anesthesia and another for the postoperative pain management. Because all of the anesthesiologists within our institution rotate between these two functions and follow established protocols, it is easier to distribute responsibility. This is not always possible when anesthesiologists and pain specialists work independently.

In this chapter, I have attempted to indicate, by means of a few examples, some of the factors that have contributed to the development of orthopaedic anesthesia into a subspecialty. There is no doubt that this subspecialty will continue to develop and to grow in stature. The data in Table 1-1 below give a clear indication of the future of orthopaedic anesthesia and acute pain relief.

CHAPTER 2

Homeostasis in Massive Multiple Trauma

John A. Myburgh

▶ INTRODUCTION

The challenges that face clinicians who manage patients with multiple trauma are among the most daunting in medicine. Trauma is a unique disease. Unlike many other diseases, there is a definitive time of onset, followed by a series of time-critical periods when the victim is vulnerable to a number of life-threatening and potentially life-threatening insults.

The survival of these patients depends on some factors that cannot be prevented, such as the degree and nature of the external force causing the injury and the physiologic reserve of the victim. There are, however, a number of preventable factors that directly affect functional survival, such as hypoxia, shock, and infection. For the successful management of traumatized patients during any of these periods, clinicians need to recognize patterns of injuries and to prioritize treatment options so that the patient is not compromised and preventable insults are not missed.

This chapter addresses the pathophysiologic basis of effective trauma management. Many of these principles apply to the management of trauma victims throughout their stay in the hospital. Some of these principles and strategies have been definitively studied in appropriate trials, so that management can be based on evidence. However, for the majority of these strategies, trial-based evidence is limited and clinicians must rely on time-honored physiologic principles and hard-earned experience.

Although this is a chapter in a textbook on orthopaedic anesthesia, it is written from the perspective of the clinician who is presented with traumatized patients during their passage through the health care system. These perspectives are unified by the aim of improving the patient's survival.

▶ EPIDEMIOLOGY OF TRAUMA

In global terms, trauma poses the greatest threat to human survival.[1] Although patterns of trauma have stabilized in developed or high-income countries, trauma levels are increasing exponentially in developing or low-income countries. This phenomenon is primarily related to increased mechanization in low-income countries, where an expanding population is becoming dependent on vehicular transport for economic survival.[2] This increase in mechanization is not occurring at the same pace as infrastructure development and access to effective health care systems. Adequacy of roads, enforcement of traffic regulations and the use of passenger restraining devices, improvements in vehicular safety, and road safety education are variable and lag behind those in developed countries. Coupled to the increasingly violent environment—owing to economic polarization, war, terrorism, religious fundamentalism, and firearm availability—that predominates in low-income countries, it is not surprising that trauma is regarded as the "silent global epidemic."[3]

In high-income countries, the incidence of trauma is decreasing, primarily due to the reversal of the adverse phenomena prevalent in low-income countries. Indeed, many regard the rate of trauma death as an index of societal stability and civility.

Globally, trauma remains predominantly a disease of the young. The majority of victims are male, and trauma is the leading cause of death in children. The cost to survivors in all societies in emotional, social, and financial terms is substantial, since the effects of the original injury may persist for many years.[4,5] Trauma is therefore a major disease confronting all societies.

▶ PATHOPHYSIOLOGIC RESPONSE TO TRAUMA

It is imperative that clinicians have a clear understanding of the pathophysiologic processes that underlie trauma and the systemic responses to these processes.

The physiologic response to trauma, infection, and inflammatory conditions (e.g., pancreatitis and burns) results in a complex neurohumoral phenomenon that has been studied extensively. Despite numerous changes in nomenclature over the last 10 years, the systemic response to injury has been recognized for the last century. This response is characterized by complex neural-endocrine-humoral effects at cellular and organ levels, and the resultant clinical response represents the teleologic reaction to ensure the organism's survival. Originally described as "fight or flight," the magnitude of this physiologic response will depend on the severity of the injury and the inherent ability of the host to mount an appropriate response. In the clinical situation, the physiologic reserve of the host will depend on associated comorbidities, medications, and secondary injuries.

Cellular and Neurohumoral Factors

The cellular response to injury results in a nonspecific cascade of numerous molecular effects.[6] The initiating triggers of this response may vary and include direct trauma causing cellular or organ damage, systemic release of toxins from invading microbes, fluctuations in temperature greater than homeostatic limits, and toxicity from drugs. Regardless of the nature of this initiating stimulus, the resultant cellular response is nonspecific and may be regarded as a coordinated endogenous response to augment protective systems that may be depressed after injury ("proinflammatory") and/or to suppress systems that may cause further cellular or systemic injury ("anti-inflammatory") (Fig. 2-1).

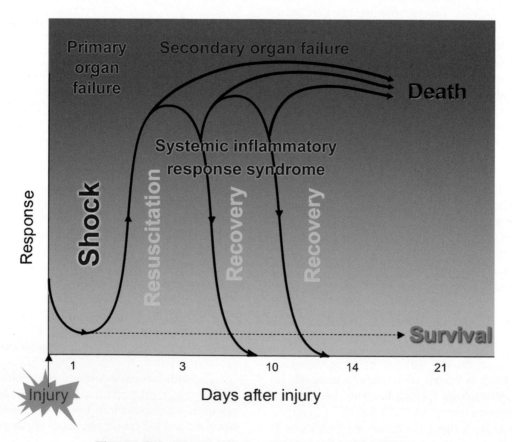

Figure 2-1. The systemic response to acute injury.

Although the distinction into pro- and anti-inflammatory mediators assists in conceptualizing this response, there is marked inter- and intraindividual variation in the effects and response of these mediators. A number of cellular systems and mediators of inflammation have been identified and studied.

Cytokines

Mediators of inflammation include cytokines, which exist in both circulating and cell-associated forms.[7,8] These include the family of interleukins (ILs), of which IL-1 and IL-6 have been extensively studied as markers of pro- and anti-inflammatory cytokine release, respectively. Tumor necrosis factors (TNF-α, β, and δ) as well as platelet-activating and inhibiting factors are primary mediators that induce the release of other cellular factors (mostly endothelial), such as nitric oxide, endothelin, and populations of eicosanoids (prostaglandins and leukotrienes). The effects of these mediators are to alter tissue and vascular permeability in order to improve regional blood flow and metabolism. Endothelin and nitric oxide are ubiquitous endothelial compounds that are integral in vasoconstriction and vasodilation, respectively. They form the basis of regional autoregulation—that is, when regional blood flow rates are kept relatively constant in the presence of altered metabolism and perfusion.

Complement

Activation of the complement cascade is a fundamental component of cell-mediated and humoral immunity. Apart from the activation of antibodies and cellular responses to injury, activated components of the complement cascade such as C3a and C5a interact with endothelial mediators to alter membrane permeability, both directly and in association with circulating activators such as bradykinin and histamine. In regional circulations, such as in the kidney, complement activation is integral in maintaining renal perfusion and defending glomerular filtration.[9,10]

Coagulation

Regulation of intravascular coagulation is a principal homeostatic mechanism. Rather than simply regarding this system as a series of chemical reactions that are activated in response to hemorrhage, the coagulation system should be regarded as a complex system in a state of fluctuating conformational change, balancing intravascular coagulation and thrombolysis. The interaction between circulating procoagulants (e.g., activated factor VII and von Willebrand factor), anticoagulant proteins (e.g., proteins C and S), opsonic glycoproteins (e.g., fibronectin), and endothelium-derived mediators form the basis for maintaining intravascular integrity and membrane stability. Depletion of these vital homeostatic factors following hemorrhage often result in subsequent coagulopathy and endothelial disruption.[11,12]

Neurohumoral Factors

Under the influence of a number of physiologic stimuli and interactions, autonomic neural control of regional and systemic vasculature and organ function is a principal homeostatic system.[13] Through a series of endogenous conversions, phenylalanine is converted to dopamine within adrenergic nerve terminals. Dopamine is converted to norepinephrine and released into the neural synapse, where it interacts with populations of adrenoreceptors. Under physiologic conditions, norepinephrine is the predominant neuroendocrine agonist. Release and reuptake of norepinephrine from adrenergic terminals is controlled by presynaptic alpha$_2$ receptors in response to changes in physiologic perturbations, such as changes in posture, altitude, and energy expenditure. Under physiologic conditions of stress or in pathologic states, norepinephrine release is augmented by the release of epinephrine from the adrenal gland via the same presynaptic alpha$_2$ systems. Teleologically, dopamine and epinephrine may be regarded as norepinephrine precursors, norepinephrine being the predominant endogenous catecholamine.[14]

Catecholamine-mediated physiological responses are complex. Agonists bind to populations of adrenergic receptors, which are largely divided into alpha and beta subgroups. Further subgroups of α- (1A, 1B, 2A, 2B, and 2C) and β-receptors (1, 2, and 3) have been identified.[15]

Signal transduction from agonist-receptor occupation to the effector cell is modulated by conformational changes in G proteins associated with these receptors. Under the additional influence of second messengers such as nitric oxide, endothelin, and eicosanoids, these conformational changes promote the release of calcium from intracellular stores and increased membrane calcium permeability. Subsequent phosphorylation of substrate proteins via protein kinases prompts third messengers to trigger a cascade of events leading to specific cardiovascular and metabolic effects.[15,16]

In addition to adrenergic regulation, other neurohumoral substances have a permissive or regulatory role in maintaining vasomotor tone. These are mediated through the renin-aldosterone-angiotensin axis and local mediators such as vasopressin and corticosteroids. Of these influences, specific vasopressinergic receptors (V_1 and V_2) have been identified in association with sympathetic terminals and may be responsible for systemic vasoresponsiveness. Similarly, the endogenous release of corticosteroids has been shown to exert an important vasoresponsive role, thereby augmenting catecholamine-mediated interactions.[17,18]

Organ Responses

The clinical expression of the physiologic response to injury and inflammation outlined above will vary considerably between and within individuals. Ultimately, the effects on the functions of vital and nonvital organs will determine a person's response to injury (Fig. 2-2).

Initially, the clinical response to injury is nonspecific. Over the last 20 years, there has been extensive debate to define the systemic inflammatory response syndrome (SIRS), usually in association with infection.[19,20]

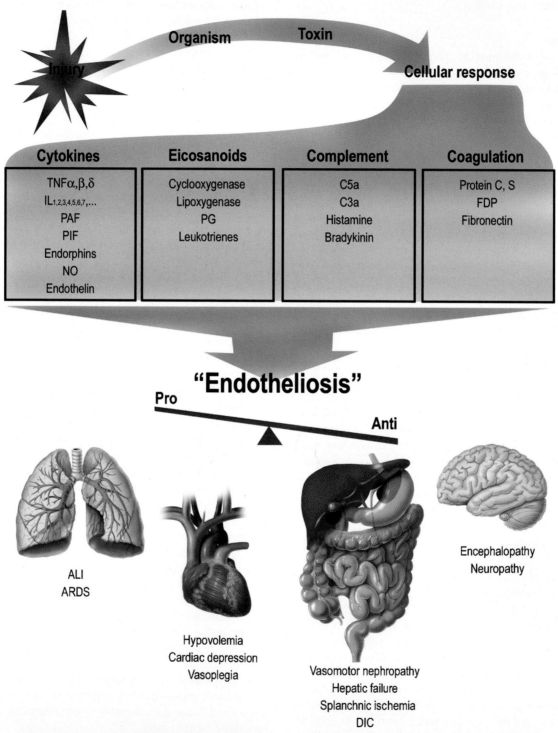

Figure 2-2. The effects on the functions of vital and nonvital organs will determine the person's response to injury. Individual variation is vast.
ABBREVIATIONS: ALI = acute lung injury; ARDS = acute respiratory distress syndrome; DIC = disseminated intravascular coagulation; FDP = fibrinogen degradation product; NO = nitric or nitrous oxide; PAF = platelet-activating factor; PIF = prolactin-inhibiting factor; TNF = tumor necrosis factor.

The impetus for this debate was to define baseline clinical features as criteria for including patients in clinical trials, although the use of these criteria has expanded into clinical practice. The SIRS criteria are generic and include at least two clinical features from a list that includes a temperature change (<36 or >38°C; <98.6 or >100.4°F), tachycardia (>90 beats per minute), tachypnea (>30 breaths per minute or an arterial carbon dioxide tension <32 mmHg), and alteration in leukocyte count (<12 or <4 $10^3/mm^3$ or >10 percent banded neutrophils). Clearly, there are numerous causes of these physiologic changes, and although they are commonly used as criteria in clinical and research practice, they have limited clinical utility.

An alternative approach is to consider the effects of injury on each organ system and to interpret the resultant changes in the light of the underlying physiologic response and the impact of external injury.

Cardiovascular System

Because of the autonomic responses outlined above, the cardiovascular effects of injury are often the most acute and clinically apparent. The endogenous sympathetic response is directed at maintaining the perfusion of vital organs. Circulatory homeostasis is predicated on the principle that cardiac output is equal to venous return.[21] The assessment and treatment of circulatory failure must consider these two processes.

Cardiac output primarily depends on the heart rate and stroke volumes.[22,23] Increasing the heart rate will increase cardiac output, so tachycardia is an inevitable sign following trauma. The absence of tachycardia after trauma is therefore always abnormal and suggests sympathetic ablation, either due to adrenergic blocking agents (beta blockers), autonomic neuropathy (e.g., severe diabetes), or high spinal injury (quadriplegia). To eject blood effectively, the heart depends on a critical ventricular mass and contractility. On rare occasions, loss of myocardial contractility after trauma may be due to severe myocardial contusion or rupture.

Although only 20 percent of the circulating blood volume is contained in the arterial (conducting) circulation, stroke volume depends primarily on the amount of blood returned to the heart at the end of diastole. The venous system contains 70 percent of the blood volume and, as such, represents an endogenous blood reservoir. Sympathetic innervation of venous conductance vessels causes venoconstriction, in both major capacitance veins and peripheral veins, resulting in an increased venous return and increased preload. This can represent up to 20 percent of the venous blood volume. This sympathetic response converting the "unstressed" venous volume into a "stressed" venous volume is one of the earliest physiologic responses to injury, and in conjunction with an increase in heart rate and contractility,

represents the endogenous cardiovascular response to injury.[23,24]

Consequently, loss of effective intravascular volume through hemorrhage represents the most common threat to hemodynamic function. An adult can usually tolerate an acute blood loss of up to 20 percent of the blood volume (about 1000 mL in an adult), but this represents the upper limit of physiologic reserve in the majority of patients. Greater blood loss requires volume replacement to maintain effective venous return and cardiac output.

Sudden sympathetic ablation, usually by anesthetic drugs or high doses of analgesics, will result in loss of stressed venous tone, thereby unmasking relative hypovolemia.

Other important physiologic factors that compromise hemodynamic function in the traumatized patient include positive intrapleural pressure (e.g., positive-pressure ventilation or tension pneumothorax), loss of atrial contraction (e.g., atrial fibrillation), and ablation of muscle tone and pump (e.g., neuromuscular blockers or quadriplegia/paraplegia). These factors primarily compromise venous return and must be promptly identified and treated.

During the later stages of trauma, superimposed infection, sepsis, or multiple organ failure will adversely affect on cardiovascular function.[25-27] Initially a hyperdynamic vasodilated state is recognized, conventionally attributed to pathologic arterial vasodilation or vasoplegia. Although arterial vasodilatation is indeed a feature, the predominant vascular dysfunction is venoplegia, whereby sympathetically mediated venoconstriction is blunted, resulting in relative inability to maintain a stressed volemic response. Consequently, cardiac output becomes dependent on heart rate, resulting in a high-output state, also described as warm shock. As septic shock progresses, sympathetic reserve progressively becomes blunted via quantitative (downregulation) and qualitative (desensitization) processes, resulting in failure to maintain cardiac output.[28,29] This is conventionally termed "low-output" or "cold" shock, but in effect represents the failure of predominantly adrenergic homeostatic mechanisms to maintain hemodynamic function. Accordingly, treatment strategies are directed at augmenting or replacing failing neurohumoral systems.

Renal System

Apart from blood purification and production of urine, the kidney is an integral homeostatic organ in the response to injury. Fundamental aspects of this response are the defense of mean arterial pressure and water retention. Glomerular filtration and urine production are under intense control by neurohumoral systems, of which the renin-angiotensin-aldosterone neuroendocrine axis is predominant. Loss of effective intravascular volume or blood pressure causes a reduction in renal perfusion pressure, which triggers the release of renin from the juxtaglomerular apparatus. Apart from converting angiotensinogen to angiotensin and aldosterone, renin augments the adrenal release of epinephrine via second-messenger systems. These powerful endocrine responses cause increased tubular absorption and production of small volumes of concentrated urine. In trauma cases, oliguria should therefore be regarded as a normal physiologic response.

Second, neuroendocrine function, particularly angiotensin-converting enzyme (ACE) and angiotensin II, is integral to maintaining mean arterial pressure.[30] By maintaining efferent arteriolar tone and water retention, the kidney is able to maintain effective renal perfusion pressure in the presence of fluctuating renal blood flow and mean arterial pressure (autoregulation).[31,32] Furthermore, the kidney has substantial reserve to tolerate ischemia and relative hypoxia. Oliguria (defined as <0.5 mL/kg/h) in the initial period after trauma (up to 48 to 72 h) should therefore not be regarded as renal failure unless urea and creatinine levels are elevated and there is evidence of loss of renal vascular integrity. However, in patients with premorbid hypertension or in those taking ACE inhibitors, endogenous renal reserve to tolerate ischemia may be reduced and renal failure may ensue at an earlier juncture.

Although oliguria after injury may be regarded as a normal clinical sign, spontaneous diuresis during the recovery phase is equally important. The neuroendocrine basis for this reflects the defervescence of the physiologic responses in the acute phase, often heralding the resolution of organ dysfunction, and may be termed a reversal of water retention. Traditionally, the acute response to injury has been described as an initial "ebb" phase, which is followed by a "flow" phase. These observations are based on the neuroendocrine fundamentals outlined above.[33]

Brain

Brain injury is the leading cause of death in traumatized patients. The majority of immediate deaths caused by trauma are attributed to lethal head injury sustained at the time of impact. Among patients who reach a hospital alive but subsequently die, the mortality due to brain injury is approximately 90 percent.[34] Of these, the majority have severe primary brain injury; i.e., injury sustained at the time of impact. Secondary brain injuries—defined as systemic insults that occur during the postinjury period—are independent determinants of adverse outcome.[35] Of these insults, hypotension and hypoxia are the most profound.[36,37] There is a sound physiologic basis for these observations.

Under physiologic conditions, the brain receives 20 percent of the cardiac output.[38] The "luxury perfusion" of the brain reflects the metabolic requirements for brain function. The brain has therefore developed autoregulatory mechanisms to maintain a relatively constant cerebral blood flow when systemic blood pressure fluctuates. In contrast to the kidney, cerebral autoregulation is based on the relative impermeability of the blood-brain barrier to exogenous vasoactive peptides, such as catecholamines; therefore intense local microvascular regulation is employed, predominantly through endothelial fluxes of endothelin and nitric oxide.

Despite its autoregulatory mechanisms, the brain is extremely vulnerable to the effects of systemic hypotension, particularly after brain injury. Patterns of abnormal cerebral blood flow have been described in these cases.[39,40] Initially, within 72 h of injury, cerebral blood flow is reduced, often to a critical level of <20 mL/100 g/min within 6 h. This is well below the autoregulatory threshold or "breakpoint" where cerebral blood flow becomes pressure-passive (35 mL/100 g/min). This breakpoint may be higher in patients with associated systemic hypertension and must be considered during resuscitation and treatment. A number of intrinsic mechanisms have been described for this reduction in cerebral blood flow. They include neurohumorally mediated vasoconstriction, microvascular thrombosis, and traumatic subarachnoid hemorrhage. Importantly, secondary ischemia, in particular hypovolemia due to extracranial trauma and the injudicious use of osmotic diuretics, may aggravate primary and secondary brain injury. Furthermore, lethal ischemic cerebral damage has been described in patients who have not sustained a primary brain injury but suffered exsanguinating hemorrhage from their injuries. Despite surviving the initial trauma, they suffered fatal ischemic damage to the brain.

The maintenance of normal systemic blood pressure and cardiac output therefore form the basis of resuscitation of the patient with head injuries. Prioritization of treatment of extracranial injuries is done by considering the injury most likely to cause extensive hemorrhage or hypotension and treating it in the first instance. In this context, "damage control" surgery is regarded as primarily hemostatic. Provided the patient remains stable, further investigation and treatment of injuries to the head and other parts can proceed.

The use of hyperventilation to reduce increased intracranial pressure in traumatic brain injury has been advocated for many years. Despite guidelines based on evidence against the use of hyperventilation,[41] it is still strongly advocated by some neurosurgeons.[42] Hypocapnia induced by hyperventilation is a potent cerebral vasoconstrictor and has been demonstrated to induce and exacerbate cerebral ischemia in the traumatized brain, particularly during the initial period after head injury. Cerebral ischemia induced by hyperventilation may be regarded as a preventable secondary brain injury.

Similarly, the use of osmotic diuretics, such as mannitol, and hypertonic crystalloid solutions has been advocated to reduce cerebral edema following traumatic brain injury. Although there is a theoretical basis for the use of these solutions, the purported benefit may be related mainly to a transient expansion of intravascular volume which increases cerebral blood flow, rather than a specific rheologic effect. Indeed, hyperosmolar states caused by the overuse of these solutions, particularly in patients with alcohol intoxication, may negate their rheologic benefit. Furthermore, osmotic diuresis may cause hypovolemia, particularly at a period of increased vulnerability of the brain to hypotension.[43]

The use of hyperventilation and osmotherapy should therefore be restricted and used only as a temporary measure in hemodynamically stable patients in whom there is a high probability of rapidly developing intracranial hypertension and for whom urgent neuroimaging or surgery is considered.[44]

Respiratory System

An open airway is fundamental to the maintenance of oxygenation. At all stages of resuscitation and management, airway patency is mandatory, and this requires constant vigilance. Because of the increased metabolic rate associated with injury, minute ventilation is increased to reduce carbon dioxide levels. Increased minute ventilation also helps to increase oxygenation, although a significant effect on arterial oxygenation is limited at ambient pressure and oxygen concentration. For this reason, all injured patients should receive oxygen at the highest inspired oxygen concentration during the initial resuscitation, since injuries such as tension pneumothorax or pulmonary contusion may cause profound hypoxia. This situation includes patients with chronic obstructive pulmonary disease. Ablation of the hypoxic drive by oxygen is rare in these patients, and the need for supplemental oxygen should always supersede this theoretical concern.[45]

Apart from direct lung injury—such as pulmonary hemorrhage, contusion, or aspiration pneumonitis—the lungs are also vulnerable to an indirect endothelial injury. The surface area of the lungs is large (>100 m²), and since it receives the entire cardiac output, presents a large endothelial area that is exposed to potential inflammatory insult. Extrapulmonary insults may therefore cause an intense inflammatory response that manifests as an acute lung injury.

Ashbaugh described "shock lung" (later termed the adult respiratory distress syndrome (ARDS)) in 1967, during the Vietnam War, as "a sudden clinical pathophysiological state characterized by severe dyspnea, hypoxia, diffuse bilateral pulmonary infiltrations and stiff lungs following massive acute lung injury, usually in persons with no previous lung injury."[46] Typically, the insult is nonhomoge-

neous and spares some areas of lung parenchyma. In damaged areas, the lung is atelectatic, edematous, and hemorrhagic. Hypoxia occurs owing to increased intrapulmonary shunting of blood caused by the loss of functional alveoli and the resultant reduction in functional residual capacity. Lung compliance is reduced (<30 mL/cmH$_2$O) and physiologic dead space is increased, resulting in hypercapnia. Progressive diffuse alveolar and interstitial infiltrates appear on the chest radiograph and have been quantified according to the severity of the injury. Microscopic examination reveals intraalveolar collections of proteinaceous fluid, red blood cells, and inflammatory cells. Microthrombi or white cell aggregates may be seen in small vessels. After 24 to 48 h, hyaline membranes line the alveoli. These are formed by fibrin that has escaped through the capillary walls. As repair of the injury occurs, fibrosis may ensue.[47]

This syndrome is characterized by an alteration in the permeability of alveolar endothelium and presents as alterations in oxygenation, defined by the ratio of arterial to fractional inspired oxygen tensions (PaO$_2$/FiO$_2$), the development of alveolar and interstitial infiltrates, and reductions in pulmonary compliance. Importantly, these physiologic derangements occur in the absence of pulmonary venous hypertension (cardiac failure). A PaO$_2$/FiO$_2$ ratio of <350 is used to define acute lung injury (ALI); if it progresses to a PaO$_2$/FiO$_2$ ratio <250 mmHg, it is defined as ARDS.[48]

Although the treatment of ALI/ARDS is largely supportive and directed at resuscitation and the underlying cause, the knowledge that lung injury may be induced by mechanical ventilation has changed the way in which patients who need mechanical ventilation for respiratory failure are managed. Increased alveolar distention associated with positive-pressure ventilation or "volutrauma" has been shown to cause endothelial disruption and acute pulmonary inflammation resulting in an acute lung injury/ARDS. This is distinct from, but often associated with, extraalveolar air or "barotrauma" induced by positive pressure, which may also result in endothelial injury and is often associated with pulmonary interstitial emphysema, subcutaneous emphysema, pneumothorax, pneumomediastinum, or pneumopericardium.[49] Accordingly, patients with evidence of ALI/ARDS or who may be at risk of developing it should be ventilated with limitations of peak airway pressures and tidal volumes.

Endocrine System

Alterations in endocrine function integrated with systemic autonomic responses after trauma have been described. Foremost of these is hyperglycemia, which may be attributed to exaggerated autonomic responses and insulin resistance during the acute-phase response. Hyperglycemia is therefore common, and there is increasing evidence suggesting that the maintenance of normoglycemia during acute illness leads to improved outcomes.[50,51] This may be because the overwhelmed endogenous insulin responses are supplemented. The physiologic effects of insulin extend beyond blood glucose homeostasis; they include improved phagocytosis by white blood cells, amino acid utilization, and improved neuronal function.

As outlined above, optimal cardiovascular function is dependent on nonadrenergic neurohormonal influences. Adrenocortical function may be impaired during acute illness; this has been attributed to adrenal medullary infarction following profound hemorrhagic shock, alterations in circulating corticoid-binding globulin, and reduced efficacy or levels of adrenocorticotropic hormone (ACTH). These changes may result in absolute or functional hypoadrenalism, which may manifest as catecholamine-resistant shock, hypoglycemia, anergy, and hypothermia.[52] In a massively traumatized patient, these signs should prompt one to consider treatment with corticosteroids or to test the adrenal response to ACTH.

Similar reductions in thyroid, posterior pituitary, and gonadal endocrine functions have been described. The clinical relevance of these changes is unclear but should be considered in anergic trauma patients and particularly in patients with preexisting endocrine illness.

▶ PRINCIPLES OF TRAUMA MANAGEMENT

On the basis of the above physiologic responses, an integrated plan for treating the traumatized patient may be arrived at. A number of highly regarded and effective management protocols have been developed, such as the Advanced Trauma Life Support (ATLS) initiative of the American College of Surgeons.[53] These protocols provide a logical and prioritized approach to the early management of patients with severe trauma and have significantly improved the education of doctors and paramedics in the handling and treatment of these patients. Importantly, these protocols direct the attention of clinicians to the most life-threatening trauma, so that correcting vital-organ homeostasis supersedes less threatening but often more dramatic injuries.

The following section is written to complement overarching ATLS principles. In this regard, the reader is encouraged to read these manuals or similar trauma management texts.

What follows is a physiologic approach based on evidence to many of these trauma management principles, providing the rationale on which they are based.

Two phases of management are considered: the initial resuscitation phase followed by the period of stabilization.

Resuscitation

The resuscitation period is the conditio sine qua non where the ATLS principles apply.

This phase begins as soon as bystanders or emergency personnel attend to the patient. It extends until the patient is stabilized and transferred to a hospital ward or the intensive care unit (ICU). During this period, the patient may be attended by many people, including paramedics, emergency personnel at the first receiving or referral hospitals, and surgeons/physicians with variable experience and expertise.

Accurate documentation of vital signs—such as blood pressure, pulse rate, oxygen saturation, respiratory rate, temperature, and neurologic function (Glasgow Coma Scale score)—during this period is critical. These signs are important in quantifying initial physiologic function and determining whether the patient has suffered secondary insults. This information is often important for subsequent prognostication. The adequacy of documentation of these early signs is often variable; therefore it should ideally be obtained as soon as possible and directly from the personnel involved.

Initial emphasis is directed at assessing and maintaining airway patency, ensuring adequate oxygenation and ventilation, establishing adequate intravenous lines, and restoring normal hemodynamic function. Neurologic assessment should follow only when cardiorespiratory function has been stabilized.

Airway Management

Loss of an open airway at any stage of management represents an acute life-threatening complication. Hypoxia is a prominent cause of secondary brain injury.

The need for an open airway may necessitate endotracheal intubation by emergency personnel under suboptimal circumstances. The intubation of traumatized patients by emergency personnel outside a hospital is a controversial issue, since its success depends on the expertise of the paramedic. The benefits of the early establishment of a definitive airway, oxygenation, and control of carbon dioxide may be offset by the complications of failed intubation, pulmonary aspiration, and delay in transfer to a hospital. Small studies have shown increased mortality in patients intubated before hospitalization, although this practice remains under evaluation.[54,55]

All traumatized patients with altered consciousness have potentially threatened airways. The emergency intervention required to clear airways will depend on the level of consciousness, adequacy of protective glottic reflexes, and the relative risk of aspiration and airway compromise.

All traumatized patients, particularly those with head injury, should be assumed to have an injured cervical spine and be immobilized in a rigid collar until such an injury is definitively excluded radiologically. During any airway intervention and until injury to the cervical spine is excluded by radiological evidence, in-line immobilization of the cervical spine by a rigid collar or by a dedicated person is mandatory.

The mouth and upper airway must be inspected for foreign bodies, hemorrhage, or dentures and cleared under direct vision using a rigid sucker. Simple maneuvers, such as a chin lift and/or a jaw thrust and the use of oropharyngeal airways or laryngeal masks may make a compromised airway functional and allow efficient oxygenation in patients who still breathe. Nasopharyngeal airways must be used cautiously in patients in whom a cribriform plate fracture is suspected, since these instruments may pass directly into the cranial cavity. They may also cause trauma to the nasal mucosa and bleeding into the nasopharynx and upper airway, leading to further airway compromise. The same caution applies to the insertion of nasotracheal and nasogastric tubes.

The decision to perform endotracheal intubation will depend primarily on the level of consciousness, the degree of respiratory failure (hypoxia or hypercapnia), and the requirements for diagnosis and surgery. The selection of intubation technique will depend on the expertise of the operator. Clearly the most experienced person must perform this lifesaving procedure.

In using anesthetic induction agents, sedation, and muscle relaxants to facilitate intubation, one must consider the effects of these agents on sympathetic tone. As described above, the acute response to injury is characterized by intense sympathetic activity. Anesthetic induction agents such as thiopentone, propofol, and benzodiazepines have a significant dose-dependent sympatholytic effect. In compromised but compensated patients, the administration of these drugs may cause profound hypotension, primarily due to ablation of autonomically mediated stressed venous capacitance as well as reduction in venous return and cardiac output. This phenomenon will be exacerbated in hypovolemic patients. Furthermore, autonomically mediated tachycardia may also be blunted by these anesthetic agents, further compromising systemic blood pressure. The worsening of hypotension due to anesthetic induction drugs must therefore be anticipated in all severely traumatized patients. To minimize the resultant hypotension, accurate measurement of systemic blood pressure (ideally via an intraarterial catheter), preemptive volume replacement, and the early use of vasoactive agents should be considered. This is discussed below.

Agitated or combative patients may best be managed initially by intubation and controlled ventilation until diagnostic and therapeutic interventions are completed.

Unconscious patients should be intubated as soon as possible, as should patients with concomitant maxillofacial trauma or upper airway obstruction due to direct laryngeal trauma. This is best performed at a location where expert anesthesiologists and procedures such as rapid induction and intubation, blind nasal intubation, fiberoptic laryngoscopy, cricothyroidotomy, and tracheostomy are available.

For patients who cannot be intubated or ventilated via a bag and mask, surgical airway access should be provided by urgent cricothyroidotomy. There is little or no role for urgent tracheostomy (either percutaneously or surgically) in this situation.

Respiratory Management

As outlined above, oxygen at the highest concentration should be administered to all traumatized patients in the initial period. For patients who still breathe, face-mask oxygen using circuits is suitable. In intubated patients, handheld or mechanical ventilating devices can reliably deliver a fractional inspired oxygen concentration of 1.0 (100%). Handheld, self-inflating devices can effectively ventilate both intubated and nonintubated patients and allow a clinical assessment of lung compliance during inflation, thereby reducing the risk of disconnecting the endotracheal tube or face mask.

Assessment of oxygenation in emergency situations may be difficult in traumatized patients, whose consciousness may be affected by head injuries, alcohol, drugs, or sedatives. All patients should be monitored using pulse oximetry. A saturation of greater than 95% is recommended, as this generally corresponds to an arterial oxygen tension (PaO_2) of at least 75 mmHg (10 kPa). These devices are unreliable in hypoperfused, hypothermic, and agitated patients. However, the demonstration of an oxygen saturation <95% and a pulse waveform even under conditions of poor perfusion indicates hypoxia until proven otherwise.

Mechanically ventilated patients should be ventilated with 100% oxygen until blood gas analysis is obtained. Thereafter, the fractional inspired oxygen concentration may be decreased provided that oxygenation is maintained at a minimum of at least 100 mmHg (13 kPa). Ventilation should be adjusted by using sufficient tidal volumes to obtain normocapnia. Initially this may require tidal volumes of 10 mL/kg, particularly right after endotracheal intubation, when patients are frequently hypercapnic. Once blood gas levels are known, the ventilator should be adjusted to achieve a normal arterial carbon dioxide tension ($PaCO_2$) (35 to 40 mmHg; 4.5 to 5.0 kPa), using peak airway pressures of less than 35 to 40 cmH$_2$O, ideally using tidal volumes of 5 to 7 mL/kg. End-tidal capnography should be used whenever possible. This not only provides an approximate $PaCO_2$ but also shows definitely that the endotracheal tube is correctly placed and allows an assessment of cardiac output.

In combative patients, nondepolarizing muscle relaxants and narcotics such as fentanyl may facilitate ventilation in the immediate postintubation period.

Circulatory Management

Prompt restoration of circulating blood volume and a euvolemic state is critical.[37,56]

The initial assessment of circulatory status may be difficult, since the blood pressure may be maintained owing to sympathetic stimulation. Tachycardia, although common in trauma patients, and reduced capillary return are cardinal signs of hypovolemia. Peripheral perfusion may be difficult to assess in hypothermic patients.

Sources of external hemorrhage must be identified and rapidly treated, usually with direct pressure. Causes of refractory hypotension in these patients include acute spinal injury, tension pneumothorax, cardiac tamponade, and severe myocardial contusion; they must be excluded early.

There is no evidence to recommend crystalloid over colloid volume resuscitation; either will suffice.[57,58] This controversy has been fueled by the conflicting results of metaanalyses of small clinical trials, often of poor quality. A recent large randomized controlled trial demonstrated that saline and albumin were equally effective for the resuscitation of critically ill patients.[57] Some 1 to 2 L of balanced salt solution (lactated Ringer's or normal saline) or an equivalent volume of synthetic colloid (Hemaccel, Gelfusin, or Hetastarch) should initially be infused in all patients through large-bore peripheral venous lines. Hypertonic saline may theoretically be useful as a small-volume resuscitation fluid, which is effective in expanding intravascular volume, with potentially beneficial effects in head-injured patients.[59] However, hypertonic saline given before the patient reaches a hospital has not been demonstrated to improve outcome.[60]

Blood transfusion must be administered to patients who have lost more than 20 to 30 percent of their blood volume or where further serious hemorrhage is anticipated.

Early and accurate measurement of arterial pressure (ideally through a central artery) and a central venous catheter are essential to guide volume replacement and administrate blood and drugs. The placement of these lines must not delay volume resuscitation.

The target for mean arterial pressure should be estimated on the basis of the patient's premorbid blood pressure, since higher pressures may be necessary in hypertensive or elderly patients. The early use of vasoactive agents may be necessary to achieve this.

Vasoactive agents such as epinephrine, norepinephrine or dopamine or vasopressors such as phenylephrine or metaraminol may be used to defend blood pressure once correction of hypovolemia is under way or achieved.[61,62] There is no evidence that any vasoactive

agent or combinations of vasoactive agents are superior to one another.

In selected patients with penetrating thoracic injury, a "permissive hypotension" strategy has been advocated during resuscitation pending definitive surgical intervention.[63] This strategy is based on the assumption that aggressive hemodynamic resuscitation may increase surgically remediable bleeding in noncompressible areas. Although there is some evidence to support this strategy, it cannot be used in patients with an associated traumatic brain injury or those with blunt trauma.

Neurologic Assessment

The assessment of neurologic function is important to quantify the severity of brain injury and provide prognostic information. The level of function may be influenced by associated injuries, hypoxia, hypotension, and drug or alcohol intoxication.

Neurologic assessment of the patient should be done frequently. During the resuscitation phase, neurologic signs should be documented before and after any major intervention (e.g., intubation, correction of blood pressure, patient transport) and at least at hourly intervals.

Neurologic assessment includes observing the best neurologic response to the least noxious stimulus. This includes simple scores such as AVPU (awake, verbal, pain, unresponsive to stimulation) or more integrated scores, such as the Glasgow Coma Scale score[64] and pupillary responses.

Secondary Survey

After the initial assessment and when resuscitation is under way, a thorough secondary survey adopting a head-to-toe approach is mandatory.

The principles outlined in the initial assessment form the basis for deciding priorities of interventions in the secondary survey. Causes of hypoxia or hypercapnia—such as pulmonary contusion, and hemothorax/pneumothorax—must be excluded and promptly treated. Hemorrhage, both external and internal, must be aggressively treated until the circulation is stable.

The approach of "damage-control surgery" outlined above is advocated in head-injured patients so as to minimize secondary insults. In the initial 24 to 48 h after injury, only life- or limb-threatening injuries should be treated. After this, patients are transferred to the ICU for stabilization and monitoring. Thereafter, semiurgent surgery such as fixation of closed fractures or delayed plastic repairs may be completed.[65] Patients with severe head injury who undergo prolonged emergency surgery should ideally have intracranial pressure monitoring begun as soon as possible.

Routine x-rays of the chest, pelvis, and cervical spine and baseline blood tests (including tests for blood alcohol and other drugs of abuse level when deemed necessary) are part of the secondary survey.

For intubated and ventilated patients, sedation in the acute phase must be titrated against the patient's hemodynamic stability. High doses of narcotics (e.g., 15 to 25 μg/kg fentanyl) and nondepolarizing muscle relaxants (e.g., vecuronium 8 to 10 mg) will provide sufficient sedation and allow control of ventilation for 1 to 2 h, during which time imaging and other investigations can be performed. Frequent assessment of consciousness is essential, because excessive sympathetic activity may potentiate raised intracranial pressure or myocardial ischemia in a paralyzed but awake patient. Sedation may need to be supplemented with intermittent doses of opiates or benzodiazepines.

Stabilization

Depending on the degree of trauma and extent of injuries, patients may be transferred to the operating theater for emergency or definitive surgery. The majority of patients with massive or multiple trauma will be transferred to a high-acuity-care area such as a trauma unit or an ICU.

This section addresses the principles of management of patients who require intensive care for stabilization following trauma resuscitation.

There is no standard or uniform method of managing traumatized patients in the ICU. Local preferences, experience, caseload, and resources determine most practices. After initial resuscitation, intensive care is regarded as a continuation of care in the emergency department or operating theatre.

Hemodynamic Management

The defense of perfusion in vital organs forms the basis of hemodynamic management, considering the physiologic principles outlined above.

▶ MONITORING

Circulatory dysfunction is commonly defined as a mean arterial pressure ≤60 mmHg for 1 h despite adequate fluid administration, although this may vary between patients and will depend on the etiology. Accurate measurement of systemic blood pressure is essential and should be done via an arterial catheter referenced to the aortic root. A large artery, such as the femoral artery, should be considered in hemodynamically unstable patients, because measurements from radial or dorsalis pedis arteries may underestimate systemic pressure in shocked patients. Given the importance of maintaining adequate systemic pressures, noninvasive measurement of blood pressure is not recommended during the acute phase of monitoring.[56]

Therapy should be titrated to mean arterial pressure in accordance with the patient's premorbid blood pressure; i.e., in older patients, higher mean arterial pressure (e.g., 80 mmHg) may be necessary.

Central venous catheters are inserted in the majority of severely traumatized patients requiring intensive care. Volume status should be assessed by electronically transduced measurements of central venous pressure and hourly measurements of urine output. Right atrial pressure monitoring via a central venous catheter provides the best assessment of volume status.[66] Accuracy may be affected by tricuspid regurgitation or pulmonary hypertension.

The response of right atrial pressure to a fluid challenge, rather than an absolute number, will yield useful information regarding the patient's volume status.

Pulmonary artery catheters allow measurement of two independent variables—cardiac output and pulmonary artery pressures—but is rarely indicated in traumatized patients unless there is associated cardiac dysfunction. Measurement of these two variables may be useful in patients with states of low cardiac output or in those with acute pulmonary hypertension, such as ALI/ARDS. Pulmonary artery occlusion pressure may be used as an indirect measurement of left atrial pressure. However, this measurement may be affected by respiratory artifact, positive airway pressure, tachycardia, hypovolemia, and poor ventricular compliance and has limited clinical utility in critically ill patients.

Derived hemodynamic variables, such as systemic vascular resistance, are frequently calculated and used as a surrogate index of afterload. However, the clinical utility of systemic vascular resistance is limited to providing a crude estimate of global vascular tone, as it does not reflect afterload, arteriolar tone, or venous return. Consequently, systemic vascular resistance should not be used as a criterion for the selection of vasoactive drug or as a titratable endpoint.[67]

Central venous catheters are a major source of nosocomial infection and cause significant morbidity and mortality. There is no agreement about how long such catheters should be left in place or the diagnosis of catheter-induced sepsis.[68,69] By puncturing the skin, these catheters provide a nidus for infection and a point of entry into the circulation for bacteria.

Generally, catheters inserted during resuscitation should be changed as soon as possible unless strict asepsis was used in their insertion. The incidence of infection increases markedly after 5 days and varies with the site of the catheter, with an increasing rate of infection in subclavian, internal jugular, and femoral venous catheters. How long catheters should be left in situ before replacement remains controversial; such decisions must consider the reason for their use and the patient's clinical state as well the risk involved in placing new catheters. Catheters should not be changed routinely and should be observed daily or until clinical evidence of infection is apparent. The development of persistent or new pyrexia, leukocytosis, and an inflamed insertion site indicate catheter sepsis and warrant a new catheter. Semiquantitative culture of the intradermal portion or tip of the catheter may determine whether an infection was present.[70]

▶ FLUID MANAGEMENT

The maintenance of a euvolemic state is essential throughout the intensive care period. This is determined by regular measurements, such as serum sodium and osmolality, urea and creatinine, pulse rate, right atrial and mean arterial pressure, and urine output.

Resuscitative fluids depend on local preferences, since there is no evidence to recommend crystalloids over colloids.[57,71] Similarly, fluids should be titrated to maintain neutral fluid balance and biochemical normality.

Hemoglobin invariably falls following an acute insult. The lower limit of tolerable hemoglobin levels in critically ill patients has been extensively debated, with increasing evidence that a restrictive transfusion strategy (hemoglobin ≤8 g/L) is associated with improved outcomes compared to a more liberal transfusion strategy (hemoglobin <10 g/L).[72] Rather than using an absolute value, acceptance of hemoglobin of 8 to 10 g/L appears to be physiologically appropriate in acutely traumatized patients, although subgroups of patients, such as those with concomitant cardiac disease, may require maintenance of higher hemoglobin levels.

▶ VASOACTIVE THERAPY

Catecholamines such as epinephrine, norepinephrine, or dopamine are frequently used to increase mean arterial pressure. Normally these drugs should be used only when volume resuscitation is actively under way or complete. However, the early use of catecholamines is increasingly being advocated to maintain homeostatic systemic pressure, often to counter the depressant cardiovascular effects of acute injury and the effects of sedation and anesthesia. On a pathobiologic basis, catecholamines are essentially used to increase endogenous mechanisms that may be failing, with norepinephrine being regarded as the principal endogenous catecholamine to defend systemic blood pressure.

Except when very small doses of vasoactive drugs are used, the mean arterial pressure of all patients who receive them should be monitored, ideally with an intraarterial catheter referenced to the aortic root. There is no conclusive evidence to recommend one vasoactive agent over another or any combination of vasoactive agents. In clinical practice, epinephrine, norepinephrine, and dopamine are most commonly used. These drugs have similar pharmacodynamic profiles with equivalent effects on mean arterial pressure and cardiac output and without significant changes in systemic vascular resistance. Increases in cardiac output are matched by increased venous return, which results in a pressor effect.[67]

Prediction of the response of an individual to a catecholamine is problematic because inter- and intraindividual responses to inotropic agents may vary markedly.

Although norepinephrine is widely used as an initial inotropic agent, epinephrine is still advocated by many as a first-line agent. However, its use may be associated with metabolic side effects such as hyperlactatemia and hyperglycemia, which may complicate metabolic management.[73,74] There is, however, no evidence that these side effects are associated with morbidity. Although dopamine is a commonly employed inotrope, its use is questioned due to significant neuroendocrine effects, particularly inhibition of posterior pituitary gland function.[75] Furthermore, the use of dopamine is associated with the highest incidence of tachyarrhythmias, which may be important in patients with ischemic heart disease.

Synthetic catecholamines, such as dobutamine, dopexamine, and isoprenaline, and agents such as milrinone and levosimendan offer little advantage over the endogenous catecholamines. These agents are predominantly vasodilators with moderate and unpredictable inotropic activity, particularly in hypovolemic patients.

Renal Protection

By increasing mean arterial pressure, vasoactive agents have an important role in preventing or lessening acute renal failure in critically ill patients. This is important in hypertensive patients, in whom higher mean arterial pressure may be required to maintain renal perfusion, particularly when these patients develop intercurrent causes of circulatory failure.

A "renal" dose of dopamine (2 μg/kg/min) has been advocated for many years as a renal-protective agent by causing renal vasodilatation. However, this has not been substantiated in controlled clinical trials in susceptible patients.[76] Its use as an adjunctive agent with other inotropes in septic shock has also not been proven.[77] In addition, the prolonged use of low-dose dopamine is associated with suppression of anterior and posterior pituitary hormonal secretion and impairment in T-cell function.[78,79] It is therefore no longer recommended. Equivalent renal protection has been demonstrated with dopamine, norepinephrine,[80] and dobutamine;[81] this effect may be primarily due to their effect in sustaining renal perfusion rather than to a specific renal effect.[82]

Diuretics should be used sparingly in traumatized patients. As outlined above, oliguria is a normal response to injury. The injudicious use of diuretics may therefore not only mask this important clinical sign but also exacerbate hypovolemia. There is no evidence to support the use of diuretics to prevent acute renal failure by inducing polyuria. Indeed, in the hemodynamically unstable patient, the use of diuretics may be regarded as potentially nephrotoxic.

The use of iodinated intravenous contrast media is associated with acute renal dysfunction, particularly in hemodynamically unstable patients. Contrast-induced nephropathy may be minimized by ensuring adequate hemodynamic resuscitation before contrast administration. Renoprotective effects of intravenous N-acetylcysteine[83] or sodium bicarbonate[84] have been described and should be considered in susceptible patients who receive contrast media.

SIRS and Septic Shock

The development of high- or low cardiac output shock will occur in a minority of traumatized patients. Noninfective causes of this syndrome include massive blood transfusion, pancreatitis, ischemic colitis, and drug reactions. Infection usually develops 72 h after injury and may be due to infected wounds, intraabdominal or intrathoracic abscesses, or nosocomial sepsis. Regardless of the cause, the hemodynamic management of this syndrome remains essentially the same.

An increasing body of literature now supports the use of norepinephrine and epinephrine as first-line agents in the systemic inflammatory response syndrome and septic shock, since they maintain tissue perfusion by effectively defending cardiac output and mean arterial pressure.[85-87] Systemic vascular resistance is not significantly altered by catecholamine infusions in septic shock.[88]

Despite their widespread recent use, the efficacy of dobutamine and isoprenaline in septic shock is questionable; it appears to add little to the efficacy of norepinephrine or epinephrine when used in combination.[89] However, the benefit attributable to a particular catecholamine in preventing mortality due to septic shock has not been established.

A proportion of patients with severe septic shock who require high doses of catecholamines to support the circulation will need less of these drugs when treated with infusions of vasopressin (0.04 u/h).[90] This phenomenon appears to be independent of any direct vasopressor effect; rather, it may be due to a supplemental "catecholamine sparing" strategy.[91] However, its impact on mortality has not been determined in conclusive clinical trials.

The role of steroid supplementation in circulatory failure has been studied for many years. Although immunosuppressive or anti-inflammatory doses have been shown to be ineffective, particularly in septic shock, stress response doses (approximately 100 to 200 mg of hydrocortisone per day) have been shown to improve vasoresponsiveness to catecholamines in patients with refractory shock.[92] Patients who respond to low doses of steroids may have biochemical evidence of hypoadrenalism, defined by a low serum cortisol level or a blunted response to intravenous adrenocorticotropin, or functional hypoadrenalism as part of the multiple organ failure syndrome.

Respiratory Therapy

AIRWAY MANAGEMENT

Patients should remain intubated only as long as necessary. In patients with head injuries, endotracheal intubation may be prolonged due to their slow recovery of consciousness and adequate glottic reflexes.

Endotracheal intubation may be performed either translaryngeally through the nose or mouth or transtracheally via a tracheostomy. The use of polyvinylchloride tubes with low-pressure, high-volume cuffs decreased the incidence of tracheal mucosal damage and ulceration from nasal or oral endotracheal tubes. Consequently the duration of translaryngeal intubation depends on the degree of underlying head injury, preexisting lung reserve, and concomitant lung function.

Oral intubation is the preferred method for emergencies and allows passage of a tube of a larger diameter (8 mm or more) with easier bronchial toilet. These tubes are more prone to movement and are more difficult to secure. The incidence of nosocomial sinusitis is significantly lower with oral intubation.[93] Nasal intubation provides good support for the endotracheal tube and patients often require less sedation to tolerate the tube. Nasal tubes are also less prone to move in the trachea and therefore cause less tracheal mucosal damage than oral tubes. However, suction through these tubes is more difficult owing to the smaller diameter of the tube and the increased distance from the nasal aditus to the end of the tube. Nasal tubes allow patients to swallow their saliva; it is therefore easier to maintain oral hygiene. Nasal intubation is, however, contraindicated in patients with fractures of the basal skull and cribriform plate.

Tracheostomy is generally indicated in patients when prolonged ventilation due to respiratory failure is anticipated for more than 7 to 10 days, or when a return to full consciousness is not expected for weeks or months. These patients usually have poor protective glottic reflexes and inadequate clearance of secretions and are predisposed to recurrent aspiration and nosocomial pneumonia. Tracheostomy tubes are more comfortable than translaryngeal tubes and allow easier tracheobronchial toilet. Tubes with a device that directs a stream of retrograde air through the larynx above the cuff site make speech possible in selected patients.

Tracheostomy should be performed only by experienced operators and when pulmonary reserve is adequate to tolerate an operation on the airway. In ventilated patients, this means a fractional inspired oxygen concentration of 0.5 or less to achieve a PaO_2 greater than 80 mmHg and peak inflation pressures of less than 30 cmH$_2$0. Clotting status should be normal.

Tracheostomy may be performed in the operating room or in the ICU.[94] A number of percutaneous dilatational tracheostomy techniques have been described that can be performed in the ICU to avoid moving the patient.[95] These procedures are quick and allow the passage of a normal 8- or 9-mm tube. Tracheal stenosis is a recognized complication of tracheostomy, but its incidence after the percutaneous procedure compared to surgical tracheostomy is unknown.[96]

Irrespective of the route of intubation, cuffed tubes must be inflated sufficiently to seal the airway in order to prevent aspiration. Cuffs may leak due to changing cuff compliance, tracheal dilatation during prolonged intubation, or tube movement. Excess cuff pressure on the tracheal mucosa may predispose to tracheal ulceration and subsequent stenosis. Frequent volumetric cuff checks and cuff pressure measurements should be performed to ensure a safe seal.

VENTILATORY MANAGEMENT

The majority of severely traumatized patients will require mechanical ventilation to ensure adequate oxygenation (PaO_2 > 75 mmHg; 10 kPa) and to maintain an arterial carbon dioxide tension between 36 and 40 mmHg (4.5 to 5.0 kPa). The need for normal oxygenation and carbon dioxide must outweigh the potential hazards of ventilation. Advances in the design of mechanical ventilators and an increased awareness of ventilator-induced lung injury and nosocomial pneumonia have improved ventilation methods and made them safer.

Positive-pressure ventilation is the routine form of mechanical ventilation in current practice. Gas is delivered under positive pressure to a preset inspiratory pressure or tidal volume. Mechanical ventilation should be regarded as lung support that is adapted to the individual patient's respiratory condition.

Complete control of ventilation is usually necessary during the resuscitation period. This requires a mode of ventilation that will override the patient's efforts to breathe. When resuscitation has been completed and cardiorespiratory and neurologic stability are achieved, the patient should be allowed to breathe spontaneously with as little respiratory support as possible. The degree of respiratory support will depend on the improvement or resolution of acute traumatic and systemic processes, level of sedation, and preexisting cardiorespiratory disease.

During the initial period when controlled ventilation is desired, modes such as assist or volume or pressure control may be employed. These modes deliver a preset tidal volume, respiratory rate, and inspiratory pressure. At this stage patients are usually heavily sedated or paralyzed with muscle relaxants. For the majority of patients with normal lungs, either mode will suffice to achieve adequate gaseous exchange. However, patients with acute lung injury (e.g., direct lung injury, aspiration pneumonitis, fat embolism syndrome, or neurogenic pulmonary edema or those with extensive bodily trauma) are at risk of developing ventilator-induced lung injury. Accordingly, a protective ventilation strategy should be considered.[97]

The distinction between volume- and pressure-based ventilatory modes is less important in modern practice. These modes deliver tidal volumes and inspiratory pressures in what is considered a safe range, which reduces the risk of ventilator-induced lung injury. Central to this strategy is the use of low tidal volumes (5 to 7 mL/kg) and limited peak inspiratory pressures (<35 to 40 cmH$_2$O). Under these conditions, mechanical ventilation has been shown to improve survival in patients with severe ALI or ARDS.[98] A consequence of this ventilatory strategy is permissive hypercapnia, in which $PaCO_2$ is allowed to increase, resulting in acute respiratory acidosis (pH 7.1 to 7.2).

Although controlled ventilation is useful in the above situations, deep sedation may be associated with accumulation of secretions, hypostatic and nosocomial pneumonia, gastroparesis, and neuromuscular weakness.

Assisted ventilation should be instituted as soon as possible. This is determined by reducing sedation requirements and allowing the patient to breathe spontaneously, with sufficient mechanical support to maintain gaseous exchange. Modes such as assist control ventilation (ACV), synchronized intermittent mandatory ventilation (SIMV), pressure support ventilation (PSV), and flow-by ventilation are suitable. These modes allow the patient to generate a small negative airway pressure or flow that activates the inspiratory cycle, the duration of which is determined either by a preset tidal volume, the ratio of inspiration to expiration (I:E ratio), or by reaching a pressure limit. The triggering mechanism must be sensitive enough to detect inspiratory efforts of the patient, increasing the work of breathing, but not so sensitive that the ventilator will cycle in response to fluctuations in airway pressure not initiated by the patient.

Weaning from ventilation should start once cardiorespiratory and neurologic homeostasis has been achieved and no major operations are scheduled. The advent of "noninvasive" modes of ventilation (i.e., positive-pressure ventilation without an endotracheal tube), such as biphasic positive-pressure ventilation (BiPAP), or continuous positive airway pressure (CPAP), has greatly facilitated the weaning of ventilated patients. Noninvasive ventilation is particularly useful in patients with postextubation stridor, moderate chronic obstructive airways disease, asthma, atelectasis, or congestive cardiac failure.

Trials of extubation should be carefully considered so that subsequent hypoxic episodes do not occur, as these are potent secondary insults.

MAINTENANCE OF VENTILATED PATIENTS

Inspired gases must be humidified for all ventilated patients because the humidifying functions of the nasopharynx are bypassed by endotracheal intubation. Ideally gas should be humidified to 75 to 100% and at a constant temperature (32 to 36°C; 89.6 to 96.8°F) and should not increase work of breathing, dead space, or resistance in either spontaneous or controlled ventilation.

Humidifiers include water baths and aerosol nebulizers or atomizers. Bacterial contamination of water reservoirs, overhydration, overheating, and electrical hazards may complicate the use of these systems. Most of these complications may be avoided by attaching heat and moisture exchangers to the endotracheal tube. These devices provide safe, efficient humidification and may be combined with a bacterial filter.[99]

Patients with reactive airways due to asthma, chronic airways disease, or acute bronchospasm from infection or pulmonary edema may benefit from nebulization of beta$_2$ agonists, such as salbutamol, to improve gas exchange and reduce inspired airway pressure. The addition of nebulized anticholinergics, such as ipratropium bromide, may be beneficial in patients with severe airflow obstruction, particularly in the weaning phase. The routine use of these agents in ventilated patients has, however, not been shown to be beneficial.

NOSOCOMIAL PNEUMONIA

Patients who require prolonged ventilation are susceptible to respiratory infections. During the later stages of trauma management, the lung is vulnerable to nosocomial infection. The causes for this association include reduced airway defense mechanisms due to endotracheal intubation, impaired mucociliary clearance, aspiration pneumonitis, and hematogenous spread of inflammatory and infective mediators to the lung. The resultant nosocomial pneumonia may induce or exacerbate an acute lung injury and increase morbidity and mortality.

Early pneumonia is defined as respiratory infection present or developing soon after intubation and may arise from aspiration of gastric contents or infection of lobar collapses in the acute stages. Late or true ventilator-associated or nosocomial pneumonia is defined as infection that first occurs 48 h after intubation.[100]

True ventilator-associated pneumonia causes significant morbidity and mortality, particularly in patients who develop an acute lung injury. In patients who need positive-pressure mechanical ventilation for more than 3 days, the incidence of pneumonia has been reported to be 35 to 70 percent. Nosocomial pneumonia prolongs ventilation and ICU stay significantly, although the incidence of mortality attributable to it remains low.[101]

Several criteria for a clinical diagnosis of nosocomial pneumonia have been reported.[102] These include radiographic evidence of a new or progressive pulmonary infiltrate, fever, leukocytosis, and purulent tracheobronchial secretions. In addition to these clinical criteria, a Gram's stain of the sputum showing >25 polymorphonuclear leukocytes and <10 squamous epithelial cells per low-power field and the presence of a significant pathogen (by stain or culture) has been advocated. In a previously healthy person, these signs almost invariably indicate pneumonia, and treatment with antibiotics should be started as soon as bacterial sensitivities have been established.

Mechanically ventilated patients frequently develop other conditions that obscure these findings or cause a similar clinical picture, which may be due in part to the systemic inflammatory response to acute injury. Moreover, purulent secretions are invariably present in patients on prolonged mechanical ventilation but are not caused by pneumonia in most. Secretions may originate from the sinuses, stomach, or oropharynx and may accumulate above the endotracheal tube cuff and be aspirated by minor manipulation. In addition, the proximal airways of ventilated patients are colonized early by potentially pathogenic organisms.

No combination of clinical variables is completely accurate in predicting pneumonia in ventilated patients. Postmortem studies have shown that pneumonia is underdiagnosed in patients with acute lung injury but overdiagnosed in acute respiratory failure from other causes.[100]

Mortality rates in patients who received antimicrobial therapy before the onset of pneumonia are significantly lower than in those who did not. However, the overuse of broad-spectrum antibiotics in patients without infection is potentially harmful because it may facilitate colonization and superinfection with highly virulent organisms.[103]

To improve the recognition of pneumonia and identify the responsible microbes, a number of techniques have been described. Although a culture from lung tissue is regarded as the gold standard in establishing this diagnosis, open lung biopsy is obviously not feasible in all patients. Numerous nonbronchoscopic and bronchoscopic methods to obtain lower respiratory secretions and various microbiologic analyses have been described but are beyond the scope of this review. Of these, quantitative cultures of tracheal aspirates and nondirected bronchoalveolar lavage are recommended for the majority of patients. Other systemic sources of infection should also be actively sought and treated. The relative risk of investigations must be balanced against the benefit to the patient, particularly when invasive investigations such as bronchoalveolar lavage are considered.

Effective pulmonary toilet, postural drainage, and the prevention of gastric aspiration is essential.[104] Increased sedation may be necessary during tracheal suctioning to prevent sympathetically mediated swings in blood pressure. Antibiotic coverage should use the least toxic bactericidal agent in appropriate doses and should be guided by monitoring its level if necessary. Antibiotics should be used only when the criteria for nosocomial pneumonia are established and bacteriologic cultures are positive. Sensitivity testing is the best guide to antibiotic choice.

ACUTE RESPIRATORY DISTRESS SYNDROME/ACUTE LUNG INJURY

As outlined above, the hallmarks of this syndrome relate to increased permeability of the alveolar-capillary endothelium.

In traumatized patients, the causes of ALI/ARDS are many and may be considered as direct or indirect insults. It is important to distinguish between these causes, since their outcomes vary. Some patients with ALI/ARDS develop dysfunction or failure of one or more organ systems sequentially or simultaneously. Other patients develop multiple organ failure without ALI/ARDS, although they may have less severe degrees of parenchymal lung injury. This suggests that ALI/ARDS is the respiratory manifestation of multiple organ failure syndrome, just as distributive or septic shock is the cardiovascular manifestation.

The treatment of patients with ALI/ARDS is supportive and aims to maintain oxygenation. The majority—80 percent—of patients with ARDS die from multiple organ failure or sepsis rather than from respiratory impairment. The underlying cause must be treated and suspected sites of sepsis need to be managed with appropriate antibiotics and surgical drainage. Volume- or pressure-limited ventilation and the effective use of positive end-expiratory pressure form the mainstays of support of these patients in the ICU. Techniques such as prone ventilation, extended- or inverse-ratio pressure-control ventilation, and selected pulmonary vasodilators such as nitric oxide and nebulized prostacyclin are used in selected patients. On rare occasions, when survival cannot be sustained with mechanical ventilation, extracorporeal techniques such as extracorporeal membrane oxygenation (ECMO) with or without low-frequency positive-pressure ventilation and extracorporeal removal of carbon dioxide (LFPPV-ECCO$_2$R) have been employed with anecdotal success.[105] No conclusive studies have demonstrated improved outcomes in ARDS with these advanced supportive techniques.

The prognosis of ALI/ARDS depends largely on the cause of the insult and the subsequent development of multiple organ failure. Fat embolism syndrome and neurogenic pulmonary edema may cause a severe but transient ALI/ARDS, which is often associated with a good outcome and probably has little influence on mortality. However, other causes, such as gram-negative sepsis and shock states, are associated with a higher incidence of multiple organ failure with an increased mortality rate on the order of 40 to 60 percent.

Metabolic Management

Routine measurement of biochemical variables is essential to keep them all within normal limits. Hyperglycemia is common after massive trauma and is usually centrally mediated and transient. Blood sugar levels should be maintained within normal limits with insulin infusions. Recent studies have demonstrated that the strict maintenance of normoglycemia in critically ill patients is associated with improved survival.[50,51] Blood sugar levels between 4.4 to 6.1 mmol/L are recommended, using infusions of insulin as required. Concomitant administration of 20% dextrose may be necessary to reduce the risk of hypoglycemia, which may go unrecognized in sedated or unconscious patients. Hypoglycemia is a recognized secondary insult and must be avoided.[106]

RENAL DYSFUNCTION

Renal dysfunction and failure is common after multiple trauma. As outlined above, oliguria is a normal physiologic response to acute injury in the initial period (up to 48 to 72 h following injury). However, in the traumatized patient, oliguria should also be regarded as a cardinal sign of hypovolemia, for which the appropriate initial treatment is a fluid challenge and/or augmentation of mean arterial pressure with a vasoactive agent. In traumatized patients, this forms the vanguard to protect renal homeostasis. In managing acute trauma, one should always consider premorbid renal function and concomitant medications, in particular ACE inhibitors and nonsteroidal anti-inflammatory agents, which may exacerbate acute renal dysfunction. Anuria is uncommon after trauma and should raise the possibility of prerenal vascular disruption or postrenal (ureteric, vesical, or urethral) obstruction. This is highly probable for injuries such as pelvic fractures, retroperitoneal hematoma, or major abdominal vascular injury.

RHABDOMYOLYSIS

Patients with significant soft tissue injury—particularly when it is associated with long bone fractures and crush injury, threatened limbs from acute arterial insufficiency, and prolonged immobility—may develop acute renal dysfunction caused by deposition of myoglobin.[107] Although this is a recognized insult, the association between myonecrosis and acute tubular necrosis is tenuous, since the associated renal deficiency is primarily due to hypotension, shock, and hypovolemia. The treatment of acute renal failure associated with crush injury is therefore directed primarily at restoration of hemodynamic function rather than the use of specific antidotes to myoglobin deposition. For the latter condition, urinary alkalinization and the use of osmotic diuretics has been advocated for many years, although there is little evidence that these agents are effective. These agents should therefore be used carefully so that hemodynamic function is not compromised.

Abdominal Compartment Syndrome

Another important and reversible cause of acute renal dysfunction after trauma is the abdominal compartment syndrome.[108] Increased intraabdominal pressure due to excessive bowel distention, intra- or retroperitoneal hematoma, or tense ascites may cause intrinsic and/or extrinsic renal compression. The resultant reduction in glomerular filtration is multifactorial and is related to a reduction in renal preload, exaggerated activation of renin, and postrenal compression. This syndrome should be suspected in susceptible patients who develop marked abdominal distention. This may be quantified by measuring intravesical pressures, for which a value of >20 mmHg suggests abdominal compartment syndrome. These clinical signs and measurements may necessitate surgical decompression of the peritoneal cavity.

Acute renal failure that requires dialysis is associated with a high mortality rate (40 to 60 percent). New continuous renal dialysis techniques such as continuous venovenous hemo(dia)filtration make it possible to provide prompt and effective dialysis without the hemodynamic and coagulation disturbances that often complicate conventional intermittent hemodialysis. The indications for dialysis in traumatized patients include clinically significant hyperkalemia, symptomatic fluid overload, and azotemia associated with hypercatabolism. There is insufficient evidence to recommend continuous renal dialysis solely to remove unwanted pro- or anti-inflammatory mediators.

▶ GENERAL HOMEOSTATIC MANAGEMENT

Sedation, Analgesia, and Muscle Relaxants

There are no standards for sedation and analgesia for traumatized patients; protocols will depend on local preferences and resources. The level of sedation and analgesia required for traumatized patients depends on the degree of coma, hemodynamic stability, and associated injuries.

During the resuscitation phase, sedation should be titrated to cause the least effect on systemic blood pressure. During this period, short-acting narcotics such as fentanyl are useful. These agents are relatively cardiostable and have the additional benefit of tempering the systemic sympathetic surges that frequently occur after injury. Intermediate acting muscle relaxants, such as vecuronium, are useful during this phase to control combative patients after intubation, ventilation, and sedation.

During the intensive care phase, requirements for sedation are different. The aim should be to sedate the patient as lightly as possible to allow clinical assessment of neurologic function and to facilitate mechanical ventilation. The level of sedation will depend on the patient's hemodynamic stability and the degree of intracranial pressure. Infusions of narcotic and benzodiazepines (e.g., fentanyl, morphine, and midazolam) are useful in providing moderate to deep levels of sedation and are effective in controlling surges of intracranial pressure. However, these agents may accumulate, resulting in a delay in the return of consciousness; if used for prolonged periods, they may be associated with the emergence of delirium.

The use of propofol as a sole sedating agent has become popular.[21] It provides deep sedation, which is effective in controlling systemic sympathetic swings. It does not accumulate, and its effects are rapidly reversible on cessation, allowing prompt assessment of neurologic status. Propofol should be used with caution in hemodynamically unstable patients, since it is a potent negative inotrope. The prolonged use of propofol is associated with tachyphylaxis and significant caloric loading from the lipid vector. Concerns have been raised about myocardial depression and sudden cardiac death, particularly if large doses are administered.[109] The routine use of muscle relaxants to facilitate sedation is not recommended. Prolonged use of nondepolarizing muscle relaxants is associated with the development of polyneuromyopathy.

Nutrition

The caloric needs of traumatized patients must be addressed as soon as possible following resuscitation. Early enteral feeding is recommended.[110]

The placement of nasogastric or enteral feeding tubes in traumatized patients is usually done via the oral route. If the cribriform plate is not fractured, postpyloric tubes via the oral, nasal, or percutaneous route are recommended, since gastroparesis is common after major trauma, particularly if there is intraabdominal injury. Formulated enteral feeds should be started as soon as possible and increased as tolerated to 1 to 2 mL/kg/h to deliver a total caloric intake of 35 to 40 kcal/kg/day.

In patients who cannot be fed enterally within 2 to 5 days of injury or for extended periods (>4 days) due to gastrointestinal pathology, parenteral nutrition may be required. A normal caloric load is administered as dextrose (2 g/kg/day at 4.1 kcal/g) and synthetic amino acids (1 g/kg of protein per day). Intravenous lipid, administered as an emulsion of fat (2 g/kg/day at 9 kcal/g) may be given as an additional caloric source and to replenish essential fatty acids.

Stress Ulcer Prophylaxis

The incidence of gastric erosions and stress ulceration has markedly decreased with better resuscitation and early enteral feeding. Traumatized patients, including those with brain injury or burns, are at no more risk than other critically ill patients for developing stress ulceration. Increased risk factors for gastric bleeding include critically ill patients who require mechanical ventilation for more than 48 h and those with an associated coagulopathy.[111]

There is no difference in the efficacy of H_2 antagonists (e.g., ranitidine) or proton-pump inhibitors. These should be used in susceptible patients until enteral feeding is established, after which they may be discontinued. Patients with a history of peptic ulceration should remain on antacid therapy for the duration of the acute phase.

Thromboprophylaxis

Traumatized patients, particularly those who require prolonged ventilation and sedation and those with pelvic or lower limb fractures, are at increased risk for developing thromboembolism. For these patients, treatment with fractionated or low-molecular-weight heparins, with or without compression stockings or calf-compressors, should be considered as soon as possible. The use of anticoagulants is, however, contraindicated for 7 to 10 days after injury in patients with intracranial hemorrhage. When intracranial pathology has stabilized; however, prophylactic anticoagulants may be considered, although there are no evidence-based standards for their use.[112] As a general rule, anticoagulants should not be used in head-injured patients with destructive intracranial pathology or hemorrhage, until a CT scan shows resolution of these processes.

Frequent surveillance of the iliofemoral veins using Doppler ultrasound in high-risk patients, such as those with pelvic fractures, should be performed. In patients who develop deep venous thrombosis but cannot be treated with anticoagulants, inferior vena caval filters should be considered.

Patient Transport

Patients with multiple trauma frequently require transportation for specialized investigations such as computerized tomography, angiography and ultrasound, or for multiple trips to the operating room. The transport of critically ill patients is associated with an increased risk of accidents and adverse events.[113,114] These include loss of airway, ventilator malfunction, temporary loss of monitoring, dislodgment of important drains and catheters, and omission of important medications. The urgency of each intended transfer must therefore be considered and transport undertaken only after the patient has been resuscitated and is hemodynamically stable. Appropriately trained personnel should attend all transported patients, particularly when they are hemodynamically unstable but require urgent transportation.

For patients who undergo multidisciplinary surgical procedures, a trauma specialist should be asked to coordinate the procedures so that life- and limb-threatening injuries receive priority. Underpinning this must be the recognition that severely injured patients, particularly those with traumatic brain injury, are vulnerable to potentially damaging secondary insults, and these must be prevented.

▶ OUTCOMES

Once the functions of vital organs recover and patients no longer require intensive support, they may be progressively weaned and organ supports removed. During this period patients require the most emotional and psychosocial support, because the period of resuscitation and intensive care is usually associated with profound retrograde amnesia. Rehabilitation as well as physical, occupational, and speech therapy should begin as soon as possible. Although these aspects only become critical after the acute period, they are often key determinants of functional survival.

Deaths from trauma are related to the degree of external force suffered by the patient. The majority of immediate deaths are due to head injury and major vascular disruption. These are usually nonpreventable and account for up to 40 percent of all deaths due to trauma. Early deaths are usually due to hypoxia secondary to airway compromise or exsanguinating hemorrhage. For patients who survive the initial injury and resuscitation, the outcome will largely depend on their injuries, the time taken to reach proper health care, and the adequacy of resuscitation and definitive treatment. Severely traumatized patients without serious brain injuries who are admitted to major hospitals survive in over 90 percent of cases. However, patients admitted to hospitals with head injuries, have a mortality rate of approximately 30 percent. Late deaths are usually due to complications of the primary injury, such as multiple organ failure, infection, and associated morbidities. Indeed, a proportion of these patients will have active treatment limited or withdrawn due to the burden of the acute injury.

Although mortality is often used as a primary measure of outcome for trauma, functional survival, particularly at 6 and 12 months after injury, is regarded as a more appropriate measure of outcome. It depends on the patient's underlying reserve and on how well injuries are repaired and heal.

In conclusion, this chapter has taken the reader through a physiologic journey from the moments of injury to recovery from massive multiple trauma. A consistent theme is that assiduous defense of vital-organ oxygenation and perfusion forms the vanguard in the management of these difficult cases. Most resuscitative and acute management strategies have been simplified and directed at augmenting the physiologic responses to injury. Where these responses are intact and the patient is compensating, close observation and preemptive support are often all that is required. When these systems begin to fail, their replacement by treatment becomes the priority, and the patient's survival will ultimately depend on his or her physiologic reserve.

REFERENCES

1. Ozanne-Smith J. Road traffic injury—A global public health scourge: A review for World Health Day 2004 (April 7). *Aust N Z J Public Health* 28:109, 2004.
2. Nantulya VM, Reich MR. Equity dimensions of road traffic injuries in low- and middle-income countries. *Inj Control Saf Promot* 10:13, 2003.
3. Goldstein M. Traumatic brain injury: A silent epidemic. *Ann Neurol* 27:327, 1990.
4. McGregor K, Pentland B. Head injury rehabilitation in the UK: An economic perspective. *Soc Sci Med* 45:295, 1997.
5. National Institute of Health. Consensus conference. Rehabilitation of persons with traumatic brain injury. NIH Consensus Development Panel on Rehabilitation of Persons with Traumatic Brain Injury. *JAMA* 282:974, 1999.
6. le Roux P. An update on the pathophysiology of sepsis. *S Afr Den J* 59:163,165, 2004.
7. Cavaillon JM, Adib-Conquy M, Fitting C, et al. Cytokine cascade in sepsis. *Scand J Infect Dis* 35:535, 2003.
8. Pawlinski R, Mackman N. Tissue factor, coagulation proteases, and protease-activated receptors in endotoxemia and sepsis. *Crit Care Med* 32:S293, 2004.
9. Blatteis CM, Li S, Li Z, et al. Signaling the brain in systemic inflammation: The role of complement. *Front Biosci* 9:915, 2004.
10. Ward PA. The dark side of C5a in sepsis. *Nat Rev Immunol* 4:133, 2004.
11. Liaw PC. Endogenous protein C activation in patients with severe sepsis. *Crit Care Med* 32:S214, 2004.
12. O'Brien JM Jr, Abraham E. Human models of endotoxemia and recombinant human activated protein C. *Crit Care Med* 32:S202, 2004.
13. Magder S, Rastepagarnah M. Role of neurosympathetic pathways in the vascular response to sepsis. *J Crit Care* 13:169, 1998.
14. Runciman WB, Morris JL. Adrenoceptor agonists, in Feldman AC, Paton W Scurr C (eds): *Mechanisms of Drugs in Anesthesia*. London: Edward Arnold, 1993:262.
15. Insel PA. Seminars in medicine of the Beth Israel Hospital, Boston. Adrenergic receptors—evolving concepts and clinical implications. *N Engl J Med* 334:580, 1996.
16. Muller-Werdan U, Werdan K. Immune modulation by catecholamines—A potential mechanism of cytokine release in heart failure? *Herz* 25:271, 2000.
17. Oppert M, Reinicke A, Graf KJ, et al. Plasma cortisol levels before and during "low-dose" hydrocortisone therapy and their relationship to hemodynamic improvement in patients with septic shock. *Intensive Care Med* 26:1747, 2000.
18. Hatherill M, Tibby SM, Hilliard T, et al. Adrenal insufficiency in septic shock. *Arch Dis Child* 80:51, 1999.
19. Alberti C, Brun-Buisson C, Goodman SV, et al. Influence of systemic inflammatory response syndrome and sepsis on outcome of critically ill infected patients. *Am J Respir Crit Care Med* 168:77, 2003.
20. Norwood MG, Bown MJ, Lloyd G, et al. The clinical value of the systemic inflammatory response syndrome (SIRS) in abdominal aortic aneurysm repair. *Eur J Vasc Endovasc Surg* 27:292, 2004.
21. Kelly DF, Goodale DB, Williams J, et al. Propofol in the treatment of moderate and severe head injury: A randomized, prospective double-blinded pilot trial. *J Neurosurg* 90:1042, 1999.
22. Guyton AC, Lindsay AW, Kaufmann BN. Effect of mean circulatory filling pressure and other peripheral circulatory factors on cardiac output. *Am J Physiol* 180:463, 1955.
23. Jacobsohn E, Chorn R, O'Connor M. The role of the vasculature in regulating venous return and cardiac output: Historical and graphical approach. *Can J Anesth* 44:849, 1997.
24. Bressack MA, Raffin TA. Importance of venous return, venous resistance, and mean circulatory pressure in the physiology and management of shock. *Chest* 92:906, 1987.
25. MacKenzie IM. The hemodynamics of human septic shock. *Anesthesia* 56:130, 2001.
26. Carpati CM, Astiz ME, Rackow EC. Mechanisms and management of myocardial dysfunction in septic shock. *Crit Care Med* 27:231, 1999.
27. Magder S, Vanelli G. Circuit factors in the high cardiac output of sepsis. *J Crit Care* 11:155, 1996.
28. Gustafsson F, Holstein-Rathlou N. Conducted vasomotor responses in arterioles: Characteristics, mechanisms and physiological significance. *Acta Physiol Scand* 167:11, 1999.
29. Silverman HJ, Penaranda R, Orens JB, et al. Impaired beta-adrenergic receptor stimulation of cyclic adenosine monophosphate in human septic shock: Association with myocardial hyporesponsiveness to catecholamines. *Crit Care Med* 21:31, 1993.
30. Watanabe T, Miyoshi M, Imoto T. Angiotensin II: Its effects on fever and hypothermia in systemic inflammation. *Front Biosci* 9:438, 2004.
31. Takenaka T, Hayashi K, Ikenaga H. Blood pressure regulation and renal microcirculation. *Contrib Nephrol* 46:143, 2004.
32. Loutzenhiser R, Bidani AK, Wang X. Systolic pressure and the myogenic response of the renal afferent arteriole. *Acta Physiol Scand* 181:407, 2004.

33. Hall TS. Euripus, or the ebb and flow of the blood. *J Hist Biol* 8:321, 1975.

34. Thurman DJ, Alverson C, Dunn KA, et al. Traumatic brain injury in the United States: A public health perspective. *J Head Trauma Rehabil* 14:602, 1999.

35. Chesnut RM, Marshall LF, Klauber MR, et al. The role of secondary brain injury in determining outcome from severe head injury. *J Trauma* 34:216, 1993.

36. Chesnut RM. Secondary brain insults after head injury: Clinical perspectives. *New Horiz* 3:366, 1995.

37. Chesnut RM. Avoidance of hypotension: Conditio sine qua non of successful severe head-injury management. *J Trauma* 42:S4, 1997.

38. Abboud FM. Special characteristics of the cerebral circulation. *Fed Proc* 40:2296, 1981.

39. Bouma GJ, Muizelaar JP. Cerebral blood flow in severe clinical head injury. *New Horiz* 3:384, 1995.

40. Martin NA, Patwardhan RV, Alexander MJ, et al. Characterization of cerebral hemodynamic phases following severe head trauma: Hypoperfusion, hyperemia, and vasospasm. *J Neurosurg* 87:9, 1997.

41. BTF Guidelines. Brain Trauma Foundation. American Association of Neurological Surgeons. Hyperventilation. *J Neurotrauma* 17:513, 2000.

42. Cruz J. The first decade of continuous monitoring of jugular bulb oxyhemoglobin saturation: Management strategies and clinical outcome. *Crit Care Med* 26:344, 1998.

43. Myburgh JA, Lewis SB. Mannitol for resuscitation in acute head injury: Effects on cerebral perfusion and osmolality. *Crit Care Resusc* 2:344, 2000.

44. BTF Guidelines. Brain Trauma Foundation. American Association of Neurological Surgeons. Mannitol. *J Neurotrauma* 17:521, 2000.

45. Gomersall CD, Joynt GM, Freebairn RC, et al. Oxygen therapy for hypercapnic patients with chronic obstructive pulmonary disease and acute respiratory failure: A randomized, controlled pilot study. *Crit Care Med* 30:113, 2002.

46. Ashbaugh DG, Bigelow DB, Petty TL, et al. Acute respiratory distress in adults. *Lancet* 2:319, 1967.

47. Bhatia M, Moochhala S. Role of inflammatory mediators in the pathophysiology of acute respiratory distress syndrome. *J Pathol* 202:145, 2004.

48. Frank JA, Matthay MA. Science review: Mechanisms of ventilator-induced injury. *Crit Care* 7:233, 2003.

49. Gattinoni L, Vagginelli F, Chiumello D, et al. Physiologic rationale for ventilator setting in acute lung injury/acute respiratory distress syndrome patients. *Crit Care Med* 31:S300, 2003.

50. Van den Berghe GH, Wouters P, Weekers F, et al. Intensive insulin therapy in the critically ill patients. *N Engl J Med* 345:1359, 2001.

51. Van den Berghe GH, Wouters PJ, Bouillon R, et al. Outcome benefit of intensive insulin therapy in the critically ill: Insulin dose versus glycemic control. *Crit Care Med* 31:359, 2003.

52. Prigent H, Maxime V, Annane D. Science review: Mechanisms of impaired adrenal function in sepsis and molecular actions of glucocorticoids. *Crit Care* 8:243, 2004.

53. American College of Surgeons Committee on Trauma. *Advanced Trauma Life Support for Doctors.* Chicago: American College of Surgeons, 1997.

54. Davis DP, Hoyt DB, Ochs M, et al. The effect of paramedic rapid sequence intubation on outcome in patients with severe traumatic brain injury. *J Trauma* 54:444, 2003.

55. Bochicchio GV, Ilahi O, Joshi M, et al. Endotracheal intubation in the field does not improve outcome in trauma patients who present without an acutely lethal traumatic brain injury. *J Trauma* 54:307, 2003.

56. Brain Trauma Foundation, American Association of Neurological Surgeons. BTF guidelines: Hypotension. *J Neurotrauma* 17:591, 2000.

57. Finfer S, Bellomo R, Boyce N, et al. A comparison of albumin and saline for fluid resuscitation in the intensive care unit. *N Engl J Med* 350:2247, 2004.

58. Clifton GL, Miller ER, Choi SC, et al. Fluid thresholds and outcome from severe brain injury. *Crit Care Med* 30:739, 2002.

59. Qureshi AI, Suarez JI. Use of hypertonic saline solutions in treatment of cerebral edema and intracranial hypertension. *Crit Care Med* 28:3301, 2000.

60. Cooper DJ, Myles PS, McDermott FT, et al. Prehospital hypertonic saline resuscitation of patients with hypotension and severe traumatic brain injury: A randomized controlled trial. *JAMA* 291:1350, 2004.

61. Alspaugh DM, Sartorelli K, Shackford SR, et al. Prehospital resuscitation with phenylephrine in uncontrolled hemorrhagic shock and brain injury. *J Trauma* 48:851, 2000.

62. Ract C, Vigue B. Comparison of the cerebral effects of dopamine and norepinephrine in severely head-injured patients. *Intensive Care Med* 27:101, 2001.

63. Bickell WH, Wall MJ Jr, Pepe PE, et al. Immediate versus delayed fluid resuscitation for hypotensive patients with penetrating torso injuries. *N Engl J Med* 331:1105, 1994.

64. Teasdale G, Jennett B. Assessment of coma and impaired consciousness. A practical scale. *Lancet* 2:81, 1974.

65. Townsend RN, Lheureau T, Protech J, et al. Timing fracture repair in patients with severe brain injury (Glasgow Coma Scale score <9). *J Trauma* 44:977, 1998.

66. Magder S. More respect for the CVP. *Intensive Care Med* 24:651, 1998.

67. Myburgh JA. Inotropic agents, in Oh TE, Bersten AD, Soni N (eds): *Intensive Care Manual,* 5th ed. London: Butterworth, 2003:841.

68. Ferretti G, Mandala M, Di Cosimo S, et al. Catheter-related bloodstream infections. Part I: Pathogenesis, diagnosis, and management. *Cancer Control* 9:513, 2002.

69. Ferretti G, Mandala M, Di Cosimo S, et al. Catheter-related bloodstream infections, Part II: Specific pathogens and prevention. *Cancer Control* 79:10, 2003.

70. O'Grady NP, Alexander M, Dellinger EP, et al. Guidelines for the prevention of intravascular catheter-related infections. *Infect Control Hosp Epidemiol* 23:759, 2002.

71. Finfer S, Bellomo R, Myburgh J, et al. Efficacy of albumin in critically ill patients. *BMJ* 326:559, 2003.

72. Hebert PC, Wells G, Blajchman MA, et al. A multicenter, randomized, controlled clinical trial of transfusion requirements in critical care. Transfusion Requirements in Critical Care Investigators, Canadian Critical Care Trials Group. *N Engl J Med* 340:409, 1999.

73. Day NP, Phu NH, Bethell DP, et al. The effects of dopamine and adrenaline infusions on acid-base balance and systemic hemodynamics in severe infection. *Lancet* 348:219, 1996.

74. Totaro RJ, Raper RF. Epinephrine-induced lactic acidosis following cardiopulmonary bypass. *Crit Care Med* 25:1693, 1997.

75. Van den Berghe GH, De Zegher FE. A senescent pattern of pituitary function during critical illness and dopamine treatment. *Verh K Acad Geneeskd Belg* 58:383, 1996.

76. Bellomo R, Chapman M, Finfer S, et al. Low-dose dopamine in patients with early renal dysfunction: A placebo-controlled randomised trial. Australian and New Zealand Intensive Care Society (ANZICS) Clinical Trials Group. *Lancet* 356:2139, 2000.

77. Bersten AD, Rutten AJ. Renovascular interaction of epinephrine, dopamine, and intraperitoneal sepsis. *Crit Care Med* 23:537, 1995.

78. Van den Berghe G., de Zegher F. Anterior pituitary function during critical illness and dopamine treatment. *Crit Care Med* 24:1580, 1996.

79. Van den Berghe GH, de Zegher F, Lauwers P, et al. Growth hormone secretion in critical illness: Effect of dopamine. *J Clin Endocrinol Metab* 79:1141, 1994.

80. Desjars P, Pinaud M, Bugnon D, et al. Norepinephrine therapy has no deleterious renal effects in human septic shock. *Crit Care Med* 17:426, 1989.

81. Duke GJ, Briedis JH, Weaver RA. Renal support in critically ill patients: Low-dose dopamine or low-dose dobutamine? *Crit Care Med* 22:1919, 1994.

82. Bersten AD, Holt AW. Vasoactive drugs and the importance of renal perfusion pressure. *New Horiz* 3:650, 1995.

83. Buller GK. Review: Prophylactic acetylcysteine reduces contrast nephropathy in chronic renal insufficiency. *ACP J Club* 140:41, 2004.

84. Merten GJ, Burgess WP, Gray LV, et al. Prevention of contrast-induced nephropathy with sodium bicarbonate: A randomized controlled trial. *JAMA* 291:2328, 2004.

85. Nasraway SA. Norepinephrine: No more "leave 'em dead"? *Crit Care Med* 28:3096, 2000.

86. Tordoff SG, Thompson JL, Williams AW. Noradrenaline as a vasoactive agent in septic shock. *Intens Care Med* 26:648, 2000.

87. Martin C, Papazian L, Perrin G, et al. Norepinephrine or dopamine for the treatment of hyperdynamic septic shock? *Chest* 103:1826, 1993.

88. Moran JL, O'Fathartaigh MS, Peisach AR, et al. Epinephrine as an inotropic agent in septic shock: A dose-profile analysis. *Crit Care Med* 21:70, 1993.

89. Martin C, Viviand X, Arnaud S, et al. Effects of norepinephrine plus dobutamine or norepinephrine alone on left ventricular performance of septic shock patients. *Crit Care Med* 27:1708, 1999.

90. Malay MB, Ashton RC Jr, Landry DW, et al. Low-dose vasopressin in the treatment of vasodilatory septic shock. *J Trauma* 47:699, 1999.

91. Rozenfeld V, Cheng JW. The role of vasopressin in the treatment of vasodilation in shock states. *Ann Pharmacother* 34:250, 2000.

92. Briegel J, Forst H, Haller M, et al. Stress doses of hydrocortisone reverse hyperdynamic septic shock: A prospective, randomized, double-blind, single-center study. *Crit Care Med* 27:723, 1999.

93. Geiss HK. Nosocomial sinusitis. *Intens Care Med* 25:1037, 1999.

94. Susanto I. Comparing percutaneous tracheostomy with open surgical tracheostomy. *BMJ* 324:3, 2002.

95. Ambesh SP, Pandey CK, Srivastava S, et al. Percutaneous tracheostomy with single dilatation technique: A prospective, randomized comparison of Ciaglia blue rhino versus Griggs' guidewire dilating forceps. *Anesth Analg* 95:1739, 2002.

96. Mittendorf EA, McHenry CR, Smith CM, et al. Early and late outcome of bedside percutaneous tracheostomy in the intensive care unit. *Am Surg* 68:342, 2002.

97. Brower RG, Rubenfeld GD. Lung-protective ventilation strategies in acute lung injury. *Crit Care Med* 31:S312, 2003.

98. The Acute Respiratory Distress Syndrome Network. Ventilation with lower tidal volumes as compared with traditional tidal volumes for acute lung injury and the acute respiratory distress syndrome. *N Engl J Med* 342:1301, 2000.

99. Bench S. Humidification in the long-term ventilated patient: A systematic review. *Intens Crit Care Nurs* 19:75, 2003.

100. Hubmayr RD, Burchardi H, Elliot M, et al. Statement of the 4th International Consensus Conference in Critical Care on ICU-Acquired Pneumonia—Chicago, Illinois, May 2002. *Intens Care Med* 28:1521, 2002.

101. Markowicz P, Wolff M, Djedaini K, et al. Multicenter prospective study of ventilator-associated pneumonia during acute respiratory distress syndrome. Incidence, prognosis, and risk factors. ARDS Study Group. *Am J Respir Crit Care Med* 161:1942, 2000.

102. Ruiz M, Torres A, Ewig S, et al. Noninvasive versus invasive microbial investigation in ventilator-associated pneumonia: Evaluation of outcome. *Am J Respir Crit Care Med* 162:119, 2000.

103. Kolleff MH. Appropriate antibiotic therapy for ventilator-associated pneumonia and sepsis: A necessity, not an issue for debate. *Intensive Care Med* 29:147, 2003.

104. Collard HR, Saint S, Matthay MA. Prevention of ventilator-associated pneumonia: An evidence-based systematic review. *Ann Intern Med* 138:494, 2003.

105. Lucey MA, Myburgh JA. Recombinant activated factor VII for exsanguinating hemorrhage post bilateral lung transplantation for extra-corporeal lung support-dependent respiratory failure. *Anesth Intens Care* 31:465, 2003.

106. Rovlias A, Kotsou S. The influence of hyperglycemia on neurological outcome in patients with severe head injury. *Neurosurgery* 46:335, 2000.

107. Holt S, Moore K. Pathogenesis of renal failure in rhabdomyolysis: The role of myoglobin. *Exp Nephrol* 8:72, 2000.

108. Balogh Z, McKinley BA, Cox CS Jr, et al. Abdominal compartment syndrome: The cause or effect of post-injury multiple organ failure. *Shock* 20:483, 2003.

109. Cremer OL, Moons KGM, Bouman ACB, et al. Long-term propofol infusion and cardiac failure in adult head-injured patients. *Lancet* 357:117, 2001.

110. Brain Trauma Foundation, American Association of Neurological Surgeons. BTF Guidelines: Nutrition. *J Neurotrauma* 17:539, 2000.

111. Cook DJ, Reeve BK, Guyatt GH, et al. Stress ulcer prophylaxis in critically ill patients. Resolving discordant meta-analyses. *JAMA* 275:308, 1996.

112. Hammond FM, Meighen MJ. Venous thromboembolism in the patient with acute traumatic brain injury: Screening, diagnosis, prophylaxis, and treatment issues. *J Head Trauma Rehabil* 13:36, 1998.

113. Reynolds HN, Habashi NM, Cottingham CA, et al. Interhospital transport of the adult mechanically ventilated patient. *Respir Care Clin North Am* 8:37, 2002.

114. Stevenson VW, Haas CF, Wahl WL. Intrahospital transport of the adult mechanically ventilated patient. *Respir Care Clin N Am* 8:1, 2002.

CHAPTER 3

Prevention of Infection in Orthopaedic Surgery

HALA H. SHAMSUDDIN

► INTRODUCTION

Before the introduction of antiseptic technique and antibiotics, life-threatening wound infections were the usual outcome of a major surgical procedure. The following quotation describes conditions in the nineteenth century: "Not a single wound healed without festering, and small wonder. In the operating theatre—to which one's nose bore witness as being the favorite retiring room of the nurses' cats—there was no appliance for washing the hands, nor was there any in the robing room opposite." The instruments lay "open for anyone to handle," and suture needles "were stuck ready in a jam pot of rancid lard." A sign over the operating room read "Prepare to meet thy God."[1]

It is appropriate to a chapter on preventing orthopaedic infections that the person credited with the introduction of aseptic principles was Joseph Lister, an orthopaedic surgeon. After Pasteur demonstrated that germs were responsible for putrefaction, Lister (in 1867) theorized that bacteria in the ambient air could cause wound infections if they gained access to tissues through the broken skin. He used carbolic acid (a phenol) directly on wounds and later started nebulizing it into the air. He "invented a donkey engine which sprayed a mist of carbolic acid through the operating room, and poisoned the microbes, the patient, and the surgeon alike."[2] Semmelweis advocated the use of antiseptics (chlorine solution) on the unbroken skin of the physician's hands to prevent them from transmitting infections. Surgical gloves were introduced in 1889. Koch described the benefits of heat in sterilizing equipment. Thus modern aseptic techniques were born.

These aseptic techniques decreased but did not eliminate bacterial contamination. After the introduction of antibiotics in the mid-twentieth century, their use in preventing infections after elective surgery was studied, with initially conflicting results. However, after Burke demonstrated the importance of timing the administration of antibiotics to maximize their efficacy, prophylactic antibiotics became standard care before certain operative procedures.[3] Antibiotics decreased but did not completely eliminate the incidence of postoperative infections; currently, surgical site infections (SSI) are the second most common cause of nosocomial infections,[4,5] with adverse consequences. The development of an SSI increases hospital stay, cost, mortality, and morbidity.[6–12]

Antimicrobial prophylaxis refers to a *critically timed brief course* of antibiotics started just before an operation begins. The value of antimicrobial prophylaxis has been clearly established for "clean" and "clean-contaminated" surgery. In "dirty" wounds, by definition, antimicrobials would be given for treatment rather than preventive purposes.

In this chapter, the principles of prophylaxis, the importance of timing, choice of antibiotics, and impact of emerging resistance patterns, with special emphasis on orthopaedic surgical procedures, are addressed.

► PRINCIPLES OF PROPHYLAXIS

To effectively prevent an infection, one must be able to:

- Identify the patients at risk.
- Identify procedures that pose risk.
- Define the pathogenesis.

- Define period of risk.
- Define spectrum of organisms involved.
- Have available safe, effective, and relatively inexpensive agents to which these organisms are sensitive.
- Use an antibiotic that carries a low risk of inducing resistance in the bacterial strains targeted.

Patients at Risk

There are patients at increased risk of SSI: patients with a coincident remote site of infection, patients known to be colonized with certain bacteria (e.g., *Staphylococcus aureus*), diabetics (especially if uncontrolled), smokers, obese people (>20 percent of ideal body weight), very old patients, patients on steroids, or those with poor nutritional status.[13–20] A risk index of three variables was developed by the National Nosocomial Infections Study (NNIS), as follows: American Society of Anesthesiology (ASA) preoperative assessment score of 3, 4, or 5; an operation lasting longer than T hours (where T depends on the procedure); and an operation classified as dirty/infected.[21,22] The index has values of 0, 1, 2, or 3. It is a better predictor of the risk of SSI than the traditional wound classification system.[23]

Staphylococcus aureus Colonization

Nasal carriage of *S. aureus* is the most significant independent risk factor for SSI due to that organism.[24–26] In a study of patients undergoing orthopaedic surgery with prosthetic implants, those who were nasal carriers of *S. aureus* had a relative risk of 8.9 of developing prosthetic infection compared with those who were not carriers.[27] Similar findings have been reported for patients undergoing neurosurgical and cardiac operations. The use of mupirocin prophylactically is addressed later in the chapter.

▶ PROCEDURES THAT POSE RISK

Surgical Wounds have been classified into *clean, clean/contaminated, contaminated,* and *dirty/infected.* The surgeon anticipates *preoperatively* the surgical wound class that would be present *postoperatively.* Antimicrobial prophylaxis is then designed accordingly.

Clean wounds are those operative wounds in which no inflammation is encountered. The respiratory, alimentary, genital, or uninfected urinary tract is *not* entered. Clean wounds are primarily closed but, if necessary, drained with closed drainage. Operative incision wounds after blunt trauma can be included in this category if they meet the criteria.

Clean/contaminated wounds are those operative wounds in which the respiratory, alimentary, genital, or urinary tract is entered under controlled conditions and without unusual contamination.

Contaminated wounds are fresh, open, accidental wounds or operations with a major break in surgical technique, gross spillage from the GI tract, or where acute nonpurulent inflammation is encountered.

Dirty/Infected wounds are those old wounds with retained devitalized tissue and those that involve existing clinical infection or perforated viscera.[18,28]

As mentioned earlier, contaminated and dirty/infected wounds would not be candidates for antibiotic prophylaxis. Antibiotics would be given for treatment instead. Antibiotic prophylaxis is recommended for all clean contaminated procedures, for the insertion of prosthetic devices, or for clean surgeries where the consequences of an infection would be catastrophic (spine surgeries, coronary artery bypass grafting, and vascular procedures).[18]

▶ PATHOGENESIS OF SURGICAL SITE INFECTIONS

Bacterial infection of any wound starts by contamination. This is inevitable even under the most stringent aseptic conditions. After contamination, the interplay of the dose and virulence of the organism and the resistance of the host determine the risk of infection. This has been described by the following equation[29]:

$$\text{Risk of SSI} = \text{dose of contaminating organism} \times \text{virulence/resistance of the host}$$

Virulence of organism: Many bacteria produce substances that can cause injury to tissue, help invade tissue, or evade host defense. These include the endotoxins of gram-negatives, exotoxins of streptococci or clostridia, glycocalyx (or slime) of coagulase-negative staphylococci, and numerous proteins and exotoxins of *S. aureus*.

Dose of the organism: The probability of a wound infection increases as the dose of bacterial contamination increases. The dose needed to cause infection, however, decreases dramatically if a foreign body is present. In one study, >100,000 organisms of *S. aureus* per gram of tissue were needed to produce a wound infection. In the presence of silk sutures, the dose decreased to <100 organisms.[30] In another model of SSI involving foreign body, the ID_{50} value was 100 colony-forming units (CFU) when polytetrafluoroethylene (PTFE) tissue cages were used,[31] 10 CFU with PTFE vascular grafts,[32] and 1 CFU for dextran microbeads.[33]

Source of Bacterial Contamination— Spectrum of Organisms Involved

The most common sources of bacterial contamination of surgical sites are the patient's endogenous skin, mucous membranes, and viscera.[34] In orthopaedic surgery, the skin is generally the source.[35] In this situation, *Staphylococcus* (*aureus* and coagulase-negative) would be the most likely pathogen. Other sources of contamination include the hands of the surgical team (and at times vaginal or rectal shedding of organisms),[36–38] contaminated equipment, contaminated host tissue, or seeding from a remote site of infection.[39]

Period of Risk—Timing of Antibiotic Administration

The critical time of contamination of clean wounds is when the skin is broken. For effective prophylaxis, the antimicrobial agent must achieve adequate concentrations in the serum and tissue to kill the bacteria anticipated at the time of incision. Timing therefore is critical. Most failures of antibiotic prophylaxis occur because of inappropriate timing (too early or too late). A Canadian survey of prophylaxis among patients with hip fractures showed that administration was too early (10 percent), too late (39 percent), or too long (78 percent).[40] A common misconception is that if a patient is already receiving antibiotics for a remote-site infection, surgical prophylaxis is not needed. This is false, since, as already mentioned, the antibiotic concentration must peak at the time of surgical incision. Patients who receive prophylaxis too early or too late have an odds ratio of developing an SSI of 4.3 and 5.8, respectively, compared to patients who receive antibiotic prophylaxis within 2 h preoperatively.[41]

Recently, the Surgical Infection Prevention (SIP) Guideline Writers Workgroup (SIPGWW) hosted by the Medicare National SIP project endorsed the national performance measure, which advocates that infusion of the first antimicrobial dose should begin within 60 min before the incision. However, when a fluoroquinolone or vancomycin is indicated, the infusion should begin 120 min before incision, so as to prevent antibiotic-associated reactions. There is no consensus on whether the infusion must be completed before the incision; but when a proximal tourniquet is required, the entire antimicrobial dose should be infused before the tourniquet is inflated.[42]

In addition to achieving adequate tissue concentration at the time of incision, adequate concentrations must be maintained throughout the surgery. Redosing intraoperatively may be indicated depending on the half-life of the antibiotic, the minimal inhibitory concentration (MIC) for the organism, the anticipated level in the tissues, and the duration of the operation (redose if the operation is still in progress two half-lives after the first dose).[18,42] For cefazolin, a second dose is indicated if the operation is longer than 3 to 4 hours[8,43]; for vancomycin or ceftriaxone, it is 6 to 8 hours. The antibiotic should also be given in an adequate dose depending on the

patient's body weight or body mass index.[18,42] A higher dose would be needed for morbidly obese patients.[44]

Choice of Agent

Cephalosporins have been the agents most studied and most frequently used in prophylaxis. Of these, cefazolin is the most frequently used. This is because it provides adequate coverage for many clean-contaminated operations, has a favorable safety profile, and is reasonably inexpensive.

However, there is increasing resistance among bacterial pathogens, especially staphylococcal species. The proportion of *S. aureus* causing nosocomial infection that is methicillin-resistant increased from 14.3 percent in 1987 to 39.7 percent in 1997.[45] In the 1997 SENTRY program, this resistant strain was isolated from 26.9, 49.8, 29, and 48 percent of hospitalized U.S. patients with bloodstream, pneumonia, wound, and urinary tract infections respectively.[46] In a study of postoperative infections in patients undergoing vascular surgery, 57.5 percent of *S. aureus* isolates were methicillin-resistant.[47] Of the coagulase-negative staphylococci, more than 80 percent are resistant to oxacillin,[48] and these organisms can cause devastating infections when prosthetic devices are implanted. For these resistant organisms, cefazolin or any of the other cephalosporins would not provide adequate coverage. Some authors have therefore advocated the routine use of vancomycin before surgeries where prosthetic devices are to be inserted. At present, the Centers for Disease Control and Prevention (CDC) does not recommend the routine use of vancomycin but does recommend its use as perioperative prophylaxis under certain circumstances, such as a cluster of methicillin-resistant *S. aureus* or methicillin-resistant coagulase-negative staphylococcal infections or high local frequency of methicillin-resistant *S. aureus* (MRSA). "The decision [to use vancomycin] should involve consideration of local frequency of MRSA isolates, surgical site infection rates for particular operations, review of infection control practices, and consultation between surgeon and infectious disease experts." However, the CDC does not define what constitutes a high rate, and a threshold has not been defined where the routine use in an institution is considered scientifically acceptable. In a decision analysis model to calculate the clinical benefits and costs associated with the use of either cefazolin or vancomycin for prophylaxis in coronary artery bypass surgery,[49] cefazolin had the advantage against susceptible organisms unless the prevalence of methicillin-resistance was >3 percent. In a study randomizing 885 patients undergoing cardiac surgery to receive either cefazolin or vancomycin as prophylaxis, there was no difference in SSI between the two groups.[50] However, patients who received cefazolin and vancomycin and later developed an SSI were more likely to be infected with MRSA. In Europe, where teicoplanin is frequently used (teicoplanin is a glycopeptide of similar spectrum to vancomycin but is not available in the United States), a study comparing teicoplanin to cefazolin in orthopaedic patients did not show significant differences in outcomes at 3 or 12 months.[51]

In the absence of firm recommendations, the use of vancomycin would be appropriate in the context of an outbreak of surgical infections due to methicillin-resistant staphylococci or for a patient known to be colonized with MRSA,[42] especially if this patient is to undergo insertion of a prosthetic device. The Society for Health Care Epidemiology of America recently recommended routine surveillance cultures at the time of admission for patients at high risk for MRSA carriage,[52] but identifying these patients in a timely manner before surgery is still problematic. The impact of routine use of vancomycin on the epidemiology of glycopeptide resistance is not entirely clear.

In patients with beta-lactam allergy, prophylaxis against gram-positive organisms can be achieved with either vancomycin or clindamycin.[18]

▶ DURATION OF PROPHYLAXIS

Most guidelines recommend that antimicrobial prophylaxis should end within 24 h after the operation,[18,53,54] and recently the SIP work group reiterated this recommendation.[42] There is no evidence that continuing antibiotics until all drains and catheters are removed will lower infection rates.[18,42] Continuing antibiotics beyond 24 h increases cost as well as the risk of bacteremia and line infections.[55]

▶ PROPHYLAXIS FOR ORTHOPAEDIC SURGERY

Most orthopaedic operations are in the category of "clean" (i.e., uninfected operative wound in which no inflammation is encountered and the respiratory, alimentary, genital, or urinary tracts are not entered, with or without insertion of hardware), or "contaminated" (trauma with open wounds). For those "clean" orthopaedic operations where any foreign material is to be implanted, antimicrobial prophylaxis should be given. In general, antimicrobial prophylaxis is recommended for joint replacement, repair of closed fractures and hip fractures, all spinal surgeries, or insertion of any prosthetic device. It is not recommended for elective surgery that does not involve prosthetic device implantation (e.g., arthroscopy).

It has been shown—by the analysis of pooled results from 22 trials in patients undergoing surgery for internal fixation or replacement arthroplasty for a closed fracture of the femur or any other long bone fracture, utilizing any regimen of systemic antibiotics administered at the time of surgery—that a single perioperative antibiotic dose with or without two or more postoperative doses reduced the incidence of an SSI as well as urinary tract and respiratory tract infections.[56] A single dose of short-acting antibiotic was inferior to multiple doses of the same antibiotic. Multiple doses of a short-acting antibiotic were equal to a single dose of a long-acting antibiotic. This reflects of the need to maintain an adequate concentration of the antibiotic throughout the surgical procedure. Multiple doses of antibiotics given over 24 h or less were equal to the same antibiotic given for a longer period.[57]

For patients undergoing total joint replacement, metaanalysis of small, randomized trials, many of which were underpowered, revealed that antibiotics given preoperatively and for 24 h to 2 weeks postoperatively reduced the rate of superficial and deep infections compared to placebo. Pooled data were of insufficient power to determine whether the shorter duration is preferable or inferior.[57,58]

For orthopaedic surgery, the preferred antibiotic in patients undergoing hip or knee replacement is cefazolin.[59,60] Vancomycin or clindamycin can be used in patients with beta-lactam allergy. However, the discussion in the previous section regarding the use of vancomycin would be particularly pertinent to orthopaedic surgery, especially if a prosthesis is to be inserted.

Use of Antibiotic Beads for Prophylaxis

Systemic aminoglycosides are seldom used for prophylaxis because of their poor tissue concentrations and toxicity profile. Beads impregnated with aminoglycosides (gentamicin and tobramycin) are widely used in orthopaedic surgery for the supplemental therapy of established infection. Two trials compared impregnated beads (one with gentamicin and one with cefuroxime) with systemic antibiotics for prophylaxis. Deep prosthetic infections occurred more frequently in the systemic group and superficial infections more frequently in the beads group.[61,62] However, beads themselves can act as a biomaterial surface on which bacteria can grow. In a report from the Netherlands, in 18 of 20 of cases of infected prostheses, bacteria were found on the beads. Negative routine cultures were found in 12 of 18 cases.[63] The role of beads in prophylaxis is not clear.

Operating Room Environment

The operating room (OR) air contains microbes, and efforts should be made to minimize that. Traffic in the OR increases the number of these microbes, so traffic should be limited. The CDC has published recommendations for maintaining airflow and pressure in the OR.[18] Since the inoculum of organisms needed to produce an SSI is considerably smaller in the presence of prosthetic material, the use of ultraclean air over the operating field for operations involving prosthesis implants has been advocated. This is done by laminar airflow, which moves particle-free air over the aseptic field at a uniform velocity (0.3 to 0.5 μm/s), sweeping away particles in its path. Laminar airflow can be directed vertically or horizontally. Recirculated air then flows through a high-efficiency particulate air (HEPA) filter.[64]

The studies with ultraclean air have been done only in orthopaedic surgery.[65] In a multicenter study of more than 8000 total hip and knee replacements, ultraclean air alone was compared to perioperative antibiotics alone or both. Ultraclean air reduced infection from 3.4 to 1.6 percent, antibiotics alone from 3.4 to 0.8 percent, and both from 3.4 to 0.7 percent. In a case-control study of more than 26,000 patients undergoing total hip or knee replacement, laminar airflow was not a significant factor in reducing infections.[66] Thus the use of ultraclean air in addition to antimicrobial prophylaxis does not seem to be of added benefit.

Ultraviolet irradiation to sterilize the air in the OR has also been used, with results comparable to those from the use of ultraclean air.[67]

▶ USE OF MUPIROCIN

Many studies have examined the role of mupirocin in preventing SSIs. In a study in orthopaedic patients undergoing prosthesis implantation nasal mupirocin was compared with placebo. The mupirocin group were less likely to develop endogenous *S. aureus* infection, but the overall rate of infection was not different.[68] In another study,[69] nasal mupirocin for 5 days and triclosan shower prior to surgery were used in orthopaedics wards. The incidence of SSIs by methicillin-resistant *S. aureus* decreased from 23 per 1000 operations to 3.3 per 1000 operations in the subsequent 6 months. The incidence of nasal carriage of MRSA decreased significantly, as did the use of vancomycin. Low-level resistance to mupirocin increased from 2.3 to 10 percent. No high-level resistance was detected. Other studies, however, have found marked increases of high-level mupirocin resistance after its widespread use.[70] In a randomized double-blind placebo-controlled trial involving 3864 patients undergoing a variety of surgical procedures, the use of mupirocin decreased the incidence of *S. aureus* SSIs in patients who were *Staphylococcus* carriers but did not significantly reduce the overall incidence of *S. aureus* SSI.[71]

As mentioned earlier, the Society for Health Care Epidemiology of America has recently recommended routine surveillance cultures at the time of admission for patients at high risk for MRSA carriage.[52] Mupirocin may be a useful adjunct in patients who are known to be carriers or at high risk of being carriers (e.g., in cases of diabetes, hemodialysis, recurrent staphylococcal infections, or residence in nursing homes).

▶ SUMMARY

Antimicrobial prophylaxis refers to a *critically timed brief course* of antibiotics started just before an operation begins. The value of antimicrobial prophylaxis has been clearly established for "clean" and "clean-contaminated" surgery. In "dirty" wounds, by definition, antimicrobials would be given for treatment rather than prevention. The choice of agent depends on the anticipated spectrum of organisms. Additional doses of the antibiotic given intraoperatively depend on the half-life of the antibiotic and the duration of surgery. Antibiotics should be stopped within 24 h of the operation. Additional measures (mupirocin, ultraclean air) can be considered for special patient populations and procedures.

REFERENCES

1. Ogston WH, Cowan HH, Smith H. Alexander Ogston: Memories and tributes of relatives colleagues and students, with some autobiographical writings. Aberdeen, Scotland: *Aberdeen University Press*, 1943.
2. Shaw GB. The collective biologist, in *Everybody's Political What's What?* New York: Dodd, Mead, 1944:234.
3. Burke JF. Effective period of preventive antibiotic action in experimental incisions and dermal lesions. *Surgery* 50:161, 1961.
4. Burke JP. Infection control: A problem for patient safety. *N Engl J Med* 348:651, 2003.
5. National Nosocomial Infections Surveillance (NNIS) report, data summary from October 1986–April 1996, issued May 1996: A report from the National Nosocomial Infections Surveillance (NNIS) system. *Am J Infect Control* 24:380, 1996.
6. Albers BA, Patka P, Haarman HJ, et al. Cost effectiveness of preventive antibiotic administration for lowering the risk of infection by 0.25% [German]. *Unfallchirurgie* 97:625, 1994.
7. Mangram AJ, Horan TC, Pearson ML, et al. Guideline for prevention of surgical site infection. *Infection Control Hosp Epidemiol* 20:247, 1999.
8. Poulsen KB, Bremmelgaard A, Sorensen AI, et al. Estimated costs of postoperative wound infections. A case-control study of marginal hospital and social security costs. *Epidemiol Infect* 113:283, 1994.

9. Vegas AA, Jodra VM, Garcia ML. Nosocomial infection in surgery wards: A controlled study of increased duration of hospital days and direct cost of hospitalization. *Eur J Epidemiol* 9:504, 1993.

10. Kirkland KB, Briggs JP, Trivette SL, et al. The impact of surgical site infections in the 1990s: Attributable mortality, excess length of hopitalization, and extra costs. *Infect Control Hosp Epidemiol* 20:725, 1999.

11. Perencevich EN, Aands KE, Cosgrove SE, et al. Health and economic impact of surgical site infections diagnosed after hospital discharge. *Emerg Infect Dis* 9:196, 2003.

12. Whitehouse JD, Friedman D, Kirkland KB, et al. The impact of surgical site infections following orthopedic surgery at a community hospital and a university hospital: Adverse quality of life, excess length of stay, and extra cost. *Infect Control Hosp Epidemiol* 23:183, 2002.

13. Cruse PJ, Foord R. A five year prospective study of 23,649 surgical wounds. *Ann Surg* 107:206, 1973.

14. Edwards LD. The epidemiology of 2056 remote site infections and 1966 surgical wound infections occurring in 1875 patients: A four year study of 40,923 operations at Rush-Presbyterian-St. Luke's Hospital, Chicago. *Ann Surg* 184:758, 1976.

15. Gordon SM, Serkey JM, Barr C, et al. The relationship between glycosylated hemoglobin (HgA1c) levels and postoperative infection in patients undergoing primary coronary artery bypass surgery (CABG) [abstr]. *Infect Control Hosp Epidemiol* 18:29, 1997.

16. Greene KA, Wilde AH, Stulberg BN. Preoperative nutritional status of total joint patients. Relationship to postoperative wound complications. *J Arthrop* 6:321, 1991.

17. Llienfeld DE, Vlahov D, Tenney JH, et al. Obesity and diabetes as risk factors for postoperative wound infections after cardiac surgery. *Am J Infect Control* 16:3, 1988.

18. Mangram AJ, Horan TC, Pearson ML, et al. Guideline for prevention of surgical site infection, 1999. Hospital Infection Control Practices Advisory Committee. *Infect Control Hosp Epidemiol* 20:250, 1999.

19. Nagachinta T, Stephens M, Reitz B, Polk BF. Risk factors for surgical wound infection following cardiac surgery. *J Infect Dis* 156:967, 1897.

20. Perl TM, Golub JE. New approaches to reduce *Staphylococcus aureus* nosocomial infection rates: Treating *S. aureus* nasal carriage. *Ann Pharmacother* 32:S7, 1998.

21. Culver DH, Horan TC, Gaynes RP, et al. Surgical wound infection rates by wound class, operative procedure, and patient risk index. *Am J Med* 91:152S, 1991.

22. Haley RW, Culver DH, Morgan WH, et al. Identifying patients at high risk of surgical wound infection: A simple multivariate index of patient susceptibility and wound contamination. *Am J Epidemiol* 121:206, 1985.

23. Gaynes R, Culver D. The National Nosocomial Infection Study: Emergence of MRSA in the United States 1987–1997. Emerging Infectious Diseases Conference, Atlanta, GA, March 8–12, 1998.

24. Kluytmans JA, Mouton JW, Ijzerman EP, et al. Nasal carriage of *Staphylococcus aureus* as a major risk factor for wound infection after cardiac surgery. *J Infect Dis* 171:216, 1995.

25. Wenzel RP, Perl TM. The significance of nasal carriage of *Staphylococcus aureus* and the incidence of postoperative wound infection. *J Hosp Infect* 31:13, 1995.

26. White A. Increased infection rates in heavy nasal carriers of coagulase positive staphylococci. *Antimicrob Agents Chemother* 3:667, 1963.

27. Kalmeijer MD, Van Nieuwland-Bollen E, Bogaers-Hofman D, et al. Nasal carriage of *Staphylococcal aureus* is a major risk factor for surgical site infections in orthopedic surgery. *Infect Control Hosp Epidemiol* 319, 2000.

28. Garner JS. CDC guideline for prevention of surgical wound infections, 1985. Revised. *Infect Control* 7:193, 1986.

29. Cruse PJ. Surgical wound infection, in Wonsiewicz MJ (ed): *Infectious Diseases*. Philadelphia: Saunders, 1992:758.

30. Noble NC. The production of subcutaneous staphylococcal skin lesions in mice. *Br J Exp Pathol* 46(3):254–262,1965.

31. Zimmerli W, Waldvogel FA, Vaudaux P, et al. Pathogenesis of foreign body infection: Description and characteristics of an animal model. *J Infect Dis* 146:487, 1982.

32. Arbeit RD, Dunn RM. Expression of capsular polysaccharide during experimental focal infection with *Staphylococcus aureus. Infect Dis* 156:947, 1987.

33. Kaiser AB, Kerndole DS, Parker RA. A low-inoculum animal model of subcutaneous abscess formation and antimicrobial prophylaxis. *J Infect Dis* 166:393, 1992.

34. Altemeier WA, Culbertson WR, Hummel RP. Surgical considerations of endogenous infections: Sources, types, and methods of control. *Surg Clin North Am* 48:227, 1968.

35. Wiley AM, Ha'eri GB. Routes of infection: A study using "tracer particles" in the orthopedic operating room. *Clin Orthop* 139:150, 1979.

36. Letts RM, Doermer E. Conversation in the operating theater as a cause of airborne bacterial contamination. *J Bone Joint Surg [Am]* 65:357, 1983.

37. Mastro TD, Farley TA, Elliot JA, et al. An outbreak of surgical wound infections due to group A streptococcus carried on the scalp. *N Engl J Med* 323:968, 1990.

38. Stamm WE, Feeley JC, Faclam RR. Wound infection due to group A streptococcus traced to a vaginal carrier. *J Infect Dis* 138:287, 1978.

39. Valentine RJ, Weigelt JA, Dryer D, et al. Effect of remote infection on clean wound infection rates. *Am J Infect Control* 14:64, 1986.

40. Zoutman D, Cahn L, Watterson J, et al. A Canadian survey of prophylactic antibiotic use among hip fracture patients. *Infect Control Hosp Epidemiol* 20:752, 1999.

41. Classen DC, Evans RS, Pestotnik SL, et al. The timing of prophylactic administration of antibiotics and the risk of surgical wound infection *N Engl J Med* 326:281, 1992.

42. Bratzler DW, Houck PM, for the Surgical Infection Prevention Guidelines Writers Work group. Antimicrobial prophylaxis for surgery: An advisory statement from the National Surgical Infection Prevention Project. *Clin Infect Dis* 38:1706, 2004.

43. Zanetti G, Giardina R, Platt R. Intraoperative redosing of cefazolin and risk of surgical site infection in cardiac surgery. *Emerg Infect Dis* 7:828, 2001.

44. Forse RA, Karam B, Maclean LD, et al. Antibiotic prophylaxis for surgery in morbidly obese patients. *Surgery* 106:750, 1989.

45. Gaynes RP, Culver D, Horan TC, et al. Surgical site infection rates in the United States, 1992–1998: The National Nosocomial Infection Surveillance System basic SSI risk index. *Clin Infect Dis* 33:S69, 2001.
46. Jones RN. Resistance patterns among nosocomial pathogens. *Chest* 119:397S, 2001.
47. Taylor MD, Napolitano LM. MRSA infections in vascular surgery: Increasing prevalence. *Surg Infect (Larchmt)* 5:80, 2004.
48. Archer GL, Climo MW. Antimicrobial susceptibility of coagulase-negative staphylococci. *Antimicrob Agents Chemother* 38:2231, 1994.
49. Zanetti G, Goldie SJ, Platt R. Clinical consequences and cost of limiting use of vancomycin for perioperative prophylaxis: Example of coronary artery bypass surgery. *Emerg Infect Dis* 7:820, 2001.
50. Finkelstein R, Rabino G, Mashiah T, et al. Vancomycin versus cefazolin prophylaxis for cardiac surgery in the setting of a high prevalence of methicillin-resistant staphylococcal infections. *J Thorac Cardiovasc Surg* 123:326, 2002.
51. Periti P, Stringa G, Mini E, et al. Comparative multicenter trial of teicoplanin versus cefazolin for antimicrobial prophylaxis in prosthetic joint implant surgery. Italian Study Group for Antimicrobial Prophylaxis in orthopedic surgery. *Eur J Clin Microbiol Infect Dis* 18:113, 1999.
52. Muto CA, Jernigan JA, Ostrowsky BE, et al. SHEA guideline for preventing nosocomial transmission of multidrug-resistant strains of *Staphylococcus aureus* and *Enterococcus*. *Infect Control Hosp/Epidemiol* 24:362, 2003.
53. Dellinger EP, Gross PA, Barrett, TL, et al. Quality standard for antimicrobial prophylaxis in surgical procedures. Infectious Diseases Society of America. *Clin Infect Dis* 18:422, 1994.
54. Antimicrobial prophylaxis in surgery. *Med Lett Drugs Ther* 43:92, 2001.
55. Namias N, Harvill S, Ball S, et al. Cost and morbidity associated with antibiotic prophylaxis in the ICU. *J Am Coll Surg* 188:225, 1999.
56. Gillespie WJ, Walenkamp G. Antibiotic prophylaxis for surgery for proximal femoral and other closed long bone fractures (Cochrane review), in *The Cochrane Library*, Issue 3. Chichester, UK: Wiley, 2004.
57. Gillespie WJ. Prevention and management of infection after total joint replacement. *Clin Infect Dis* 25:1310, 1997.
58. Genny AM, Song F. Antimicrobial prophylaxis in total hip replacement: A systematic review. *Health Technol Assess* 3(21):1–57, 1999.
59. American Society of Health-System Pharmacists. ASHP therapeutic guidelines on antimicrobial prophylaxis in surgery. *Am J Health Syst Pharm* 56:1839, 1999.
60. Page CP, Bohnen JM, Fletcher JR, et al. Antimicrobial prophylaxis for surgical wounds: Guidelines for clinical care. *Arch Surg* 128:79, 1993.
61. Josefsson G, Gudmundsson G, Kolmert L, et al. Prophylaxis with systemic antibiotics versus gentamicin bone cement in total hip arthroplasty: A five-year survey of 1988 hips. *Clin Orthop* 253:173, 1990.
62. McQueen M, Littlejohn A, Hughes SP. A comparison of systemic cefuroxime and cefuroxime loaded bone cement in the prevention of early infection after total joint replacement. *Int Orthop* 11:241, 1987.
63. Neut D, van de Belt H, Stokroos I, et al. Biomaterial-associated infection of gentamicin-loaded PMMA beads in orthopaedic revision surgery. *J Antimicrob Chemother* 47:885, 2001.
64. Hambraeus A. Aerobiology in the operating room: A review. *J Hosp Infect* 11:68, 1988.
65. Lidwell OM, Elson RA, Lowbury EJ, et al. Ultraclean air and antibiotics for prevention of postoperative infection. A multicenter study of 8,052 joint replacement operations. *Acta Orthop Scand* 58:4, 1987.
66. Berbari EF, Hanssen AD, Duffy MC, et al. Risk factors for prosthetic joint infection: Case-control study. *Clin Infect Dis* 27:1247, 1998.
67. Berg M, Bergman BR, Hoborn J. Ultraviolet radiation compared to an ultra-clean air enclosure. Comparison of air bacteria counts in operating rooms. *J Bone Joint Surg Br* 73:811, 1991.
68. Kalmeijer MD, Coertjens H, van Nieuwland-Bollen, et al. Surgical site infections in orthopedic surgery: The effect of mupirocin nasal ointment in a double-blind, randomized, placebo-controlled study. *Clin Infect Dis* 35:353, 2002.
69. Wilcox MH, Hall J, Pike H, et al. Use of perioperative murpirocin to prevent methicillin-resistant *Staphylococcus aureus* (MRSA) orthopaedic surgical site infections. *J Hosp Infect* 54:196, 2003.
70. Miller MA, Dascal A, Portnoy J, et al. Development of mupirocin resistance among methicillin-resistant *Staphylococcus aureus* after widespread use of mupirocin ointment. *Infect Control Hosp Epidemiol* 17:811, 1996.
71. Perl TM, Cullen JJ, Wenzel RP, et al. The risk of *Staphylococcus aureus* study team. *N Engl J Med* 346:1871, 2002.

CHAPTER 4

Thromboprophylaxis in Orthopaedic Surgery

ANTHONY G. BEETON/ANDRÉ P. BOEZAART

► INTRODUCTION

Venous thromboembolism (VTE) encompasses acute thrombotic events such as symptomatic and asymptomatic deep venous thrombosis (DVT), pulmonary embolism (PE), and chronic sequelae such as recurrent VTE, postthrombotic syndrome (PTS), and the manifestations of chronic pulmonary thromboembolic disease.[1,2] Certain major orthopaedic surgical procedures such as total hip arthroplasty (THA), total knee arthroplasty (TKA), hip fracture surgery (HFS), and major pelvic surgery represent situations with a particular risk for VTE.[1,3]

► NORMAL HEMOSTASIS

Hemostasis is a complex process designed to defend and preserve the integrity and patency of the vascular system. It involves interactions between the vascular endothelium, platelets, clotting factors, and the fibrinolytic system.[4,5]

The endothelium has an array of functions in hemostasis. It releases endothelin in response to injury, provoking intense vasoconstriction. This reduces bleeding and results in sustained contact between the damaged endothelium, platelets, and coagulation factors, thereby promoting clotting. It also modulates the degree of coagulation, producing not only procoagulant agents such as tissue factor (TF) and von Willebrand factor (vWF) but also anticoagulants (nitric oxide, endothelium-derived relaxant factor, thrombomodulin, and tissue factor pathway inhibitor) and fibrinolytic system components (tissue plasminogen activator).[5]

Platelets are responsible for the formation of the initial plug at the site of vascular injury. They have surface receptors for interaction with other platelets, von Willebrand factor (vWF), fibrinogen, and collagen and form the nidus for formation of the primary clot. They also produce the phospholipids required for normal coagulation.[5]

The coagulation pathway is designed to produce thrombin (factor IIa), the key enzyme in hemostasis.[6] Thrombin catalyzes the conversion of soluble fibrinogen to fibrin, which is the major component of the clot.[7] Fibrin then forms cross-links to produce a stable clot.[5] These steps represent the common coagulation pathway. Thrombin is formed via the intrinsic and extrinsic coagulation pathways.[8] The intrinsic pathway is the major source of thrombin generation and is activated by exposure of blood to subendothelial connective tissue. It produces a massive, focused burst of thrombin synthesis.[5,7,8] The smaller extrinsic pathway produces a smaller amount of thrombin in response to contact between blood and TF. Its action is more rapid than that of the intrinsic pathway and serves to augment it.[7]

The extent of clotting is controlled by circulating regulators of coagulation and by the fibrinolytic system. Several activators convert plasminogen to plasmin, the major fibrinolytic protein.[5] Antithrombin (AT) is the major circulating inhibitor of clotting factors. It forms complexes with these factors, notably factor Xa and thrombin, allowing rapid hepatic clearance. The activity of AT is accelerated 5000 to 10,000-fold by heparin.[5,7]

Other circulating anticoagulants include tissue factor pathway inhibitor (TFPI) and proteins C and S.[7–9] The last mentioned serves mainly as a cofactor for protein C. Proteins C and S strongly inhibit or inactivate several coagulation factors, accelerating their normal rate of inactivation up to 20,000-fold.[5] TFPI may mediate some of the antithrombotic effects of unfractionated heparin (UFH) and low-molecular-weight heparin (LMWH) as it is released from the vascular endothelium in response to therapeutic doses of these agents.[9] Thrombomodulin is an endothelial receptor that binds circulating thrombin and prevents clot formation in undamaged vessels.[7]

▶ RISK FACTORS FOR VENOUS THROMBOEMBOLISM

The risk for VTE is a composite of various demographic and comorbid factors that make up the *predisposing risk* and factors related to the surgical procedure that form the *exposing risk.* [4,5,10–12] The major risk factors are tabulated below. These are additive, although some (e.g., age, malignancy, and previous VTE) may carry more weight than others.[13] Patients may therefore be classified into risk categories ranging from lowest to highest risk. The patients at greatest risk for VTE are those who undergo major orthopaedic surgery of the lower limbs and victims of major trauma or acute spinal cord injury.[5,10,12] Risk stratification for other orthopaedic patients depends largely on age, duration of surgery, and the presence of additional risk factors (Table 4-1).[5]

Predisposition to VTE is based on disturbances in one or more components of Virchow's triad: the vascular endothelium, blood coagulability, and blood flow (stasis).[4,6] Major hip and knee surgeries (THA, TKA, and HSF)

cause significant and sustained alterations in all of these components.[5,7,14]

The vascular endothelium has been shown by intraoperative venography to be damaged or disrupted by direct surgical trauma.[14] In addition, twisting and folding of the common femoral vein during hip dislocation produces distention and breakage of endothelial intercellular bridges and exposure of collagen and tissue factors.[4,13] Retractors (e.g., the posterior tibial retractor in TKA) may have similar effects.[4] The heat generated by the polymerization of methyl methacrylate also causes endothelial injury (see Chap. 33).[4] The consequences of these injuries are platelet adherence and aggregation, initiation of coagulation, and decreased endothelial function.

Hypercoagulability, as evidenced by circulating markers of thrombosis, commences at the time of femoral canal reaming, peaks at insertion of the cemented stem, and continues for up to 5 weeks postoperatively.[7,11,13] Noncemented prostheses appear to be less thrombogenic.[13] Hypercoagulability results from bone marrow destruction and the release of TF.[4] Bone cement increases thrombin activity. Fibrinolytic failure contributes to the risk of thrombosis.

Intraoperative venography has also shown a significant reduction in venous blood flow and stasis in lower limb orthopaedic surgery. This is related to venous obstruction in all cases and to the use of a tourniquet in TKA (see Chap. 11).[14] The immobilization and bed rest associated with these procedures exacerbates stasis.[4] Reduced venous flow affects both the operated and the contralateral limb. Reduced venous blood flow may last for up to 6 weeks after surgery.[5,7,8,11,14]

In TKA, the majority of DVT starts in the calf veins but may propagate proximally in 15 percent of cases.[14] In hip surgery and trauma, DVT may arise primarily in

▶ TABLE 4-1. RISK FACTORS FOR VENOUS THROMBOEMBOLISM (VTE)

Predisposing Risk Factors	Exposing Risk Factors
Increasing age	Nature of surgery (pelvic and lower limb surgery,
Prolonged immobility	cancer surgery, abdominal surgery)
Previous VTE	Duration of surgery
Malignancy	Type of anesthesia
Obesity	Degree of immobilization
Varicose veins	Presence of infection
Cardiac disease	Trauma to spine, pelvis and lower limbs
Thrombophilic disorders	
Others (pregnancy, hormone replacement therapy, nephrotic syndrome, inflammatory bowel disease, psychotropic drugs, prolonged travel)	

VTE = venous thromboembolism.
Sources: Adapted from Geerts et al.,[1] Offord and Perry,[5] Samama et al.,[10] and Geerts et al.[12]

the proximal veins.[15] Pulmonary embolism is usually preceded by proximal DVT, the majority of which is clinically silent.[8,16] It is impossible to predict which distal thrombi may progress to pulmonary embolism.[17] Therefore, any venographic DVT is accepted as a valid surrogate measure of potentially symptomatic VTE.[12,15,17]

▶ INCIDENCE AND IMPACT OF VTE IN ORTHOPAEDIC SURGERY

Symptomatic DVT and PE represent a small fraction of the total incidence of venographically confirmed VTE. The vast majority of VTE events are clinically silent.[5,15,18] It is estimated that for every 100 silent cases of DVT, there are 10 clinically detected DVTs and one fatal PE.[1,15] Bilateral venography has shown that between 7 to 14 days after operation, 41 to 85 percent of patients who undergo lower limb arthroplasty and HFS develop VTE in the absence of thromboprophylaxis.[1,8] A substantial proportion of VTE (20 to 87 percent) presents during the second and subsequent postoperative weeks, much of it after hospital discharge.[8,19] Major lower limb orthopaedic surgery is not a homogeneous entity, and differences exist between the procedures in terms of the incidence, distribution, and onset time of VTE events (Table 4-2).[16]

Following major orthopaedic surgery, VTE is usually silent, but it may present as acute DVT or PE or as a delayed PTS or a recurrent VTE.[20–22a] The use of virtually any thromboprophylactic protocol reduces the risk of VTE by half or more.[3,15] With the possible exception of dextran infusion (which reduces PE selectively), the reduction is in all components of VTE. Proximal DVT is more likely to be clinically apparent than distal DVT and is also more likely to produce PE. Only 5 to 20 percent of total thrombotic events are, however, clinically apparent.[24,25] It is therefore clear that the majority of radiologically demonstrated venous thrombosis resolves spontaneously.

In major orthopaedic surgery, only 20 percent of fatal thrombotic events are suspected before death[24] and only 12 percent of patients present with clinically apparent DVT before the onset of pulmonary embolism.[15]

There has been a substantial reduction in the incidence of clinically apparent VTE associated with major orthopaedic surgery in the last 30 years.[4,5] This is attributable only partly to the use of thromboprophylaxis.[12] Improvements in surgical technique, general perioperative care, mobilization, analgesia, anesthetic technique, and duration of bed rest/hospitalization have also contributed.[4,5,11] This has led to the perception among some orthopaedic surgeons that VTE (particularly fatal PE) is an overemphasized problem and that routine prophylaxis is not indicated. This perception is enhanced by the clinically silent nature of the majority of VTE cases and by the fact that many occur after discharge and frequently present to other specialties.[5,8,11,12,25,26]

Venous thrombosis, however, remains a massive problem in major orthopaedic surgery. It is the most common complication of TKA and the likeliest cause of readmission.[16] It is the second most frequent cause of death associated with THA (causing 18 percent of deaths)[5,11,12] and ranks third or fourth in HFS (14 percent).[3,4,11] In 1990, there were an estimated 1.7 million hip fracture procedures worldwide, resulting in about 17,000 deaths due to VTE.[11] In addition, it is likely that failure to detect VTE during autopsy may cause underestimation of its role as a cause of death.[11,24] In major orthopaedic surgery, the occurrence of a DVT increases the risk of death 2.5-fold, while PE produces a 20-fold rise.[27] It is expected that HFS will increase to 6 million worldwide by 2050,[11] while THA is projected to increase by 25 to 50 percent by 2020 and TKA by 30 percent by 2030.[2,6,12] At the same time, the population undergoing these procedures is aging. The median age for THA rose by 2 years between 1996 and 2001, and that for TKA by 1 year.[28] Patients' increasing age along with their likelihood of having more comorbid diseases will increase the risk of VTE in the future.[4,29]

Venous thrombosis is also responsible for a substantial amount of morbidity.[6] Recurrent VTE occurs in 20 percent of patients within the 2 years after initial presentation and in 30 percent within 10 years.[18] Chronic lower limb venous insufficiency follows in 50 to 60 percent of cases of symptomatic proximal DVT and 30 percent of symptomatic calf DVT.[20] Postthrombotic syndrome (PTS) has an incidence of 8.5 percent 1 year after DVT, rising to 24.1 percent at 20 years (and 36.1 percent after proximal DVT).[30] Venous ulcers complicate 3.7 percent of DVT by 20 years after the initial event.[21,29]

The economic impact of VTE is enormous. It is estimated that VTE costs the U.S. health care system $3.2 billion per year.[31] The impact of VTE on various aspects of health economics is summarized in Table 4-3.

▶ **TABLE 4-2.** EPIDEMIOLOGY OF VENOUS THROMBOEMBOLISM WITHOUT PROPHYLAXIS SINCE 1980

	THA	TKA	HFS
Total DVT (%)	42–57	41–85	46–60
Proximal DVT (%)	18–36	5–22	23–30
Contralateral DVT (%)	20	14	
PE (%)	0.9–28	1.5–10	3–11
Fatal PE (%)	0.1–2	0.1–1.7	2.5–7.5
Mean time to VTE (days)	17	7	17

DVT = deep venous thrombosis; HFS = hip fracture surgery; PE = pulmonary embolism; THA = total hip arthoplasty; TKA = total knee arthroplasty; VTE = venous thromboembolism.

▶ **TABLE 4-3.** IMPACT OF VENOUS THROMBOEMBOLISM ON HEALTH ECONOMICS IN MAJOR ORTHOPAEDIC SURGERY

	Mean Hospital Stay (Days)	Mean ICU Stay (Days)	Total Inpatient Cost ($)
No VTE	5.4	0.2	9,345
DVT	11.5	1.7	17,114
PE	12.4	2.7	18,521

DVT = deep venous thrombosis; PE = pulmonary embolism; VTE = venous thromboembolism.
Sources: Adapted from Paiement,[4] Agnelli et al.,[19] and Anderson et al.[27]

▶ OPTIONS FOR THE PREVENTION OF VENOUS THROMBOEMBOLISM

There is ample evidence that routine prophylaxis during hospitalization is more effective than screening and treatment in this group of patients.[4,21,30,32] It is unclear at present what the cost-benefit ratio is of long-term postdischarge prophylaxis. Evidence for efficacy of long-term prophylaxis (4 weeks) is, however, abundant.[21,33] In view of the high incidence of venous thrombosis in major orthopaedic surgery, a thromboprophylactic strategy is mandatory.[16] This strategy may be nonpharmacologic or pharmacologic or, ideally, may combine both modalities. In general, prophylaxis has a lower success rate in knee arthroplasty than in hip surgery, possibly because many of the thrombi formed are small and distal.[3,14,16]

Nonpharmacologic methods include improved surgical technique (noncemented prostheses, pulsed lavage, minimally invasive surgery, limited use of tourniquet); anesthetic interventions (neuraxial anesthesia, optimal analgesia for early mobilization); autologous blood donation and transfusion; and physical measures (elevation of the foot of the bed, active and passive ankle exercises, early mobilization).[1,4,13] Mechanical methods are graded elastic stockings, intermittent pneumatic calf compression, sequential compression detection devices, and pneumatic plantar plexus compression.[1,4,14] Anesthetic interventions are discussed further in a subsequent section. All of the listed nonpharmacologic methods have been shown to reduce venous thrombosis under specific circumstances, but it is questionable whether any or combination of them provide adequate prophylaxis in high-risk orthopaedic surgery.[1,5,12] They should rather be seen as adjuvant to pharmacologic prophylaxis except when anticoagulants are contraindicated (e.g., for excessive bleeding risk).[1,5] Mechanical methods do not cause increased bleeding and are therefore considered to be safe.[1] They may be limited by high acquisition cost, and compliance tends to be incomplete owing to their discomfort. It is not possible to perform properly "blinded" trials to determine their true efficacy, and concerns have been expressed about observer bias.[1,5,12]

Graded elastic stockings have a pressure gradient decreasing from 15 to 18 mmHg at the foot to 5 mmHg at the proximal thigh. They increase peak femoral venous blood flow velocity by 50 percent and reduce stasis. They have no impact on de novo proximal DVT formation in hip surgery and consequently no protective effect against pulmonary embolism. Their cost-effectiveness has not been studied.[1,4]

Intermittent pneumatic compression (IPC), sequential compression detection (SCD) devices, and pneumatic plantar plexus compression increase the velocity of venous blood flow and stimulate fibrinolysis.[4,14] They decrease the DVT risk by 20 to 60 percent but have little impact on proximal DVT. They appear to be most effective in knee arthroplasty, but less so than anticoagulants.[1,4]

Dextran infusions are effective in preventing fatal PE in general surgical patients.[34] Dextran enhances blood flow characteristics, decreases platelet adhesion to the endothelium, and increases the lysability of fibrin clots. Its utility in major orthopaedic surgery is unknown. Drawbacks include bleeding, anaphylactic reactions, and cost.[1,34]

Aspirin is not a first-line drug in prophylaxis against venous thrombosis.[1,30] It may protect against fatal pulmonary embolism and postoperative cardiovascular mortality but is less effective than first-line agents for VTE prevention.[1,35] In addition, it poses a high risk of bleeding and gastrointestinal side effects.[5,35]

Except where the bleeding risk is prohibitive, pharmacologic prophylaxis is the cornerstone of the prevention of venous thrombosis in high-risk orthopaedic patients.[1,8] Specific agents are considered in the following section, but certain general rules apply:

1. Each major orthopaedic procedure has unique patient demographics, consequent comorbidities, and balance of thrombotic and bleeding risk. Data from one case are not necessarily applicable to another.[2]
2. Comparison of agents within and between pharmacologic groups is rendered difficult by variations in kinetics as well as recommended dosages and regimens, particularly the time between drug administration and surgery and speed of onset of anticoagulant effect.[3,25,36] Rapid-onset drugs

administered close to the time of surgery will produce the best antithrombotic effect.

3. Nevertheless, there appear to be differences between agents and regimens in respect to antithrombotic efficacy and bleeding risk at recommended doses.[16,25]

4. Drug costs vary from one country to another and depend on many factors. However, the cost-effectiveness of routine pharmacologic prophylaxis is not in question.[30,32,37,38] The most efficacious drugs perform most cost-effectively.[30]

5. The ideal agent would be easy to administer (oral; long dosage interval), efficacious, require no monitoring, be suitable for outpatient use, and have minimal side effects (i.e., bleeding, thrombocytopenia, osteoporosis, liver enzyme elevation).[2,9,15]

6. Administration in close proximity to surgery confers better antithrombotic protection but carries a significantly increased bleeding risk.[25,36]

7. For best antithrombotic effect, there appears to be a window of opportunity from about 2 h preoperatively until 6 to 8 h after the operation. Starting drug therapy 6 to 8 h postoperatively carries no increased bleeding risk compared with traditional regimens and is generally compatible with neuraxial anesthesia.[25,36,39]

8. Bleeding risk is a composite of the intensity of the anticoagulant effect (depends on drug and dose), patient factors such as age >75 years, and the use of concomitant drugs with impact on coagulation.[2,9,25,36]

9. Substantial evidence exists for the continuation of in-hospital prophylaxis for a total of 4 weeks, particularly in hip surgery patients.[5,6,17,19,21,32]

A recent audit of American arthroplasty practice based on a voluntary registry revealed that 99 percent of patients received at least one form of prophylaxis.[3,28] Elastic stockings were used in 58 to 61 percent of patients (usually in combination with another modality). Other options employed were warfarin (53 to 56 percent); LMWH (38 to 40 percent); IPC (23 to 25 percent), and aspirin (4 to 7 percent in hospital and 20 to 21 percent after discharge).[28] Prophylaxis was in compliance with the guidelines of the American College of Chest Physicians (ACCP) in 94 percent of THA patients.[3] In more than 50 percent of patients, prophylaxis was continued for at least 21 days postoperatively.[28]

▶ PHARMACOLOGY OF ANTITHROMBOTIC MEDICATIONS

Major orthopaedic surgery is an ideal model for the assessment of drugs that affect coagulation and bleeding, since it carries a substantial risk of both thrombosis and hemorrhage.[6] Pharmacologic prophylaxis will always be a tradeoff between preventing venous thrombosis and bleeding risk. The risk of major or critical bleeding with most prophylactic regimens is around 3 percent.[4,5,40] Three major groups of drugs are recommended and utilized for thromboprophylaxis[1,7]:

1. Oral anticoagulants (warfarin/Coumadin)
2. Indirect thrombin inhibitors
   - Unfractionated heparin (UFH)
   - Low molecular weight heparin (LMWH)
   - Pentasaccharides
3. Direct thrombin inhibitors (DTI)
   - Irreversible—hirudin and recombinant hirudins
   - Reversible—melagatran/ximelagatran

The traditional agents for prophylaxis are warfarin, UFH, and LMWH. However, all have limitations that make them less than optimal drugs. The major limitation is inadequate efficacy, and up to 20 percent of THA patients (and up to 50 percent in TKA and HFS) may still develop venous thrombosis.[6,34] Safety issues, the need for monitoring, and difficulty of administration have given impetus to the search for drugs that are more effective, safer, and easier to administer, particularly in outpatients.[6,9,15,17,34,36]

Oral Anticoagulants (Warfarin/Coumadin)

Warfarin is the most frequently used thromboprophylactic agent for major orthopaedic surgery in the United States.[3] It is commenced on the night before surgery or the night of surgery.[4] It has numerous indications in the prevention and treatment of arterial, cardiac, and venous thrombosis.[1,5] It is a vitamin K antagonist, producing depletion of vitamin KH_2, the essential substrate for the γ carboxylation of the vitamin K–dependent clotting proteins (factors II, VII, IX, and X as well as proteins C and S).[41,42] The factors produced are deficient and unable to chelate calcium and bind to platelet phospholipids during the clotting process.[41,42] Warfarin's onset of action requires the initial clearance of normal clotting factors. Factor VII has a half-life ($t_{1/2}$) of 6 to 7 h; the onset of anticoagulation may therefore be as early as 24 h.[41,42] However, a full anticoagulant effect is not achieved until 72 to 96 h because of the longer $t_{1/2}$ of the other clotting factors.[1,4,12,41,42] For the same reason, anticoagulation may persist for up to 96 h after stopping warfarin despite a prompt recovery in levels of factor VII.[41,42] Protein C is rapidly depleted; this may result in an initial thrombogenic phase for the first 48 h of warfarin therapy.[2,5,41,42]

Warfarin has a predictable onset and duration of action but a variable dose-response relationship.[1,4,42] It is also subject to numerous drug and dietary interactions.[6,42] As such, its anticoagulant effect must be monitored, using the international normalized ratio (INR).[4,42] The target INR for prophylactic anticoagulation in major orthopaedic surgery is 2 to 3.[1,2,6,42] This may take some days to achieve from its recommended immediate preoperative or early postoperative commencement.[2,41,42] This delay in the onset of an anticoagulant effect may explain the marginally inferior performance of warfarin compared with LMWH or adjusted-dose heparin in some trials of VTE prophylaxis in THA. It nonetheless produces a 59 percent relative risk reduction (RRR) versus placebo in THA.[1,42] Warfarin appears to be substantially less effective than heparin in TKA but equally effective in HFS.[3,22,34] These differences reflect different risks for DVT associated with different operations.[12] Because it is an oral drug, warfarin is ideal for postoperative outpatient use for prolonged prophylaxis, but it requires ongoing INR monitoring and possible dose adjustments. The major complication of warfarin is bleeding, but this appears to be no more common than with other anticoagulants at 1 to 3 percent.[4,42] Warfarin has been largely abandoned as a prophylactic anticoagulant in Europe because of its delayed onset of action, interpatient variation, inferior efficacy compared to LMWH, drug interactions, and need for frequent monitoring and dose adjustment to maintain the target INR.[1,42]

Indirect Thrombin Inhibitors

Unfractionated heparin (UFH) is a mixture of polysaccharide chains whose molecular weight (MW) varies from 3 to 30 kDa (10 to 50 saccharides in length).[43] The active pentasaccharide moiety, present on about one-third of the molecules, binds to AT to increase its thrombin inhibitory action some 5000 to 10,000-fold.[4,43] The larger molecules (>18 saccharides in length) have predominant antithrombin (anti-IIa) activity and are responsible for the platelet binding and interactions of heparin.[4,43,44] Smaller molecules are unable to bind AT and thrombin simultaneously and have more anti-Xa activity. Unfractionated heparin has an Xa:IIa affinity ratio of around 1 (3 for LMWH).[8,44] Heparin can then dissociate from AT and be reutilized. At very high doses, UFH may also inhibit IIa via binding with heparin cofactor II.[43,44] The use of UFH for more than 5 days may lead to nonimmune thrombocytopenia in 1 to 3 percent of patients. This is usually trivial and resolves spontaneously.[5,6,43–45] A much more feared complication is the immunologically mediated heparin-induced thrombocytopenia (HIT), where antibodies are formed against heparin-platelet factor 4 (PF4) complexes.[6,43,45] This is seen in 0.1 to 1 percent of patients and results in platelet aggregation and destruction. This, in turn, causes thrombocytopenia and potentially fatal thrombotic events in 10 to 15 percent of patients. Many of these patients will die or require amputation because of arterial or venous thromboses.[5,45] This condition is then termed heparin-induced thrombocytopenia

thrombosis (HITT). HIT is an emergency, necessitating the withdrawal of all sources of heparin and switching to alternative antithrombotic therapy.[12,45] A history of HIT contraindicates any future heparin therapy, including LMWH.[44,45] All patients receiving heparin should have their platelet counts monitored from the fourth or fifth day of therapy. The other complications of heparin therapy include bleeding, heparin resistance, and osteoporosis. Bleeding may be more significant than with equiefficacious doses of other anticoagulants.[15,45]

Unfractionated heparin has an onset time of 2 h after subcutaneous administration and a $t_{1/2}$ of 2 h (versus 30 min and 1 h for intravenous administration).[8,43] The clinical duration of prophylaxis is 4 to 6 h. It is 30 percent bioavailable and may be administered as fixed dose (5000 U/8 to 12 h) or as adjusted doses according to partial thromboplastin time (PTT).[43] The fixed-dose regimen is more effective than no prophylaxis (27 percent RRR for total DVT in THA) but less effective than other prophylactic anticoagulants.[8,46] Adjusted-dose UFH (usually by constant intravenous infusion) aims to maintain PTT at or slightly above normal. This technique is highly effective, producing a 74 percent relative risk reduction for overall DVT compared with placebo, but the regular testing is expensive and the technique too labor-intensive for routine use.[1] For this reason it is no longer recommended by the ACCP.[1] There is some evidence that a single dose of 1000 U of heparin given intravenously at the time of medullary canal reaming produces a significant reduction in VTE.[13,14]

Low-molecular-weight heparins (LMWHs) are derived from the same animal sources as heparin, by chemical or enzymatic depolymerization.[44] A range of agents is available with MW of 4 to 6 kDa.[4,43] Their polysaccharide chains range from 13 to 22 saccharides in length. As such, they have greater anti-Xa than antithrombin activity.[44] This results in little or no impact on PTT.[1,4] LMWHs have more favorable pharmacokinetic profiles than unfractionated heparin, with 90 to 100 percent bioavailability and half-lives of 2 to 4 h, resulting in a duration of clinical effect of around 12 h.[8,44] They achieve peak anticoagulation 3 to 4 h after subcutaneous administration and are cleared renally. Doses should be adjusted where renal function is impaired.[8,44] The risk-benefit ratio (bleeding versus thromboprophylaxis) is superior to that of UFH and the low-molecular-weight forms produce significantly less HIT and osteoporosis than the UFHs and less bleeding complications at equiefficacious doses.[4]

LMWHs perform as well as or better than warfarin or UFH across the range of major orthopaedic procedures.[3,7,12,16,25,32,37,38] The advantage is likely due to a more rapid onset of anticoagulant effect. They reduce the risk of DVT by 70 percent in THA, 52 percent in TKA, and 44 percent in HFS.[1,4,14] These figures are obtained with once- or twice-daily regimens (e.g., 40 mg enoxaprin daily starting 12 h preoperatively or 30 mg twice daily starting 12 to 24 h postoperatively). Preoperative initiation of LMWH therapy is no more effective than early postoperative commencement.[3,25] There is little increase in the antithrombotic benefit of the 60-mg daily dose but an increased bleeding risk.[3,8] It would therefore appear that a 40-mg daily dose is optimal in terms of risk-benefit ratio. There is good evidence that a further improvement in antithrombotic effect can be achieved without an increase in bleeding risk if the initial dose of LMWH is administered within 6 to 8 h of skin closure at half of the normal high-risk dose followed by a full dose daily thereafter.[12,25,39,47] Earlier postoperative or immediate preoperative administration is associated with an unacceptable bleeding risk.[39,47] Current recommendations for prophylaxis are a fixed daily dose of LMWH for 7 to 10 days after major orthopaedic surgery (up to 4 weeks after hip surgery).[1,19,21] Monitoring is not required.[1,16] Should it become necessary, PTT will usually be unaffected and anti-Xa activity may be measured. It is prudent to decrease LMWH doses in elderly patients with impaired renal function and in those weighing less than 50 kg.[8,48,49]

Pentasaccharides, of which the prototype is fondaparinux, are synthetic molecules with pure anti-Xa effect mediated entirely via reversible binding to AT.[15,17,50] Fondaparinux increases AT activity 300-fold.[50] The fondaparinux-AT complex binds irreversibly with Xa and inhibits its action. Fondaparinux then dissociates from the complex and is free to activate another AT molecule.[50] This represents a catalytic reaction compared to the stoichiometric mechanism of action of direct thrombin inhibitors (DTI), in which each molecule can inhibit only a single thrombin molecule.[50] Factor Xa is the pivotal step in the coagulation pathway, the junction of intrinsic and extrinsic pathways. One molecule of Xa activates 50 molecules of thrombin.[50] Factor Xa inhibition results in linear, dose-dependent, and predictable inhibition of thrombin formation.[51] Fondaparinux can inhibit both free and clot bound Xa; it therefore prevents de novo clot formation and growth of existing thrombi.[50,51] It does, however, permit the formation of a certain amount of normal thrombin, which may allow effective primary hemostasis, normal wound healing (where thrombin is thought to have a role), and activation of endogenous protein C via thrombin—thrombomodulin binding.[50] Hence, endogenous anticoagulant activity is preserved.[15,50] In addition, fondaparinux does not bind to platelets, cause thrombocytopenia, or cross-react with sera of HIT patients.[15,52] It does not inhibit osteoblasts or cause elevation of liver enzymes.[50–52] The risk of major bleeding at a fixed daily dose of 2.5 mg is not different from that associated with UFH or LMWH, but its long half-life and lack of reversibility imply that bleeding with fondaparinux may be more difficult to manage than with heparin.[2,51]

Fondaparinux is fully absorbed from a subcutaneous injection. Onset of action is 1 to 3 h after administration, and the $t_{1/2}$ is about 17 h. The kidneys excrete it almost entirely. There is minimal intra- and intersubject variability; therefore routine monitoring and dose adjustments are not necessary unless creatinine clearance is less than 30 mL/min.[8,15,17] It is not registered for use in patients under 50 kg. The drug is given as a single daily dose of 2.5 mg, starting 6 to 8 h after the operation for best balance of antithrombotic effect and bleeding risk.[15,17] It is currently registered for up to 9 days of postoperative use, but there is overwhelming evidence of further benefit if therapy is prolonged up to 4 weeks postoperatively. A 4-week prophylactic regimen produces a 96 percent reduction in VTE compared with 1 week of fondaparinux followed by 3 weeks of placebo.[11,17,23,53] The overall risk reduction for fondaparinux versus conventional enoxaparin regimens is 55.2 percent, with no clinically important increase in bleeding.[15,17,23] Idraparinux is a derivative of fondaparinux that is currently under investigation for long-term prophylaxis.[9,17] It has a $t_{1/2}$ of 130 h and is administered as a 2.5-mg subcutaneous injection once weekly. At this dose, it appears to cause less bleeding complications than warfarin, adjusted to an INR of 2 to 3. Bleeding management poses the same problems that apply to fondaparinux.[9,17]

Direct Thrombin Inhibitors

These drugs bind irreversibly (hirudin and recombinant hirudins; e.g., desirudin) or reversibly (melagatran/ximelagatran, dabigatran etexilate) to the active catalytic site of thrombin.[6,15] All the physiologic functions of thrombin are inhibited, including conversion of fibrinogen to fibrin, fibrin cross-linking, feedback activation of clotting cascades, protein C and platelet activation, and inhibition of fibrinolysis.[2,6] Direct thrombin inhibitors can inhibit both free and clot-bound thrombin, especially the smaller molecules like melagatran, which inhibit them in a ratio of 1:1.[2,6,15] They therefore prevent growth of existing clots and inhibit de novo thrombus formation.[6,15] The reversible agents allow periods of normal thrombin activity to facilitate normal hemostasis.[6] The action of DTIs is a direct stoichiometric inhibition of thrombin, which does not require AT; they are therefore effective in AT deficiency.[6,15] The antithrombotic efficacy of DTI is at least as good as that of LMWH or warfarin, and some trials point to a 20 to 30 percent advantage over warfarin. They do not produce HIT and are therefore indicated for anticoagulation in patients with a history of HIT.[2,6] At doses producing equivalent antithrombotic effect, bleeding is less than with UFH or warfarin.[6] The drugs are predominantly excreted by the kidneys and dose adjustment is required in severe renal impairment.[2] Transient elevation of liver transaminases is seen in 6 to 13 percent of patients; a twofold elevation in this variable is an indication to discontinue DTI and use another anticoagulant.[2,6]

The two DTIs that have undergone extensive testing for prophylaxis against thrombosis in major orthopaedic surgery are desirudin and melagatran/ximelagatran.[6,54] Desirudin is given as a twice-daily fixed dose of 15 mg subcutaneously. It has a $t_{1/2}$ of 4 to 8 h. Monitoring of its anticoagulant effect is not indicated. When started 30 min before surgery, it resulted in a threefold reduction in thrombosis versus UFH and a 25 percent advantage over 40 mg of enoxaparin daily.[6,54] Part of this advantage may be due to the more efficient anticoagulant effect of the DTI, but the administration very soon before surgery probably also plays a role.[6,54] Owing to its high cost, desirudin is usually reserved for prophylaxis in HIT patients. Melagatran is a small, reversible parenteral DTI, which is also available as an oral prodrug, ximelagatran.[2,54] It has a $t_{1/2}$ of 4 to 5 h and is administered twice daily. It acts rapidly after oral or subcutaneous administration.[2,6,54] This, and the short $t_{1/2}$, means that anticoagulation can be reversed rapidly in cases of excessive bleeding, but it can also be reestablished quickly.[2,6] Diuresis promotes clearance and offset of action.[6] Various regimens are used for thrombosis prophylaxis and all are comparable or superior to warfarin.[2,6] High-dose regimens, especially where prophylaxis is started soon before surgery, have achieved a 25 percent reduction in VTE compared with LMWH, but at the cost of increased noncritical bleeding.[2,6] In Europe, treatment with subcutaneous melagatran (2 mg) is started 4 to 8 h postoperatively, followed by 3 mg 12 h later and then 24 mg of ximelagatran orally twice daily.[2,6] In the United States, oral ximelagatran 24 to 36 mg is administered twice daily, starting 12 to 24 h postoperatively.[2,6] The 24-mg dose reduces VTE rates to a similar extent as adjusted doses of warfarin (but less so than LMWH), and the 36-mg dose shows a 20 to 30 percent improvement over warfarin.[2] Ximelagatran has a substantially wider therapeutic range than warfarin. No monitoring of anticoagulant effect is required.[2,15]

▶ RECOMMENDATIONS FOR THROMBOPROPHYLAXIS IN MAJOR ORTHOPAEDIC SURGERY

Routine prophylaxis has been standard in major orthopaedic surgery for more than 15 years.[8] This is not surprising, since without prophylaxis VTE rates are unacceptably high. Even with current prophylaxis, 1.5 to 10 percent of patients suffer symptomatic venous thrombosis within 3 months of surgery. Some occur after silent DVT already present in the hospital, but many occur primarily after discharge. It is thus impossible to predict,

with routine screening on discharge, which patients will develop VTE.[8,16,17] The following recommendations for prophylaxis are those of the seventh ACCP consensus conference.[1] They are based on an exhaustive analysis of almost 800 published trials for which the strength of evidence for benefit or risk, and the methodologic quality of the studies was taken into account. Where there is certainty of benefit or risk, the evidence is classified as grade 1 and a "recommendation" is made. Where evidence is less certain, it is termed grade 2 and a therapeutic "suggestion" is made. Randomized controlled trials with consistent results are classified as grade A, while those with less consistent results or methodologic flaws are designated grade B. Data from observational studies or extrapolated from a group in a randomized trial to another similar group of patients are labeled grade C. Where the grade C observations or data are particularly compelling or secure, they are classified as grade C+. Grade C+ recommendations are regarded as stronger than grade B. Overall, therefore, recommendations may fall anywhere from grade 1A to grade 2C, with progressively declining validity and strength.[55]

For THA, the following list of prophylactic antithrombotics constitutes a grade 1A recommendation (see Chap 10).[1] Any one of the following three regimens can be used:

1. LMWH at the usual high-risk dose (e.g., enoxaparin 30 mg twice daily or 40 mg daily). Administration is started 12 h preoperatively or 12 to 24 h postoperatively. Alternatively, a half dose (e.g., dalteparin 2500 IU) may be administered 4 to 6 h postoperatively and the full dose continued daily thereafter.[1,39,47]
2. Fondaparinux 2.5 mg subcutaneously daily, commencing 6 to 8 h postoperatively.[1,5]
3. Warfarin, starting preoperatively or the evening after surgery to a target INR of 2 to 3.[1]

The recommendations carry equal weight, since the prophylactic advantages of fondaparinux and LMWH are balanced by a slightly higher bleeding risk. Grade 1A recommendations are made against the use of aspirin, dextran, low-dose unfractionated heparin, graded elastic stockings, IPC, and plantar plexus compression as sole prophylactic options.[1]

In TKA, the incidence of symptomatic and proximal DVT is lower despite the higher overall incidence of venous thrombosis seen by venography (see Chap. 11).[5] Prophylaxis is less effective than in THA,[12] although a substantial benefit exists for fondaparinux over LMWH and for LMWH over warfarin.[1] This must be balanced by the potential severity of the consequences of local bleeding. The same grade 1A recommendations made for hip arthroplasty apply to TKA.[1] However, optimal use of IPC as a sole option receives a grade 1B recommendation where anticoagulants cannot be used. Aspirin and UFH are not recommended (grade 1A). The same applies to plantar plexus compression (grade 1B). Knee arthroscopy requires no drug prophylaxis. Early mobilization is sufficient unless the patient has other risk factors, in which case LMWH is recommended.[1]

Hip fracture surgery has the highest risk of major symptomatic venous thrombosis and PE (see Chap 16).[1] Routine prophylaxis is mandatory in all cases. Unlike THA and TKA, the thrombogenic event has already occurred preoperatively, and preoperative prophylaxis is recommended unless immediate surgery is planned (grade 1C+).[56] The prophylactic recommendations are fondaparinux (grade 1A), LMWH (grade 1C+), warfarin (grade 2A), and low-dose UFH (grade 1B).[1] Where anticoagulants are contraindicated, properly applied mechanical prophylaxis is a grade 1C+ recommendation.[1,5]

The ACCP have also formulated recommendations for other orthopaedic procedures.[1] They recommend against prophylaxis in elective spinal surgery (grade 1C) unless additional risk factors exist (e.g., malignancy or previous thrombosis) (see Chap. 14). Should these be present, they make a grade 1B recommendation for the use of UFH, LMWH, or IPC alone.[1] With acute spinal cord injury, however, routine prophylaxis is a grade 1A recommendation because of the excessive thrombotic risk posed by this lesion. Until primary hemostasis has been achieved, this should be with mechanical methods. Thereafter, LMWH is the method of choice.[1,12] Extended prophylaxis is advised during rehabilitation (grade 1C). This can be achieved with either long-term LMWH or warfarin.[1]

In isolated lower limb fractures other than the hip, no prophylaxis is recommended (grade 2A) (see Chap. 16).[1] In trauma, routine prophylaxis is a grade 1A recommendation if the patient has one or more VTE risk factors (see Chaps. 2 and 16).[1,12] LMWH is the agent of choice once adequate hemostasis is established. In the interim, mechanical methods can be employed (grade 1B). Prophylaxis should be continued until discharge (grade 1C).[1]

Recommendations have also been made for the initiation, timing, and duration of prophylaxis and the use of predischarge screening.[1] There appears to be little advantage to starting prophylaxis preoperatively, although the regimen remains an acceptable one. The best prophylaxis is achieved when it is started between 2 h preoperatively and 6 to 8 h after the operation. The latter time may offer the best tradeoff between efficacy and bleeding risk. If LMWH is used, the dose administered at this time is half of the normal high-risk dose. With fondaparinux, current recommendations are that the full 2.5-mg prophylactic dose be administered. Patients at particularly high risk for bleeding should receive the first dose of anticoagulants between 12 and 24 h after surgery. In this case, reduced prophylactic efficacy is balanced by a reduced risk of bleeding.[1]

There is consensus in the ACCP that there is no clinical or cost benefit in routine screening, particularly Doppler examinations, at or after discharge to determine in which patients prophylaxis should be continued.[1,12] It is known that a substantial proportion of patients leave the hospital with a clinically silent DVT and that the risk of new thrombus formation persists for 4 to 12 weeks after hip surgery (shorter with TKA).[5,11,12] About 45 to 80 percent of thromboses associated with hip and knee arthroplasty occur after discharge. The major factors that predict rehospitalization with thrombosis are a previous history of venous thrombosis, obesity, and advanced age.[1,12] Extended thromboprophylaxis (28 to 35 days), especially in hip surgery, results in a risk reduction for symptomatic thrombosis of about 60 percent.[5,30] Economic studies have indicated that extended prophylaxis after discharge may be cost-effective compared with only in-hospital prophylaxis.[33] The current grade 1A recommendations for all major orthopaedic procedures are for 10 days of prophylaxis with current agents.[1] With THR and HFS, this should be continued until 28 to 35 days postoperatively.[5,19,21] The agents of choice for THR are LMWH or warfarin (recommendation for both grade 1A) or fondaparinux (grade 1C+). For hip fracture surgery, fondaparinux is a grade 1A recommendation; LMWH and warfarin are grade 1C+.[1,17] At the time of the ACCP consensus conference, ximelagatran was not yet registered for prophylaxis, therefore no recommendations were made for its use.[1,17]

▶ IMPACT OF ANESTHESIA ON VENOUS THROMBOEMBOLISM

Neuraxial anesthesia (spinal or epidural) has been associated with consistent and substantial reductions in DVT incidence in major orthopaedic surgery (see Chap. 30).[3] This is most evident when other prophylactic measures are not used.[57] Reductions of 50 percent in proximal DVT have been confirmed venographically in patients who underwent TKA or THA under epidural anesthesia (see Chaps. 10 and 11).[57,58] The impact on overall DVT in TKA patients is less significant, possibly because the use of a tourniquet counteracts the beneficial effect of neuraxial anesthesia on venous blood flow.[58] Neuraxial anesthesia is the only intervention that is associated with reduced DVT and reduced perioperative bleeding and transfusion requirements.[57]

Various mechanisms are postulated to explain the impact of neuraxial anesthesia on thrombosis. These include a beneficial effect on arterial and venous blood flow in the lower limbs due to sympathetic block, an endothelial protective effect, and direct inhibition of coagulation or platelet function by absorbed local anesthetic.[13,57] However, a significant direct anticoagulant or antiplatelet effect is unlikely, because the plasma concentrations of local anesthetic, even during constant epidural infusions, are lower than those required to produce in vitro anticoagulation. In addition, the reduced bleeding associated with neuraxial anesthesia is incompatible with a clinically important anticoagulant effect.[57] However, epidural anesthesia prevents the hypercoagulable state associated with THA completely. This is probably due to an inhibition of the release of the inflammatory mediators involved in initiating the hypercoagulable state.[57]

Hypotensive neuraxial anesthesia with the administration of intravenous vasopressors for maintenance of adequate perfusion pressures is associated with reduced VTE rates. The reasons proposed include reduced blood loss, reduced surgical time, diminished tissue factor production, and less inhibition of antithrombin formation.[13,14]

Neuraxial anesthesia has demonstrated benefits in preventing DVT and other morbidity in high-risk patients.[8,59] Consequently its use has grown steadily in recent years. Between 1996 and 2001, the use of neuraxial anesthesia increased by more than 10 percent in THA and TKA, being utilized in 46 and 54 percent of these cases respectively.[59] However, the thromboprophylactic efficacy of neuraxial anesthesia alone is insufficient to qualify it as the sole means to prevent venous thrombosis. It is therefore generally viewed as an adjunct to anticoagulants.[3,12,59]

▶ IMPLICATIONS OF PROPHYLAXIS ON CHOICE OF ANESTHESIA

The hemorrhagic complications of anticoagulant prophylaxis are not restricted to the surgical site.[40] Bleeding may be caused by other invasive procedures. As mentioned, a significant proportion of major orthopaedic operations are performed under neuraxial anesthesia.[59] This may be continued postoperatively by local anesthetic infusions through a catheter. Many other patients receive plexus or peripheral nerve blocks with or without indwelling catheters.

Vertebral canal hematoma (VCH) is defined as symptomatic bleeding within the spinal neuraxis.[40] It is a rare but catastrophic complication of neuraxial anesthesia, anticoagulation, and the combination thereof. These hematomas present an average of 3 days after anticoagulant therapy is started.[40] Almost 70 percent of cases present with a new progressive sensory or motor block.[8,41] Only 38 percent of patients have a good or fair outcome after VCH.[40,59] This figure increases to 75 percent when surgical decompression is done within 8 h of the onset of symptoms.[40] Hematomas of the vertebral column account for 50 percent of spinal injuries associated with anesthesia.[40,59] Spinal injuries were the leading cause of legal claims against anesthesiologists in the United States in the 1990s. Anesthetic care in cases of VCH was judged adequate in only 7.5 percent of cases, and settlements were generally high.[40]

The incidence of VCH is difficult to determine because of regional differences in thromboprophylactic drug use and protocols, varying levels of compliance with guidelines, and the likelihood of underreporting.[40] VCH was rare worldwide, with an incidence not exceeding 1 per 150,000 for epidural and 1:220,000 for spinal anesthesia, until the release of LMWH in North America in the early 1990s.[2] Since that time, over 80 cases have been reported to the Medwatch system, most of them in the first 5 years of this period.[8,40] The estimated incidence of VCH at this time was about 1:3000 in epidural anesthesia and 1:40,000 in spinal anesthesia.[40] Since 1998, there appears to have been a slowing of reports. This may represent increased compliance with guidelines for the concomitant use of neuraxial anesthesia and anticoagulants.[40] The most recent of these guidelines were formulated by the Second American Society of Regional Anesthesia (ASRA) Consensus Conference on Neuraxial Anesthesia and Anticoagulation of 2002.[40]

There are several risk factors identified for the development of VCH:

1. Elderly women undergoing major orthopaedic surgery under neuraxial anesthesia account for 75 percent of cases of VCH.[2,8,59]
2. Hemostatic abnormalities were present in 68 percent of cases. These included administration of excessive doses of anticoagulants, administration close to the time of neuraxial procedures, combinations of anticoagulant drugs, and use of these drugs in patients with hepatic or renal impairment.[3,8,28,40,59,60]
3. Difficulties with needle placement: traumatic insertion or bleeding on insertion were encountered in half of the patients. A combination of this factor plus a hemostatic abnormality was seen in 87 percent of cases.[40]
4. Epidural anesthesia accounts for about 75 percent of cases and spinal anesthesia for 25 percent. In Europe, spinal anesthesia is used about four times as often as epidural anesthesia, but epidural anesthesia still accounts for the majority of VCH cases.[59]
5. Two-thirds of cases were associated with neuraxial catheter techniques.[59]
6. Fully 47 percent of VCH cases followed catheter removal. This is therefore no less risky than the initial neuraxial puncture.[8]
7. Many patients received other drugs with an effect on clotting in addition to their prophylactic anticoagulants. Nonsteroidal anti-inflammatory agents and antiplatelet agents were most commonly implicated.[2,59]

8. The choice and dose of anticoagulant and timing with respect to the neuraxial puncture or catheter removal are of critical importance.[59]

There have been five case reports of VCH associated with UFH and four in patients who received warfarin.[8,41,59] All of the latter occurred when the epidural catheter was removed. However, the vast majority of cases of VCH (more than 80) have been reported to be associated with LMWH prophylaxis.[40] There appears to be no advantage of one LMWH preparation over any other in terms of risk for VCH.[40] The majority of VCH cases have occurred when LMWH was given twice a day.[3] This means that many of patients had unsafe levels of anticoagulation when catheters were removed, since no true nadir in anticoagulant level could occur.[40,60] These patients receive 50 percent more LMWH than patients on a once-daily regimen. There appears to be no major advantage in starting prophylaxis preoperatively. Neuraxial puncture can therefore be performed entirely in the absence of anticoagulation.[40]

There is much controversy about the impact of antiplatelet agents on VCH. It appears that aspirin or nonsteroidal anti-inflammatory drugs (NSAIDs) in themselves do not pose a risk for VCH.[40,59] When they are combined with other anticoagulants, however, the risk of VCH increases by an unspecified amount.[40,59] Such combinations are not prohibited, but they make it mandatory to follow dosing guidelines closely. Other antiplatelet agents—such as thienopyridines (clopidogrel, ticlopidine) and platelet glycoprotein IIb/IIIa inhibitors (abciximab, eptifibatide, tirofiban)—have more profound and multimodal antiplatelet activity. They must be discontinued 5 to 14 days before surgery [59] and, although specific guidelines are lacking, are probably incompatible with other anticoagulants for safe surgery or neuraxial anesthesia.[40]

No case reports or recommendations exist at present for the DTI melagatran/ximelagatran, although it has been used in conjunction with neuraxial anesthesia in major orthopaedic surgery in over 2000 patients.[2,40] Fondaparinux has not been associated with VCH in more than 3600 neuraxial blocks for major orthopaedic surgery.[17,40,52,61] In these trials, single-injection neuraxial anesthetics were employed; scrupulous attention was paid to exclude patients with traumatic blocks and to dosing initiation and intervals. At this stage, it is impossible to confirm the safety of catheter techniques with this drug.[40]

The ASRA consensus conference of 2002 has produced guidelines to maximize safety when neuraxial anesthesia/analgesia is used concomitantly with anticoagulants[40]:

1. Unfractionated heparin at low doses is compatible with neuraxial anesthesia and catheter techniques. It should, however, be delayed for at least an hour after the neuraxial procedure. Catheter removal should occur 2 h or more after a preceding dose and at least 1 h before one. A bloody tap may indicate that surgery should be postponed, but decisions should be made on an individual basis. Platelet counts should be checked on day 5 of UFH therapy.[8,40]

2. There is virtually no evidence that a once-daily LMWH regimen started at least 6 to 8 h or more after the operation places the patient at increased risk for VCH.[8,59] Indwelling catheters are safe provided that they are removed no sooner than 10 to 12 h after the previous dose of LMWH and at least 2 h before the next dose.[59] Should preoperative LMWH be used, it must be given at least 10 to 12 h before the neuraxial procedure.[59] If twice-daily LMWH administration is planned, it should be started no sooner than 24 h after surgery and at least 2 h after removal of the epidural catheter.[59] Twice-daily regimens are not safe with indwelling neuraxial catheters.[3,59] Traumatic insertion or a bloody spinal tap does not make it necessary to postpone surgery but requires delay of the first dose of LMWH for 24 h.[59]

3. Warfarin has been associated with VCH only when started preoperatively.[41] All cases occurred on removal of the epidural catheter and all had INR values of >1.5.[40] It is advisable to check the INR before performing a neuraxial block if warfarin has been started more than 24 h preoperatively because of the unpredictability of its dose-response relationship. Likewise, INR should be measured while an indwelling neuraxial catheter is in place or before its removal.[41] An INR of >3 requires withholding of warfarin until it has fallen to 1.5. The latter value corresponds with a factor VII level of 40 percent of baseline.[40] At this level, the catheter can be removed safely.[59] Since the target INR level for prophylaxis is 2 to 3, warfarin prophylaxis is not readily compatible with the use of indwelling neuraxial catheters.[40,41]

Because VCH is so rare, it is not possible to perform a prospective study of sufficient power to guide practice.[40,59] We therefore, must rely on a consensus derived from the collective experience of experts in the field. This consensus cautions the practitioner to weigh decisions to combine neuraxial techniques and anticoagulation on an individual basis.[8] Every attempt should be made to ensure that all neuraxial interventions are carried out when the coagulation status is normal or nearly normal.[59] This is best achieved by adherence to guidelines, giving particular attention to factors that may enhance anticoagulant effect. These are advanced age; low body mass; hepatic, renal, or cardiac disease; drug interactions; and concomitant use of other drugs with a potential for anticoagulant effects.[2,59] Should the safety of neuraxial anesthesia be uncertain in a particular patient, it is prudent to err on the side of caution and to avoid neuraxial blockade.[8,59] Should a neuraxial block be indicated by the patient's medical condition and the coagulation status be questionable, a single injection spinal block with a small-gauge needle is the technique of choice.[41,59] In all patients in whom anticoagulation is used concomitantly with any neuraxial technique, monitoring is mandatory until at least 24 h after the termination of the block or catheter removal.[2,59] Any symptoms or signs of cord compression dictate emergency radiologic investigation to confirm or exclude VCH, followed by immediate compulsory decompression in all cases.[40,59] Using the lowest effective concentration of local anesthetic so as to avoid motor block facilitates monitoring during continuous infusion of local anesthetic via an indwelling catheter. Motor function can then be monitored on an ongoing basis.[8]

The precise risk associated with *plexus and peripheral nerve blocks* in the presence of anticoagulants is unclear.[40] The frequency and severity of hemorrhagic complications is unknown.[40] Case reports have confirmed the possibility of major, critical, and even fatal bleeding in this situation.[62] The bleeds have been associated with UFH, LMWH, and thienopyridine drugs.[40] All such reports relate to psoas compartment or lumbar sympathetic block.[40] Significant bleeds requiring transfusion are possible, since the psoas compartment can accommodate up to 3 L of blood.[40] Neurologic deficits are usually minimal and reversible within a maximum of 6 to 12 months. Since most nerve sheaths do not lie in nonexpandable compartments, the likelihood of irreversible neural ischemia is far smaller than in the spinal cord.[63] At this stage, consensus statements regarding neuraxial anesthesia are applied to deep plexus blocks. It is unclear at present whether this policy is too restrictive.[40]

REFERENCES

1. Geerts WH, Pineo GF, Heit JA, et al. Prevention of venous thromboembolism. The Seventh ACCP Conference on Antithrombotic and Thrombolytic Therapy. *Chest* 126:338S–400S, 2004.
2. Rosencher N. Ximelagatran, a new oral direct thrombin inhibitor, for the prevention of venous thromboembolic events in major elective orthopaedic surgery: Efficacy, safety and anesthetic considerations. *Anesthesia* 59:803–810, 2004.
3. Gallus AS. Applying risk assessment models in orthopaedic surgery: Overview of our clinical experience. *Blood Coagul Fibrinolysis* 10:S53–S61, 1999.
4. Paiement GD. DVT Prophylaxis: DVT prophylaxis after total joint arthroplasty. *Medscape Orthop Sports Med* 2:3036–3046, 1998.
5. Offord R, Perry D. *Anticoagulation.* London: Science Press, 2002.
6. Eriksson BI, Dahl OE. Prevention of venous thromboembolism following orthopaedic surgery: Clinical potential of direct thrombin inhibitors. *Drugs* 64:577–595, 2004.
7. Brenkel IJ. DVT prophylaxis in patients undergoing total hip arthroplasty. *Curr Orthop* 15:356–363, 2001.
8. Hawkinberry DW II, Broadman LM. The best approaches to prophylaxis against DVT formation when using a combination of neuraxial anesthesia and heparins, in Fleisher LA (ed): *Evidence-Based Practice of Anesthesiology.* Philadelphia: Saunders, 2004:292–304.
9. Weitz JI, Hirsh J, Samama MM. New anticoagulant drugs. The Seventh ACCP Conference on Antithrombotic and Thrombolytic Therapy. *Chest* 126:265S–286S, 2004.
10. Samama MM, Dahl OE, Quinlan DJ, et al. Quantification of risk factors for venous thromboembolism: A preliminary study for the development of a risk assessment tool. *J Hematol* 88:1410–1421, 2003.
11. Warwick DJ. Venous thromboembolism following major orthopaedic surgery: Does it really matter? *Second International Expert Session on Selective Factor Xa Inhibition,* 10–12, 2003.
12. Geerts WH, Heit JA, Clagett GP, et al. Prevention of venous thromboembolism. *Chest* 119:132S–175S, 2001.
13. Salvati EA. Multimodal prophylaxis of venous thrombosis. *Am J Orthop* 1:4–11, 2002.
14. Miric A, Lombardi P, Sculco TP. Deep vein thrombosis prophylaxis: A comprehensive approach for total hip and total knee arthroplasty patients. *Am J Orthop* 29:269–274, 2000.
15. Hyers TM. Management of venous thromboembolism: Past, present and future. *Arch Intern Med* 163:759–768, 2003.
16. Howard AW, Aaron SD. Low molecular weight heparin decreases proximal and distal deep venous thrombosis following total knee arthroplasty: A meta-analysis of randomized trials. *Thromb Hemost* 79:902–906, 1998.
17. Turpie AGG, Eriksson BI, Bauer KA, Lassen MR. New pentasaccharides for the prophylaxis of venous thromboembolism: Clinical studies. *Chest* 124:371S–378S, 2003.
18. Heit JA, Mohr DN, Silverstein MD, et al. Predictors of recurrence after deep vein thrombosis and pulmonary embolism: A population based cohort study. *Arch Intern Med* 160:761–768, 2000.
19. Agnelli G, Mancini GB, Biagini D. The rationale for long-term prophylaxis of venous thromboembolism. *Orthopaedics* 23(6):S643–S646, 2000.
20. Blanchard J, Meuwly JY, Leyvraz PF, et al. Prevention of deep-vein thrombosis after total knee replacement: Randomized comparison between a low-molecular-weight heparin (Nadroparin) and mechanical prophylaxis with a foot pump system. *J Bone Joint Surg (Br)* 81-B:654–659, 1999.
21. Haentjens P. Venous thromboembolism after total hip arthroplasty: A review of incidence and prevention during hospitalization and after hospital discharge. *Acta Orthop Belg* 66:1–8, 2000.
22. Fitzgerald RH, Spiro TE, Trowbridge AA, et al. Prevention of venous thromboembolic disease following primary total knee arthroplasty: A randomized, multicenter, open-label,

parallel-group comparison of enoxaparin and warfarin. *J Bone Joint Surg* 83:900–906, 2001.

22a. Eriksson BI. The clinical evaluation of fondaparinux in the prevention of venous thromboembolism after major orthopaedic surgery. *Second International Expert Session on Selective Factor Xa Inhibition. Thromb Haemost* 90:13–16, 2003.

23. Sandler DA, Martin JF. Autopsy proven pulmonary embolism in hospital patients: Are we detecting enough deep vein thrombosis? *J R Soc Med* 82:203–205, 1989.

24. Hull RD, Pineo GF, Francis C, et al. Low-molecular-weight heparin prophylaxis using dalteparin in close proximity to surgery vs. warfarin in hip arthroplasty patients: A double-blind, randomized comparison. *Arch Intern Med* 160:2199–2207, 2000.

25. Douketis JD, Eikelboom JW, Quinlan DJ, et al. Short-duration prophylaxis against venous thromboembolism after total hip or knee replacement: A meta-analysis of prospective studies investigating symptomatic outcomes. *Arch Intern Med* 162:1465–1471, 2002.

26. Ollendorf DA, Vera-Llonch M, Oster G. Cost of venous thromboembolism following major orthopaedic surgery in hospitalized patients. *Amer J Health Syst Pharm* 59:1750–1754, 2002.

27. Anderson FA, Hirsh J, White K, et al. Temporal trends in prevention of venous thromboembolism following primary total hip or knee arthroplasty 1996–2001: Findings from the hip and knee registry. *Chest* 124:349S–356S, 2003.

28. Heit JA. Venous thromboembolism epidemiology: Implications for prevention and management. *Semin Thromb Hemost* 28:4–13, 2002.

29. Davidson BL, Sullivan SD, Kahn SR, et al. The economics of venous thromboembolism prophylaxis: A primer for clinicians. *Chest* 124:393S–396S, 2003.

30. Bick RL. Therapy for venous thrombosis: Guidelines for a competent and cost-effective approach. *Clin Appl Thromb Hemost* 5:2–9, 1999.

31. Anderson DR, O'Brien BJ. Cost effectiveness of the prevention and treatment of deep vein thrombosis and pulmonary embolism. *Pharmacoeconomics* 12:17–29, 1997.

32. Hull RD, Pineo GF, Francis C, et al. Low-molecular-weight heparin prophylaxis using dalteparin extended out-of-hospital vs in-hospital warfarin/out-of-hospital placebo in hip arthroplasty patients: A double-blind randomized comparison. *Arch Intern Med* 160:2208–2215, 2000.

33. Haas S. Limitations of established antithrombotic strategies. *Blood Coagul Fibrinolysis* 10:S11–S18, 1999.

34. Patrono C, Coller B, FitzGerald GA, et al. Platelet-active drugs: The relationships among dose, effectiveness and side effects. The Seventh ACCP Conference on Antithrombotic and Thrombolytic Therapy. *Chest* 126:234S–264S, 2004.

35. Raskob GE, Hirsh J. Controversies in timing of the first dose of anticoagulant prophylaxis against venous thromboembolism after major orthopaedic surgery. *Chest* 124:379S–385S, 2003.

36. Hull RD, Raskob GE, Pineo GF, et al. Subcutaneous low-molecular-weight heparin vs warfarin for prophylaxis of deep vein thrombosis after hip or knee implantation: An economic perspective. *Arch Intern Med* 157:298–303, 1997.

37. Botteman MF, Caprini J, Stephens JM, et al. Results of an economic model to assess the cost-effectiveness of enoxaprin, a low-molecular-weight heparin, versus warfarin for the prophylaxis of deep vein thrombosis and associated long-term complications in total hip replacement surgery in the United States. *Clin Ther* 24:1960–1986, 2002.

38. Hull RD, Pineo GF, Stein PD, et al. Timing of initial administration of low-molecular-weight heparin prophylaxis against deep vein thrombosis in patients following elective hip arthroplasty: A systematic review. *Arch Intern Med* 161:1952–1960, 2001.

39. Horlocker TT, Wedel DJ, Benzon H, et al. Regional anesthesia in the anticoagulated patient: Defining the risks (The Second ASRA Consensus Conference on Neuraxial Anesthesia and Anticoagulation). *Reg Anesth Pain Med* 28:172–197, 2003.

40. Broadman LM. Vitamin K antagonists and spinal axis anesthesia, in Fleisher LA (ed): *Evidence-Based Practice of Anesthesiology.* Philadelphia: Saunders, 2004:305–311.

41. Ansell J, Hirsh J, Poller L, et al. The pharmacology and management of the vitamin K antagonists. The seventh ACCP conference on antithrombotic and thrombolytic therapy. *Chest* 126:204S–233S, 2004.

42. Hirsh J, Raschke R. Heparin and low-molecular-weight heparin. The Seventh ACCP Conference on Antithrombotic and Thrombolytic Therapy. *Chest* 126:188S–203S, 2004.

43. Hirsh J, Warkentin TE, Shaughnessy SG, et al. Heparin and low-molecular-weight heparin: Mechanisms of action, pharmacokinetics, dosing, monitoring, efficacy and safety. *Chest* 119:64S–94S, 2001.

44. Warkentin TE, Greinacher A. Heparin-induced thrombocytopenia: Recognition, treatment and prevention. The Seventh ACCP Conference on Antithrombotic and Thrombolytic Therapy. *Chest* 126:311S–337S, 2004.

45. Leyvraz PF, Bachmann F, Hoek J, et al. Prevention of deep vein thrombosis after hip replacement: Randomized comparison between unfractionated heparin and low molecular weight heparin. *Br Med J* 303:543–548, 1991.

46. Hull RD, Pineo GF, MacIsaac S. Low-molecular-weight heparin prophylaxis: Preoperative versus postoperative initiation in patients undergoing elective hip surgery. *Thromb Res* 101:V155–V162, 2001.

47. Mismetti P, Laporte-Simitsidis S, Navarro C, et al. Aging and venous thromboembolism influence the pharmacodynamics of the anti–factor Xa and anti-thrombin activities of a low-molecular-weight heparin (Nadroparin). *Thromb Hemost* 79:1162–1165, 1998.

49. Vitoux JF, Aiach M, Roncato M, Fiessinger JM. Should thromboprophylactic dosage of low molecular-weight heparin be adapted to patient's weight? *Thromb Hemost* 59:120, 1988.

50. Bauersachs R. Factor Xa inhibition: A unique approach to thrombin modulation. *Second International Expert Session on Selective Factor Xa Inhibition. Thromb Hemost* 5–7, 2003.

51. Bauer KA. New pentasaccharides for prophylaxis of deep vein thrombosis: Pharmacology. *Chest* 124:364S–370S, 2003.

52. Kwong LM. Fondaparinux (Arixtra) in day-to-day practice. *Second International Expert Session on Selective Factor Xa Inhibition. Thromb Hemost* 17–19, 2003.

53. Eriksson BI, Lassen MR. Duration of prophylaxis against venous thromboembolism with fondaparinux after hip fracture surgery: A multicenter, randomized, placebo-controlled, double-blind study. *Arch Intern Med* 163:1337–1342, 2003.

54. Evans HC, Perry CM, Faulds D. Ximelagatran/melagatran: A review of its use in the prevention of venous thromboembolism in orthopaedic surgery. *Drugs* 64:649–678, 2004.

55. Guyatt G, Schunemann HJ, Cook D, et al. Applying the grades of recommendation for antithrombotic and thrombolytictherapy. The Seventh ACCP Conference on Antithrombotic and Thrombolytic Therapy. *Chest* 126:179S–187S, 2004.

56. Zufferey P, Laporte S, Quenet S, et al. Optimal low-molecular-weight heparin regimen in major orthopaedic surgery. *Thromb Hemostasis* 90:654–661, 2003.

57. Hollmann MW, Wieczorek MS, Smart M, et al. Epidural anesthesia prevents hypercoagulation in patients undergoing major orthopaedic surgery. *Reg Anesth Pain Med* 26:215–222, 2001.

58. Sharrock NE, Haas SB, Hargett MJ, et al. Effects of epidural anesthesia on the incidence of deep-vein thrombosis after total knee arthroplasty. *J Bone Joint Surg* 73A:502–506, 1991.

59. Horlocker TT. Low molecular weight heparin and neuraxial anesthesia. *Thrombosis Res* 101:V141–V154, 2001.

60. Douketis JD, Kinnon K, Crowther MA. Anticoagulant effect at the time of epidural catheter removal in patients receiving twice-daily or once-daily low-molecular-weight heparin and continuous epidural analgesia after orthopaedic surgery. *Thromb Hemost* 88:37–40, 2002.

61. Cannavo D. Use of neuraxial anesthesia with selective factor Xa inhibitors. *Am J Orthop* 31:21–23, 2002.

62. Weller RS, Gerancher JC, Crews JC, et al. Extensive retroperitoneal hematoma without neurological deficit in two patients who underwent lumbar plexus block and were later anticoagulated. *Anesthesiology* 98:581–585, 2003.

63. Ben-David B, Joshi R, Chelly JE. Sciatic nerve palsy after total hip arthroplasty in a patient receiving continuous lumbar plexus block. *Anesth Analg* 97:1180–1182, 2003.

CHAPTER 5
Fat Embolism

ANDRE R. COETZEE

► INTRODUCTION

Fat embolism (FE) is the partial obstruction of multiple blood vessels by fat globules.[1] This is usually a temporary phenomenon. The fat embolism syndrome (FES) is the clinical manifestation of FE.

► HISTORY

In initial experiments, milk injected into the circulation of dogs produced FE. This was followed by oil-injection studies in the nineteenth century.[2,3] However, the pathology and clinical picture were appreciated only in 1862, when fat was detected in the lungs of trauma patients.[2,3] Zenker postulated that the fat in the lung was aspirated, but Wagner showed that fractures of bones released fat into the circulation.[2,3]

The clinical manifestation of FE, that is, FES, was described in 1873 by Bergman,[3] and 350 cases were described in 1913.[2] In a review, Lehman and Moore in 1927[4] postulated a metabolic mechanism to explain the FES, while Sevitt drew a distinction between systemic and pulmonary fat emboli.[1] Peltier concluded that the morbidity associated with FE was caused by fatty acids and associated inflammation.[5]

► INCIDENCE

Fat emboli in the lungs of patients with skeletal trauma are common.[6] Analysis of blood taken from the pulmonary artery of patients with long bone or pelvic fractures demonstrated that 7 percent of patients had fat emboli.[7] Long bone fractures, of the lower extremities in particular, seem to cause fat emboli.[8,9]

However, the presence of fat emboli is not synonymous with FES and, because of under reporting, differences in diagnostic criteria, and studies in different populations, the reported incidence of FES varies from 0.25 to 29 percent.[10–12] Perioperative FES, after immediate fixation of fractures, has a reported incidence of 0 to 5 percent.[9,13] A report on more than 900 cases of surgery for lower extremity fracture gave an incidence of 0.2 percent.[3]

► PATHOLOGY

The etiology of FE and FES is classified as traumatic and nontraumatic.

Traumatic

The essential pathology is the entrance of marrow fat into veins. This process is enhanced by

Multiple fractures
Unstable fractures
Increased pressure in the medullary cavity
Shock, hypoxia, and stress, although this will not cause FES by itself[14]

The attachment of veins to bone prevents their collapse; even during episodes of low venous pressure, such as circulatory shock.[15] Fractures of bones with a higher density of vessels, such as the isthmus of the proximal femoral shaft, are more likely to cause the release of fat into the circulation.[9]

Mechanics dictate that if the medullary pressure is raised when veins are torn, more fat will enter the circulation. Hence closed fractures result in more fat emboli.[9,16] Reaming of medullary spaces during surgery and nailing of prostheses (which raises the medullary pressure to 500 mmHg) tend to cause more fat emboli.[17,18] Venting of the medullary cavity before inserting instruments therefore decreases the incidence of fat emboli.[19] Young men are more prone than others to develop FES.[20]

Burns and soft tissue injury can also result in FES,[21] but it is less common, even though fat emboli are common.

Nontraumatic

These are rare causes of FES and they are classified as follows[3]:

Procedure-Related

This group includes intraosseous fluid administration, intraoperative autotransfusion, and lipid-soluble radiocontrast.

Disease-Related

Sickle cell hemoglobin C, pancreatitis, fat necrosis of the omentum, and immunosuppressive disease are typical examples.

Drug-Related

Intravenous hyperalimentation, intraarterial cisplatinum, and long-term steroid administration are included here.

▶ PATHOPHYSIOLOGY

Three main hypotheses have been put forward to explain FES:

Mechanical hypothesis
Biochemical hypothesis
A combination of mechanical and biochemical mechanisms

Mechanical Hypothesis

This hypothesis proposes that the embolized fat causes mechanical obstruction of the pulmonary and systemic capillaries. Fat has been demonstrated in the circulation soon after injury,[22] and fat in the lungs of animals has been shown to originate from the bone marrow.[22–24] Experiments in rabbits have demonstrated that raising the intramedullary pressure at a fracture site increased the extravasation of marrow fat.[23] In humans, significant amounts of fat have been found in the ipsilateral femoral vein of a fractured femur during surgery.[25,26]

The lung capillaries are prominently affected in FE, and there appears to be a relationship between the decrease in arterial PaO_2 in FES and compressed closed fractures.[27] Hypoxia was less common in patients with decompressed fractures.[9]

Neutral fat (not free fatty acids) can obstruct the pulmonary arterial system, causing acute pulmonary artery hypertension and acute right ventricular failure.[28–31] The resultant decrease in cardiac output together with inflammatory changes in the lung will worsen hypoxia.

Obstruction of capillaries is not restricted to the lung but occurs in the myocardium, brain, kidney, and other organs when fat enters the systemic circulation. The mechanisms by which fat enters the systemic circulation are either through a patent foramen ovale, which opens once the right atrial pressure is raised (because of acute pulmonary hypertension associated with acute lung injury or mechanical obstruction), or through the pulmonary capillaries. Patent foramina ovale were, however, not found in many patients with FES, and this supports the capillary transit theory.[32] Another way in which fat may enter the systemic circulation is via pulmonary-bronchial anastomoses if the obstruction of the pulmonary bed results in reverse flow.

Chylomicrons are small (1 μm in diameter) but, under the influence of mediators, coalesce into 10- to 40-μm fat globules,[4] which are thought to obstruct the capillaries in the lung and the systemic capillary bed.[33] One study demonstrated a significant increase in cholesterol in fat obtained from the pulmonary capillaries of patients with FES,[34] but this observation has not been confirmed.

Biochemical Hypothesis

This hypothesis proposes that the fat globules in the systemic and pulmonary circulation originate from fat normally present in the blood, presumably altered by physical and more probably biochemical factors, resulting in either toxic or obstructive pathology.[33]

The toxic hypothesis suggests that fat is broken down to free fatty acids (FFA), which cause injury to capillaries and pneumocytes. The resultant clinical picture is similar to that of acute lung injury with hemorrhagic lung injury to the pulmonary interstitium, edema, and pneumonitis.[5,35,36] The effects of FFA on the pulmonary tissue have been confirmed and there is a correlation between serum FFA levels and hypoxia.[37,38] However, this association does not necessarily imply causation. In addition, there is uncertainty about the origin of the FFA, with one group postulating that it is formed in the lung by the activity of pulmonary lipase on fat, while others postulate that it originates from the body fat.[5,35,36]

Trauma and catecholamines do result in FFA release, but whether this is important in the development of FES is uncertain.[39,40] If one considers the number of surgical procedures performed and/or trauma cases managed annually, the relatively low incidence of FES argues against this theory as a sole explanation for FES. Some studies have suggested that the serum albumin neutralizes the effect of FFA on the systemic circulation.[41–43] There is also a suggestion that FFA is raised more in patients with decreased liver function. This hypothesis has some credibility, since shock, hypoxia, and anesthesia decrease liver blood flow. Under these circumstances, together with raised catecholamines, FE may well become a clinical entity.

Combined Mechanical and Biochemical Hypothesis

Because mechanical and biochemical hypotheses separately do not appear to completely explain the FES, a combination of the two has been proposed.[5,34] The fat embolization of the capillaries by marrow is the initiating event and thereafter biochemical factors come into play.

Other Theories

Neutral fat has a thromboplastic effect, which activates the clotting cascade and could lead to disseminated intravascular coagulation (DIC) and eventually depletion of clotting factors. The end result is spontaneous bleeding.[44] This tendency, coupled with the suppression of the fibrinolytic system by trauma, results in the accumulation of red blood cells, platelets, leukocytes, and fibrin in the microvascular bed, including the lung.[45–47] The aggregates and clots will be filtered in part by the lung, and this contributes to the clinical picture of pulmonary parenchymal dysfunction often associated with FES. An inverse relationship has been demonstrated between platelet count and the degree of pulmonary dysfunction in these patients.[48]

DIC is not always associated with FES; in the author's practice, however, it does seem to occur regularly, albeit more often as subtle DIC patterns.

Another hypothesis is that trauma depresses the immune system, but the evidence for this as a cause of the FES is scanty.[49]

▶ CLINICAL PRESENTATION

FES usually presents in one of three degrees of severity[3]:

Subclinical
Nonfulminant subacute
Fulminant

Subclinical Form

The clinical signs are nonspecific and often confused with postoperative symptoms ascribed to pain, discomfort, or the postoperative inflammatory process. Tachypnea (defined as a breathing rate in excess of 25/min), elevated temperature (>37.8°C; 100.4°F) and tachycardia (>100 beats per minute) occur in the majority of patients with the subacute and mild form of FES.[50] Approximately 50 to 90 percent of patients with lower extremity fractures suffer from some degree of hypoxia (defined as a PaO_2 <80 mmHg; 10.6 kPa),[50–52] and FES is viewed as the most likely explanation for the recorded desaturation of the arterial blood. Increased alveolar ventilation, resulting in various degrees of hypocapnia, also occurs in patients with subclinical FES.[48] The latter study demonstrated a 48 percent incidence of thrombocytopenia (platelet count less than 200,000/µL), which has been regarded as an important indicator for FES[48] and suggested to be linked to the lung injury in FES. However, some of the conclusions in this regard rest on indirect evidence ($AaDo_2$) and are uncertain, since the $AaDo_2$ is affected by numerous factors and does not correlate well with the calculated shunt (Qs/Qt).[53]

An echocardiographic study showed marrow particles in the right atrium in 60 percent of patients in whom bones had been manipulated during surgery.[54]

Nonfulminant Form (Subacute Form of FES)

This is the more classic and well-known mode of presentation.

Patients often have *petechial rashes* on the anterior upper portion of the chest, especially in the areas adjacent to the axillae. Other areas commonly affected are the shoulders, mucous membranes (mouth), and conjunctiva.[35,41,55] These rashes usually appear 12 to 96 h after the injury and may last from hours to a week. It is important that an active search be made for these telltale signs of FES. It has been suggested that the upper areas of the body are more affected because fat is lighter than blood, but this is at best an uncertain explanation. Histology of the skin lesions shows occlusion and distention of the capillaries with fat globules and increased permeability of the capillaries.[56]

Neurologic signs are present in up to 86 percent of patients with FES.[55,57] These vary in severity and include confusion, stupor, coma, and even decerebrate rigidity. Confusion is the more common presenting symptom and convulsions have been reported. Signs are nonlateralizing and are usually progressive, starting with confusion and progressing to more severe encephalopathy in many patients. Localizing signs such as hemiplegia, apraxia, visual scotomata, and conjugate eye deviation occur but are rare.[57] The pathophysiology of neurologic dysfunction is thought to be the direct result not of cerebral hypoxia but rather of embolization. Cerebral edema may be induced by the FFA causing vascular disruption.[10,58]

The *respiratory system* is often also involved in FES, and this syndrome is among the causes of acute lung injury (ALI), the severe form of which is called acute respiratory distress syndrome (ARDS). The clinical picture includes tachypnea, cyanosis or some degree of arterial hemoglobin desaturation, and a respiratory alkalosis.

The pathophysiology of the acute lung injury is that of poor pulmonary compliance resulting in tachypnea, low ventilation/perfusion ratios, either Qva/Qt or Qs/Qt causing hypoxia, and an increased Vd/Vt. This is accompanied by various degrees of pulmonary hypertension, which jeopardize right ventricular function and cardiac output, resulting in mixed venous blood desaturation. The latter will be aggravated by the raised temperature that commonly occurs in patients with FES. The combination of mixed venous blood desaturation and pulmonary shunt will further depress the arterial oxygenation.

The pulmonary effects of FES usually have a relatively benign course, and by the third day—barring new fat emboli or infection—the lung parenchyma starts to improve rapidly.

There are reports of patients who had FES without pulmonary involvement.[59–61] The retina is affected in approximately 50 percent of patients.[62] In 4 percent of patients with long bone fractures, retinopathy presents subclinically.[63] Eye lesions, consisting of cotton-wool spots and flame-like hemorrhages, are indistinguishable from the Purtscher retinopathy described in extraocular trauma.[63,64] The cotton-wool areas are microinfarcts in the nerve fiber layer of the eye[63] and the pathophysiology is the same as in other organs—i.e., capillary engorgement and loss of endothelial integrity. This results in hemorrhage, edema, and microinfarction. The lesions disappear in weeks but permanent central scotomata have been described.

Fulminant FES

This form of FES contains all the elements of nonfulminant FES but is more severe. It has been described after the release of limb tourniquets, reaming of the femur, insertion of intramedullary prostheses, closed reductions of fractures, and manipulation of a deformed hip. However, it can also occur in the absence of surgery and several hours after surgery.[28,58,65] In the anesthetized patient, it may present as sudden hypotension, wheezing, tachycardia or bradycardia, poor lung compliance, pulmonary edema, cyanosis, or unexplained bleeding. Failure to regain consciousness after orthopaedic surgery and anesthesia should raise the possibility of cerebral FES.

In the unanesthetized patient, the signs and symptoms of the nonfulminant type occur, including more severe cerebral symptoms such as agitation, choreoathetosis, seizures, psychosis, or coma. These may precede fever, acute respiratory distress, significant hemodynamic instability, oliguria, renal failure, and clotting disorders.[3]

The lungs are affected in various ways: lung edema (even in the upper lung lobes) as well as reduced compliance and poor gas transfer resulting in hypoxia. Involvement of the upper lobe is explained by the hypothesis that fat is lighter than blood and hence will affect the upper zones. What argues against this idea is that the toxic effects of FFA damage the endothelium of the vasculature; hence areas with higher perfusion, such as the dependent parts of the lung, will be affected more. Another explanation for the upper lobe edema is the acute pulmonary hypertension associated with acute lung injury. This will increase perfusion of the upper lobes and may highlight the edema seen in those areas of the lung that are normally less well perfused (because of gravity). The picture can progress to a full-blown ARDS with all the clinical signs and symptoms of severe acute lung injury requiring respiratory support.

The right heart is severely affected by acute increases in the afterload. Acute lung injury is virtually always associated with ARDS, and data show that by the time the patient is admitted to the intensive care unit with a diagnosis of ARDS, acute pulmonary hypertension is already present.[66] The patient will have tachycardia, raised jugular venous pressure, and raised right ventricular end-diastolic pressure. Acute cor pulmonale results in systemic hypotension, intraventricular septal shift, and low cardiac output. The arterial pressure will swing with the ventilator (pulsus paradoxus) because of the low left ventricular end-diastolic volume; but because of the septal shift, the end-diastolic pressure in the left ventricle is raised, and this will aggravate the tendency to lung edema. Left ventricular ischemia occurs because of the low arterial pressure, and the risk of ischemic right and left ventricular failure is significant.[67] The resultant low cardiac output, especially in the presence of fever, results in low mixed venous hemoglobin oxygen saturation. This, together with the shunt or low V/Q lung units, aggravates arterial hypoxia, which cannot be corrected with mechanical ventilation or increased inspiratory fraction of oxygen. Angina has been reported, which is presumed to result from emboli in the coronary arteries or cor pulmonale.[68]

Acute renal failure occurs relatively seldom and it is thought that less neutral fat emboli enter the kidneys than other organs. In acute circulatory failure, as in cor pulmonale, the neurohumoral response of the body significantly decreases the renal blood flow, decreasing the number of renal emboli.[69]

We have observed acute and severe diffuse intravascular coagulation and clotting disorder (DIC) during surgery on long bones. This occurred without other prodromata of the FES. The patient started to bleed spontaneously, and special examinations showed raised D-dimers, low fibrinogen and platelets, raised international normalized ratio (INR) and partial thromboplastin time (PTT), and excessive levels of fibrinogen breakdown products. Some degree of clotting disorder is, in the author's experience, very common in patients with the fulminant form of FES.

▶ SPECIAL EXAMINATIONS

The FES is a syndrome and the diagnosis is therefore primarily a *clinical* one. Special examinations can help to confirm it and indicate the degree of organ dysfunction.

The arterial blood gases, more often than not, show a low PaO_2, and this is often described as a diagnostic criterion. However, there are many other reasons for a low PaO_2, and the absence of a reduction in arterial oxygen tension does not exclude the diagnosis.[13,60,61,70] Hypoxia is usually accompanied by a respiratory alkalosis, but once mechanical respiratory failure occurs, the $PaCO_2$ increases because of alveolar hypoventilation, which results from respiratory muscle fatigue.

X-rays of the lungs are nonspecific and lag behind the clinical syndrome. In the presence of FES, the typical x-ray findings are useful and help to confirm the diagnosis. The typical pattern is that of a "snowstorm."[71–73] Bilateral patchy infiltrates occur mainly in the perihilar and basilar areas, usually sparing the apices. This classic picture can be modified by pulmonary edema, which can occur because of the septal shift associated with acute pulmonary hypertension and the resultant raised left atrial pressure or primary (usually ischemic) left ventricular failure.

Dilatation of the right heart (acute cor pulmonale) can sometimes be seen.

Computed tomography (CT) scans of the lungs show the subsegmental perfusion defects and ventilation/perfusion scans confirm the ventilation/perfusion mismatch. Indeed, CT and V/Q scan findings can be diagnostic when radiologic findings are negative.[74]

A CT scan of the brain may show the absence of cortical sulci and compressed lateral ventricles due to brain edema. Hemorrhagic brain infarcts have been recorded.[58]

Acute cor pulmonale patterns and/or myocardial ischemia may be revealed by an electrocardiogram (ECG), depending on the severity of the FES and its effects on the pulmonary and coronary circulation.

Coagulation disorders, although not specific for FES, require quantification for effective treatment, since the INR, PTT, fibrinogen, D-dimer, fibrinogen breakdown products, and platelet count will identify either accelerated clotting and/or clot lysis.[75] Fibrinogen, an acute-phase protein that should be increased because of the trauma and stress, is often decreased or may be normal because of the activation of the coagulation system. As the patient improves, the fibrinogen usually increases (within 3 to 5 days).

A progressive fall in hemoglobin has been reported,[76] with a 30 percent decrease over 48 h in 75 percent of patients with FES. This is thought to be the result of intraalveolar hemorrhage.[5] However, this hypothesis is uncertain, since a similar aggressive decrease in hemoglobin does not regularly occur in patients with other causes of ARDS.

Cytologic examination of urine and sputum could be useful in confirming the clinical diagnosis. Sudan red staining will detect free fat globules in the macrophages. This procedure takes about 2 to 3 h, but its value is questionable, since it has given negative results in a group of patients with a positive diagnosis of FES.[77] This highlights the point that FES is primarily diagnosed clinically, and the value of confirmatory tests is subject to their specificity and sensitivity.

The cryostat test can be used to identify fat globules in blood. Peripheral blood is rapidly frozen and the clot sectioned for microscopic examination.[50,78] This test has a limitation in that most of the fat will be found in the veins draining the source area and not in the peripheral blood. Because the fat globules are trapped in the pulmonary capillaries, a blood sample from a pulmonary artery catheter in a wedged position would increase positive results for the test.[49,78] Bronchoalveolar lavage (BAL) may contain cells with fat droplets.[79] This was seen in 31 percent of patients with FES but in only 2 percent of those without FES.

Blood lipids do not correlate with the severity of FES.[10] Activated complement (C5a) increases in FES, but this increase is not specific for this syndrome.[77]

▶ DIAGNOSIS

The only pathognomic sign for fat embolism is the petechiae. Other clinical signs and symptoms and most of the readily available special examinations are nonspecific. However, FES is a syndrome, and the diagnosis rests on a constellation of findings. If all the signs and symptoms are present, the diagnosis is usually not difficult; but if some of them are lacking, the diagnosis may be uncertain.

For patients with lower body skeletal trauma, Gurd and Wilson[10] have compiled the following diagnostic criteria:

> One of the *major* manifestations; i.e., petechiae and pulmonary or cerebral involvement
> Four of the five *minor* manifestations; i.e., pyrexia, tachycardia, jaundice, renal or retinal changes, and fat macroglobulinemia

The approach of Gurd and Wilson is limited by the absence of arterial blood gas findings and other lung pathology descriptors. Lindeque[70] therefore expanded on the Gurd and Wilson approach by including the following:

PaO_2 < 60 mmHg (8 kPa) on a FiO_2 of 0.21

$PaCO_2$ > 55 mmHg (7.3 kPa) or a pH < 7.3

Respiratory rate >35 breaths per minute (even after sedation)

Increased work of breathing as manifest by dyspnea, use of accessory muscles, and a tachycardia

As can be seen from the above, the criteria for diagnosis are fairly nonspecific except for petechiae. Even the inclusion of the lung descriptors does not make criteria more specific, since the latter could signify lung injury without FES.[3]

Based on individual organ dysfunction, which can occur in FES, there is an extensive list of differential diagnoses that should be considered.[3] However, the key issues in diagnosing the syndrome remain a high degree of suspicion, petechiae and other organ involvement. The timing of the clinical signs may also assist in the diagnosis. For example, the development of petechiae soon after bone manipulation or injury would very likely suggest FES; on the other hand, if it occurs after 3 days and after stabilization of the fractures, the diagnosis is less likely (although not excluded).

The clinical picture may differ in patients under general anesthesia as well as muscle relaxation and mechanical ventilation, since the telltale cerebral and pulmonary signs can obviously not be observed in them.

▶ TREATMENT

There is no specific treatment for FES; the only option is to continue life support until the patient recovers.

The management of shock is very important in the outcome of FES. Data indicate that mortality was higher in patients with systolic blood pressure <100 mmHg and a heart rate in excess of 120 beats per minute.[53] Because this was a retrospective study and it is not ethical to do a trial in which hypovolemia and incipient shock is not treated, it is not known whether the increased mortality was due to FES and incipient shock or hypovolemia and shock alone. It was most likely the latter. Hemodynamic shock alone can cause acute lung injury, and this could well be aggravated by FES. In addition, hypovolemia in the presence of acute pulmonary hypertension could have a significant effect on the cardiac output.

Excessive fluid loading is detrimental to the thin-walled right ventricle in the presence of an acute increase in afterload. Intravascular fluid restoration should therefore be done cautiously and monitored closely. A central venous catheter is valuable, since it will give indirect guidance as to the volume status and also indicate whether the right ventricle is under strain. The latter can

be gauged from the central venous pressure response to a small fluid load, abnormal a or c waves, and the appearance of acute tricuspid incompetence. In severe FES, a pulmonary artery catheter is necessary to determine right ventricular failure. The latter is diagnosed by critically evaluating the right ventricular stroke work (RVSW) against the pulmonary artery pressure. If RVSW remains normal or does not increase as the pulmonary artery pressure increases, right ventricular failure is occurring. This implies that the function of the right ventricle changes from maximal efficiency to maximum stroke work. This is indicated by lower than expected RVSW in the presence of a raised pulmonary artery pressure. It is mandatory to support right ventricular function with inotropes and to maintain the systemic pressure so as to prevent hypotension and right ventricular ischemic failure. The choice of inotrope depends on the systemic blood pressure: if the perfusion pressure is still normal, dobutamine is useful. If the perfusion pressure is low, an alpha agonist is required and epinephrine or norepinephrine is a more appropriate choice. Pulmonary vasodilators are singularly unsuccessful, and since drugs like isoproterenol will cause systemic hypotension and increase the pulmonary shunt, they should not be used. The same can be said for all of the other generally available nonspecific vasodilators. The role of inhaled nitric oxide has not been established, and in view of the mechanical theory of obstruction, it is doubtful that it would be helpful.[80] If there is significant pulmonary vasoconstriction in addition to the capillary obstruction, then there would be reason to expect that nitric oxide could help in unloading the right ventricle (and improving arterial oxygenation).[81]

Studies indicate that albumin should be used for volume restoration because, in addition to this, it binds the FFA and thereby reduces the potential for lung injury.[82,83] Excessive fluid will, as in all cases of acute lung injury (ALI), increase the amount of interstitial fluid in the lungs and could worsen the venous admixture or pulmonary shunt.

Ventilatory support is often mandatory to restore arterial oxygenation. The decision to support oxygenation and ventilation rests on known criteria. These maneuvers include additional inspired oxygen, noninvasive and invasive ventilation. Given that the basic pulmonary pathology is that of low ventilation/perfusion units resulting from a reduction in the functional residual capacity, the judicious application of positive end-expiratory pressure with or without lung recruitment is valuable. The management of mechanical ventilation and alveolar pressure is guided by the current knowledge of volume trauma, and protective ventilatory strategies should be employed when dealing with these patients.[84,85]

Of all the causes for acute lung injury, fat embolism is one of the more benign etiologies. The acute ventilatory difficulty usually lasts for approximately 3 days, after which the patient often improves and can be weaned from ventilatory support. Unfortunately associated problems—such as acute renal failure, right ventricular failure, or pulmonary infection—can intervene and will obviously modify the course of the disease.

Although cardiac and pulmonary fat embolectomy has been performed, it is of little value, since the emboli are in the capillaries.[86]

High doses of corticosteroids have not been shown to be of value in ALI.[87] Because FES is often an isolated problem and generally has a less malignant course than, for instance, ALI caused by sepsis, it has nevertheless been suggested that steroids, given early in the course of the disease, could be beneficial.[76,88–91]

Aprotinin has been administered because it decreases platelet aggregation and the release of serotonin. A retrospective study demonstrated an increased recovery and decreased mortality when aprotinin was used in FES.[10] Another study confirmed that aprotinin will lessen the reduction in platelet count but does not prevent the pulmonary effects of FES.[51]

For the prevention and treatment of diffuse intravascular clotting disorder, heparin should be used. For prevention 300 U of unfractionated heparin per hour administered intravenously was successful in preventing thrombin-induced DIC in baboons.[92] For treatment of established DIC, it is mandatory to know whether the DIC is in the accelerated clotting phase, clot-lysis phase, or both. This can be achieved by means of a complete coagulation scan. Heparin dosage can then be titrated against the pathology, and once the accelerated clotting is controlled, clotting factors can be given to replace those used in the process.

There is a theoretical argument that heparin may be detrimental because it raises the FFA significantly. However, the need to prevent or treat DIC in these patients, outweighs this possible negative effect, and the author elects to use heparin as described.

▶ PREVENTION

Early stabilization of fractures is important in an effort to prevent the FES; this will reduce its incidence and decrease the incidence of septic and pulmonary complications (see Chap. 16).[7,13,93–97]

Intraoperative drilling of a venting hole before inserting a prosthesis reduces the intramedullary pressure but does not prevent the FES in every patient.

The use of a tourniquet has been proposed as a method of preventing the fat from reaching the systemic circulation. However, once the tourniquet is released, the fat will still reach the systemic circulation. In addition, the accumulated fat could cause severe FES; this method is therefore not recommended.[28,35]

The only drug that seems to have some (still debatable) value is corticosteroid. There is great variation in the suggested dose, from 9 mg/kg over 2 days to 90 mg/kg over 4 days.[77,89]

▶ PROGNOSIS

The general mortality rate associated with FES is 10 to 20 percent.[6,69,98] However, it appears that early fixation of fractures reduces the mortality to less than 10 percent (see Chap. 16).[9]

There are, however, publications suggesting higher and lower mortalities. Whereas Burgher[99] reported a mortality of 33 percent, Guenter[100] reported no deaths in 54 patients.

Death is more often than not the result of respiratory insufficiency, but it is difficult to collect accurate data, since there may be many intervening problems that can be fatal.

Permanent cerebral injury can occur, especially in young patients with the fulminant variant of the disease.

REFERENCES

1. Sevitt S. The significance and pathology of fat embolism. *Ann Clin Res* 9:173, 1977.
2. Warthin AS. Traumatic lipemia and fatty embolism. *Int Clin* 4:171, 1913.
3. Capan LM, Miller SM, Patel KP. Fat embolism. *Anesthesiol Clin North Am* 11:25, 1993.
4. Lehman EP, Moore RM. Fat embolism: Including experimental production without trauma. *Arch Surg* 14:621, 1927.
5. Peltier LF. Fat embolism III. The toxic properties of neutral fat and free fatty acids. *Surgery* 40:665, 1956.
6. Peltier LF. Fat embolism syndrome: A current concept. *Clin Orthop* 241:241, 1969.
7. Lozman J, Deno C, Feustel PJ, et al. Pulmonary and cardiovascular consequences of immediate fixation or conservative management of long bone fractures. *Arch Surg* 121:992, 1986.
8. Duis HJT, Nijsten MW, Klasen JH, et al. Fat embolism in patients with an isolated fracture of the femoral shaft. *J Trauma* 28:383, 1988.
9. Fabian TC, Hoots AV, Stanford DS, et al. Fat embolism syndrome: Prospective evaluation in 92 fracture patients. *Crit Care Med* 18:42, 1990.
10. Gurd AR, Wilson RI. The fat embolism syndrome. *J Bone Joint Surg* 56(B):408, 1974.
11. De Vries J, Oosterhuis JW, Oldhoff J. Bone marrow embolism following cryosurgery of bone. An experimental study. *J Surg Res* 46:200, 1989.
12. Moore P, James O, Saltos N. Fat embolism syndrome. Incidence, significance and early features. *Austr NZ J Surg* 51:546, 1981.
13. Riska EB, Myllynen P. Fat embolism in patients with multiple injuries. *J Trauma* 22:891, 1982.

14. Cotev S, Rosenmann E, Eyal Z. The role of hypovolemic stress in the production of fat embolism in rabbits. Morphologic alterations in the lung. *Chest* 69:523, 1976.

15. Orlowski JP, Julius CJ, Petras RE, et al. The safety of intraosseous infusions. Risk of fat and bone marrow emboli to the lungs. *Ann Emerg Med* 18:1062, 1989.

16. Manning JB, Bach AW, Herman CM, et al. Fat release after femur nailing in the dog. *J Trauma* 23:322, 1983.

17. Kallos T, Enis JE, Gollan F, et al. Intramedullary pressure and pulmonary embolism of femoral medullary content in dogs during insertion of bone cement and prosthesis. *J Bone Joint Surg* 56(A):1363, 1974.

18. Byrick RJ, Forbes D, Waddel JP. A monitored cardiovascular collapse during cemented total knee replacement. *Anesthesiology* 65:213–216, 1986.

19. Cailloutte JT, Anzel SH. Fat embolism syndrome following the intramedullary alignment guide in total knee arthroplasty. *Clin Orthop* 251:199, 1990.

20. Mokkhavesa S, Shim SS, Patterson FP. Fat embolism: Clinical and experimental studies with emphasis on therapeutic aspects. *J Trauma* 9:39, 1969.

21. Emson HE. Fat embolism in 100 patients dying after injury. *J Clin Pathol* 11:28, 1958.

22. Morton P, Kendall MJ. Fat embolism: Its production and source of fate. *Can J Surg* 8:214, 1965.

23. Hausberger FX, Whitenack SH. Effect of pressure on intravasation of fate from the bone marrow cavity. *Surg Gynecol Obstet* 134:931, 1972.

24. Sherr S, Gertner SB. Production and recovery of pulmonary fat emboli in dogs. *Exp Mol Pathol* 21:63, 1974.

25. Allardyce DB, Meek RN, Woodruff B, et al. Increasing our knowledge of the pathogenesis of the fat embolism: A prospective study of 43 patients with fractured femoral shafts. *J Trauma* 14:955, 1974.

26. Herndon JH, Bechtol CO, Crickenberger DP. Fat embolism during total hip replacement: A prospective study. *J Bone Joint Surg* 56(7):1350, 1974.

27. Collins JA, Gordon WC, Hudson TL, et al. Inapparent hypoxemia in casualties with wounded limbs: Pulmonary fat embolism? *Ann Surg* 167:511, 1968.

28. Hagley SR. The fulminant fat embolism syndrome. *Anaesth Intens Care* 11:167, 1983.

29. Hagley SR. The fulminant fat embolism syndrome. *Anaesth Intens Care* 11:162, 1983.

30. Weber KT, Janicki JS, Shroff SG, et al. The right ventricle: Physiology and pathophysiologic considerations. *Crit Care Med* 11:323, 1983.

31. Fourie P, Coetzee A, Bolliger CT. Pulmonary artery compliance: Its role in right ventricular-arterial coupling. *Cardiovasc Res* 26:839, 1992.

32. Nijlsten MW, Hamer JP, Ten Huis HJ, et al. Fat embolism in patients with patent foramen ovale. *Lancet* 1:1271, 1989.

33. Levy D. The fat embolism syndrome. *Clin Orthop* 261:281, 1990.

34. Lequire VS, Sharpiro JL, Lequire CB, et al. A study of the pathogenesis of the fat embolism based on human necropsy material and animal experiments. *Am J Pathol* 35:999, 1959.

35. Peltier LF. Fat embolism: The prophylactic value of a tourniquet. *J Bone Joint Surg* 38(A):835, 1956.

36. Peltier LF: The diagnosis of fat embolism. *Surg Gynecol Obstet* 121:371, 1965.

37. Parker FB, Wax SD, Kutsajima K, et al. Hemodynamic and pathological findings in experimental fat embolism. *Arch Surg* 108:70, 1974.

38. Riseborough EJ, Herndon JH. Alterations in pulmonary function, coalgulation and fat embolism in patients with fractures of the lower limbs. *Clin Orthop* 115:248, 1976.

39. Warner WA. Release of fatty acids following trauma. *J Trauma* 9:692, 1969.

40. MacNamara JJ, Molot M, Dunn R, et al. Lipid metabolism after trauma. Role in the pathogenesis of fat embolism. *J Thorac Cardiovasc Surg* 63:968, 1972.

41. Bergentz SE. Fat embolism. *Prog Surg* 175:128, 1968.

42. Moylan JA, Birnbaum M, Katz A, et al. Fat emboli syndrome. *J Trauma* 16:341, 1976.

43. Moylan JA, Evenson MA. Diagnosis and treatment of fat embolism. *Annu Rev Med* 28:85, 1977.

44. Saldeen T. Intravascular coalgulation in the lungs in experimental fat embolism. *Acta Chir Scand* 135:653, 1969.

45. Keith RG, Mahoney LJ, Garvey MB. Disseminated intravascular coalgulation: An important feature in the fat embolism syndrome. *Can Med Assoc J* 105:634, 1971.

46. Rammer L, Saldeen T. Inhibition of fibrinolysis in posttraumatic death. *Thromb Hemost* 24:68, 1970.

47. Rennie AM, Ogston D, Cooke RJ, et al. The fibrinolytic system after trauma and in patients with fat embolism. *J Bone Joint Surg* 56(B):421, 1974.

48. McCarthey B, Mammen E, LeBlanc LP, et al. Subclinical fat embolism: A prospective study of 50 patients with extremity fractures. *J Trauma* 13:9, 1973.

49. Hutchins PM, Macnicol MF. Pulmonary insufficiency after long bone fractures: Absence of circulating fat or significant immunodepression. *J Bone Joint Surg* 67(B):835, 1985.

50. Chan KM, Tham KT, Chow YN, et al. Post-traumatic fat embolism: Its clinical and subclinical presentation. *J Trauma* 24:45, 1984.

51. Sari A, Micauchi Y, Yamashita S, et al. The magnitude of hypoxia in elderly patients with fractures of the femur neck. *Anesth Analg* 65:892, 1986.

52. Tachakra SS, Sevitt S. Hypoxia after fractures. *J Bone Joint Surg* 57(B):197, 1975.

53. Coetzee A, Swanevelder J, Vd Spuy G, et al. Gas exhange indices, how valid are they? *S Afr Med J* 85(Crit Care Suppl):1227, 1995.

54. Heinreich H, Kremer P, Winter H, et al. Transesphageal two-dimensional echocardiography during total hip replacement. *Anaesthetist* 34:118, 1985.

55. Pazell JA, Peltier LF. Experience with sixty three patients with fat embolism. *Surg Gynecol Obstet* 135:77, 1972.

56. Kaplan RP, Grant JN, Kaufman AJ. Dermatologic features of the fat embolism syndrome. *Cutis* 38:52, 1986.

57. Jacobson DM, Terrance CF, Reinmuth OM. The neurological manifestations of fat embolism. *Neurology* 36:847, 1986.

58. Meek RI, Fitzpatrick GJ, Phelan DM. Cerebral edema and the fat embolism syndrome. *Int Care Med* 13:291, 1987.

59. Findlay JE, DeMajo W. Cerebral fat embolism. *Can Med Assoc J* 131:755, 1984.

60. Bolesta MJ. Fat embolism syndrome without adult respiratory distress syndrome. *NC Med J* 47:257, 1986.

61. Font MO, Nadal P, Betran A. Fat embolism syndrome with no evidence of pulmonary involvement [letter]. *Crit Care Med* 17:108, 1989.

62. Thomas JE, Ayyar DR. Systemic fat embolism: A diagnostic profile of 24 patients. *Arch Neurol* 26:517, 1972.

63. Chuang EL, Miller FS, Kalina RE. Retinal lesions following long bone fractures. *Ophthalmology* 92:370, 1985.

64. Roden D, Fitzpatrick G, O'Donoghue H, et al. Purtscher's retinopathy and fat embolism. *Br J Ophthalmol* 73:677, 1989.

65. Van Miert M, Thornington RE, Van Velzen D. Cardiac arrest after massive acute fat embolism. *Br J Med* 303:396, 1991.

66. Coetzee A, Rousseau H, Lahner D. Acute pulmonary hypertension and right ventricular failure in adult respiratory distress syndrome. *S Afr Med J* 86(Cardiovasc Suppl):C148, 1996.

67. Vlahakes GJ, Turley K, Hoffman JE. The pathophysiology of failure in acute right ventricular hypertension: Hemodynamic and clinical observations. *Circulation* 63:87, 1981.

68. Schwartz DA, Finkelstein SD, Lumb GD. Fat embolism and the cardiac conduction system associated with sudden death. *Hum Pathol* 19:116, 1998.

69. Roger JA, Stirt JA. Fat embolism syndrome. *Semin Anesth* 6:176, 1987.

70. Lindeque BG, Schoeman HS, Dommisse GF, et al. Fat embolism and the fat embolism syndrome: A double blind therapeutic study. *J Bone Joint Surg* 69(B):128, 1987.

71. Horne RH, Horne JH. Fat embolism prophylaxis. *Arch Intern Med* 133:288, 1974.

72. Greenberg HB. Roentgenographic signs of post-traumatic fat embolism (editorial). *JAMA* 204:540, 1968.

73. Maruyama Y, Little JB. Roentgen manifestations of traumatic pulmonary fat embolism. *Radiology* 79:945, 1962.

74. Park HM, Ducret RP, Brindley DC. Pulmonary imaging in fat embolism syndrome. *Clin Nucl Med* 11:521, 1986.

75. Gossling HR, Pelligrini VD. Fat embolism syndrome: Review of the pathophysiology and physiological basis of treatment. *Clin Orthop* 165:68, 1982.

76. Rokkanen P, Lahndensuu M, Kataja J, et al. The syndrome of fat embolism: Analysis of thirty consecutive cases compared to trauma patients with similar injuries. *J Trauma* 10:299, 1970.

77. Schonfeld SA, Ploysongsang Y, Dilisio R, et al. Fat embolism prophylaxis with corticosteroids: A prospective study in high risk patients. *Ann Intern Med* 99:438, 1983.

78. Masson RG, Ruggieri J. Pulmonary microvascular cytology: A new diagnostic application of the pulmonary artery catheter. *Chest* 88:908, 1985.

79. Chastre J, Fagon J, Soler P, et al. Bronchoalveolar lavage for rapid diagnosis of the fat embolism syndrome in trauma patients. *Ann Intern Med* 113:583, 1990.

80. Luyt S, Coetzee A, Lahner D, et al. Nitric oxide has little effect on the acute pulmonary hypertension and right ventricular function during acute respiratory distress syndrome. *S Afr Med J* 87:639, 1997.

81. Frostell CG, Blomqvist H, Hedenstierna G, et al. Inhaled nitric oxide selectively reverses human hypoxic pulmonary vasoconstriction without causing systemic vasodilation. *Anesthesiology* 78:427, 1993.

82. Nixon JR, Brock-Utne JG. Free fatty acids and arterial oxygen changes following major injury: A correlation between hypoxia and increase in free fatty acid levels. *J Trauma* 18:23, 1978.

83. Liljedahl SO, Westermark L. Aetiology and treatment of fat embolism: Report of five cases. *Acta Anaesthesiol Scand* 11:177, 1967.

84. Amato MB, Barbas CS, Medeiros D, et al. Effect of a protective ventilation strategy on mortality in the acute respiratory distress syndrome. *N Engl J Med* 338:447, 1998.

85. Acute Respiratory Distress Syndrome Network: Ventilation with lower tidal volumes as compared with traditional tidal volumes for acute lung injury and the acute respiratory distress syndrome. *N Engl J Med* 342:1301, 2000.

86. Nelson CS: Cardiac and pulmonary fat embolectomy. *Thorax* 29:134, 1974.

87. Bernard GR, Luce JM, Sprung C, et al. High dose corticosteroids in patients with the adult respiratory distress syndrome. *N Engl J Med* 317:1565, 1987.

88. Fischer JE, Turner RH, Herndon JH, et al. Massive steroid therapy in severe fat embolism. *Surg Gynecol Obstet* 132:667, 1971.

89. Kallenbach J, Lewis M, Zaltzman M, et al. Low dose corticosteroid prophylaxis against fat embolism. *J Trauma* 27:1173, 1987.

90. Kreis WR, Lindenauer SM, Dent TL. Corticosteroids in experimental fat embolism. *J Surg Res* 14:238, 1973.

91. Shier MR, Wilson RF, James RE, et al. Fat embolism prophylaxis. A study of four treatment modalities. *J Trauma* 17:621, 1977.

92. Du Toit H, Coetzee A, Charlton D. Heparin treatment in thrombin induced disseminated intravascular coagulation in the baboon. *Crit Care Med* 19:1195, 1991.

93. Svenningsen S, Nesse O, Finsen V, et al. Prevention of fat embolism syndrome in patients with femoral fractures. Immediate or delayed operative fixation? *Ann Chir Gynecol* 76:163, 1987.

94. Talucci RC, Manning J, Lampard S, et al. Early intramedullary nailing of femoral shaft fractures: A cause of fat embolism syndrome. *Am J Surg* 146:107, 1983.

95. Seibel R, LaDuca J, Hassett JM, et al. Blunt multiple trauma (ISs36), femur traction and pulmonary failure: Septic state. *Ann Surg* 202:283, 1985.

96. LaDuca JN, Bone LL, Seibel RW, et al. Primary open reduction and fixation of open fractures. *J Trauma* 20:580, 1980.

97. Johnson KD, Cadambi CF, Reinmuth OM. The neurologic manifestations of fat embolism. *Neurology* 25:375, 1985.

98. Malik AB. Pulmonary microembolism. *Physiol Rev* 63:1114, 1983.

99. Burgher LW, Dines DE, Linscheid RL, et al. Fat embolism and the adult respiratory distress syndrome. *Anesth Analg* 53:664, 1974.

100. Guenter CA, Braun TE. Fat embolism syndrome: Changing prognosis. *Chest* 79:143, 1981.

CHAPTER 6

The Dysmorphic Child and Other Pediatric Issues

Adrian T. Bösenberg

▶ INTRODUCTION

It is not uncommon for a child with bone or joint disorders of a genetic dysmorphic syndrome or a generalized metabolic disorder to require orthopaedic surgery. Many of these disorders are rare, and anesthetic practice in these cases has depended on evidence that is often based on anecdotal reports; small, uncontrolled retrospective studies usually over a prolonged period; or pathophysiologic reasoning.

Many disorders may have a progressive direct or indirect effect on the airway and/or on cardiopulmonary, neuromuscular, hepatic, or renal function. The surgical procedure may complicate the pathophysiology and compound the problem. In addition, patient positioning, temperature control, prolonged anesthesia and tourniquet time, and fluid management in association with significant blood loss all need to be considered.

The aim of this chapter is not to provide an exhaustive list of hereditary and metabolic disorders but rather to offer a general guide to orthopaedic anesthesia in dysmorphic children by using a few specific examples illustrating the problems an anesthesiologist may encounter in managing a dysmorphic child. The examples range from abnormalities of sensory input through the motor cortex to effector end organs, muscles, joints, and bone. Appropriate knowledge of any disease process is essential before any plan of anesthesia can be formulated. The reader is therefore encouraged to make use of relevant texts[1,2] or to visit some of the many helpful websites to research a specific disorder.[3,4]

▶ ANESTHETIC CONSIDERATIONS IN GENERAL

The basic principles of anesthesia should be applied to any dysmorphic child presenting for surgery. A thorough preoperative assessment is vital and an anesthetic plan that includes the postoperative management should be formulated. Many procedures can be performed as day-stay cases, but each affected child should be evaluated individually. For some procedures, postoperative intensive care may be needed and should be arranged accordingly.

Basic monitoring guidelines must be adhered to. Capnography and temperature monitoring are particularly important in orthopaedic anesthesia. Cool laminar-flow operating rooms can cause rapid body cooling unless adequate provision is made for maintaining the temperature of an exposed infant or child. Conversely, hyperthermia may be detected in a variety of orthopaedic disorders. Malignant hyperthermia (MH) is life-threatening and requires immediate management while ongoing investigations are done to confirm or exclude the diagnosis. Invasive monitoring should be used when indicated.

Pain should be managed using all available modalities if necessary. The choice and management of analgesia may be dictated by hospital protocol and the facilities available. Continuous opiate infusions or continuous neuraxial or peripheral nerve blockade may necessitate a high level of care. The combination of single-injection nerve blocks and subsequent immobilization in casts generally requires very little additional analgesia, whereas major surgery (hip, spine) may require patient- or nurse-controlled analgesia or continuous opiate or local anesthetic infusions. The use of these modalities is expensive in terms of human resources and time. Patients of an appropriate age and staff require ongoing education, and the necessary facilities must be provided.

Some of the more important aspects to be addressed in pediatric orthopaedic anesthesia are the risk of regurgitation, the tourniquet time, airway management, and the associated medical conditions that may be present.

Aspiration Risk

Preoperative fasting for elective procedures on healthy children should be based on the recommendations of the American Society of Anesthesiologists (ASA),[5] which advocate a minimum fast of 2 h after the ingestion of clear fluids, 4 h after breast milk, and 6 h after the ingestion of infant formula, nonhuman milk, and solids. A short fast clearly has many advantages. These include compliance by the patient and parent as well as comfort and a reduction in the incidence of hypoglycemia, dehydration, and metabolic acidosis (ketosis), particularly in infants and toddlers.

Despite the guidelines for fasting in healthy children, studies have shown that up to 76 percent of children fulfill the risk criteria of a gastric pH of <2.5 and a residual gastric volume of greater than 0.4 mL/kg.[6] Longer fasting does not reduce this percentage. Either the risk factors are incorrect and not applicable to children or children are at lower risk of aspiration after regurgitation. The latter seems to be the case, since large retrospective[7] and prospective studies[8,9] have shown that the incidence of clinically significant aspiration is extremely low, and when aspiration does occur, the consequences are less serious than in adults.[8]

Although it is generally accepted that these guidelines for fasting are applicable to all children, dysmorphic or syndromic children have not been studied. Fasting prescriptions should therefore take into account the patient's age, gastric emptying time, and underlying pathology as well as the risk of reflux.

Another consideration in pediatric orthopaedic anesthesia is that many children need surgery for injuries. Trauma and pain delay gastric emptying, children tend to swallow air when crying, and opiate analgesia further delays gastric emptying. The urgency of the surgery must also be taken into account. Bleeding, arterial spasm, or a threatened limb may warrant urgent surgery. The residual gastric volume is in part related to the time between the last food intake, the type of food ingested, and the time of injury. Those who had eaten 4 h before the injury had similar residual gastric volumes as healthy children who had undergone a standard fast.[10] Evidence suggests that gastric fluid volume is greater in children when they are operated on within 4 h of admission than when surgery

is delayed for 4 h or more after admission. In the latter cases, the residual gastric volumes are reduced to the same volumes as in fasted children who present for elective surgery.[11] Other factors that need to be addressed include the extent of the injury, associated pathology, and drugs administered. Risks are never eliminated and all precautions to prevent aspiration should be instituted.

Tourniquet

A tourniquet is applied to minimize blood loss and to improve surgical visual exposure. A pressure-controlled tourniquet is conventionally inflated to 100 mmHg above systolic blood pressure.[12] Such a device is far more accurate than an elastic Esmarch bandage.[12]

Systemic effects of tourniquets are related to their inflation and deflation, whereas the local effects and complications are caused by direct pressure on the underlying tissues or ischemia in tissues distal to the tourniquet. The duration of tourniquet time should be as short as possible but limited to 90 to 120 min in healthy children; in the event of more prolonged surgery, the tourniquet should be deflated for at least 10 min, to allow reperfusion of tissue beneath and distal to the tourniquet, before reinflating. Although studies have not been performed on children, it is unlikely that shorter reperfusion times would be better tolerated.[13]

Hemodynamic changes associated with inflation or deflation are proportional to the blood volume of the exsanguinated limb(s). These changes are minimal in healthy children but may not be tolerated by those with poor cardiac function or sepsis.

Metabolic disturbance occurring on deflation and its severity is related to the duration of tourniquet time. A mild lactic acidosis develops during inflation and increases transiently on release. It is manifest as a transient increase in end-tidal CO_2, a minor rise in serum K^+, and a fall in pH.[14] Generally these metabolic changes are well tolerated and without serious consequence in healthy children. But the greatest decrease in pH occurs with simultaneous deflation of bilateral tourniquets, and cardiac arrest has been reported. Simultaneous deflation should therefore be avoided.[14] It may also cause a significant rise in intracranial pressure in children with head injuries. The potential secondary brain damage can be prevented by providing hyperventilation at the time of deflation.[15]

Tourniquets are also associated with temperature changes in children. Tourniquet times extending beyond 75 min, particularly in the case of bilateral tourniquets, are associated with an exponential rise in core temperature,[16,17] which may be confused with MH. These temperature changes may be obtunded by sympathetic blockade.[18]

Tourniquet deflation may be associated with a fall in temperature proportional to the size of the occluded limb. This decrease is caused by cooling of the blood when it perfuses the hypothermic limb.[19]

Difficult Airway

The anatomy of the normal child's airway, particularly that of a neonate or infant, can make intubation difficult. Congenital anomalies or chromosomal defects may further compound the problem by causing unique anatomic and pathophysiologic derangements of the upper airway.

Unlike the case in adults, classifications such as Mallampati have not been devised to assess or predict which children may be difficult to intubate. An understanding of embryologic development of the upper airway, head, and neck will help the anesthesiologist to recognize a difficult airway. For example, the ear is derived from the same branchial arches as the mandible and maxilla; anomalies of the ear may therefore indicate an airway abnormality. In addition, airway anomalies are often associated with other defects affecting the central nervous system or cardiorespiratory systems. An awareness of these defects may influence the management and outcome of intubation. Other anomalies, such as muscle disorders, may influence the choice of drug used to facilitate intubation.

The majority of airway anomalies can be managed by applying the "difficult airway" algorithm and using simple maneuvers to facilitate laryngoscopic intubation. When this is not possible, the anesthesiologist may have to use alternative techniques to establish an airway or to intubate the child successfully. The best technique may not be one that requires the most sophisticated equipment. Most modern anesthesiologists would consider fiberoptic-assisted intubation as first-line of management, but this is not always possible or even helpful. Furthermore, in many institutions, fiberoptic equipment of appropriate size is not always available.

When a difficult intubation is anticipated or occurs unexpectedly, consider whether intubation is necessary or whether alternative methods [Laryngeal Mask Airway (LMA), mask, regional anesthesia alone] can suffice. The choice of airway should therefore depend on the child's underlying disorder, the experience of the anesthesiologist, the availability of equipment, intraoperative access to the patient's airway, the position of the patient, the duration of surgery, and expected intraoperative blood loss.

If intubation is difficult but absolutely necessary or the only option, a planned approach is essential. Innovation and improvisation may then be necessary, particularly outside the controlled environment of the operating theater.

Even in the operating room, an unplanned attempt may lead to a disaster. In applying an institutional difficult-airway algorithm, all available options to minimize the risk of a catastrophic loss of airway control should be considered. Should any of the planned steps fail, flexibility within a formulated plan is the key to success. The anesthesiologist should never be too proud to seek advice or assistance.

Every anesthesiologist should be aware of as many strategies for endotracheal intubation as possible and should develop the expertise to use these strategies in order to maintain airway patency at all times. Some of the specific problems that need to be addressed in dysmorphic children include the risk of aspiration, the stability of the cervical spine, cardiopulmonary reserve, and hematologic factors.[20]

Cervical Instability

Cervical instability may contribute to the "difficult airway," and in such instances uncontrolled attempts at endotracheal intubation may have a disastrous outcome. The cervical vertebrae and base of the skull have common embryologic origins with the upper airway and cardiovascular system. Airway abnormalities associated with cardiovascular defects are not uncommon.

Various craniovertebral anomalies may contribute to instability of the cervical spine. These include stenosis of the foramen magnum, occipitalization of C1 (axis), odontoid hypoplasia, atlantoaxial instability, and fusion of cervical vertebrae. Ligamentous laxity, infiltration, or even infection may worsen the situation.

Craniovertebral abnormalities may occur with or without subtle or overt signs of spinal cord compression. Subtle signs without physical neurologic signs include a history of cyanosis after crying or feeding, respiratory difficulties, poor head control, fatigue, and reduced effort tolerance. Muscle weakness of the upper and lower extremities is a sign of central cord compression and myelopathy.

Fusion of the cervical vertebrae may also place the child at significant risk and is the hallmark of Klippel-Feil syndrome (Fig. 6-1A to C). Two configurations (1) fusion of the occiput with C1 in combination with a long fused segment from C2-3 extending distally or (2) a single open interspace between two long segments are particularly dangerous.

Manipulation of the cervical spine during anesthesia, particularly intubation with the aid of muscle relaxants, may lead to massive pyramidal tract signs. Cervical spine radiography can provide useful information but does not necessarily exclude pathology. Computed tomography or magnetic resonance imaging may be necessary to exclude cord compression in some instances.

Management of an unstable but asymptomatic cervical spine is fraught with danger. The child should be carefully positioned and intubation must be done with great care. The head should be kept in a neutral position and flexion or extension minimized. If necessary, a fiberoptic device should be used to minimize manipulation of the neck

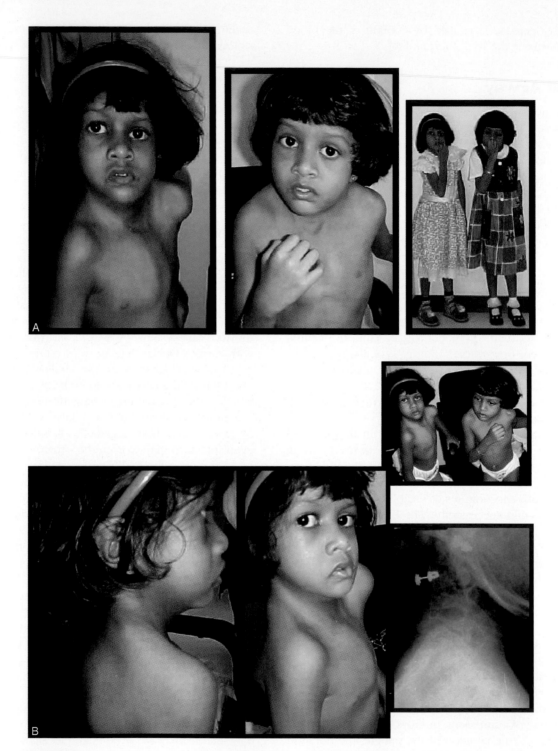

Figure 6-1. A. Twin sisters with Klippel-Feil syndrome. B. These twin girls had fused cervical vertebra, severely restricting neck movement. A Sprengel shoulder is obvious in one. C. Chest radiograph shows additional absent ribs and cardiac anomaly.

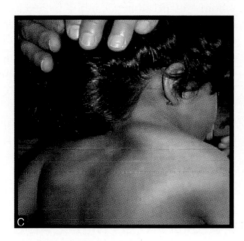

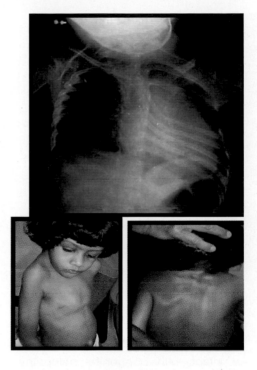

Figure 6-1. (*Continued*)

and airway. The orthopaedic surgeon should help to control neck movement while the anesthesiologist's focus is on the airway.

Malignant Hyperthermia

Susceptibility to MH is an inherited disorder of calcium metabolism within skeletal muscle. In this disorder, a rapid sustained increase in myoplasmic calcium can be triggered by the potent inhalational agents (halothane, enflurane, isoflurane, sevoflurane, and desflurane, but not xenon) and the depolarizing muscle relaxant suc-cinylcholine.[21–24] The abnormality in the skeletal muscle is at the ryanodine receptor (RyR1). This receptor makes calcium stored in the sarcoplasmic reticulum available for electromechanical coupling and contraction.[21] Mutations in the amino acid sequence of this channel receptor can lead to dysfunction of calcium regulation and thus can cause a potentially fatal reaction when triggered, usually by general anesthesia but also by fever or stress.

The predisposition to MH is a dominantly inherited disorder of *RyR1* gene with variable penetrance. The gene is situated on chromosome 19 (19q13.1 locus), although sporadic mutations around the *RyR1* gene locus may occur.[22] The incidence of MH in children is on the order of 1:15,000 cases of general anesthesia. However, the incidence is probably higher in orthopaedic surgery, since many children with underlying myopathies present for orthopaedic procedures.

A predisposition to MH is found in children with central core disease, King-Denborough syndrome (Fig. 6-2), and congenital myopathy (Fig. 6-3). More information is needed about possible associations between the phenotypic expression and the genotype.[24] It is debatable

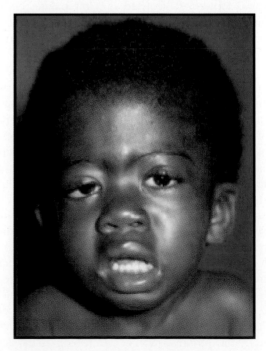

Figure 6-2. King-Denborough syndrome. This disorder has been linked with malignant hyperthermia.

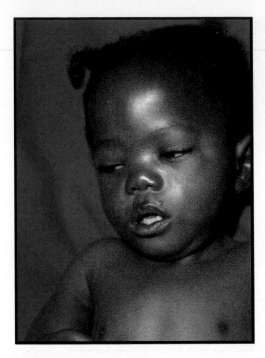

Figure 6-3. An infant with congenital myopathy showing the typical myopathic facies: expressionless, with a fish-like mouth. She previously had a cleft palate repair. She developed malignant hyperthermia, which responded to dantrolene.

whether various musculoskeletal abnormalities (scoliosis, hernias, cryptorchidism, strabismus, ptosis)[23] are associated with MH or merely indicate an underlying muscle weakness. However the triad of cleft palate, clubfoot, and myopathic facies (expressionlessness and fish mouth) (Fig. 6-3) is highly suspicious in this author's experience.[25]

The laboratory diagnosis of MH is at present cumbersome, expensive, and controversial. However, when properly conducted, the caffeine-halothane contracture test can predict susceptibility to MH with an acceptable sensitivity and specificity.[24] Chromosomal studies are expensive and have not fulfilled their early anticipated promise. To date multiple mutations at multiple gene loci have been identified (chromosomes 19, 17, 7, 3, 1, and 5) in individuals susceptible to MH.

An MH crisis is manifest by metabolic and respiratory acidosis, tachycardia, cardiac arrhythmias, skeletal muscle rigidity, hyperthermia (which may occur only late), and rhabdomyolysis.[21–24] The clinical course is highly variable from mild to fulminant. If an episode is survived, creatine kinase (CK) levels and muscle swelling and edema may take 2 weeks to resolve.[23]

Early diagnosis is essential, and the crisis can be averted by the administration of dantrolene (initial dose of 2 to 3 mg/kg), in addition to cooling and correction of life-threatening hyperkalemia and acid-base disturbances.

Supportive measures should include ventilatory support, since dantrolene per se can cause weakness and increase the weakness of the underlying muscle disorder. Recrudescence occurs in approximately 10 percent of cases, usually between 4 and 8 h later, although it may occur up to 36 h later.

In children who are susceptible to MH and those in whom the possibility cannot be excluded—an undiagnosed myopathy, for example—a "trigger free" anesthetic should be given. Propofol infusions combined with regional anesthesia are suitable for most orthopaedic procedures. Remifentanil may be a useful adjuvant. Practically, this may be more challenging than it seems, since venous access can be particularly difficult in susceptible individuals. Suitable sedation (midazolam, rectal thiopentone or methohexitone, nitrous oxide inhalation) and topical local anesthetic agents [eutectic mixture of local anesthetic (EMLA), amethocaine] should facilitate intravenous access with the least stress.

▶ ASSOCIATED MEDICAL CONDITIONS

Pulmonary

A variety of pulmonary problems may contribute to the difficulty of administering anesthesia. These problems may form part of a particular syndrome or disorder or may occur as a consequence of an underlying weakness or metabolic problem. Tracheomalacia, bronchomalacia, chest wall deformities, kyphoscoliosis, and restrictive lung disease may be part of a progressive illness or may occur in isolation. Rarely, pulmonary hypoplasia may form part of the syndrome. Aspiration pneumonia is commonly associated with cerebral palsy and neuromuscular disorders. Pulmonary hypertension and cor pulmonale may be a complication of chronic lung disease.

Cardiac

Structural cardiac defects, atrial and ventricular septal defects (ASDs and VSDs), patent ductus arteriosus, and even more complex cardiac anomalies may be seen in a variety of congenital syndromes and disorders. These must be assessed preoperatively and prophylactic antibiotic cover given as indicated. Cardiomyopathy may occur as a result of abnormal myocytes, coronary insufficiency, or deposits in the myocardium. Pulmonary hypertension and cor pulmonale may occur secondary to kyphoscoliosis, restrictive lung disease, or even obesity associated with obstructive sleep apnea.

Renal

Renal disease may be the cause of the underlying orthopaedic problem or may worsen it. Rickets (Fig. 6-4) may be due to renal tubular insufficiency (excess phosphate

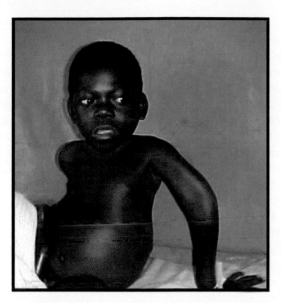

Figure 6-4. Rickets. The typical curved bones and "rickety rosary" are visible in this child with rickets, who had undergone corrective osteotomies of both tibias.

or loss of calcium), renal tubular acidosis, chronic renal failure, and hypophosphatemia.

Hematologic

Anemia may be present in a variety of disorders. Platelet dysfunction (impaired aggregation, defective release of platelet factor III, or drug-induced), capillary fragility, or reduced clotting factors must be considered in some disorders. Patients with osteogenesis imperfecta, for example, are particularly at risk of postoperative bleeding. Absence of the radius should alert the anesthesiologist to the possibility of the rare thrombocytopenia–absent radius (TAR) syndrome.

Limb Contractures

The causes of limb contractures range from injuries to the cerebral motor cortex (cerebral palsy), to neuromuscular disorders, joint involvement (arthrogryposis), and bone abnormalities. These contractures affect the anesthesiologist's ability to perform well-known regional nerve blocks, so that alternative and perhaps lesser-known approaches to specific nerve blocks may be required. Nerve mapping, nerve stimulators, or ultrasound may facilitate success (see Chap. 31).

Some limb contractures may also make intravenous access difficult, particularly when the overlying skin is smooth and featureless, as in patients with arthrogryposis syndromes or even cerebral palsy. Positioning for surgery is important; particular attention should be paid to pressure points to prevent further injury.

▶ SPECIFIC DISORDERS

In selecting the following examples, a disorder that affects each component of the motor reflex arc has been chosen. These conditions range from a common problem (cerebral palsy) to a rare abnormality of sensory input (familial dysautonomia). Neuromuscular disorders and abnormalities of the effecter organs—namely muscle (muscular dystrophy), bone (osteogenesis imperfecta) and joints (arthrogryposis syndromes)—are represented. All these disorders are likely to require significant orthopaedic surgery at some point and confront the anesthesiologist with various difficulties.

Cerebral Palsy

Cerebral palsy is a nonprogressive disorder of motion and posture, but almost all affected individuals will have at least one additional disability attributable to CNS damage. These disabilities include cognitive impairment, sensory loss (vision or hearing), seizures, behavioral and emotional disturbances, and difficulties with communication.[26,27] Other systems are secondarily involved, presenting gastrointestinal (constipation, reflux), respiratory (aspiration, pneumonia), and orthopaedic (contractures, kyphoscoliosis) problems.

The causes of cerebral palsy are numerous. There is increasing evidence that birth asphyxia may not be as common as was previously thought. Antenatal events may result in fetal complications that manifest as cerebral palsy at birth. These include antenatal infections, neuronal migration disorders, and endocrine dysfunction (hypothyroidism). Postnatal causes include meningitis, viral encephalitis, hydrocephalus, trauma, and surgical lesions.[26,27] Although the cerebral lesion is static, the clinical picture is variable and evolves over time. The type of disability depends on the site and extent of the cerebral damage: spasticity (motor cortex), athetosis (basal ganglia), and ataxia (cerebellum).

Spastic cerebral palsy is the commonest type, accounting for approximately 70 percent of cases. Affected individuals develop contractures over time, especially at the elbows, wrists, hips, knees, and ankles. Surgical intervention is aimed at releasing these contractures to improve or achieve function. In general, the more severe the motor impairment, the greater the intellectual impairment, but this is by no means universal. Epilepsy is more common in spastic cerebral palsy. When there is bulbar muscle involvement, there may be poor control of the mouth, tongue, and pharynx, resulting in feeding difficulties and a risk of aspiration.

Dyskinetic cerebral palsy (10 percent) is less common, since the incidence of kernicterus, formerly a major cause, has been reduced. Affected individuals generally have a low to normal IQ, but communication may be particularly difficult when deafness or dysarthria coexist. Individuals with ataxic cerebral palsy (10 percent) may also have intellectual impairment and speech disorders besides an impaired balance. Seizures are common in both types.

Anesthetic Considerations

In view of their various disabilities, these children require special consideration. Their feelings and emotions must be treated with sensitivity and understanding. Communication may be difficult and patience is therefore important. The assistance of the parents or caregiver may prove invaluable in this respect. The choice of premedication and the anesthetic plan should take these cognitive, communicative, and behavioral problems into account over and above the child's medical problems and drug therapy.

A number of systems may be involved and should be considered in any anesthetic plan for these children. Gastroesophageal reflux is common and may cause respiratory problems, especially in severely affected individuals. Contributing factors include esophageal dysmotility, abnormal function of the lower esophageal sphincter, esophageal stricture, feeding gastrostomy, and spinal deformities. Some may simply fail to thrive because of poor chewing or swallowing. Curtailment of nasogastric or gastrostomy feeding should be addressed, and electrolyte disturbances due to malnutrition and laxative use may require preoperative correction.

The airway may be difficult to manage because of dental caries, loose teeth, gum hyperplasia, and temporomandibular joint dysfunction. These need to be considered when the airway is being secured with an endotracheal tube or laryngeal mask.

Aspiration, recurrent infections, and a background of chronic lung disease place these children at significant perioperative risk. An ineffective cough and poor nutritional status are additional risk factors. Perioperative physiotherapy, bronchodilators, or antibiotics may be required. Physical therapy may prove difficult, given that patient cooperation is needed.

Cerebral palsied children have impaired temperature control secondary to hypothalamic dysfunction; therefore intraoperative hypothermia is common. Poor nutrition as well as the lack of muscle and fat compound the problem. These patients are particularly vulnerable to unintentional exposure.

Anticonvulsant therapy should be continued up to and including the day of surgery. Therapy should be restarted as soon as possible in the postoperative period. These patients may be on a variety of other drugs—such as antispasmodics, antireflux agents, anticholinergics, antacids, laxatives, or antidepressants—that need to be considered.

Baclofen, botulinum toxin, and clonidine have become popular in the management of spastic cerebral palsy.[28] Baclofen acts as an agonist at the gamma-aminobutyric acid (GABA) receptors in the dorsal horn of the spinal cord; it is used to reduce the pain associated with muscle spasms and in order to delay the development of contractures. Baclofen may be given intrathecally, epidurally, or orally. Abrupt withdrawal may result in seizures. Botulinum toxin produces reversible muscle denervation and results in a temporary reduction in muscle tone. It is indicated when spasticity interferes with function and may delay/prevent surgery. Systemic effects of botulinum toxin are rare; their treatment is supportive.

Postoperative analgesia is an essential part of the management. Inadequate analgesia compounded by difficulty with pain assessment in these children can lead to a vicious cycle of increased muscle tone and spasms, worsening pain, and anxiety. Regional anesthesia is particularly effective in this situation. Clonidine as an adjuvant for epidural local anesthetic infusions may reduce these muscle spasms.

Considering the communication difficulties with these children, the use of an effective validated pain scale is fraught with difficulty. A parent or caregiver is probably most able to convey the child's pain. Careful observation and vigilance should ensure that a compartment syndrome is not missed, particularly when a regional anesthetic technique has been used.

Muscle Disorders

Muscular Dystrophy

The muscular dystrophies are rare, genetically determined degenerative disorders. The most important of these diseases in children are the Duchenne and Becker types.[29–31] Both have been associated with genetic mutations resulting in abnormal or absent dystrophin, a sarcolemma protein. Dystrophin attaches the cytoskeleton to a protein complex that anchors muscle cells to the extracellular matrix. Inadequately tethered muscle fibers degenerate and are progressively replaced by connective tissue (pseudohypertrophy) (Fig. 6-5).[29,30]

Duchenne or pseudohypertrophic muscular dystrophy is characterized by progressive skeletal and smooth muscle weakness and wasting, which appear in early childhood and lead to death from cardiac or respiratory failure by late adolescence. It is the commonest childhood dystrophy, with an incidence of 1 per 3500 male births. Transmission of the gene is X-linked recessive; thus males are primarily affected, although a milder type has been observed in female carriers. Becker muscular dystrophy has a similar clinical appearance, but symptoms are milder and the clinical course is more protracted.

The muscles of the leg and pelvis are affected initially, followed by the thorax and upper limbs. Most affected individuals are wheelchair-bound by 8 to 11 years

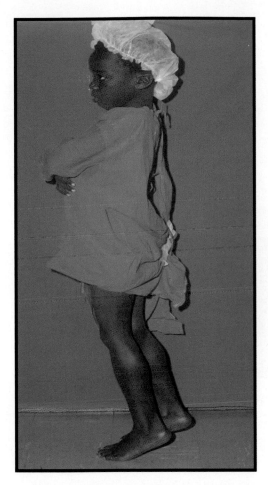

Figure 6-5. Duchenne muscular dystrophy. The pseudohypertrophy of the calves is clearly seen in this otherwise normal-looking boy.

of age, and 90 percent develop a spinal curvature of more than 20 degrees within 3 to 4 years.

Respiratory muscle weakness is the forerunner to the deterioration in respiratory function. Expiratory muscle function is affected first, reflecting the early onset of abdominal muscle weakness. Inspiratory muscle function, particularly diaphragmatic function, is spared initially but rapidly declines as the diaphragmatic musculature deteriorates. Other contributing factors include altered chest wall and lung mechanics (kyphoscoliosis), modifications in the distribution of surfactant, microatelectasis, and local fibrosis caused by recurrent chest infections. Respiratory failure inevitably occurs in the late teens or early twenties. Most of these children will require postoperative ventilatory support, particularly if the forced vital capacity is less than 40 percent predicted.

Changes in the myocardium are initially subclinical and start at about the time of skeletal muscle dysfunction. Myocardial cell death and subsequent fibrosis occur typically in the posterobasal and lateral walls of the left ventricle. By 15 years of age, 50 percent of affected individuals have some evidence of dilated cardiomyopathy with a reduced ejection fraction. Subclinical coronary insufficiency is difficult to detect in view of the decreasing physical activity of these individuals and may be revealed only as adverse cardiac events under the stress of anesthesia.

Corticosteroids, introduced into the medical management of muscular dystrophy two decades ago, significantly reduce the progressive deterioration of peripheral, respiratory, and possibly cardiac function. Corticosteroids improve muscle function by preventing muscle breakdown. Unfortunately they have significant side effects that include growth inhibition, weight gain, glucose intolerance, hypertension, and osteoporosis.

Anesthetic considerations revolve around pulmonary dysfunction and cardiomyopathy. Preoperative electrocardiography, echocardiography, and pulmonary function tests should be performed. Corticosteroids should be continued for major surgery.[29,30]

Potent volatile anesthetic agents have been linked with significant elevations in CK, myoglobinuria, and cardiac arrest that mimic MH. Although patients with Duchenne muscular dystrophy were thought to be at high risk for developing MH, current evidence suggests that the risk is no different from that in the general population. Nevertheless, succinylcholine is contraindicated because it can cause an acute rhabdomyolysis, hyperkalemia, and cardiac arrest.

Total intravenous anesthesia associated with regional anesthesia is probably the modality of choice. However, regional techniques, particularly neuraxial blockade, may be technically difficult to perform. There is no evidence that the use of a nerve stimulator and stimulation of an isolated muscle will cause a significant increase in extracellular potassium; nerve stimulation is therefore not contraindicated. The response to nondepolarizing muscle relaxants is prolonged; if these are required, lower doses should be used.

Osteochondrodysplasias

The osteochondrodysplasias (Figs. 6-6 and 6-7) constitute three major groups and include most of the numerous forms of disproportionately short stature (dwarfism).[20] Achondroplasia is the most common form, while the disorders of complex carbohydrate metabolism [e.g., mucopolysaccharidoses (Figs. 6-8 and 6-9)] form another significant group. A number of anesthetic problems are common to these syndromes, including craniovertebral abnormalities, cardiopulmonary dysfunction, and neurologic abnormalities.

Specific craniovertebral abnormalities that may occur will depend on the type of disorder, the age of the child,

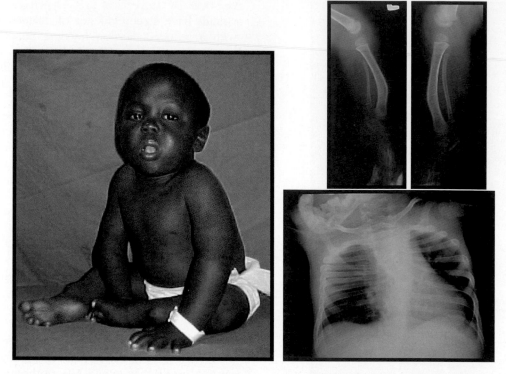

Figure 6-6. Campomelic dysplasia. This child was mildly affected but demonstrates the typical tibial prominence. The chest radiograph shows hypoplasia of the lungs, horizontal ribs, and early kyphoscoliosis.

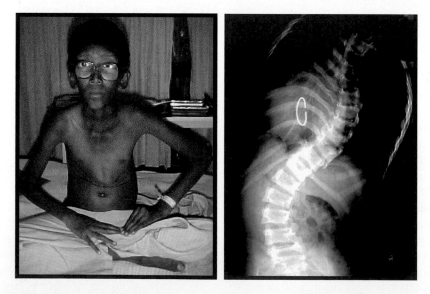

Figure 6-7. Beals syndrome—an osteochondrodysplasia—showing typical features: arachnodactyly, crumpled ear, and pectus carinatum. The chest radiograph demonstrates severe thoracolumbar kyphoscoliosis and evidence of a mitral valve replacement.

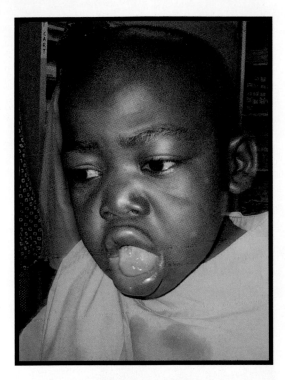

Figure 6-8. Mucopolysaccharidosis: Hunter's syndrome, showing the typical facies and macroglossia. Cervical instability and recurrent chest infections are common.

and associated pathology. Children may present with or without subtle or overt signs of spinal cord compression. A neck radiograph may show abnormalities in the bony elements (Klippel-Feil, Fig. 6-1) or soft tissue (trisomy 21, Down's syndrome) (Fig. 6-10). In children, the normal atlanto-dens interval is on the order of 1.7 mm, while in Down's it measures 2.6 mm. In 15 percent of cases it will measure 5 mm or more.

Tracheomalacia, bronchomalacia, chest wall anomalies, kyphoscoliosis, and restrictive lung disease are often seen in the osteochondrodysplasias. An enlarged liver (mucopolysaccharidoses) may restrict diaphragmatic excursion further. Cardiac anomalies include septal defects, patent ductus arteriosus, and more complex cardiac lesions.

Children with osteochondrodysplasia generally have normal intelligence and should be treated in a manner that befits their age and not their size. In some children, deafness [osteogenesis imperfecta (Fig. 6-11), some mucopolysaccharidoses] may make communication difficult. Macrocephaly, hydrocephalus, and seizures may be present. The effect of antiepileptic drugs on the anesthetic or the effect of withdrawing the drugs perioperatively should be taken into account. Positioning may be difficult in some patients. Care should be taken to prevent injury or fracture of brittle bones.

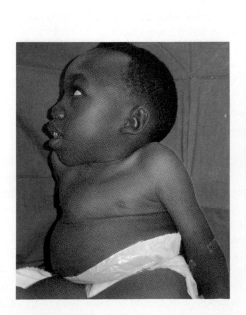
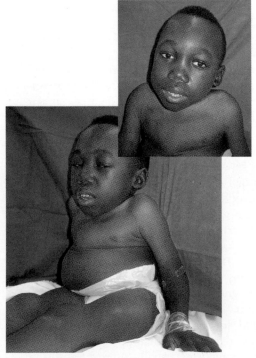

Figure 6-9. Morquio's syndrome. Hepatomegaly and severe kyphoscoliosis are clearly evident.

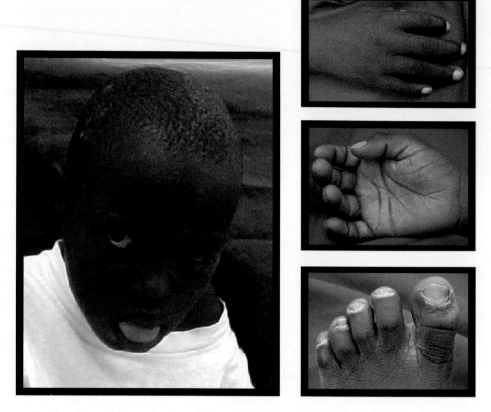

Figure 6-10. Down's syndrome. This child presented with arthritis of the knee and unilateral conjunctivitis. Clinical features shown in "sandal gap" between first and second toe, simian crease on palm and short fifth digit on the hand.

Joint Disorders

Arthrogryposis Syndromes

Arthrogryposis is a descriptive term meaning "abnormal curvature" or "persistent contracture." It refers to a variety of uncommon syndromes that have features similar to those of the classic arthrogyposis multiplex congenita but that may have different genetic origins.[32,33] The common factor in these syndromes is a lack of fetal movement, which may be caused by a neuropathy that affects the brain, the spinal cord, or the peripheral nerves. It may also be caused by abnormalities of the muscles, such as myasthenia gravis, congenital muscular dystrophies, or mitochondrial cytopathies; diseases of the connective tissues; or conditions that limit the space within the uterus.[33] The diagnosis is often made by the associated symptoms and signs and sometimes by tests such as electromyography and muscle biopsy.[33]

The phenotypic expression of these syndromes includes deformed fusiform limbs, smooth creaseless skin, and stiff or rigid joints that are present from birth.[32–34] Multiple joints are usually affected, causing adduction and internal rotation of the shoulders, fixed flexion or extension contracture of elbows and knees,

and flexion, abduction, and external rotation of the hips. The wrists and feet may also be involved.

Classically, individuals with arthrogryposis multiplex congenita have normal intelligence, a typical facial appearance, no visceral involvement, and a negative family history. The underlying muscle disorder is classically amyoplasia (infiltration with fibrofatty tissue) and involves all four limbs. Similar phenotypic expression of muscle disorders associated with MH may explain why some authors view arthrogryposis multiplex congenita as a risk for MH.

Anesthetic considerations include venous access, positioning, difficult-airway management, and cardiopulmonary function. The joint contractures and smooth, featureless skin combine to make venous access difficult. Endotracheal intubation may be a further difficulty. Mouth opening may be limited if the temporomandibular joint is affected, and neck movements may be limited by a torticollis. Contractures may also make positioning for regional blocks and surgery difficult. Protection of pressure points is essential. The risk of MH exists only because a wide spectrum of neuromuscular disorders, including MH-related disorders, have similar "arthrogrypotic features." Careful monitoring is therefore

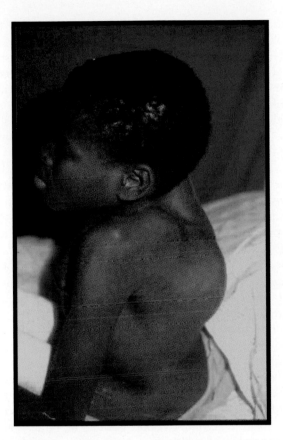

Figure 6-11. This child with osteogenesis imperfecta has had numerous fractures and osteotomies in attempts to improve function. She is short in stature and wheelchair-bound; she also has significant kyphoscoliosis.

essential. Respiratory support is indicated, particularly in older children with scoliosis and impaired respiratory function.

Bone Dysplasias

Osteogenesis Imperfecta

Osteogenesis imperfecta (OI) is a clinically heterogeneous disorder characterized by clinical anomalies of the type I collagen-containing tissues, including bone, ligaments, tendons, skin, sclera, and dentin (Fig. 6-11).[35] Approximately 80 to 90 percent of patients with osteogenesis imperfecta who fit into the type I to IV categories of the Sillence classification[36] have mutations of one of the two type I collagen genes. Hundreds of unique mutations have been identified in individuals with OI, and very few individuals or families share the same mutation. The cause of the other 10 to 20 percent remains unclear.

OI type III is the best known to orthopaedic surgeons because it is a progressive form of the disease. Standing and walking are virtually impossible for these patients because of their severe osteoporosis, progressive

deformities, and recurring fractures. Affected individuals are short in stature because of spinal compression fractures, progressive scoliosis deformities of the limbs, and disruption of the growth plate. Their teeth are usually severely affected and hearing impairment is common. The sclerae are bluish at birth but become white later in childhood. Survival is limited by the progressive kyphoscoliosis and repeated chest infections (Fig. 6-11).

Type IA OI is the classic autosomal dominant form, characterized by gray-blue sclera, osteoporosis with mild to moderate skeletal fragility, ligamentous laxity, normal dentition, and premature hearing loss. Type IB is similar, but the teeth are affected. Affected individuals have a normal life expectancy. Fractures first occur when the child starts to walk and bear weight. Although fractures seem to cease in adolescence, they may recur after inactivity, childbirth, breast-feeding, and menopause.

Type II refers to a severely affected heterogeneous group who usually die in the perinatal period. All bones are likely to be fractured and in various stages of healing. Survival is dependent on the integrity of the thorax.

Children with type IV OI vary in their clinical presentation; the severity of their condition ranges between that of types I and III. Basilar impression due to the descent of the skull on the cervical spine, with consequent brainstem compression, may occur in 70 percent of children with type IV OI, but it is less frequent in other types.

The aim of treatment in patients with OI is to increase bone mass and strength. Until recently the correction of deformities, intramedullary rodding of long bones, orthotic support, muscle strengthening, and wheelchairs were the mainstays of treatment. Two methods of improving bone mass are currently in use. Bisphosphonates, synthetic analogs of pyrophosphate, are potent inhibitors of bone resorption and are highly effective in improving bone mass in children with severe forms of OI. Children who previously had a reduced life expectancy are becoming increasingly mobile and are even able to walk and run.

The second approach is to use bone marrow transplantation to introduce mesenchymal stem cells, which have the capacity to differentiate into normal osteoblasts. However, many obstacles, principally graft-versus-host reactions, must be overcome before this method can be considered safe and as effective as bisphosphonates.

Previously, corrective osteotomies and intramedullary rodding were done to prevent progressive deformities and recurrent fractures in children with severe forms of OI. The surgical technique of fragmentation and rodding has been modified to lesser corrective osteotomies done through small incisions to preserve the blood supply to the bone and maximize healing. Progressive spinal deformities and basilar impression are two major problems that are difficult to manage because of the severity of the deformities and the fragility of the spine.

Anesthetic considerations include difficult-airway management and restrictive pulmonary function (kyphoscoliosis). The mobility and stability of the cervical spine must be assessed and basilar impression excluded. Mouth opening and the condition of the teeth must be addressed. In severe cases, fractures may be caused by rough handling or positioning of patients or by tourniquets, laryngoscopy, and even succinylcholine fasciculations. These children are at risk for respiratory infections and should be closely monitored. Careful physiotherapy, bronchodilator therapy, and antibiotics may be indicated.

A number of OI patients have developed tachycardia, tachypnea, and a rise in temperature associated with normocarbia during surgery.[37] The pyrexia is related to the duration of surgery and intraoperative blood loss and may persist for as long as 72 h after surgery. The postulated cause is an increase in basal metabolic rate induced by elevated thyroxine levels. The temperature is easily controlled by surface cooling. The association with MH is tenuous but must be excluded.

Heterotopic Bone Formation

Myositis Ossificans

Myositis ossificans or fibrodysplasia ossificans progressiva[38,39] is a rare autosomal dominant disorder that involves progressive ossification of skeletal muscle and connective tissue; that is, heterotopic bone formation. Heterotopic ossification usually progresses from proximal to distal and cranial to caudal.

Ossification can involve skeletal muscles, tendons, ligaments, or fascia at any anatomic site. The neck, shoulders (scapula, axilla), spine, chest, and abdominal wall may be involved, but the large muscles of the thigh or upper arm are the commonest sites on initial presentation.

The majority of children with this condition present between 4 and 5 years. In the early stages, there is increasing pain and swelling in a muscle, which is suggestive of a soft tissue infection or tumor. A history of trauma is not always forthcoming, particularly as minor trauma is usually forgotten. Blood tests show no signs of inflammation. The histologic appearance varies, but in the early stages it can mimic fibro- or myosarcoma.[38] Peripheral bone formation takes 6 to 8 weeks to develop and ossification is complete in 5 to 6 months. No effective treatment is at present available; surgical removal of heterotopic bone is ineffective and usually leads only to exacerbation of the disease.

The shoulder, elbow, hip, knee, and spine often become ankylosed, eventually confining affected individuals to a wheelchair. The diaphragm, larynx, tongue, and extraocular muscles are fortunately spared. Severe

restrictive pulmonary disease develops as result of thoracolumbar spinal involvement, costovertebral ankylosis, and ossification of the chest wall. Lung volumes are severely restricted, and respiratory infections are common because of an ineffective cough and atelectasis. Right ventricular dysfunction may develop as a consequence of pulmonary hypertension. Muscles of mastication become progressively fused, leading to limited mouth opening.

The most important of the anesthetic considerations[39] is to avoid precipitating any further ossification. Intravenous placement must be achieved with minimal trauma and dysfunctional intravenous infusions removed immediately so as to reduce the risk of heterotopic bone formation. Regional anesthesia may not only be technically difficult but is best avoided because of the danger of tissue trauma. Intramuscular injections, although less often used in children nowadays, are also contraindicated.

Endotracheal intubation may be difficult in view of the limited mouth opening and neck movement. Topical anesthesia should be used to facilitate fiberoptic intubation, since it carries the least risk of airway trauma. Nerve blocks of the airway or transtracheal injection of local anesthetic should be avoided because the trauma could exacerbate heterotopic bone formation. Tracheotomy may be technically difficult as a consequence of the rigid neck flexion but should also be avoided because calcification of the stoma may be triggered. Vigorous chest physiotherapy should be avoided. Steroids may be useful for flareups. Proper positioning and padding are essential.

Nerve Disorders

Familial Dysautonomia

Familial dysautonomia is a rare neurodevelopmental genetic disorder transmitted via an autosomal recessive gene. The disease affects the central nervous system and is characterized by pathologic deficits in peripheral autonomic and sensory neurons (decreased unmyelinated and small-fiber neurons). Progressive multiorgan dysfunction occurs secondary to demyelination in the brainstem and posterior columns of the spinal cord as well as degeneration of the autonomic ganglia.

Familial dysautonomia, which was first described in 1959, is also known as Riley-Day syndrome (named after an early-twentieth-century American pediatrician and physician) or HSAN—hereditary sensory and autonomic neuropathies. The condition has been described only in children of Ashkenazi Jews.[40]

These inherited autonomic neuropathies are a rare group of disorders associated with sensory dysfunction. Each is caused by a different genetic error on the long arm of chromosome 9.[40,41] In recent years, identification of specific genetic mutations for some disorders has aided both diagnosis and classification, which is ongoing.[42] Phenotypic expression varies and overlaps between different entities and makes the classification difficult.

The best-known and most intensively studied of the HSANs are familial dysautonomia (Riley-Day syndrome or HSAN type III) and congenital insensitivity to pain with anhidrosis (HSAN type IV). Diagnosis of the HSANs depends primarily on clinical examinations and specific sensory and autonomic assessments.[42]

Clinical features,[40–42] which first appear in early childhood, reflect widespread involvement of sensory and autonomic neurons. Sensory loss includes poor perception of pain and temperature. The sensory impairment affects peripheral sensation but not visceral or peritoneal sensation. Autonomic features include dysphagia, vomiting crises, blood pressure lability with hypertension and profound sweating, postural hypotension, and excessive vagal reflexes. Central dysfunction includes emotional lability, poor motor coordination, and ataxia. Intelligence is normal, although affected children may behave immaturely. Speech development may also be delayed.

Cardiovascular problems are related to both sympathetic and parasympathetic instability. Profound fluctuations in vasomotor response and blood pressure have been described, particularly under anesthesia.[43] Despite the impaired peripheral pain perception, appropriate pain management is essential. Epidural analgesia, previously considered contraindicated, has been shown to prevent the paroxysmal hypertension and exaggerated vasovagal responses.[43]

Affected individuals are also prone to recurrent respiratory infections that may lead to chronic lung disease or bronchiectasis. The causes are multifactorial. Initially, recurrent aspiration plays a major role and many of these children present for antireflux procedures (Nissen fundoplication). Hypotonia and kyphoscoliosis are compounding factors that develop as the disease progresses.

Spinal deformity is a common orthopaedic problem; it begins at approximately 4 years of age, with a prevalence of 80 percent by 15 years.[44,45] Patients with FD have a higher prevalence of fractures than do their peers.[44] The fracture pattern is also different, with a higher incidence of proximal femoral fractures. Neuropathic joints are common and occur secondary to the peripheral sensory neuropathy.

Despite the apparent insensitivity to pain, it is essential to provide adequate anesthesia to reduce the surgical stress and the "dysautonomic" events. These children have an increased sensitivity to endogenous or exogenous catecholamines.[43] A variety of anesthetic techniques have been described with varying degrees of success. Morbidity is high.

In a recent publication, Challands found that epidural anesthesia contributed to the cardiovascular and autonomic stability of three children who required a revision of their antireflux procedure. Furthermore, postoperative pain management was substantially better and respiratory complications fewer. These children had received opiate-based general anesthetic for the initial procedures, which were remarkable for the resulting hemodynamic instability, poor pain control, and respiratory complications.[43]

Premedication should be considered against a background of the emotional lability, cardiovascular lability, and the risk of respiratory depression. These children may have a blunted response to hypoxia and hypercarbia and are therefore sensitive to opiates.

Careful management of hydration is necessary. Patients may become dehydrated secondary to swallowing difficulties, excessive sweating, and episodes of diarrhea and vomiting (gastrointestinal manifestations of autonomic instability). Prolonged preoperative starvation may compound the problem. These children may not respond to hypovolemia appropriately, and hemodynamic lability may add to the confusion. Cardiac arrest has been described in response to profound hypotensive episodes and dysautonomic crises.[43] Diazepam has been used for the management of the latter and is considered the drug of choice.

Affected children have an impaired gag reflex, impaired esophageal motility, and gastric distention, and are prone to reflux. All the necessary precautions should be taken on induction, during extubation, and postoperatively to prevent aspiration. There are no specific contraindications to muscle relaxants including suxamethonium. Reduced doses should be considered in those who are hypotonic.

Respiratory support and pulmonary protection should form an essential part of the management. Perioperative physiotherapy, antibiotics, and the judicious use of opiate analgesia are important considerations. Epidural analgesia is ideal but may be difficult to administer in patients with kyphoscoliosis.

Eye protection is essential, since affected individuals lack tears and have no corneal reflexes; they are therefore vulnerable to corneal injuries[46] whether or not they are under anesthesia. Temperature regulation is also impaired. Both hypo- and hyperthermia have been reported.[43] Temperature must be monitored and controlled as far as possible.

Postoperative complications mainly center on autonomic lability and respiratory dysfunction. Persistent vomiting, orthostatic hypotension, paroxysmal hypertension, and hyperthermia may have to be addressed. Respiratory problems include aspiration, hypoventilation, and hypoxemia and are a cause for concern.

Human Immunodeficiency Virus (HIV)

Acquired immunodeficiency syndrome (AIDS), caused by the human immunodeficiency virus (HIV), is a worldwide epidemic affecting children of all ages. Children born with HIV are increasing in number, particularly in sub-Saharan Africa, Southeast Asia, eastern Europe, and the Asian subcontinent. In these developing countries, access to medical care is often inadequate. Access to highly active antiretroviral therapy (HAART) is limited and malnutrition is rife. As a result, the spectrum of disease in children living with HIV and on HAART is vastly different from that of the majority of HIV/AIDS sufferers who are not receiving treatment or, at best, limited prophylactic treatment.

AIDS has radically changed orthopaedic practice in those areas where its prevalence is highest. Delayed healing or nonunion of fractures, increased infection rates in compound fractures, or fractures requiring internal fixation have necessitated the revision of management strategies.[47]

Children with HIV/AIDS present with a wide range of infections that affect the central nervous system, gastrointestinal system, and/or respiratory tract.

The musculoskeletal system may also be affected, but with less frequency. Musculoskeletal manifestations usually correlate with low CD4 cell counts. The diagnostic difficulty lies in determining the extent of the tissue involvement, which may range from a simple subcutaneous infection to full-blown life-threatening osteomyelitis.[48]

Tuberculosis (TB) presents early in the disease and is almost synergistic with HIV. Tuberculosis mostly affects the pulmonary system but may affect extrapulmonary sites in 20 percent of cases. The most common site of musculoskeletal TB is the vertebrae, but it may also involve joints as well as other bone and soft tissue.

Since the advent of potent antiretroviral therapy, the survival of people infected with HIV has been prolonged. The incidence of opportunistic complications has decreased, but osteoporosis, osteopenia, and, less commonly, osteonecrosis have emerged as the most common bone disorders.[49] The resultant loss of bone density and deterioration in microarchitecture predisposes the bone to fracture, although an increased fracture rate in children has not been reported.[49] The pathogenesis of bone loss is probably multifactorial, and whether it is the direct effect of the potent antiretroviral therapy or a manifestation of the disease is a matter of debate.[49,50]

The effect of HIV or HAART on children with metabolic or osteopenic bone disorders has not been reported. An effect is virtually inevitable, but the alteration in the subsequent course of the disease is open to conjecture.

▶ CONCLUSION

For many anesthesiologists, particularly the occasional pediatric anesthesiologist, the spectrum and variety of congenital syndromes and genetic disorders remain an enigma. Various texts classify these disorders in different ways.[51] However, as the human genome is unraveled, patterns emerge. Many of these disorders are caused by anomalies in single or multiple genes or a chromosomal defect that can be linked to a structural, developmental, cell regulatory, or enzyme function or specifically to nerve and muscle function. Disorders in each particular category share similar clinical manifestations. Unfortunately there is still much heterogeneity among the various disorders and the phenotypic expression of different genetic disorders may be similar, as, for example, in the case of arthrogryposis.

As the genetic etiology of these disorders is uncovered and better understood, novel therapies based on modulating the abnormal gene function can be expected. This may radically change the clinical manifestations of these disorders in children. The need for orthopaedic intervention is also likely to change.

Those are prospects to look forward to. Still, to this day the anesthesiologist may not have the comfort of a definitive diagnosis at the time of surgery. For that reason a simple, safe anesthetic approach is desirable. By applying basic principles and focusing on the cardiopulmonary status, the airway, and the stability of the neck, the anesthesiologist can circumvent many problems. A multidisciplinary approach may be in the best interests of the child with diminished cardiopulmonary reserve. Regional anesthesia, although occasionally difficult to perform, has significant benefits, particularly when opiates could compromise cardiorespiratory reserve. If there were any possibility or suspicion that the child might be susceptible to MH, it would be prudent to use a nontriggering anesthetic.

REFERENCES

1. Jones KL. *Smith's Recognizable Patterns of Human Malformation*, 4th ed. Philadelphia: Saunders, 1992.
2. Baum VC, O'Flaherty JE. *Anesthesia for Genetic, Metabolic, and Dysmorphic Syndromes of Childhood*. Philadelphia: Lippincott Williams & Wilkins, 1999.
3. Online Mendelian Inheritance in Man. www.ncbi.nlm.nih.gov/Omim/
4. US Office of Rare Diseases. http://rarediseases. info.nih.gov
5. Practice guidelines for preoperative fasting and the use of pharmacologic agents to reduce the risk of pulmonary aspiration: Application to healthy patients undergoing elective procedures: A report by the American Society of Anesthesiologists Task Force on Preoperative Fasting. *Anesthesiology* 90:896–905, 1999.
6. Cote CJ. Preoperative fasting: Is the answer clear. *J Pediatr* 132:1077–1078, 1998.
7. Olsson GL, Hallen B, Hambraeus-Jonzon K. Aspiration during anesthesia: A computer-aided study of 185,358 Anesthetics. *Acta Anaesthesiol Scand* 30:84–92, 1986.

8. Tiret L, Desmonts JM, Hatton F, et al. Complications associated with anesthesia: A prospective survey in France. *Can Anaesth Soc J* 33:336–344, 1986.

9. Warner MA, Warner ME, Warner DO, et al. Perioperative pulmonary aspiration in infants and children. *Anesthesiology* 90:66–71, 1999.

10. Bricker SR, McLuckie A, Nightingale DA. Gastric aspirates after trauma in children. *Anaesthesia* 44:721–724, 1989.

11. Schurizek BA, Rybro L, Boggild-Madsen NB, et al. Gastric volume and pH in children for emergency surgery. *Acta Anaesthesiol Scand* 30:404–408, 1986.

12. Lieberman JR, Staneli CT, Dales MC. Tourniquet pressures on pediatric patients: A clinical study. *Orthopaedics* 20:1143–1147, 1997.

13. Kam PCA, Kavanaugh R, Yoong FFY. The arterial tourniquet: Pathophysiological consequences and anesthetic implications. *Anaesthesia* 56:534–545, 2001.

14. Lynn AM, Fischer T, Brandford HG, et al. Systemic responses to tourniquet release in children. *Anesth Analg* 65:865–872, 1986.

15. Townsend HS, Goodman SB, Schurman DJ, et al. Tourniquet release: Systemic and metabolic effects. *Acta Anaesthesiol Scand* 40:1234–1237, 1996.

16. Bloch EC, Ginsberg B, Binner RA, et al. Limb tourniquets and central temperature in children. *Anesth Analg* 74:486–489, 1992.

17. Goodarzi M, Shier NH, Ogden JA. Physiological changes during tourniquet release in children. *J Pediatr Orthop* 12:510–513, 1992.

18. Goodarzi M, Shier NH, Grogan DP. Does sympathetic blockade prevent the physiologic changes associated with tourniquet use in children? *J Pediatr Orthop* 17:289–292, 1997.

19. Sanders BJ, D'Alessio JG, Jernigan JR. Intraoperative hypothermia associated with lower extremity tourniquet deflation. *J Clin Anesth* 8:504–507, 1996.

20. Berkowitz ID, Raja SN, Bender KS, et al. Dwarfs: Pathophysiology and anesthetic implications. *Anesthesiology* 73:739–759, 1990.

21. Baraka AS, Jalbout MI. Anesthesia and myopathy. *Curr Opin Anaesthesiol* 15:371–376, 2002.

22. Hopkins PM. Malignant hyperthermia: Advances in clinical management and diagnosis. *Br J Anaesth* 85:118–128, 2000.

23. Jurkat-Rott K, McCarthy T, Lehmann-Horn F. Genetics and pathogenesis of malignant hyperthermia. *Muscle Nerve* 23:4–17, 2000.

24. Levitt RC, Meyers D, Fletcher JE, et al. Molecular genetics and malignant hyperthermia. *Anesthesiology* 75:1–3, 1991.

25. Bosenberg AT, Madaree A, Osborn I, et al. Malignant hypothermia associated with cleft palate, clubfoot and myopathy. *Pediatr Anesth* 12:92, 2002.

26. Nolan J, Chalkiades GA, Low J, et al. Anesthesia and pain management in cerebral palsy. *Anaesthesia* 55:32–41, 2000.

27. Wongprasartsuk P, Stevens J. Cerebral palsy and anesthesia. *Paediatr Anaesth* 12:296–303, 2002.

28. Mooney JF, Koman A, Smith BP. Pharmacologic management of spasticity in cerebral palsy. *J Pediatr Orthop* 23:679–686, 2003.

29. Stevens RD. Neuromuscular disorders and anesthesia. *Curr Opin Anaesthesiol* 14:693–698, 2001.

30. Ames WA, Hayes JA, Crawford MW. The role of corticosteroids in Duchenne muscular dystrophy: A review for the anesthetist. *Pediatr Anesth* 15:3–8, 2005.

31. Morris P. Duchenne muscular dystrophy: A challenge for the anesthetist. *Pediatr Anesth* 7:1–4, 1997.

32. Gordon N. Arthrogryposis multiplex congenita. *Brain Dev* 20:507–511, 1998.

33. Hall JG. Arthrogryposis multiplex congenita: Etiology, genetics, classification, diagnostic approach, and general aspects. *J Pediatr Orthop B* 6:159–166, 1997.

34. Bernstein RM. Arthrogryposis and amyoplasia. *J Am Acad Orthop Surg* 10:417–424, 2002.

35. Cole WG. Advances in osteogenesis imperfecta. *Clin Orthop Rel Res* 401:6–16, 2002.

36. Sillence DO, Rimoin DL, Danks DM. Clinical variability in osteogenesis imperfecta: Variable expressivity and gene heterogeneity. *Birth Defects Orig Artic Serv* 15:113–129, 1979.

37. Ghert M, Allen B, Davids J, et al. Increased postoperative febrile response in children with osteogenesis imperfecta. *J Pediatr Orthop* 23:261–264, 2003.

38. Gindele A, Schwamborn D, Tsironis K, et al. Myositis ossificans traumatica in young children: Report of three cases and review of literature. *Pediatr Radiol* 30:451–459, 2000.

39. Singh A, Ayyalapu A, Keochekian A. Anesthetic management in fibrodysplasia ossificans progressiva: A case report. *J Clin Anesth* 15:211–213, 2003.

40. Axelrod FB. Familial dysautonomia. *Muscle Nerve* 29:352–363, 2004.

41. Slaugenhaupt SA, Gusella JF. Familial dysautonomia. *Curr Opin Genet Dev* 12:307–311, 2002.

42. Axelrod FB, Hilz MJ. Inherited autonomic neuropathies. *Sem Neurol* 23:381–390, 2003.

43. Challands JF, Facer EK. Epidural anesthesia and familial dysautonomia (the Riley Day syndrome). Three case reports. *Paediatr Anaesth* 8:83–88, 1998.

44. Laplaza FJ, Turajane T, Axelrod FB, et al. Non spinal orthopaedic problems in familial dysautonomia (Riley-Day syndrome). *J Pediatr Orthop* 21:229–232, 2001.

45. Bar-On E, Floman Y, Sagiv S, et al. Orthopaedic manifestations of familial dysautonomia. A review of one hundred and thirty-six patients. *J Bone Joint Surg Am* 82-A:1563–1570, 2000.

46. Francois J. The Riley-Day syndrome. Familial dysautonomy, central autonomic dysfunction. *Ophthalmologica* 174:20–34, 1977.

47. Jellis J. Orthopaedic surgery and HIV disease in Africa. *Int Orthop* 20:253–256, 1996.

48. Tehranzadeh J, Ter-Oganesyan, Steinbach LS. Musculoskeletal disorders associated with HIV infection and AIDS. Part 1: Infectious musculoskeletal conditions. *Skeletal Radiol* 33:249–259, 2004.

49. Glesby MJ. Bone disorders in human immunodeficiency virus infection. *Clin Infect Dis* 37:S91–S95, 2003.

50. Arpadi S, Horlock M, Shane E. Editorial: Metabolic bone disease in human immunodeficiency virus–infected children. *J Clin Endocrinol Metab* 89:21–23, 2004.

51. Alman BA. A classification for genetic disorders of interest to orthopaedists. *Clin Orthop Rel Res* 401:17–26, 2002.

PART II

Operative Orthopaedic Procedures

CHAPTER 7

The Shoulder Joint

R. Kumar Kadiyala/André P. Boezaart

▶ INTRODUCTION

Although shoulder arthroplasty is dealt with extensively in this chapter, some anesthetic considerations of subacromial decompression and "frozen shoulder" are also discussed. Sport injuries to the shoulder and related topics, including rotator cuff repair, are extensively discussed in Chap. 17.

With the incidence of arthritic deformities in the aging population approaching 20 percent, shoulder arthroplasty has become an increasingly commonplace procedure to treat maladies of the glenohumeral joint's articular surfaces. While shoulder arthroplasty is similar in concept to arthroplasty procedures of the hip or knee, there are unique anatomic, biomechanical, surgical, and rehabilitative considerations that must be taken into account to ensure optimal patient outcomes.

▶ BIOMECHANICS

Motion of the shoulder is achieved through a complex integration of actions between the sternoclavicular, acromioclavicular, scapulothoracic, and glenohumeral joints. The soft tissue restraints of ligamentous structures and the dynamic motor of the rotator cuff and periscapular muscles control the concerted interactions of all these structures.

Elevation of the shoulder requires concomitant motion of the scapula on the thorax, rotation of the clavicle at the acromioclavicular and sternoclavicular joints, and motion of the humeral head within the glenoid (glenohumeral motion). To achieve full overhead elevation of the arm, the rotation that occurs at either end of the clavicle ranges from 10 to 30 degrees, and the ratio of overall glenohumeral to scapulothoracic motion averages 2:1.

Despite its appearance of a ball-and-socket joint, intrinsic motion within the glenohumeral joint cannot be described as rotation of the spherical humeral head within the shallow dish of the glenoid. Actually, the intrinsic motion of the glenohumeral joint is a combination of rotation, rolling, and translation (sliding) of the humeral head on the glenoid.

The stability afforded by the shallow glenoid is not similar to that provided by the deeper acetabulum for the hip joint. Therefore ligamentous attachments between the glenoid and humerus (glenohumeral ligaments) provide a degree of static stability to the shoulder joint, and the rotator cuff and periscapular muscles provide dynamic stability to keep the humeral head centered within the glenoid as active motion of the shoulder occurs (Fig. 7-1).

▶ PATHOPHYSIOLOGY

Alteration of the integrity of the articular cartilage of the shoulder joint leads to bone-on-bone contact, loss of subchondral bone support of the joint surface, development of osteophytes and loose bodies, soft tissue contracture, and muscular atrophy, with concomitant loss of motion and onset of pain. The arthritic process affects all facets of shoulder motion: bony congruity is altered, ligamentous balancing is disrupted, soft tissue adhesions develop, and rotator cuff and periscapular muscle strength is reduced.

Etiology

Glenohumeral arthritis can be linked to a variety of causes, including congenital, inflammatory, traumatic, septic, and vascular diseases as well as the most common

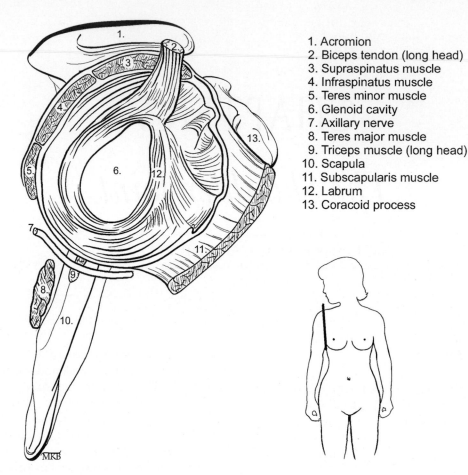

1. Acromion
2. Biceps tendon (long head)
3. Supraspinatus muscle
4. Infraspinatus muscle
5. Teres minor muscle
6. Glenoid cavity
7. Axillary nerve
8. Teres major muscle
9. Triceps muscle (long head)
10. Scapula
11. Subscapularis muscle
12. Labrum
13. Coracoid process

Figure 7-1. Schematic anatomy of the glenohumeral joint.

degenerative or osteoarthritic process. It can also be seen in postsurgical cases when soft tissue balance of the shoulder has been altered, and with chronic rotator cuff tears (rotator cuff arthropathy). While the arthritic changes typically affect articular surfaces of both the glenoid and humeral head, changes can be isolated to one side of the joint, such as osteonecrosis of the humeral head after long-term corticosteroid use.

Epidemiology

Glenohumeral arthritis is typically seen in the elderly population, with an incidence approaching 20 percent in that age group. Shoulder arthroplasty procedures are becoming more common, but only at a frequency of 1/30 that of total knee replacements. The impact of glenohumeral arthritis on overall health status is comparable to congestive heart failure, coronary artery disease and diabetes.

▶ ANATOMIC CONSIDERATIONS

Developmental Anatomy

By the fifth week of gestation, limb buds, precursors to the upper and lower extremities, can be identified in the human embryo. Under the influence of the apical ectodermal ridge, an inductive cascade of growth and differentiation factors promotes growth and development of the shoulder and upper extremity from the upper limb bud. By the eighth week of gestation, the main components of the shoulder girdle are well defined. These include the brachial plexus, clavicle, glenohumeral joint, scapula, periscapular muscles, pectoralis muscles and rotator cuff.

Surgical Anatomy

Awareness of the muscles about the shoulder girdle and their respective innervation is necessary for proper evaluation and treatment. Branches of the brachial plexus innervate all the major muscles of the shoulder girdle. Exceptions are the spinal accessory nerve (cranial nerve XI), innervating the trapezius muscle; the dorsal scapular nerve (direct branch of C5 nerve root), innervating the rhomboid muscles; and the long thoracic nerve (branches from C5, C6 and C7 roots), innervating the serratus anterior muscle.

Branches of the upper trunk of the brachial plexus typically provide sensory innervation to the shoulder. Branches of the cervical plexus innervate the superior aspect of the shoulder and the supraclavicular area.

Surgical approaches for arthroplasty of the gleno-humeral joint typically exploit the deltopectoral interval: the internervous plane between the deltoid (axillary nerve innervation) and the pectoralis muscles (medial and lateral pectoral nerve innervation) (Fig. 7-2). Occasionally, a muscle-splitting approach through the deltoid is utilized. These intervals are extensively used; however, recognition of key neurovascular structures is important to prevent iatrogenic injury.

The conjoined tendon's attachment to the coracoid process marks a safe lateral border to the neurovascular structures about the shoulder. Medial to this lie the cords of the brachial plexus and the axillary artery. The musculocutaneous nerve innervates the coracobrachialis muscle 1 to 5 cm from the tip of the coracoid. Excessive retraction of the conjoined tendon and coracobrachialis must be avoided to prevent musculocutaneous nerve palsy. The axillary nerve branches off the posterior cord of the brachial plexus, traveling along the inferior glenoid neck, caudal to the subscapularis muscles, before traversing the quadrilateral space and curving around the posterior aspect of the neck of the humerus. Dissection inferior to the glenoid and intradeltoid dissection more

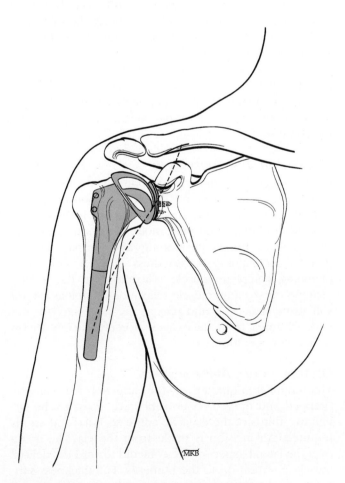

Figure 7-2. Total shoulder arthroplasty.

than 5 cm from the edge of the acromion places the axillary nerve at risk. The suprascapular nerve is 1 to 2 cm from the superior glenoid rim after it passes beneath the suprascapular ligament. Excessive soft tissue release along the superior glenoid and dissection medial to the base of the coracoid places the suprascapular nerve at risk of injury.

► SURGICAL PROCEDURE

Patient Selection

Patients who are candidates for shoulder arthroplasty have painful functional limitations due to destructive changes within the glenohumeral joint. The loss of articular cartilage, with development of osteophytes and loss of motion, can readily be treated with hemiarthroplasty or total shoulder arthroplasty. The ideal candidates have good bone stock to accept and keep the prosthetic components stable. They also have well-functioning muscles about the shoulder girdle and are motivated to participate in a postoperative physiotherapy program. Satisfactory results are also possible with mild to moderate deficits in bone, motion, and strength recognized preoperatively. The patient's overall health status must obviously be evaluated before surgery. The systemic stress from shoulder arthroplasty is usually well tolerated, and intraoperative blood loss rarely requires a transfusion. Strict contraindications to shoulder arthroplasty are a nonfunctioning deltoid muscle, active infection, severe destructive bone loss, and severe injury to the brachial plexus. Those disorders are better treated with shoulder arthrodesis.

Patients 50 years of age or older with arthritic changes of the humeral head and glenoid are ideal candidates for total shoulder arthroplasty. This can include replacement of the humeral head as well as resurfacing of the glenoid. An intact rotator cuff is necessary to perform a total shoulder arthroplasty successfully. If a rotator cuff tear is noted, a sound repair must be made to obtain a successful outcome.

Patient Profile

The typical patient presenting for shoulder arthroplasty is in his or her sixth, seventh, or eighth decade of life, though successful long-term results have been reported for active patients under the age of 50. The chief complaint is pain that limits routine activities. Pain when the shoulder is used and difficulty in reaching into kitchen cupboards, reaching behind the back, dressing, and participating in work and leisure activities are invariably present. Patients have already exhausted measures such as rest, physiotherapy, injections, and oral analgesic medications. Radiographs confirm the diagnosis of glenohumeral arthritis, but the decision to operate is based on the amount of pain and disability the patient is experiencing.

Positioning on the Operating Table

Patient positioning is the key to avoid intraoperative struggles. The patient is usually placed in the semireclining or full sitting beach-chair position. Sequential compression devices are placed on the lower extremities to prevent deep venous thrombosis. The head and neck are safely stabilized. In the elderly kyphotic female, care must be taken to avoid a hyperextension force to the cervical spine. Any arthritic or existing deformities of the lumbar spine, hip, or knee must also be addressed during positioning. The unaffected arm is comfortably placed into a padded arm holder, ensuring that there is slight flexion and abduction of the shoulder so as to avoid brachial plexus stretch. The bony prominences of the medial epicondyle and wrist are protected to prevent ulnar or radial sensory nerve palsy. A padded brace is placed against the lateral chest wall of the affected side to stabilize the thorax during surgery. Before prepping and draping, the shoulder is manipulated to ensure that excessive traction will not be exerted on the cervical spine during the operation. Full abduction, elevation, extension, and rotation of the arm are necessary during the surgery.

The entire forequarter of the affected extremity must be draped free for access during surgery. All tubing and leads must come off the field to the opposite side. The lateral two-thirds of the clavicle is within the sterile field. If interscalene catheters are used, they must be tunneled away subcutaneously from the surgical field.

Surgical Technique

Options

The options for arthroplasty are total shoulder arthroplasty, hemiarthroplasty, resection arthroplasty, and arthrodesis.

The modern prosthetic implants used in shoulder arthroplasty consist of the modular humeral component and a high-density polyethylene glenoid liner. The humeral component is made of a metallic alloy with an intramedullary stem and an interchangeable hemispheric head component designed to recreate the normal anatomy of the shoulder. The intramedullary stem can be press-fitted into the intramedullary canal of the humerus or cemented into place with methylmethacrylate (see Chap. 33). The glenoid component is commonly cemented into place or secured with a metal back plate and bone screws. To obtain proper soft tissue tension and joint kinematics, the normal anatomy of the joint is duplicated with the prosthetic implants as much as possible. Replacement of both the humeral and glenoid surfaces constitutes a total shoulder arthroplasty. Replacement of the humeral component is a hemiarthroplasty. The deltopectoral approach is the most common one used for arthroplasty procedures (Fig. 7-2).

If the arthritic process mainly involves the humeral head and leaves a congruent glenoid surface, hemiarthroplasty (replacement of the humeral head) can be performed. Hemiarthroplasty does not provide the same degree of pain relief as total shoulder arthroplasty. It may be appropriate in the younger patient who is physically very active to allay concern about long-term wear of the polyethylene glenoid component. Hemiarthroplasty is technically easier to perform than total arthroplasty; it can be done with the standard endoprosthesis stem placed in the medullary canal of the humerus or with a resurfacing arthroplasty, in which a metallic cup is placed onto the molded humeral head.

Patients with painful arthritic changes and a chronic rotator cuff tear are also candidates for hemiarthroplasty. Total shoulder arthroplasty in these patients will become unstable and polyethylene wear will be rapid due to loss of soft tissue balance secondary to the rotator cuff tear.

Recently a new type of shoulder prosthesis has received FDA approval for treatment of arthropathy associated with rotator cuff tear. This new prosthesis, called the reverse shoulder prosthesis, has a spherical component implanted onto the glenoid and a cupped stem placed into the humerus. Early European clinical results show promise for the use of the new device in this subset of patients.

Resection arthroplasty of the humeral head is limited to patients with active infectious processes not treated with joint debridement. Glenohumeral arthrodesis is generally reserved for paralytic problems involving the shoulder.

The Surgeon's Technique

Proper surgical technique and optimal outcome require a knowledge of normal and abnormal anatomy, with the ultimate goal of restoring normal anatomic relationships, soft tissue tension, and joint motion. Keys to achieving this include proper positioning and draping of the patient, maintaining a bloodless surgical field, and obtaining complete muscle relaxation. In the elderly osteoporotic patient, muscle relaxation as well as careful soft tissue dissection and release are necessary to prevent fractures from excessively forceful manipulation during the operation.

DELTOPECTORAL APPROACH

The entire forequarter of the affected extremity is prepped and draped. Unencumbered access to the lateral two-thirds of the clavicle, entire scapula, and arm is required. An incision is made from the clavicle, going over the lateral aspect of the coracoid toward the deltoid muscle insertion on to the humerus. Full-thickness subcutaneous flaps are developed, exposing the deltoid and pectoralis muscles. A fatty layer overlying the cephalic vein often marks the deltopectoral interval. The plane between the deltoid and pectoralis muscles is bluntly dissected from the clavicle to the humerus, retracting the cephalic vein laterally and superiorly with the deltoid and the pectoralis muscles medially. Blunt dissection beneath the deltoid muscle over the humeral head and into the subacromial space is performed to release soft tissue adhesions. The clavipectoral fascia overlying the conjoined tendon and the humeral head is excised superiorly to the level of the coracoacromial ligament, and the superior centimeter of the pectoralis insertion onto the humerus is released for soft tissue mobilization. The subscapularis muscle is now clearly exposed. The conjoined tendon is retracted medially with a handheld retractor (use of a self-retaining retractor is avoided to prevent musculocutaneous nerve injury). The subscapularis tendon is released from its insertion on the greater tuberosity and then reflected medially with the associated anterior joint capsule.

Blunt dissection along the inferior capsule is performed to identify and protect the axillary nerve. The anesthesiologist can assist with identification of the axillary nerve in the nonparalyzed patient by nerve stimulation. Using a nerve stimulator probe and a current of approximately 0.5 mA, the surgeon can confirm the position of the axillary and musculocutaneous nerves by deltoid and biceps muscle contractions respectively.

HEMI-SHOULDER ARTHROPLASTY

A careful excision of the anteroinferior capsule is done to gain proper soft tissue mobilization. Osteophytes about the humeral head are then removed, followed by controlled adduction, extension, and external rotation of the arm to remove the humeral head from the glenoid. The humeral head is resected, utilizing the appropriate guides from the chosen arthroplasty system. The insertions of the supra- and infraspinatus muscles onto the greater tuberosity are protected, as is the biceps tendon within the intertubercular groove. Appropriate sizing of the intramedullary implant is performed, and a decision whether to proceed with a press-fit implant or to use methylmethacrylate cement is made (see Chap. 33). A humeral head prosthesis to restore the normal anatomy of the original head is also chosen.

If a hemiarthroplasty procedure has been done, the surgery is completed by securely reattaching the subscapularis muscle to the greater tuberosity and routine subcutaneous and skin closure. The limb is then placed into a shoulder immobilizer.

TOTAL SHOULDER ARTHROPLASTY

To continue with a total shoulder arthroplasty (Fig. 7-2), exposure of the glenoid is begun. A humeral neck retractor is placed into the depth of the shoulder joint to move the humerus laterally. A soft-tissue release of the subscapularis muscle along the anterior rim of the glenoid is performed, as well as excision of any remnants of the glenoid labrum. Soft tissue release of the anteroinferior capsule, and at times of the posterior capsule, may be needed to see the entire glenoid clearly. This is typically the most difficult part of the surgery. Reaming or burring of the glenoid surface is performed to accept the polyethylene prosthetic liner, which is then fixed in the glenoid with methylmethacrylate cement or bone fixation screws.

The shoulder is then reduced and range of motion is evaluated, followed by secure repair of the subscapularis muscle to the greater tuberosity. Routine subcutaneous and skin closure is performed, and the arm is placed into a shoulder immobilizer.

▶ ANESTHETIC CONSIDERATIONS FOR SHOULDER SURGERY

General Comments

Shoulder surgery is one of the areas in which an understanding of the surgery and participation by the anesthesiologist is vital to the outcome of the surgery. This applies to preoperative evaluation of the patient and avoidance of nerve blocks in certain circumstances as much as it does to doing nerve blocks for others, positioning on the operating table, management of the surgical field, and postoperative pain management. Understanding in which surgical procedures motor function is important and in which operations it is not is also important.

Preoperative

ASSOCIATED MEDICATION

Shoulder arthroplasty is usually limited to the older population with osteoarthritis, although rheumatoid arthritis is a common comorbidity (see Chap. 9). Patients frequently receive nonsteroidal anti-inflammatory drugs (NSAIDs), with side effects on platelet function and blood clotting (see Chap. 4). Drugs associated with rheumatoid arthritis are discussed in Chap. 9.

Elderly patients often receive a plethora of different drugs, most with anesthetic implications. These include diuretics (associated with hypo- and hyperkalemia), digitalis (for cardiac dysrhythmias), beta-adrenergic antagonists (for bradycardia, bronchospasm, and cardiac failure), and oral hypoglycemics (for hyperglycemia); they may also use alcohol.

ASSOCIATED COMORBIDITIES

The most common comorbidities associated with shoulder joint arthroplasty are rheumatoid arthritis (see

Chap. 9) and advanced age. Diseases that often accompany aging include essential hypertension, ischemic heart disease, cardiac conduction disturbances, congestive heart failure, chronic pulmonary disease, diabetes mellitus, subclinical hypothyroidism, rheumatoid arthritis, and osteoarthritis.

It is outside the scope of this book to discuss each of the above conditions exhaustively. Suffice it to state that in the preoperative evaluation of the elderly patient's functional reserve as well as all the organ systems and airway, one should consider the changes characteristic of aging. These include stiffened myocardium and vasculature, blunted responsiveness of beta-adrenergic receptors, and impaired reflex control of the autonomic nervous system. The potential presence of vestibulobasilar arterial insufficiency can be evaluated by determining the effects of extension and rotation of the patient's head on orientation. Elderly patients are often volume-depleted, and perioperative fluid management should be carefully calculated. Finally, senile skin atrophy, with collagen loss and decreased elasticity, makes the skin more sensitive to injury from adhesive tape and monitoring electrodes.

Premedication

It is customary to continue with the medication that a patient is using during the perioperative period. It may be necessary to adjust or continue anticoagulation therapy and any other specific therapy, depending on the reason for using it. For example, it may be unwise to discontinue warfarin that a patient has been using because of a heart valve replacement (see Chap. 4). It may be considered necessary to change longer-acting irreversible drugs for shorter-acting reversible ones. The use of anxiolytic agents in the elderly patient is controversial, but it is customary to use these drugs in smaller dosages or directly preoperatively by intravenous injection.

Nerve Block

Shoulder arthroplasty is very painful, while other shoulder operations, such as arthroscopic subacromial decompression (ASAD), may be less painful. Some operations cause pain for only a limited time, while others cause severe pain for some days after surgery. Furthermore, in some surgical procedures, for "frozen shoulder," for example, it may be important to provide analgesia without motor blockade to allow the patient to participate in his or her physical therapy. In other situations, for example, rotator cuff repair, it may be advantageous to have no motor function in affected muscles for a few days postoperatively. It is therefore important to match the nerve block to the surgical situation.

It may be inappropriate to offer a continuous nerve block to a patient scheduled for ASAD, since the pain associated with this operation is short-lived and not severe; it is probably caused by the subcutaneous extravasation of the irrigation fluid. On the other hand, it may be equally inappropriate not to offer a continuous nerve block to a patient scheduled for rotator cuff repair (RCR) or shoulder arthroplasty.

Arthroscopic Subacromial Decompression (ASAD)

This is typically not very painful surgery and a continuous block is usually not indicated. Some shoulder surgeons even question the existence of the subacromial impingement syndrome. Brachial plexitis may well be the cause of the shoulder pain in more patients than is commonly realized. This condition may be greatly underdiagnosed, since specific and reliable diagnostic tests are unavailable. Blocks should therefore be used sparingly and with great caution in these patients.

Patients who undergo ASAD normally require only a single injection block that provides analgesia for a few hours postoperatively (see Chap. 23). We prefer to use general anesthesia and no block for the surgery until the shoulder pathology becomes clear after diagnostic arthroscopy. If a patient suffers severe pain after ASAD, it is usually due to subcutaneous fluid extravasation and swelling; all that is usually required is a single-injection brachial plexus block in the recovery room. For this a cervical paravertebral or interscalene block with 20 mL (0.2 to 0.5%) bupivacaine is usually all that is necessary. The cervical paravertebral block can be guided by loss of resistance to air only (see Chap. 23).

If, however, a rotator cuff tear was found and repaired, a continuous cervical paravertebral block can be placed. This can be done in the operating room utilizing loss of resistance to air and before waking the patient or in the recovery room after the patient has emerged from general anesthesia. The choice depends on the institutional protocol and the anesthesiologist's preference. Nerve stimulation should be avoided for postoperative blockade after rotator cuff repair (RCR) because muscle contractions could damage the freshly repaired tendons and it would be severely painful in unanesthetized patients. See discussion of rotator cuff tear below.

Shoulder Arthroplasty, Shoulder Stabilization, and Rotator Cuff Repair

The continuous cervical paravertebral block (CCPVB) (see Chap. 23) is ideally suited for total or hemi-shoulder arthroplasty, shoulder stabilization procedures, and RCR, although continuous interscalene block (CISB) (see Chap. 23) is the "gold standard" block for this surgery. We suspect that this will change as CCPVB becomes more widely used. A relatively large volume of local anesthetic (20 to 40 mL) is injected as a bolus. This usually blocks all the brachial plexus roots, making it ideal for this type of surgery. It should be kept in mind that the onset of action of the CCPVB is slower than that with interscalene block, probably because of the dural sheath surrounding the roots more distally.

A continuous infusion of 5 mL/h of a lower concentration of the drug (for example ropivacaine 0.2%) with patient-controlled regional anesthesia (PCRA) boluses of 10 mL of the same drug at a lockout time of 1 h seems to be ideal for this application. Some authors suggest that PCRA without continuous infusion is satisfactory (see Chap. 21).

With CCPVB, the motor block is denser in the proximal parts of the upper limb than in the distal parts when using a bolus injection of 30 mL of 0.5% ropivacaine and a continuous infusion of 0.2% ropivacaine at 0.1 mL/kg/h (see Chap. 23). The distal motor block can also be expected to subside earlier than the proximal block, and the sensory block usually outlasts the motor block (see Chap. 23). This makes this block ideal for shoulder surgery, since it provides a dense sensorimotor block in the early postoperative period, while motor function returns to the hand after approximately 36 h and only after 60 h in the shoulder area. The sensory block and analgesia are present for as long as the infusion is used. The motor block virtually "tapers off" as the need for it subsides over time.

The administration of local anesthetic can be reduced after 1 or 2 days of continuous infusion, as the need for motor function increases and the need for analgesia decreases. The progressive decrease of the infusion rate and concentration of local anesthetic agent not only decreases the risk of local anesthetic toxicity but also lowers the need to refill the infusion reservoir. Another way of achieving this tapering effect, especially if increased motor function is required for physical therapy, would be to refill the half-empty reservoir with saline after every 24 h so that the concentration of local anesthetic is halved every day. This method has not yet been formally evaluated in clinical studies.

Other major shoulder operations, such as sinovectomy and debridement, are managed in a similar way.

"FROZEN SHOULDER"

Patients with primary adhesive capsulitis or primary frozen shoulder pose special problems. Frozen shoulder is a chronic fibrosing condition of the shoulder joint capsule. Its histologic pathology and biochemical pathway are similar to those of Dupuytren's disease, which lead to Dupuytren's contracture. The latter is, however, a progressive condition, while primary frozen shoulder is a self-limiting disorder that resolves fully with time. There is also evidence that primary frozen shoulder is a sympathetic dystrophy, having the characteristics of an algoneurodystrophic process similar to that of complex regional pain syndrome (CRPS).

Whatever the cause or association, there is anecdotal evidence that anesthesiologists should be cautious in dealing with primary frozen shoulder. In a yet unpublished series of 4700 continuous interscalene blocks for shoulder surgery, we encountered 14 patients who developed postoperative neuropathic pain. Of these 14 patients, 10 had received continuous interscalene blocks for arthroscopic capsulotomy for primary frozen shoulder. A theoretical explanation for this may be that the shoulder "freezes" in the neutral position of abduction, flexion, and internal rotation while the patient carries the arm at the side. This causes the scapula to rotate and cause a condition of "pseudowinging of the scapula." Because the distance between the coracoid process and the cervical vertebrae, where the brachial plexus is relatively "fixed," increases, it causes chronic traction on the brachial plexus. This, in turn, will cause shoulder pain due to ischemia and irritation of the brachial plexus, which may be especially vulnerable where the nerves cross the first rib. Although this is speculative, it may be conceivable that this point of maximum irritation also happens to be where the catheter for continuous interscalene block is placed. The additional volume here is thought to cause further irritation or ischemia of the already irritated nerves. Since we started using CCPVB for adhesive capsulitis, we have not encountered this postoperative course again.

The CCPVB is placed more proximal and away from the area of stress, which may explain why postoperative neuropathy has not yet been encountered when the CCPVB is used for primary frozen shoulder.

In the rehabilitation of primary frozen shoulder, it is essential that the patient be totally free of pain and that there be no or very little motor block, so that the patient can participate in physical therapy. For that reason low concentrations (0.1%) of ropivacaine should be used. We use low infusion rates varying from 1 to 3 mL/h of 0.1% ropivacaine and allow 5- to 10-mL PCRA boluses at a 60 min lockout time. This gives excellent analgesia with no or very little motor block.

Intraoperative

SURGICAL REQUIREMENTS

The positioning of the patient on the operating table should be done carefully. Nerve injury due to brachial plexus traction is probably more common than is appreciated. The surgeon needs complete access to the shoulder, and it is important to supply muscle relaxation with neuromuscular blocking agents or a dense sensorimotor nerve block.

ANESTHETIC TECHNIQUE

There are numerous approaches to anesthesia for shoulder surgery, and each technique should be tailored to the surgical and patient requirements. Short operations performed by confident and dexterous surgeons can easily be done under nerve block only, while longer operations usually require general anesthesia. It is important to remember that, for shoulder surgery, the airway cannot be reached should it be "lost" during heavy sedation. We therefore use regional anesthesia with only very light sedation or formal general anesthesia.

Our practice is to place appropriate blocks before the induction of anesthesia, although some authorities place blocks after general anesthesia has been induced. It is debatable if this should be done or not, but our argument is that the placement of blocks should not be painful or uncomfortable, and it is therefore not necessary to have patients unconscious for this purpose. Anxiety is probably the most important reason for pain with the placement of blocks, and unless painful conditions, such as fractures, are present, we make liberal use of anxiolytic drugs like midazolam or alprazolam to place blocks.

We typically induce anesthesia with propofol and maintain it with a continuous infusion of propofol. To maintain normocapnia, we ventilate the patient's lungs with intermittent positive-pressure ventilation (IPPV) with air in oxygen via a laryngeal mask airway (LMA). If there is any doubt about the suitability of the LMA for a particular patient, we insert an endotracheal tube.

If a nerve block was not placed for some reason, we use a continuous infusion of remifentanil in addition to the above regimen. Among the many anesthetic techniques that are appropriate for shoulder surgery, we have found that the above approach gives us excellent results.

CONTROL OF THE SURGICAL FIELD

Arthroscopic shoulder surgery is one of the situations where the anesthesiologist can greatly help to improve the quality of the surgical field and ultimately the outcome of surgery.

For *"open" shoulder surgery*, intraoperative bleeding is mainly from veins and capillaries. We use the beach-chair position to promote venous drainage, while the propofol and remifentanil combination decreases the cardiac output slightly and therefore reduces blood flow to the tissue. This may cause a drop in blood pressure, and the flow through the tissue can be reduced further by causing peripheral vasoconstriction with a continuous infusion of small doses of phenylephrine. The combination of propofol and remifentanil reduces cardiac output and, combined with peripheral vasoconstriction, will provide excellent bloodless surgical conditions while normotension is maintained. The same effect can be achieved if the propofol and remifentanil are replaced by isoflurane and fentanyl, for example.

A short acting beta-adrenergic blocking agent, such as esmolol, can also be used to achieve the same results.

Continuous infusion of esmolol, a beta$_1$-selective antagonist with no intrinsic sympathomimetic activity and zero membrane-stabilizing activity, decrease cardiac output, and this will initiate a peripheral alpha-adrenergic response with precapillary arteriolar constriction via the baroreceptor mechanism. The resulting and slight controlled cardiac depression and peripheral vasoconstriction are similar to that achieved with propofol/remifentanil combined with phenylephrine or isoflurane/fentanyl combined with phenylephrine. The cerebral vasculature has very few alpha-adrenergic receptors; under normotensive conditions and with the patient's head elevated in the beach-chair position, this technique should increase the cerebral blood flow (decrease intracranial pressure due to upright position and normotension).

In elderly patients it may be disadvantageous to decrease the cardiac output even slightly. It is therefore our practice to monitor the cardiac output continuously if this technique is employed. A HemoSonic (Arrow International, Reading, PA) transesophageal or other noninvasive cardiac output-monitoring device is ideal for this purpose. As long as the cardiac output remains normal, the cardiac afterload can safely be increased with drugs like phenylephrine.

During *arthroscopic shoulder surgery* it may be necessary to reduce the systolic arterial pressure slightly. Morrison and coworkers have demonstrated that the visual clarity of the surgical field during shoulder arthroscopy is based on the pressure at which bleeding is observed from trabecular bone or the soft tissue capillaries. They found a direct correlation between the systolic blood pressure (SBP), subacromial space pressure (SASP), and the clarity of the visual field. Maintaining a pressure difference between SBP and SASP of 49 mmHg or less prevented bleeding and permitted good visualization. With a greater differential, significant bleeding occurred. Furthermore, the use of relative systolic hypotension permitted lower irrigation pressures and significantly reduced the risk of fluid extravasation into the subcutaneous tissue of the shoulder. The intraarticular pressure during arthroscopic shoulder surgery is typically kept between 70 and 100 mmHg. We therefore maintain the systolic pressure at or around 120 mmHg during arthroscopic shoulder surgery if the condition of the patient permits it. Communication between surgeon and anesthesiologist here, as in so many other situations, is essential. This can make a big difference in the surgical outcome.

Postoperative

ANALGESIA

Apart from the usual postoperative care, postoperative analgesia by continuous or single-injection nerve blocks is optimal (see Chaps. 20, 21, and 23). If it is not possible for some reason to place a nerve block, intravenous patient-controlled analgesia (PCA) with morphine sulfate or another suitable agent should be used at a minimum. Patients who have undergone shoulder surgery are ideal candidates for ambulatory continuous nerve blocks (see Chap. 21).

▶ POSTOPERATIVE PROTOCOL

Nursing Requirements

A main advantage of performing shoulder procedures under regional anesthesia (or a combined technique) is the rapid recovery and functioning of patients. Most patients can be treated on a 23-h observation basis; in some centers, outpatient arthroplasty procedures are being performed. Patients can be rapidly mobilized to sitting, eating, and independent ambulation. While the extremity is anesthetized and immobilized, care must be taken to avoid undue pressure on the medial epicondyle and wrist and the associated ulnar, superficial radial, and median nerves. Placing a pillow or soft pad about these areas will prevent such injuries. The arm should be positioned so that the elbow is kept anterior to the midaxillary line so as to prevent excessive strain of the anterior soft tissues of the shoulder. A simple pillow under the elbow while the patient is supine will prevent this.

Ambulation

Immediate ambulation once the patient is alert is encouraged so as to prevent atelectasis and deep venous thrombosis. As long as the arm is in the shoulder immobilizer, walking activities are not limited. If the patient uses a wheelchair or walker, the operated extremity cannot be used for weight bearing.

Physiotherapy

The postoperative rehabilitation program in many ways is just as important as the surgical procedure itself. Within the first 24 h, passive exercises of the shoulder, such as pendulum motions, are started. The presence of a brachial plexus nerve block does not preclude this. Passive elevation of the shoulder is also started 1 to 7 days after surgery, and active motion of the elbow, wrist, and hand is started immediately. Active motion of the shoulder is usually limited for the first month, particularly external rotation. In general terms, the first month of rehabilitation concentrates on passive motion of the shoulder, the second month on active motion, and the third month on strengthening exercise of the shoulder. Most patients undergo some form of supervised therapy program for 3 to 6 months after surgery.

▶ COMMON COMPLICATIONS

Fortunately, the majority of series have indicated a high success rate with shoulder arthroplasty procedures, with greater than 90 percent excellent results achieved at 5-year follow-up. Component loosening of the glenoid has been noted radiographically and occurs over time in as many as 30 percent of patients, but this has been a clinical problem in only a small fraction. Periprosthetic fractures have occurred at a rate of 2 percent in elderly osteoporotic patients, as noted intraoperatively and after falls in the postoperative period. As with other major joint replacements, infection occurs less than 1 percent of the time. Nerve injuries of the axillary, musculocutaneous, ulnar, radial, and median nerves have been reported. The incidence is much less than 1 percent and is typically related to excessive traction or intraoperative retraction of soft tissues. The majority of these problems resolve within 6 months.

SUGGESTED FURTHER READING

Azar FM, Wright PE II. Arthroplasty of the shoulder and elbow, in Canale ST (ed): *Campbell's Operative Othopaedics*, 10th ed. Philadelphia: Mosby, 2003:483–533.

Craig EV. The shoulder, in *Master Techniques in Orthopaedic Surgery,* 2d ed. Philadelphia: Lippincott Williams & Wilkins, 2004.

Morrison DS, Schaefer RK, Friedman RL. The relationship between subacromial space pressure, blood pressure, and visual clarity during arthroscopic subacromial decompression. *Arthroscopy* 11(5):557–560, 1995.

Rockwood CA, Matsen FA III. *The Shoulder,* 2d ed. Philadelphia: Saunders, 1998.

CHAPTER 8

The Elbow Joint

BRIAN D. ADAMS/ANDRÉ P. BOEZAART

▶ INTRODUCTION

Elective elbow surgery is usually an outpatient procedure except for more complex reconstructions performed for arthritis or posttraumatic conditions. Common outpatient procedures include ulnar nerve transposition for cubital tunnel syndrome, procedures for lateral epicondylitis, olecranon bursectomy, arthrotomy with radial head resection or other joint debridement for arthritis, and arthroscopy for loose-body removal and joint debridement. Complex procedures that require postoperative hospitalization include capsule release for joint contractures, corrective osteotomy for malunion, and joint replacement. The duration of outpatient procedures range from 30 min to 2 h. The majority of patients undergoing these procedures are healthy. Conversely, some patients undergoing complex elbow surgery may be debilitated from rheumatoid arthritis and/or advanced age.

Biomechanics of the Elbow Joint

The elbow joint is essentially a hinge, with the primary articulation between the trochlea of the distal humerus and the olecranon of the ulna, which allows approximately 140 degrees flexion. The elbow also includes the proximal articulation between the radius and ulna and that between the radius and the capitellum of the distal humerus. These articulations in combination with the distal radioulnar joint allow forearm rotation, which is about 160 degrees. Because the elbow's articulations are highly congruous, this joint is particularly prone to stiffness from articular damage due to trauma or arthritis. Ligament complexes on the medial and lateral aspects of the elbow provide additional joint stability. Powerful muscles originating from the humerus and shoulder region drive elbow motion. These muscles include the biceps, brachialis, and triceps. Other muscles that originate from the distal humerus contribute to both elbow and forearm movement, including the brachioradialis and the forearm flexor and extensor muscle wads. Although less common than stiffness, joint instability from cumulative ligamentous injury (especially of the medial collateral ligament) is a well-recognized condition in throwing athletes.

▶ ANATOMIC CONSIDERATIONS OF ELBOW SURGERY

Surgical Anatomy

The ulnar, median, and radial nerves that supply both motor and sensory innervation to the forearm and hand cross the elbow joint at different locations (Fig. 8-1). Several cutaneous nerves also cross the elbow or terminate near it. The terminal branches of the medial, lateral, and posterior brachial cutaneous nerves supply cutaneous sensation about the elbow. In addition, branches of the medial, lateral, and posterior antebrachial cutaneous nerves may have early branches about the elbow. Thus, there is abundant and redundant cutaneous innervation to the elbow region. Following Hilton's law that any nerve crossing a joint innervates the joint, the elbow joint is also abundantly supplied, with the potential for any of the above-named nerves to supply branches to the joint.

The ulnar nerve has minimal protection by soft tissue at the elbow. It lies behind the medial intermuscular septum in the midarm and then passes through a fibroosseous groove behind the medial epicondyle. The depth of the when the patient uses immunosuppressive drugs. Regional anesthesia is typically preferred to reduce the overall anesthetic risk and improve postoperative pain management. A continuous nerve block is used during the initial postoperative period and extended throughout the hospitalization, which is typically 48 h.

For capsule resection and extensive joint debridement, the patient is supine with the extremity either positioned on a hand table or flexed over the chest, depending on the surgical approach and surgeon's preference.

Elbow Arthroplasty

Surgical Options

Interpositional and implant are the two types of arthroplasty used. *Implant arthroplasties* are engineered as "constrained," "semiconstrained," and "unconstrained," depending on the rigidity with which the humeral component is fixed to the ulnar component. Because of the tendency to loosen and break, the constrained prosthesis is rarely used. *Interpositional arthroplasty* refers to the placement of fascia between the articular or surfaces of the joint, which is usually the triceps fascia or fascia lata.

The primary indications for total elbow arthroplasty are pain, instability, and bilateral elbow ankylosis. Another indication is rheumatoid arthritis with roentgenographic evidence of joint destruction that is too far advanced to benefit from radial head excision and sinovectomy, especially in patients whose activities are limited by painful instability and stiffness. Deformity or dysfunction without pain are not indications for arthroplasty. Similarly, weakness and discomfort due to instability are relative indications, especially in patients with posttraumatic arthritis.

Authors' Technique

Total elbow joint replacement (Fig. 8-2) is usually performed with the patient supine, a small pad placed under the ipsilateral scapula, and the extremity positioned over the chest. A dorsal surgical approach is used. During the initial dissection, the ulnar nerve is released and transposed anterior to the medial epicondyle. Division, lifting, or splitting of the triceps tendon exposes the joint. The collateral ligaments are released and the joint is dislocated to complete the exposure. Using special cutting guides, the distal humerus and proximal ulna are cut. The medullary canals of the two bones are prepared with broaches. Implant trials are inserted and the joint is tested for range of motion and stability. Additional soft tissue releases may be needed to achieve maximum motion. The final implant is inserted with cement (see Chap. 33), which is typically impregnated with antibiotic. Cementation for elbow replacement is rarely associated with blood pressure reductions, as reported for total hip replacement. The triceps tendon is

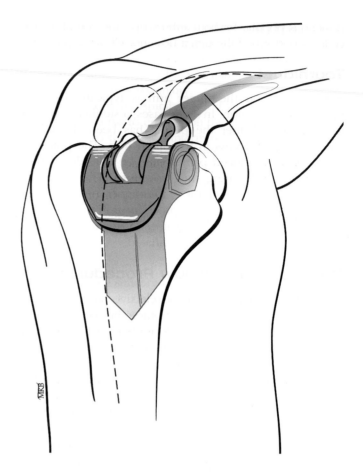

Figure 8-2. Total elbow arthroplasty.

repaired and the skin closed. A suction drain is inserted to prevent hematoma formation; however, overall blood loss does not usually exceed 250 mL. A bulky sterile dressing incorporating a plaster splint is applied.

▶ ANESTHETIC CONSIDERATIONS

Preoperative

Many patients suffer from rheumatoid arthritis and multiple organ system involvement. Side effects of drugs used to treat rheumatoid arthritis must be appreciated in planning the anesthesia, which include the effects of steroid and nonsteroidal anti-inflammatory therapy on coagulation and adrenal function. Methotrexate can cause bone marrow suppression and liver cirrhosis. Anticytokine therapy may cause inhibition of tumor necrosis factor but does not have any implications for anesthesia. Corticosteroids are frequently used and can subject the patient to higher risks of osteoporosis, infection, myopathy, and poor wound healing. The immunosuppressive agents cyclophosphamide and azathioprine are also frequently used to treat rheumatoid arthritis and may also lead to a higher incidence of infection.

Airway management may be difficult in these patients. Flexion deformity of the cervical spine may lead to airway obstruction during induction of anesthesia, while atlantoaxial subluxation may increase the risk of cervical spinal cord compression or interfere with blood flow in the vertebral artery. Furthermore, limited temporomandibular joint mobility may impair visualization of the vocal cords during direct laryngoscopy. Cricoarytenoid inflammation and arthritis may obstruct the view of the glottic opening during direct laryngoscopy and cause postextubaton laryngeal obstruction. Fiberoptic intubation in the awake patient, a laryngeal mask airway (LMA), or regional anesthesia with or without mild sedation may have to be considered.

Preoperative pulmonary function tests and blood gas and pH analysis may be necessary if severe lung disease due to rheumatoid arthritis is suspected. The need for postoperative ventilatory support should be anticipated if a patient has severe restrictive lung disease.

Nerve Block

Elbow surgery is very often performed under regional anesthesia alone, for which many blocks of the brachial plexus have been promoted (see Chaps. 23, 24, and 25). It should, however, be kept in mind that for complete surgical anesthesia of the elbow, complete block of the entire brachial plexus is required. If a tourniquet is used, the branches of the intercostobrachial nerve to the inner upper arm must also be blocked. It is therefore our practice to use a single injection infraclavicular block of all three brachial plexus cords (see Chap. 24) for minor surgery to the elbow. Supraclavicular block (see Chap. 23) is also useful, and in both instances the branches of the intercostobrachial nerve usually have to be blocked separately, although this may not be necessary with the supraclavicular block.

Single-injection blocks should probably not be used routinely for major elbow surgery since they do not contribute anything to the relief of postoperative pain, which is usually severe. Arguably, single-injection blocks may even worsen situations, because the patient may awake alone in the middle of the night following surgery and with severe unmanageable pain. Readmission for pain management is common in these situations and counterproductive if cost-effective surgery and pain management are goals of ambulatory surgery. Continuous supraclavicular block may be of value, but again, it is important to block the entire brachial plexus to achieve anesthesia and analgesia for major surgery to the elbow. Our experience is that distal brachial plexus blocks (supraclavicular, infraclavicular and axillary blocks) provide excellent surgical anesthesia after the initial large bolus dose of local anesthetic agent. However, when used as a continuous block, the catheter settles on one of the cords or terminal branches of the brachial plexus and provides incomplete analgesia during the days after the surgery, since small volumes and lower concentrations

of local anesthetic agents are infused. Our practice is therefore to use a continuous cervical paravertebral block (see Chap. 23) for major elbow surgery, which blocks all roots of the brachial plexus, to provide anesthesia for the procedure and postoperative analgesia.

Intraoperative

Intraoperatively, special care should be taken to protect vulnerable nerves against compression by using appropriate padding, since this surgery can last for 3 to 4 h. Furthermore, the eyes and pressure points of patients with rheumatoid arthritis should receive special attention.

If the surgery is anticipated to last a long time, general anesthesia or deep sedation is considered. Our practice when the surgery is to last longer than 2 h is to use an infusion of propofol with a LMA and controlled ventilation in the presence of a solid cervical paravertebral block. In case of poor pulmonary compliance due to restrictive lung disease, tracheal intubation is used. For shorter operations, a block of the entire brachial plexus with or without sedation will provide excellent surgical conditions. For sedation, our practice is to use varying doses of midazolam in combination of small doses of meperidine. In addition to the usual monitoring, the patient's respiration should be monitored throughout by capnography via a divided cannula. Modern noise-cancellation headphones with soothing music of the patient's choice go a long way toward comforting the patient during surgery.

Because a tourniquet is used during most or all of the surgery, it is not necessary for the anesthesiologist to participate in controlling the quality of the surgical field.

Postoperative

Patients who have undergone day-case ambulatory surgery under peripheral nerve block anesthesia should be instructed in how to care for the anesthetized limb and to prevent trauma to vulnerable nerves (see Chap. 32). They should also be instructed to start taking oral analgesic medication before the effects of the block wear off. If severe pain follows the surgery and discharge from the hospital, single-injection blocks are inappropriate treatment. Instead, patients are discharged with continuous blocks in place (see Chap. 21).

A main feature of modern orthopaedic anesthesia is the treatment of acute postoperative pain with continuous nerve blocks. There are very few instances in which this cannot be offered. If such cases do occur, intravenous patient-controlled morphine sulfate should be offered as an absolute minimum. Continuous peripheral nerve blocks should be adjusted continuously to the patient's analgesic and physical therapy needs on an individual basis and should be discontinued only when the patient no longer requires the continuous block (see Chap. 21).

▶ POSTOPERATIVE PROTOCOL (ARTHROPLASTY)

After total elbow arthroplasty, patients are hospitalized for 48 h for pain control, antibiotics, bandage change, and initial rehabilitation. The bandages are changed on the morning of the second postoperative day, after which the patient is seen in the physiotherapy department for fabrication of a thermoplastic elbow splint and instruction in gentle exercises. When an anesthetic catheter is used for regional anesthesia, it is typically retained until the second day, at which time the patient's analgesic regimen is converted to oral analgesics.

The goals of reconstructive elbow surgery are to restore function through the relief of pain and the restoration of motion and stability.

▶ COMMON COMPLICATIONS

Excessive swelling with persistent drainage are the most common problems after elbow arthroplasty in the first week. Wound dehiscence can occur if swelling is severe and aggressive motion is started too early. Stiffness of the elbow is sometimes prolonged, requiring formal rehabilitation. Light use of the hand is allowed within a few days. Depending on the condition of the triceps tendon, general use of the arm begins after 6 weeks. Implant loosening is the greatest long-term concern. The infection rate for elbow replacement is slightly higher than for other major joint replacements.

SUGGESTED FURTHER READING

Ayoub CM, Rizk LB, Yaacoub CI, et al. Music and ambient operating room noise in patients undergoing spinal anesthesia. *Anesth Analg* 100:1316–319, 2005.

Dellon AL. Review of treatment results for ulnar nerve entrapment at the elbow. *J Hand Surg* 14A:688–700, 1989.

Morrey BF, Adams RA. Semiconstrained elbow replacement for rheumatoid arthritis. *J Bone Joint Surg* 74A:479, 1992.

Nirschl RP, Pettrone F. Tennis elbow: The surgical treatment of lateral epicondylitis. *J Bone Joint Surg* 61A:832, 1979.

O'Driscoll SW, Morrey BF. Arthroscopy of the elbow: Diagnostic and therapeutic benefits and hazards. *J Bone Joint Surg* 74A:84–94, 1992.

CHAPTER 9

The Wrist Joint

BRIAN D. ADAMS/ANDRÉ P. BOEZAART

▶ INTRODUCTION

Wrist surgery typically involves outpatient procedures performed on healthy people. The most common procedures are performed for the treatment of ganglion cysts, benign tumors, and tendinitis. The surgical time in these cases is usually less than 1 h. Complex procedures are typically done for fractures and arthritis, which last from 1 to 4 h and may require postoperative hospitalization for pain control, neurovascular monitoring, and antibiotic administration. The occasional patient undergoing wrist surgery may be debilitated, with the most common associated condition being systemic arthritis from rheumatoid disease.

▶ BIOMECHANICS OF THE WRIST JOINT

The wrist joint is a complex articulate structure involving the distal radius, distal ulna, and seven carpal bones plus the pisiform bone. It comprises multiple intercarpal joints as well as the distal radioulnar joint. The stability of these articulations is provided by a multitude of small ligaments, some of which must withstand strong forces during strenuous activities. The primary function of the wrist is to provide a movable yet stable platform for the hand. Twenty-four tendons cross the wrist to supply stability, power, and movement to it and the fingers. There is little soft tissue coverage for the important neurovascular structures as they cross the wrist into the hand. Because of its demanding functional requirements and constant exposure to extreme conditions, the wrist is particularly susceptible to injury in all age groups.

▶ ANATOMIC CONSIDERATIONS OF WRIST SURGERY

Surgical Anatomy

The wrist joint and its surrounding soft tissues are abundantly innervated by the median, ulnar, radial, and lateral antebrachial cutaneous nerves, including their major branches, which are the anterior interosseous, posterior interosseous, dorsal branch of the ulnar nerve, and superficial radial nerve (Fig. 9-1). Anesthesiologists who perform peripheral nerve blocks for wrist surgery or postoperative pain relief, even for a simple ganglion excision, should recognize that the entire brachial plexus is involved in the innervation of the wrist and, for that matter, all major joints of the upper limb. Thus, there is no place for selective peripheral nerve blocks in surgery of the wrist joint or any other major joint of the upper limb.

The superficial branch of the radial nerve (SRN) emerges from beneath the dorsal edge of the brachioradialis tendon approximately 6 cm proximal to the radial styloid. It begins branching immediately, with several sensory branches proceeding to the dorsal aspects of the thumb, first web space, and index finger. Although primarily a cutaneous sensory nerve, it sends branches to the radiocarpal joint and the first and second carpometacarpal joints to a variable extent.

The posterior interosseous nerve (PIN) is also a branch of the radial nerve, which lies on the posterior surface of the interosseous membrane in the distal forearm. All of its motor branches, which supply the extensors of the wrist and fingers, are given off within the proximal two-thirds of the forearm. After crossing the midline of the wrist joint dorsally, the PIN gives branches to the radiocarpal, intercarpal, and the second, third, and

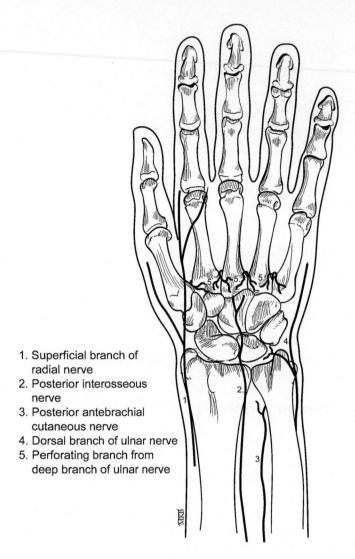

1. Superficial branch of radial nerve
2. Posterior interosseous nerve
3. Posterior antebrachial cutaneous nerve
4. Dorsal branch of ulnar nerve
5. Perforating branch from deep branch of ulnar nerve

Figure 9-1. Nerves around the wrist joint.

fourth carpometacarpal joints. The PIN is the main articular nerve on the dorsal aspect of the wrist.

The median nerve emerges from beneath the flexor digitorum superficialis in the distal forearm and then passes through the carpal tunnel. The palmar cutaneous branch takes off from the nerve proper approximately 4 to 6 cm proximal to the wrist crease. It supplies sensibility to variable extents to the proximal aspects of the thenar eminence and midpalm and may occasionally send a branch to the region of the distal scaphoid. The median nerve does not have direct articular branches.

The anterior interosseous nerve (AIN) is a branch of the median nerve, which lies on the anterior surface of the interosseous membrane. It supplies branches to the digital flexors in the proximal and midforearm and the pronator quadratus muscle in the distal forearm. Terminal branches of the AIN supply the distal radius bone and the radiocarpal and distal radioulnar joints.

At approximately the pisiform bone, the ulnar nerve divides into the deep motor branch, the sensory branch, and a small articular branch to the pisotriquetral joint. The sensory branch provides sensibility to the ulnar third of the palm and the palmar surfaces of the small finger and ulnar half of the ring finger. The motor branch innervates multiple intrinsic muscles of the hand, including the hypothenar, interosseous, two ulnar lumbricals, and adductor pollicis. The dorsal branch of the ulnar nerve branches from the ulnar nerve proper approximately 6 to 8 cm proximal to the wrist. It provides sensibility to approximately the ulnar third of the dorsal aspects of the hand and wrist, including the dorsum of the entire small finger and the ulnar half of the ring finger. Despite being considered primarily a sensory nerve, it has articular branches to the articulation between the carpus and the distal ulna, the distal radioulnar joint, and the fourth and fifth carpometacarpal joints.

The lateral antebrachial cutaneous nerve is a branch of the musculocutaneous nerve. It emerges from the lateral margin of the biceps tendon near the elbow and passes through the forearm toward the middorsal wrist. Its cutaneous supply on the dorsum of the wrist and hand is quite variable but is usually radial to the branches of the superficial radial nerve. There are consistent articular branches to the radiocarpal and first carpometacarpal joints.

The medial antebrachial cutaneous nerve is a direct branch from the medial cord of the brachial plexus. Although its branches usually terminate in the forearm, they occasionally extend to the ulnar aspect of the wrist, including articular branches.

The posterior antebrachial cutaneous nerve is a direct branch from the posterior cord of the brachial plexus. Its branches typically terminate in the posterior aspect of the forearm but occasionally extend to posterior aspect of the wrist, including radiocarpal articular branches.

▶ SURGICAL PROCEDURES

Positioning on the Operating Table

Wrist surgery is performed with the patient's arm on a hand table, which requires shoulder abduction and elbow extension. This position may be difficult or uncomfortable for some patients.

Tourniquet

A tourniquet placed on the upper arm or forearm is nearly always used in wrist surgery to improve visualization. The position of the tourniquet often depends on the surgeon's preference. Many surgeons prefer a tourniquet on the forearm for simple procedures of short duration because patients report less discomfort at this site. Regardless of the tourniquet site, the patient will often complain of pain fairly quickly when it is inflated if the regional anesthesia does not extend to this level. The generally accepted safe duration for an upper extremity tourniquet is 2 h.

Common Basic Wrist Procedures

Common indications for basic surgery of the wrist are ganglion cysts, benign tumors, and tendinitis. Arthroscopy is also a common procedure that is minimally invasive. Because these are elective and ambulatory procedures, patients rarely have unstable medical problems. In fact, if the preoperative evaluation reveals substantial medical problems, the procedure should probably be postponed.

The surgical tissue penetration may extend to or through the joint capsule, but it is limited to small areas and does not involve bone. Thus, the intraoperative and postoperative analgesia requirements are usually predictable and straightforward. Depending on the extent and duration of the operation and the patient's comorbidities, some surgeons use a single dose of prophylactic antibiotics, usually cephazolin. When regional anesthesia is used, excessive sedation should be avoided so that the patient does not become disoriented and uncooperative. Less sedation also allows more rapid discharge from the postsurgical recovery unit. Many surgeons and anesthesiologists prefer ketorolac in the immediate postoperative period for young healthy patients.

When wrist arthroscopy is being performed, the patient's arm is typically held by a traction device, sometimes referred to as the traction tower, which is placed on top of the hand table. The upper arm is strapped to the base of the traction tower, the elbow is flexed 90 degrees, and the hand is held in vertical position by finger traps applied to two or more digits. Wrist joint distraction is applied by mechanisms built into the device, allowing the scope and other instruments to be inserted through small portals in the dorsum of the wrist. Various instruments are used to perform debridement or repair damaged tissue. Depending on the anesthetic method, local anesthetic can be administered by the surgeon at the portal sites and within the joint as needed. Postoperative management depends on specifics of the procedure. If only debridement was performed, a soft dressing or simple plaster splint is applied. When a ligament repair is done, a more encompassing plaster splint is often applied to the limb.

Analgesics given on the patient's discharge range from ibuprofen to oral narcotics, sometimes in combination with mild sedatives such as hydroxyzine. Discharge instructions include elevation of the arm for 2 to 5 days, limitation of grasp, and limitation of repetitive use of the hand. However, light use of the hand for daily activities

and clerical work is often permitted by the second postoperative day. Patients return after 10 to 14 days for wound inspection, removal of sutures, and instructions for progressive use of the hand. If oral analgesics are still used, they are weaned at this time. Formal rehabilitation is rarely necessary.

Complex Wrist Procedures

Complex wrist surgery is most commonly performed for trauma and arthritis (see Chaps. 8 and 16). Trauma involves all age groups, with causes ranging from simple falls in the elderly to severe industrial injuries in young adults. Many wrist injuries are emergency cases, including open fractures with contamination and crush injuries or deep lacerations with vascular compromise of the hand. Although elderly patients with wrist fractures have in the past been treated nonoperatively, there is a modern trend toward open reduction and internal fixation of fractures in this age group as well because these individuals are increasingly requesting treatment that will allow them to resume a relatively high level of activity. Since they often have comorbidities and yet the injury requires modestly urgent operative treatment, their preoperative evaluation and management must be expedited. In some cases, this urgency necessitates compromises that are not made in elective surgery. Younger patients with wrist injuries can be difficult due to lack of medical compliance, both pre- and postoperatively.

In the younger age group, distal radius fractures are classically high-energy injuries resulting from motor vehicle accidents. Although a case may be scheduled in an ambulatory surgical setting, other serious injuries may compromise the patient's overall medical condition. Young and middle-aged people are more prone than older people to attempt suicide by deep wrist lacerations. If vascular compromise of the hand is apparent, emergency care is required. However, in attempted suicides, the possibility of altered mental and physical states due to an overdose of medications, illicit drugs, or alcohol must be recognized.

Arthritis is the other common broad indication for wrist surgery, the most common procedures being joint denervation, resection of the proximal row of carpal bones, fusion of a portion of the carpus, fusion of the entire wrist, or wrist joint replacement. Although wrist joint replacement has in the past been prone to early failure, new implant designs have shown durability similar to those of hip and knee prostheses (Fig. 9-1). Because wrist procedures for arthritis can be lengthy, proper precautions to protect against nerve compression and pressure points should be taken. Patients with arthritis may find it difficult or impossible to have their arm positioned optimally for surgery. A semirecumbent or semilateral decubitus position may be necessary for proper positioning of the wrist and the patient's comfort. Alternatively, the surgeon can compromise by operating with the wrist elevated on top of a sterile bolster. Arthritic patients are usually taking anti-inflammatory medications, which pose potential risks of excessive bleeding during surgery and anesthetic procedures. In addition, these patients often have morbidities associated with systemic arthritis and general debilitation due to older age.

Wrist Arthroplasty

Although total wrist replacement (Fig. 9-2) is perhaps the most complex elective wrist procedure, the perioperative anesthesia and surgical care are similar to those used in other extensive wrist procedures. The indication for wrist replacement is severe arthritis in a patient with relatively low physical demands who wishes to retain wrist motion but is willing to accept permanent restrictions on

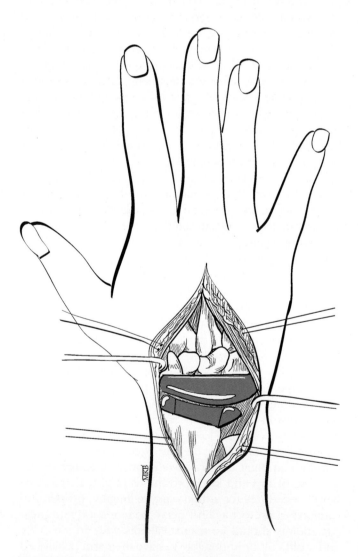

Figure 9-2. Total wrist arthroplasty.

activity. These patients often have severe generalized arthritis from rheumatoid disease, which is associated with many comorbidities including instability of the cervical spine (see Chap. 8). Preoperative radiographs of the neck in flexion-extension are therefore recommended, as is careful management of the neck during surgery, especially if intubation is required. Patients may need additional padding on the operating table to reduce the risk of pressure sores. Special needs related to the chronic use of corticosteroids should be recognized and managed by additional dosage given perioperatively. Preoperative prophylactic antibiotics are nearly always employed, especially when the patient uses immunosuppressive medication. Regional anesthesia is typically preferred to reduce the overall anesthetic risk and improve postoperative pain management.

Authors' Technique

The procedure is performed through a dorsal skin incision, which is about 4 in. long. The extensor retinaculum is reflected to allow retraction of the tendons. The entire dorsal capsule is raised to provide a wide exposure of the joint. Using special jigs and instruments under fluoroscopic control, the articular surfaces of the distal radius and a portion of the carpus are resected. Dedicated drill guides and broaches are used to prepare the bones to accept the implant's stems and screws. The implant may be inserted with or without cement, depending on bone quality and the surgeon's preference. When bone cement is used, the amount is very small, and it is not subjected to the high intramedullary pressures, that have been reported to cause blood pressure reductions (see Chap. 33). After implantation, joint stability and range of motion are tested. The joint capsule is repaired, the tendons and retinaculum are replaced, and the skin is closed. A suction drain is inserted to prevent hematoma formation. Overall blood loss is usually minimal. A bulky sterile dressing incorporating a plaster splint is applied. The patient is transferred to recovery with special care to support the wrist and provide strict elevation of the hand. The patient is hospitalized for 48 h for pain control, administration of antibiotics, bandage change, and initial rehabilitation. The bandages are changed on the morning of the second postoperative day, after which the patient is seen by the physiotherapist for fabrication of a thermoplastic wrist splint and instruction in gentle motion exercises. When a continuous peripheral nerve block is used, it is usually removed after the morning of the second day if the pain can be managed with oral medication, usually an oral analgesic (see Chap. 21).

Insufficient pain control and excessive swelling are the most common problems in the first week. Infection is rare. Stiffness of the hand and wrist is sometimes prolonged, requiring formal rehabilitation. Like other joint replacements, implant loosening is the greatest long-term complication of total wrist replacement.

▶ ANESTHETIC CONSIDERATIONS

Preoperative

These patients usually suffer from rheumatoid arthritis and multiple organ involvement. Its anesthetic implications and the drugs commonly used are discussed in Chap. 8.

Airway management may be difficult in these patients and is similar to that discussed for elbow surgery in Chap. 8.

Preoperative pulmonary function tests and blood gas and pH analysis may be necessary if severe lung disease due to rheumatoid arthritis is suspected. Postoperative ventilatory support is very rarely needed but should be anticipated if severe restrictive lung disease is present preoperatively.

Nerve Block

Wrist surgery is commonly performed under regional anesthesia alone. Many blocks of the brachial plexus have been promoted (see Chaps. 23, 24, and 25); however, it must be recognized that for complete surgical anesthesia of the wrist a complete block of the brachial plexus is required. Moreover, if a tourniquet is used, the branches of the intercostobrachial nerves to the inner upper arm must be blocked. It is therefore our practice to use a single injection infraclavicular block of all three brachial plexus cords (see Chap. 24) for basic surgery to the wrist. Supraclavicular block (see Chap. 23) is also useful, but in both instances the intercostobrachial nerves must be blocked separately.

Single-injection blocks should not be done for complex wrist surgery, since they do not contribute anything to the alleviation of postoperative pain, which is usually severe. Single-injection blocks may even complicate situations where severe pain is present since the patient may be alone in the middle of the night and wake up with severe, unmanageable pain. Readmission for pain management is common in these instances which is counterproductive if a goal of ambulatory surgery and acute pain management is to be cost-effective. Continuous supraclavicular block may be of value, but again, it is important to block the entire brachial plexus in order to achieve anesthesia and analgesia for major wrist surgery. It is our experience that distal brachial plexus blocks (supraclavicular, infraclavicular, and axillary blocks) provide excellent surgical anesthesia after the initial large bolus dose of local anesthetic. However, use of a continuous infraclavicular catheter may result in incomplete postoperative analgesia because the catheter may be placed

against only one of the cords or terminal branches of the brachial plexus, and the smaller volumes and lower concentrations of the local anesthetics will only block that cord or branch. It is therefore our practice to use a continuous cervical paravertebral block (see Chap. 23), which blocks all roots of the brachial plexus, for surgery and for postoperative analgesia.

Intraoperative

Because surgery can last 2 to 4 h or more, care should be taken to protect vulnerable nerves against compression by using appropriate padding. Furthermore, the eyes and pressure points of the patients with rheumatoid arthritis should receive special attention.

If the surgery is expected to last more than 2 h, general anesthesia or deep sedation is considered. In such cases, we use an infusion of propofol, a cervical paravertebral block with a laryngeal mask airway and controlled ventilation. In cases of poor pulmonary compliance due to restrictive lung disease, tracheal intubation is used. For shorter operations, a block of the entire brachial plexus with or without sedation will provide excellent surgical conditions. For sedation, we use varying doses of midazolam combined with small doses of meperidine. Sedation with propofol may be problematic, since light sedation may make patients uncooperative, while with deep sedation the airway may be compromised.

In addition to the usual monitoring, the patient's respiration should be monitored throughout by capnography via a divided cannula. Modern noise-cancellation headphones with soothing music of the patient's choice go a long way toward comforting the patient during surgery.

Because most or all of the surgery is done under tourniquet control of bleeding, it is not necessary for the anesthesiologist to participate in controlling the quality of the surgical field.

Postoperative

Patients who undergo day-case ambulatory surgery under peripheral nerve block anesthesia should be instructed in caring for the anesthetized limb and preventing trauma to the vulnerable nerves (see Chap. 32). They should also be instructed to start taking oral analgesic medication before the effects of the block wear off. If severe pain is experienced after the surgery and discharge from the hospital, single-injection blocks are probably inappropriate. Rather, patients can be discharged from the surgical facility or hospital with continuous blocks in place (see Chap. 21).

A main feature of modern orthopaedic anesthesia is the treatment of acute postoperative pain with continuous nerve blocks. There are very few instances in which this cannot be offered. In these rare cases, patient-controlled intravenous morphine sulfate should be offered at an absolute minimum. Continuous peripheral nerve blocks should constantly be adjusted to the patient's analgesic and physical therapy needs on an individual basis and should be discontinued when the patient no longer requires the continuous block (see Chap. 21).

SUGGESTED FURTHER READING

Divelbiss BJ, Sollerman C, Adams BD. Early results of the universal total wrist arthroplasty in rheumatoid arthritis. *J Hand Surg [Am]* 27:195–204, 2002.

Fukumoto K, Kojima T. An anatomic study of the innervation of the wrist joint and Wilhelm's technique for denervation. *J Hand Surg [Am]* 18:484–489, 1993.

CHAPTER 10
The Adult Hip Joint

MICHAEL R. O'ROURKE/JOHN J. CALLAGHAN/ANDRÉ P. BOEZAART

▶ INTRODUCTION

The goals of adult reconstructive surgery are to maintain optimal function, minimize disability, and remove pain. Diseases that affect the ability to walk obviously have a tremendous impact on our independence, ability to be productive, and general quality of life. In addition to locomotion, the hip joint has an important role in allowing other normal functions such as sitting, standing, bending to the floor, lifting objects, and dressing. Reconstructive surgery of the hip in adults encompasses surgical procedures to restore optimal function of the hip joint. The most common and successful surgical intervention has been total joint arthroplasty for arthritis of the hip; that is the primary focus of this chapter.

▶ ANATOMIC CONSIDERATIONS

Joint Anatomy

Developmental Anatomy
The acetabulum develops from the confluence of the ilium, pubis, and ischium. These three bones contribute to the triradiate cartilage, which forms the primary growth center of the acetabulum. Normal growth and development of the socket requires the presence of a round femoral head. If the femoral head is partially or completely dislocated, the acetabulum will be shallow and/or malformed. The proximal femur has a single epiphysis at birth that differentiates into the proximal femoral epiphysis (femoral head) and trochanteric apophysis (greater trochanter). The terminal branch of the medial circumflex artery (called the lateral ascending cervical artery) provides the primary blood supply to the femoral head. The hip joint is formed by the 11th week of gestation. The femoral epiphysis secondary ossification center is usually evident by 4 to 7 months of age and fuses to the femoral diaphysis on average at age 14 to 15 months in females and 17 to 18 months in males. The majority of the acetabular growth occurs by 8 years of age.

Capsule/Labrum/Synovium

The capsule of the hip joint is a specialized structure that allows motion and assists in stability of the hip joint. The normal hip joint has a suction effect created by the conformity between the articular surfaces, the labrum, and the hydrostatic forces of the synovial fluid layer. The capsule is composed of the iliofemoral ligament, pubofemoral ligament, ischiofemoral ligament, and zona orbicularis. The iliofemoral ligament (ligament of Bigelow) is a capsular thickening in the shape of an inverted Y that resists extension of the hip and is reported to be the strongest ligament in the body. In the arthritic hip, these ligamentous structures are abnormal and contribute to its limited motion. Traditionally, nearly the entire hip capsule was resected with the transtrochanteric approach to the hip. Resection of the hip capsule affects the stability of the hip after joint arthroplasty; therefore most modern approaches strive to preserve some portion or the complete capsule. In the posterior approach, repair of the capsulotomy has been associated with a decreased dislocation rate. In the anterolateral or anterior approach to the hip, dislocation is a less common problem and many surgeons remove the anterior capsule as part of the exposure of the hip joint.

Blood Supply

The obturator artery has three branches that supply the acetabulum. These include the acetabular artery (cotyloid fossa), preacetabular artery (pubis), and infraacetabular artery (inferior acetabular rim). The superior gluteal artery supplies the ilium through the supraacetabular artery branch as well as through the attachments from the gluteal muscular origins. The retroacetabular artery branches from the inferior gluteal artery to supply the posterior wall and ischium. There is a rich anastomotic network between the inferior gluteal artery, superior gluteal artery, medial and lateral circumflex arteries, and obturator artery.

The blood supply to the femoral head is more limited and is at risk during operative treatments and injuries of the hip. The medial circumflex artery (MCA) branches from the posteromedial aspect of the profunda femoris artery and courses between the pectineus muscle and iliopsoas muscle, emerging on the posterior aspect of the hip between the obturator externus and the quadratus femoris muscles. The MCA travels posteriorly to the obturator externus muscle insertion and penetrates the joint capsule between the obturator externus muscle and conjoint tendon. The lateral ascending cervical branches travel in the subsynovial fold to the intraarticular subcapital arterial ring and supply the blood flow to the femoral head. In the adult, when the epiphysis fuses to the neck, there is a medullary blood supply to the femoral head. The lateral circumflex artery has multiple penetrating arterioles into the metaphysis of the proximal femur and also supplies the greater trochanter.

Nerve Supply to the Hip Joint

Peripheral Nerve Contributions to the Hip Joint

The nerve supply to the hip joint is provided by the obturator, inferior gluteal, and superior gluteal nerves. The innervation of the capsule and synovium varies and is altered in pathologic conditions of the hip. The greatest concentration of nerve endings is in the anteroinferior aspect of the hip capsule. Some orthopaedic surgeons have proposed obturator nerve ablation for patients with refractory hip pain, but nociceptive innervation contributions also come from the superior and inferior gluteal nerves. In addition to the innervation of the periosteum, somatic and autonomic nerve fibers transverse the haversian canals of bone, with the highest concentration in the metaphyseal regions.

Obturator Branches

The obturator nerve is formed from the anterior division of L2 to L4 nerve roots. It travels with the obturator artery and vein medial to the quadrilateral plate and the obturator internus muscle, exiting the pelvis at the superolateral aspect of the obturator foramen.

Superior Gluteal Nerve

The superior gluteal nerve is formed from the posterior divisions of the L4 to L5 nerve roots. It exits the pelvis through the sciatic notch superior to the piriformis muscle and travels between the gluteus medius and gluteus minimus muscles approximately 4 to 5 cm superior to the greater trochanter. Articular branches supply the superior and anterior aspect of the hip joint capsule and acetabulum.

Inferior Gluteal Nerve

The inferior gluteal nerve is formed from the posterior divisions of the L5 to S1 nerve roots and exits the pelvis through the sciatic notch inferior to the piriformis muscle. It innervates the gluteus maximus muscle and the posterior aspect of the hip capsule and acetabulum.

Sciatic Nerve

The sciatic nerve is formed from the anterior (tibial) and posterior (peroneal) branches of the L4 to S3 nerve roots and usually courses anteriorly and medially to the piriformis muscle. There is a spatial orientation of the two common divisions (common peroneal and tibial), with the common peroneal nerve located laterally. The common peroneal division of the sciatic nerve is more susceptible to injury because it has two fixation points (sciatic notch and fibular head) and larger funiculi with less connective tissue. This makes it susceptible to traction injury.

Femoral Nerve

The femoral nerve is composed of the posterior divisions of the L2 to L4 nerve roots and travels between the iliacus and psoas muscles proximally and overlying the iliopsoas muscle, exiting the pelvis on the lateral side of the femoral triangle.

▶ SURGICAL ANATOMY

Approaches

Anterior

The anterior surgical approach is the only internervous anatomic approach to the hip joint. The advantages of this approach are exposure without violation of muscles, a relatively thin subcutaneous fat layer, and excellent visualization of the acetabulum for primary surgery. The disadvantages of the approach are increased difficulty in seeing the femur for preparation, inability to prepare the femur axially, potential injury of the lateral femoral cutaneous nerve, difficulty in performing reconstructions of the posterior column of the acetabulum, and a surgical scar that may be cosmetically unacceptable. This surgical approach can be utilized to perform both the acetabular and femoral reconstruction or for the acetabular reconstruction alone in combination with accessory approaches for the femoral reconstruction.

Placement of the surgical incision varies: longitudinal or shorter oblique. The incision is often made approximately 2 to 3 cm lateral to the anterosuperior iliac spine (ASIS) directed distally toward the lateral border of the patella for approximately 8 cm. The superficial interval is between the tensor fascia lata (TFL) muscle and the sartorius muscle. The superficial lateral femoral cutaneous nerve (LFCN) exits the fascia medial to this interval approximately 2 to 5 cm distal to the inguinal ligament and has several branches. By incising the fascia overlying the tensor fascia lata muscle and retracting the muscle belly laterally within its compartment, one will minimize the potential to injure the lateral femoral cutaneous nerve. The deep interval is between the rectus femoris muscle (femoral nerve) and the gluteus medius muscle (superior gluteal nerve). The hip capsule is immediately evident at this stage and can be either excised or incised. Exposure of the femur is enhanced with external rotation, adduction, and extension of the hip. Matta uses a fracture table with a specialized femoral hook to elevate the femur (controlled by the anesthesiologist) in order to achieve the femoral positioning.

Modified Anterolateral/Direct Lateral

The direct lateral or modified anterolateral approach for joint arthroplasty typically requires partial interruption of the gluteus medius/minimus insertion on the greater trochanter (typically one-third of the tendon). The advantages of the anterolateral/lateral approaches to the hip are the ability to perform the procedure from both the supine and lateral positions, ease of acetabular and femoral exposure, and greater protection from postoperative dislocation. The disadvantages of the approach are the interruption of the abductor muscle mechanism and the prolonged limp after surgery which this causes. The anterior portion of the superior gluteal nerve supplying the anterior one-third of the gluteus medius and the TFL can be injured if the dissection continues for more than 3 to 4 cm into the abductor muscle.

The surgical incision is directly lateral and the iliotibial band is split between the TFL and the gluteus maximus muscle. There are several variants of the modified anterolateral approach to the hip; however, all entail a release of the anterior one-third to one-half of the abductor insertion onto the greater trochanter with or without a small portion of the anterior trochanter. With the anterior portion of the abductor released, the anterior hip capsule is excised or incised and both the acetabulum and femur can be easily visualized. Axial preparation of the femur is possible with this approach. The abductors are repaired to the trochanter prior to closure.

Posterolateral

The advantages of the posterolateral approach are excellent extensile exposure of the femur and the acetabulum, protection of the abductor mechanism, full access to the femur for axial preparation, ability to perform extended trochanteric osteotomies, and access to the entire posterior column of the pelvis for complex reconstructions. The disadvantages are the potential for an increased rate of posterior dislocation.

A curvilinear incision is made over the lateral aspect of the femur extending posteriorly in line with the posterosuperior iliac spine (PSIS). The iliotibial band is incised and the gluteus maximus muscle fibers are split. The piriformis, conjoined tendon, and obturator externus muscles are released at their insertions on the femur, often with the capsule as one. The capsulotomy may be rectangular (attached medially) or T-shaped. After the arthroplasty, the posterior capsule is repaired so as to minimize rates of dislocation.

"Minimally Invasive" Surgery Compared with "Standard" Surgical Procedures for Joint Arthroplasty

So-called minimally invasive surgical techniques have become popular in all surgical fields, and joint replacement surgery is no exception. Several authors have suggested that there are potential benefits to less invasive surgical procedures, such as earlier recovery, improved cosmetic results, shorter hospital stays, and less pain. Interpreting the literature in this area is difficult because many variables affect short-term outcome (expectations, motivation, comorbidities, anesthetic technique, pain control, restrictions, and surgical invasiveness), and these are difficult to control with randomized trials. Many of the reports on the advantages of minimally invasive surgery suffer from a large selection-bias effect. Furthermore, our measurements for short-term outcomes are neither sensitive nor specific, and many are subjective.

The definition of minimally invasive surgery is not clear. Some authors have utilized more traditional approaches (modified anterolateral or posterolateral) through smaller incisions with a modification of the degree of release in the deeper planes. This technique is achieved with improved instruments (specialized retractors, fiberoptic lighting, offset acetabular reamers and inserters, etc.). Generally speaking, minimally invasive exposures are considered less than 12 cm.

Others have utilized more than one surgical approach (anterior for the acetabulum and posterior for the femur) in an attempt to minimize the need for soft tissue retraction and manipulation of the limb. Although some have suggested that no muscle is injured with these multiple incision techniques, others have shown that the abductor mechanism and the short external rotators are injured. Anatomically, it stands to reason that a percutaneous femoral preparation requires violation of the abductor mechanism. It is not known what effect this has on abductor function compared with retraction of the muscle, as with a posterolateral approach.

Concerns about minimally invasive surgery relate to possible surgical errors that could lead to poorer long-term outcome (implant positioning, bone surface preparation, and third-body wear) or a rate of higher early complications (infection, dislocation, and fracture). Woolson et al. reported the results of three surgeons who selected patients for minimally invasive posterolateral hip replacements ($N = 50$) and compared them to patients in whom standard incisions were performed through the same approach. Despite the fact that patients in the minimally invasive group were selected as ideal candidates (thinner and healthier), there was no statistically significant improvement in this group's short-term outcome measures, such as surgical time, blood loss, length of hospital stay, or disposition at discharge. In fact, the minimally invasive group had a significantly higher rate of wound complication, poor positioning of the acetabular cup, and undersized femoral components.

▶ BIOMECHANICS OF THE JOINT

The normal hip has about 130, 45, 20, and 65 degrees of flexion, abduction, internal rotation, and external rotation, respectively. The hip movements needed for activities of daily living is 120 degrees of hip flexion, 20 degrees of abduction, and 20 degrees of external rotation. Bipedal locomotion is a complex interplay of central motor planning and peripheral motor control. *In vivo* measurements of peak joint reactive force in the hip during walking and climbing stairs range from two to three times body weight. The gait cycle consists of single stance phase and a double stance phase. The center of gravity passes through the near center of the pelvis, creating an adductor moment in the stance phase hip while the contralateral limb is in swing phase. During single-limb stance phase, the pelvis is maintained level to the floor through the abductor moment created in part by the gluteus medius and minimus muscles. A Trendelenburg gait results when the abductor muscle mechanism (strength and/or lever) is unable to support the pelvis level to the floor during the single-stance phase of gait.

The goals of joint reconstruction surgery are to restore the hip mechanics, optimize abductor function, restore equal leg lengths, and minimize the risk of dislocation. The lever arm of the abductor mechanism is optimized through inferior, medial, and anterior placement of the hip center combined with restoration of offset of the femur. The normal hip center is approximately 1 cm superior from the interteardrop line [line connect-ing the most inferior aspects of the teardrop on the anteroposterior (AP) pelvis]. Restoration of the offset, in addition to the effects on the lever arm, restores the working length of the abductor muscle fibers to improve force generation (Starling's muscle-length curve). Inferomedial placement of the hip rotation center also decreases the joint reaction force, which may affect the wear and durability of the reconstruction.

▶ COMMON COMORBIDITIES

Osteoarthritis

Arthritis affects about 65 million Americans and is the second most common cause of disability in people over the age of 65 years. Osteoarthritis is the most common form of arthritis; it is characterized by the progressive noninflammatory deterioration of the hyaline cartilage in diarthrodial joints, causing pain, limited motion, and deformity. It is manifest by cartilage fissuring, focal erosive changes, cartilage loss, sclerosis/eburnation of the subchondral bone, osteophyte formation, subchondral cyst formation, and thickening of the joint capsule.

Osteoarthritis does not have a single cause and most commonly presents as a condition without a known cause—primary osteoarthritis. Several secondary causes for osteoarthritis are associated with metabolic, developmental, neurologic, or traumatic conditions. Causes of secondary osteoarthritis include trauma, dysplasia, osteonecrosis, acromegaly, Gaucher's disease, Paget's disease, Ehlers-Danlos syndrome, Stickler's syndrome, calcium pyrophosphate dihydrate deposition disease (CPPD), ochronosis, hemochromatosis, hemophilia, neuropathy, and infection.

Primary osteoarthritis is more common in the elderly, with more than 60 percent of those older than 65 years being affected. Primary osteoarthritis is not a normal result of aging. Age-related changes in the articular cartilage include a decreased chondrocyte density, decreased water content, decreased large proteoglycan content, increased collagen cross-linking, and increased collagen fibril diameter. Osteoarthritic changes include initial chondrocyte proliferation, decreased proteoglycan content and proportion of aggregated proteoglycan, increased water content, and progressive loss of collagens.

Dysplasia

The incidence of developmental dysplasia of the hip is 1.5 per 1000 births. Risk factors for its development are female, firstborn, primigravida, and breech presentation. Dysplasia is defined by femoral head uncoverage (lateral center edge angle less than 20 degrees in the adult); subluxation is defined as a break in Shenton's line on the AP radiograph. The prognosis of subluxation is worse than that of dysplasia alone. Clinical symptoms often predate radiographic change by 10 years. The true natural history of dysplasia cannot be predicted. Secondary osteoarthritis in dysplasia is often present by the sixth to seventh decades of life and third to fourth decades of life with subluxation. Some authors have reported that a large proportion of patients with primary hip osteoarthritis have some degree of hip dysplasia that was unrecognized. Acetabular reorientation osteotomies may be indicated for patients with symptoms but no significant degenerative changes and with good hip congruity.

Joint arthroplasty for a subluxated or dislocated hip is more complex. The goals of surgery are to restore the normal hip center when possible and achieve adequate host bone preparation to achieve durable fixation. Restoration of the normal hip center usually requires lengthening of the leg and may increase the risk of a traction nerve injury if more that 3 cm of lengthening occurs. Subtraction osteotomy of the femur may be necessary in cases with a high degree of dislocation.

Slipped Capital Femoral Epiphysis/Acetabulofemoral Impingement

Slipped capital femoral epiphysis generally occurs during the adolescent growth spurt and is more common in overweight males. These patients are treated by stabilizing the epiphysis. The long-term outcome of this condition is related to the degree of residual deformity and avoidance of a complication (osteonecrosis or chondrolysis). Higher degrees of slippage (stages III to IV) are associated with a higher incidence of osteoarthritis, requiring joint replacement.

Ganz has popularized the notion that acetabulofemoral impingement is a source of hip pain and limited motion. These patients may have developmental abnormalities in proximal femoral epiphyseal growth, subtle slipped capital femoral epiphysis, or acetabular retroversion. The pain may be due to impingement of the femoral neck on the rim of the acetabulum, leading to labral pathology, chondral injury, and premature osteoarthritis. The surgical treatments for this have included femoral neck osteoplasty (to recreate adequate femoral head-neck offset using an open transtrochanteric hip dislocation approach, direct anterior approach, or with hip arthroscopy), anterior acetabular debridement, and/or acetabular reorientation osteotomies.

Legg-Calvé-Perthes Disease

Legg-Calvé-Perthes disease is a condition of childhood that affects boys from 4 to 10 years of age. These children present with pain, limp, and limited range of motion. Treatment goals are to treat the pain and restore motion. The role of surgical treatment is highly controversial. Prognosis is based on the age of onset, residual femoral head deformity, and residual congruency of the hip joint. The potential of the acetabulum to be remodeled decreases significantly after the age of 8 years. McAndrew and Weinstein found that 50 percent of patients at an average age of 56 years had a joint arthroplasty or severe disabling pain.

Osteonecrosis

Osteonecrosis of the femoral head is a relatively common condition, accounting for approximately 10 to 12 percent of hip replacements in the United States. This condition can affect all age groups and can be the result of trauma (dislocation or femoral neck fracture). Atraumatic osteonecrosis can be associated with alcoholism, steroid use, organ transplantation, systemic vasculitis, or pancreatitis; it can also be idiopathic. Idiopathic osteonecrosis accounts for approximately 25 to 30 percent of cases. The etiology of osteonecrosis is unknown; however, it may be related to embolic phenomena (fat or thrombotic), venous hypertension, fat metabolism, or chemical cytotoxic effects. The chances that the disease will progress are high in symptomatic patients.

Surgical treatment options for patients without collapse include percutaneous core decompression (with or without supplemental procedures such as bone grafting or bone marrow injection), proximal femoral osteotomy, and vascularized or nonvascularized fibular grafting. Arthroplasty is often indicated for patients with refractory symptoms and those with collapse. Premature wear (due to the young age of these patients) and instability are issues of concern with total joint arthroplasty (owing to inherent range of motion).

Inflammatory Arthritis

Inflammatory arthritis can be related to infection or systemic inflammatory conditions, including rheumatoid arthritis and ankylosing spondylitis. Native hip sepsis is rare and is treated as an emergency, with irrigation and debridement to prevent secondary arthritis. Most of the inflammatory arthritides lead to osteoporosis and narrowing of concentric joint space; they may cause the development of protrusion acetabuli. During the perioperative period, the systemic manifestations of these inflammatory conditions require special attention. Many of these patients are using immunomodulating medications that may cause wound-healing problems and infection. Patients with ankylosing spondylitis may have spinal abnormalities that make neuraxial anesthesia difficult. Finally, it is important to rule out instability of the atlantoaxial or subaxial cervical spine before surgery.

▶ SURGICAL PROCEDURE

Arthroplasty

History

The management of hip arthritis has historically included joint fusion, resection arthroplasty, denervation, osteotomy, interpositional arthroplasty (fascia lata, bladder, etc.), and cup arthroplasty. Prosthetic replacements utilizing a variety of implants have been attempted with variable results. Sir John Charnley developed and implemented the concept of low-friction arthroplasty (LFA) in the 1960s. He ultimately used a polyethylene acetabular component and stainless steel cement femoral stem with a 22-mm head through a transtrochanteric approach.

The success of the LFA gradually led to its worldwide use, including the United States starting in 1969. The transtrochanteric approach provided excellent exposure, allowing complete capsulectomy and tensioning of the abductor mechanism as part of the repair. However, the incidence of trochanteric nonunion caused surgeons to seek exposures without the osteotomy. Today, the transtrochanteric approach is generally reserved for selected patients. In addition, concerns about the durability of cemented implants spurred the development of uncemented implants for both the acetabular and femoral sides. Despite some early design difficulties with femoral components in the 1980s, uncemented reconstructions continued to grow in popularity and use during the 1990s, particularly for younger patients.

The overall success of joint arthroplasty in terms of restoring pain-free function to patients with disabling hip pain has led to the use of the technique in a broader patient population earlier in the course of disease and at younger ages. As the expectations of patients and surgeons increased, so did the interest in minimally invasive surgery during the early 2000s. Minimally invasive surgical techniques were promoted as a means to enable patients to return to routine daily activities earlier. For the first time since the introduction of joint arthroplasty, short-term outcomes have become an important measure of success. But many are concerned that the focus on short-term outcomes may distract from striving for the optimal long-term durability that has made joint replacement such a success.

▶ INDICATIONS/PATIENT PROFILE

The indication for total joint arthroplasty is end-stage arthritis of the hip joint that causes pain and disability. The typical patient has a history of gradually worsening pain in the groin, which radiates to the knee with activity and with positions outside the range of allowable motion. Often pain during rest or at night will awaken the patient.

The patient also finds it difficult to tolerate normal daily activities such as walking, climbing stairs, rising from a chair, and putting on shoes. Disease-specific questionnaires to measure pain and function are the Iowa hip rating, Harris hip score, and Western Ontario and McMaster Universities Index Questionnaire (WOMAC) score.

The success of hip arthroplasty has led to broadening of the surgical indication. There is evidence that the patient's function may ultimately be better if the arthroplasty is performed in the earlier stages of disease.

▶ POSITIONING ON THE OPERATING TABLE

Lateral Position

With lateral positioning of the patient, the surgeon can access the hip joint using an anterolateral, direct lateral, or posterolateral exposure. Lateral positioning is required for the posterior approach, which has many advantages, as described above. A disadvantage of the lateral position is difficulty in achieving and maintaining the appropriate pelvic position. This may cause variation nonanatomic landmarks when the acetabular component is placed in position. There is a tendency for the pelvis to tilt anteriorly, flex, and rotate (coronal plane) during the patient's positioning on the table. Furthermore, with retraction for acetabular exposure, forces are exerted on the pelvis, which may change the patient's orientation during surgery.

The surgeon must take account of these tendencies so as to prevent errors in positioning the acetabular component. These factors include modification of the table tilt, table positioning in the room, rigid immobilization of the pelvis with lateral positioners, and control of the torso. Using lateral positioners to minimize motion of the pelvis during surgery is critical. A variety of lateral positioners are available; most aim to achieve contact with the pubic symphysis and the sacrum. Pain in the pubic symphysis can occur because of positioner placement. Care must be taken to prevent compression injuries to the contralateral sciatic nerve when vertical pegs are used to stabilize the pelvis. If the posterior peg is placed distal to the gluteal cleft, the sciatic nerve on the nonoperative side is at risk of injury. The down-limb femoral neurovascular structures are also at risk of compression with lateral retractors if placed to low. The tendency for the torso to tilt forward with lateral positioning must be countered with a positioner placed on the ventral chest wall. Constrictive positioners on the torso can cause pain or discomfort to the patient receiving regional or spinal anesthesia. The brachial plexus of the down upper arm must be protected with a roll placed on the lateral aspect of the chest wall (not in the axilla). The ulnar nerve must be protected from compression against positioning devices and other sources of compression. Many patients who undergo joint replacement (particularly those with rheumatoid arthritis) have multiple joint contractures that must be protected from further injury. Place pillows between the arms while the patient is in the lateral position to prevent the torso from tilting forward.

Supine Position

Supine positioning is more physiologic and reduces potential positioning errors. In addition, this position makes it easier for the surgeon to compare limb lengths. The supine approach is not suitable when a postero-lateral exposure is used, and exposure of the femur is more difficult without a trochanteric osteotomy (particularly if axial preparation is desired).

Matta has repopularized the use of a fracture table when total hip arthroplasty is performed through a direct anterior exposure. With this technique, the patient is placed supine on the fracture table with both legs in boot traction. A peroneal post is used to maintain the position of the pelvis while intermittent traction is exerted on the operated extremity. The nonoperated extremity is also placed in a boot traction device, but no traction is exerted on it. The purpose of the fracture table is to allow external rotation, extension, and adduction of the operated extremity for proximal femoral exposure through the anterior approach. In addition, a femoral hook (elevator) is used to maintain support for the proximal femur during preparation. Use of this table requires assistance from a circulator and the anesthesiologist to control the positioning of the limb and the femoral hook mechanisms. Clear communication between the surgeon and the people controlling the table is critical to prevent injury to the patient.

▶ SURGICAL TECHNIQUE

Primary

Options

The surgical approach for a primary hip replacement depends on the surgeon's preference, as outlined above in the discussion of surgical anatomy. Most surgeons do not perform a complete capsulectomy for primary arthroplasty; however, it is often necessary to release the retained capsular structures partially if significant contractures are present (Fig. 10-1). Capsular retention and repair with the posterolateral approach has led to a reduction in the rate of postoperative dislocation.

The acetabulum is prepared with hemispheric reamers corresponding in size and shape to the acetabular implants. Specialized retractors are generally placed on the anterior wall, posterior wall, and obturator foramen. The medial wall of the acetabular fossa, pubis, and the obturator foramen are important anatomic landmarks for

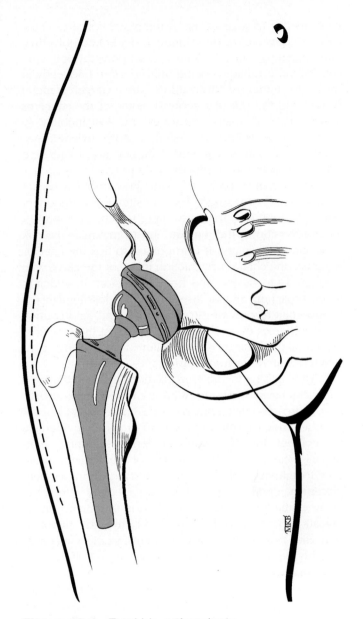

Figure 10-1. Total hip arthroplasty.

correct placement of the acetabular component to restore normal biomechanics of the hip. There is usually a medial osteophyte overlying the pulvinar fat, which must be removed with osteotomes or reamers. Removal of the osteophyte and pulvinar fat allows correct orientation in preparing the acetabulum.

The options for acetabular fixation include cemented fixation with an all-polyethylene cup or biological fixation with an uncemented modular acetabular component. Initial implant stability to allow bone ingrowth can be achieved with press-fit techniques, screws, spikes, or some combination of these. Most uncemented acetabular components have modular bearing inserts. There are several options for the bearing surface, with different advantages and disadvantages. Since the formation of particles due to wear is one of the major concerns, a so-called alternative bearing (highly cross-linked polyethylene, metal on metal, ceramic on polyethylene, and ceramic on ceramic) is being utilized more frequently in order to minimize dislocation rates (larger femoral heads) and the risk of osteolysis. Some of the concerns about these alternative bearings are susceptibility to fatigue failure (highly cross-linked polyethylene), systemic metal ion levels and lymphocyte proliferation (metal on metal), and implant fracture (ceramics).

The femur is prepared with the combined use of broaches and/or reamers. Limb positioning is important during femoral preparation in order to achieve appropriate anteversion of the implant and to minimize the risk of sciatic nerve injury. It is important to flex the knee to minimize the chance of a traction injury of the nerve with combined hip flexion and knee extension. In addition, when broaching and/or inserting cementless implants, it is important to provide support to the limb and counter the axial forces exerted in the femur when these devices are hammered into position. Failure to do so may contribute to nerve traction injuries.

The options for femoral fixation include cemented and cementless implants. With cemented femoral fixation, a broach-only technique is desirable so as to maintain the stable cancellous bone and provide the interface for cement interdigitation. Modern cementing techniques include porosity reduction of the cement, measures to minimize blood in the interface during cement placement, distal plugging of the femoral canal, retrograde filling of the femur, and pressurization to enhance interdigitation. There have been reports of hypoxia, hypotension, and cardiac arrest with cement insertion; this may possibly be due to monomer toxicity or embolization of bone marrow.

There are varieties of uncemented femoral designs that have provided successful results. The options include anatomically designed proximal fixation with circumferential coating, tapered designs, modular stems, and extensively coated distal fixation stems. The preparation concepts for all of these designs are beyond the scope of this chapter; however, the goal is to provide axial and rotational stability of the implant through the use of a combination of broaching and reaming techniques.

Revision

Options

Revision hip arthroplasty varies in complexity from exchanging a polyethylene liner to a complete revision, which necessitates additional femoral exposure techniques, a long femoral stem, and acetabular reconstruction for bone loss. The variety of options available to the reconstructive surgeon has increased.

Hip exposure in revision operations generally is through a posterolateral approach for extensile acetabular exposure and axial preparation of the femoral diaphysis. Management of scar tissue may require either a partial or complete capsulectomy, depending on the circumstances. Exposure techniques such as an extended trochanteric osteotomy (cutting off the trochanter with an approximate 12- to 15-cm portion of the lateral third of the proximal femur, keeping the abductor mechanism and vastus lateralis muscle in continuity) have been very helpful in femoral reconstructions with extensively coated long stems (8- and 10-in. bowed stems). Modular femoral stems with tapered designs (Wagner type) have also been useful for difficult femoral arthroplasty revisions.

A hemispheric uncemented acetabular component is the workhorse in socket reconstruction. Structural bone grafts, cages, and modular porous metals are available to solve problems of bone loss when necessary. Some of the more complex acetabular procedures require partial elevation of the abductors from the lateral ilium.

Special Considerations in the Revision Patient

In revision operations, greater blood loss is expected due to the complexity and duration of the surgery. In addition to the greater complexity of their hip reconstruction, many of these patients are older and frailer than those in whom primary hip arthroplasties are done. It is therefore critical for the surgeon and the anesthesiologist to anticipate blood loss and have open and frequent communication.

Comorbidities

Since the prevalence of arthritis increases with increasing age, many of the patients undergoing joint arthroplasty have comorbidities that affect their perioperative management. Medical optimization before surgery minimizes the risk of perioperative complications. There is evidence that medical comanagement of these patients decreases cost, minimizes complications, and improves patient outcomes.

Some of the comorbidities commonly seen in these elderly patients include coronary artery disease, atrial fibrillation, chronic obstructive pulmonary disease (COPD), diabetes mellitus, and systemic inflammatory conditions. Alcoholism, a history of steroid use, and solid-organ transplants are commonly encountered in patients with osteonecrosis. Joint arthroplasty is often a treatment option for malignancies involving the hip. This may affect the choice of anesthetic if the chemotherapy regimen had cardiopulmonary effects.

Many of these patients have arthritis or replacements in other joints, which require care during positioning of the nonoperated extremities. Special care is necessary in patients with rheumatoid arthritis; cervical spine risk factors must also be evaluated when they are being positioned.

Thromboprophylaxis

Thromboprophylaxis is an important and controversial area. This topic has been fully discussed in Chap. 4. Almost all patients undergoing hip replacement are receiving some form a thromboprophylaxis (mechanical and/or chemical prophylaxis). There must be a balance between the risk of fatal pulmonary embolism and that of surgical bleeding. Chemical prophylaxis is often started on the day of surgery. Warfarin requires approximately 48 h to take effect. Anesthetic techniques can play a large role in reducing the risk of thromboembolism. Neuraxial anesthesia decreases the risk of deep venous thrombosis and pulmonary embolism.

Antibiotics

The use of preoperative prophylactic antibiotics has been shown to decrease infection rates. Antibiotics should be administered for 1 h before and up to 24 h after surgery (see Chap. 3).

Heterotopic Ossification

Heterotopic ossification is the formation of bone in the soft tissue around the hip, and it may limit motion. The most common location is in the gluteus minimus and medius muscles. Patients at risk are those with a history of heterotopic ossification, trauma to the abductor muscles during surgery, hypertrophic osteoarthritis, and males. The majority of heterotopic ossifications (Brooker I and II) do not cause functional limitation of movement. For patients at high risk, prophylaxis of heterotopic ossification calls for with a single dose of external radiation (700 cGy, shielding the prosthesis) or a 2- to 4-week course of indomethacin (50 mg bid) or celecoxib (200 mg bid for 2 to 3 weeks). There is some evidence that irradiation within 24 h preoperatively may be more effective than postoperative administration.

► ANESTHETIC CONSIDERATIONS

Preoperative

Patients presenting for hip arthroplasty often fall into the older age groups; therefore comorbidities associated with advanced age, including rheumatoid arthritis and obesity, should be considered (see Chaps. 7, 8, and 12).

Surgical Requirements

Optimal anesthetic techniques for lower extremity joint arthroplasty are those that provide analgesia of the operated extremity, adequate relaxation for retraction, the ability to monitor nerve function postoperatively, and avoidance of additional risks. The experience of the anesthesiologist and the hospital environment may dictate the safest and most effective anesthetic technique.

Techniques that minimize central "hangovers" are optimal for recovery and initiation of physical therapy. Preemptive pain control (oral narcotics and COX II nonsterodial anti-inflammatory agents) and antiemesis measures are desirable. To improve the patient's transition from the operating theater to physical therapy, many surgeons utilize local administration of long-acting anesthetics at the time of wound closure.

Block

Neuraxial anesthetic techniques have several advantages. They decrease blood loss, minimize the effects of central inhalational agents, and help to prevent thromboembolism by up to 55 percent. Experience and attentiveness are critically important to minimize the risk of cardiopulmonary consequences with anesthetic techniques involving hypotension. Unilateral blocks for major proximal lower limb surgery are generally not optimal, since the nonoperated leg can become very uncomfortable for the patient; the patient may then move this leg and distract the surgeon.

Our choice of anesthetic for hip arthroplasty is a spinal-epidural block (CSE) combined with sedation (see Chap. 30). The type and amount of sedation depends on the requirements of the patient. Continuous infusion of propofol is often used at various infusion rates, although we prefer to use midazolam in varying dosages with or without small doses of meperidine, depending on the patient's requirements. We also provide patients with noise-cancellation headphones and music of the patient's choice.

A common anesthetic technique is, however, still general anesthesia, although it is not optimal. Its use depends on the choice of the patient, the experience of the anesthesiologist, and the choice of anticoagulation agent and its timing (see Chaps. 4 and 30).

New long-acting opiate epidural solutions for postoperative pain relief are currently being introduced. Practitioners should, however, be cautious, for although the duration of the analgesic effects may be increased, the duration of the adverse effects will also be increased. Preliminary reports show these agents to have an unacceptable profile of adverse effects, including long-lasting hypoxia, nausea and vomiting, and pruritus in a large percentage of patients. Long-term analgesia is usually not necessary for primary hip replacement.

Postoperative pain associated with primary hip arthroplasty is variable, and many patients have more preoperative than postoperative pain. Analgesic coverage is most essential for the first 24 h. We usually cover that period with the continuous epidural part of the CSE and remove the epidural catheter the morning after surgery, before the full effect of the warfarin sets in.

Neuraxial anesthesia decreases the central venous pressure by dilating the capacitance vessels. This is thought to reduce the bleeding from venous sinuses in bone and therefore the blood loss. As described in Chaps. 7 and 14, the anesthesiologist can play a significant role in decreasing operative blood loss by keeping the venous pressure low. If the epidural is used for this, it is essential to keep the cardiac output normal or elevated. This further lowers the venous pressure, which decreases the bleeding but also keeps the arterial blood pressure normal. Sherrock et al. demonstrated that blood loss is substantially less with this technique than with normotensive general anesthesia, and the cardiac output is maintained with a low-dose infusion of epinephrine. This has the added advantage of stimulating the $beta_1$ adrenergic receptors in the cerebral vasculature, which, in addition to causing a normal arterial blood pressure, increases cerebral blood flow.

In contrast to primary arthroplasty, revision hip arthroplasty can be very painful postoperatively. A revision operation is therefore a good indication for continuous lumbar plexus (psoas compartment) block (see Chap. 29). If a continuous epidural block is used, the timing of its removal must be carefully considered in patients using anticoagulants (see Chap. 4).

Communication between the surgeon, anesthesiologist, and acute pain physician is absolutely critical to minimize complications and optimize the efficiency of joint arthroplasty procedures.

▶ POSTOPERATIVE PROTOCOL

The postoperative protocol varies and is based on the surgeon's preferences, surgical approach, patient's age and comorbidities, and implant choice. Interest in short-term outcomes with minimally invasive surgical techniques has led to more proactive perioperative pain control and accelerated rehabilitation.

Nursing for the patient with total hip arthroplasty includes monitoring of pain and vital signs, advancement of oral intake, management of urinary catheter if present, and reinforcement of "total hip precaution" protocols.

Physical therapy is initiated on the day of surgery or the day after surgery. The goals of therapy are to instruct the patient on appropriate total hip precautions, safe transfers, and walking with crutches. Occupational therapy instructs the patient in the use of aids (such as reachers, toilet elevators, and assistive devices to put on socks) and getting into a car. Preoperative physical therapy improves functional recovery after surgery.

Weight bearing may be protected, restricted, or assisted based on the surgeon's preference, the complexity of the procedure, quality of bone, implants used, and surgical approach. Protected weight bearing with a walker and/or crutches for 6 weeks is usually preferable with uncemented implants. The purpose of these restrictions is to minimize micromotion of the implant, which would increase the risk of fibrous fixation, and to avoid worsening of an unrecognized fracture. Postoperative protocols that encourage tolerable weight bearing have become more common.

Potential Complications

Dislocation

Dislocations should occur in a low percentage of patients. With an anterolateral/direct lateral approach, the rate ranges from 0.6 to 2.6 percent. Without a capsular repair, the posterolateral approach had a reported higher dislocation rate; however, this rate is similar to that reported rate for anterolateral approaches when a posterior capsular repair is performed. Factors contributing to dislocation are increased range of motion, poor compliance with precautions, failure to achieve appropriate offset and leg length, use of skirted femoral head components, neuromuscular disorders affecting the abductor mechanism, and poor component position.

Fracture

Periprosthetic fractures can occur during broaching or insertion of uncemented components. If detected intraoperatively, a femoral fracture can be treated with cerclage wiring or the placement of a longer stem if necessary. Fractures noted on the postoperative radiograph can be treated with restricted weight bearing if they are not displaced. With an extensively coated femoral stem, a fracture involving the posterior cortex is at greater risk of displacement.

Fat Embolism

Fat embolism can occur during the broaching of the femoral canal and has been documented with intraoperative transesophageal echocardiography (see Chap. 5).

Nerve injury

SCIATIC NERVE

The incidence of clinically detected sciatic nerve injury is 0.2 to 2 percent. These injuries can occur during retractor placement, manipulation of the dislocated hip (particularly when hip flexion is combined with knee extension), traction during broaching or affecting extensively coated implants, limb lengthening, or postoperative hematoma. A large percentage (approximately 50 percent) have an unrecognized cause. Electromyographic and nerve conduction abnormalities are common during routine total hip replacements. The initial evaluation of sciatic nerve palsy must include an assessment of hematoma formation and placement of the limb in a position to decrease the traction on the sciatic nerve (hip extension and knee flexion). Only a small percentage of patients acquire full function of the nerve after injury. The most common and problematic residual effect is neuropathic pain. In general, compression injuries fare better than traction injuries. Therefore prevention of these injuries is critical. Preventive measures are meticulous retractor placement, support of the limb during broaching and implant placement, keeping the knee flexed when the hip is flexed, dissecting the nerve out in cases of heterotopic ossification resection, and prevention of lengthening more than 3 cm.

FEMORAL NERVE

Femoral nerve palsy is less common than sciatic nerve injuries and generally has less residual deficits. They are most commonly associated with aberrant anterior retractor placement. If nerve function does not recover, the residual quadriceps motor weakness is debilitating.

Hip Arthroscopy

Patient Selection/Indications

Hip arthroscopy has become a more commonly performed procedure for synovial conditions, labral pathology, certain traumatic fractures of the femoral head, and the diagnosis of cartilage lesions. Some surgeons have expanded the use of arthroscopy for the treatment of acetabulofemoral impingement caused by an inadequate femoral head-neck offset.

Positioning on the Operating Table

The patient is positioned in the lateral decubitus position or supine. Distraction of the hip joint is necessary and requires both a lateral and distally directed force. A fracture table is utilized when the patient is in the supine position and a specialized distraction device is necessary when the lateral position is chosen. The choice depends on the surgeon's experience and familiarity. The lateral decubitus position may allow better access for posterior portals.

Surgical Technique

OPTIONS

The working portals for hip arthroscopy are direct anterior, anterolateral, and posterolateral portals. A C-arm fluoroscopic unit is used for the placement of portals. The first portal placed is usually the anterolateral one positioned at the level of the anterolateral tip of the trochanter and directed toward the superior articular surface of the hip joint. A distraction force is applied to the limb by boot traction. The fluoroscope is used to confirm distraction (typically a nitrogen air layer will form in the joint from the negative pressure created). A spinal needle is inserted into the joint through the anterolateral portal. The entry of air generally breaks the intraarticular negative pressure and cause increased distraction. Most hip arthroscopy equipment sets have cannulated trochars that can be passed over a wire. The wire is introduced through the spinal needle, followed by cannulated dilators. The anterior portal is placed using a similar technique under direct visualization from a camera placed in the anterolateral portal. The starting point for the anterior portal is approximately 6 to 8 cm distal to the ASIS (generally at the level of the superior aspect of the pubic symphysis).

Most of the evaluation of the hip joint is performed through these two portals. The most common location of labral pathology is in the anterosuperior portion. Occasionally accessory portals, such as the posterolateral portal, are necessary.

Anesthetic Considerations

Although these patients are generally young and healthy and general anesthesia is appropriate, subarachnoid block is ideal for this surgery. Anesthetic considerations are generally similar to those for hip arthroplasty; continuous nerve block is usually not necessary for the treatment of postoperative pain. If it does prove to be necessary, lumbar plexus block is well indicated here (see Chap. 29).

Antimicrobial Prophylaxis

The risk of infection with joint arthroscopy is generally low, and hip arthroscopy is no exception (see Chap. 3).

Common Complications

Complications are usually related to the patient's positioning and the need for joint distraction. Peroneal nerve palsies have been reported. Adequate padding and placement of the perineal post and minimizing the duration of traction are important in decreasing the risk of the complications. The anterior portal can cause injury to branches of the lateral femoral cutaneous nerve. Aberrant anterior portal placement poses a potential risk for branches of the femoral nerve, and the posterolateral portal puts the sciatic nerve at risk.

SUGGESTED FURTHER READING

Archibec, MJ, White RE Jr. Learning curve for the two-incision total hip replacement. *Clin Orthop Relat Res* 429:232–238, 2004.

Berger RA, Duwelius PJ. The two-incision minimally invasive total hip arthroplasty: Technique and results. *Orthop Clin North Am* 35:163–172, 2004.

Bergmann G, Deuretzbacher G, Heller M, et al. Hip contact forces and gait patterns from routine activities. J Biomech 34: 859–871, 2001.

Calvo W, Forteza-Vila J. On the development of bone marrow innervation in new-born rats as studied with silver impregnation and electron microscopy. *Am J Anat* 126:355–371, 1969.

Carney BT, Weinstein SL, Noble J. Long-term follow-up of slipped capital femoral epiphysis. *J Bone Joint Surg Am* 73:667–674, 1991.

Chung SM. The arterial supply of the developing proximal end of the human femur. *J Bone Joint Surg Am* 58:961–970, 1976.

Coleman CR, Slager RF, Smith WS. The effect of environmental influence on acetabular development. *Surg Forum* 9:775–780, 1958.

Cooper RR. Nerves in cortical bone. Science 160:327–328, 1968.

Dorr LD. Comparison of primary total hip replacements performed with a standard incision or a mini-incision. *J Bone Joint Surg Am* 87:675; author reply 675–676, 2005.

Edwards BN, Tullos HS, Noble PC. Contributory factors and etiology of sciatic nerve palsy in total hip arthroplasty. *Clin Orthop Rel Res* 218:136–141, 1987.

Fortin PR, Penrod JR, Clarke AE, et al. Timing of total joint replacement affects clinical outcomes among patients with osteoarthritis of the hip or knee. *Arthritis Rheum* 46:3327–3330, 2002.

Ganz R, Gill TJ, Gautier E, et al. Surgical dislocation of the adult hip a technique with full access to the femoral head and acetabulum without the risk of avascular necrosis. *J Bone Joint Surg Br* 83:1119–1124, 2001.

Gilbey HJ, Ackland TR, Wang AW, et al. Exercise improves early functional recovery after total hip arthroplasty. *Clin Orthop Rel Res* 408:193–200, 2003.

Goldstein WM, Gleason TF, Kopplin M, et al. Prevalence of dislocation after total hip arthroplasty through a posterolateral approach with partial capsulotomy and capsulorrhaphy. *J Bone Joint Surg Am* 83-A (Suppl 2, Pt 1):2–7, 2001.

Harris WH. Etiology of osteoarthritis of the hip. *Clin Orthop Rel Res* 213:20–33, 1986.

Healy WL, Lo TC, DeSimone AA, et al. Single-dose irradiation for the prevention of heterotopic ossification after total hip arthroplasty. A comparison of doses of five hundred and fifty and seven hundred centigray. *J Bone Joint Surg Am* 77:590–595, 1995.

Hole A, Terjesen T, Breivik H. Epidural versus general anaesthesia for total hip arthroplasty in elderly patients. *Acta Anaesthesiol Scand* 24:279–287, 1980.

Huddleston JM, Long KH, Naessons JM, et al. Medical and surgical comanagement after elective hip and knee arthroplasty: A randomized, controlled trial. *Ann Intern Med* 141:28–38, 2004.

Johanson NA, Pellicci PM, Tsairis P, et al. Nerve injury in total hip arthroplasty. *Clin Orthop Rel Res* 179:214–222, 1983.

Johnston RC, Brand RA, Crowninshield RD. Reconstruction of the hip. A mathematical approach to determine optimum geometric relationships. *J Bone Joint Surg Am* 61:639–652, 1979.

Johnston RC, Smidt GL. Hip motion measurements for selected activities of daily living. *Clin Orthop Rel Res* 72:205–215, 1970.

Kennon RE, Keggi JM, Wetmore RS, et al. Total hip arthroplasty through a minimally invasive anterior surgical approach. *J Bone Joint Surg Am* 85-A (suppl 4):39–48, 2003.

Lafont ND, Kostucki WM, Marchand PH, et al. Embolism detected by transesophageal echocardiography during hip arthroplasty. *Can J Anaesth* 41:850–853, 1994.

Mardones R, Nemanich J, Trousdale R, et al. Muscle damage after THA done with the 2-incision minimally invasive and miniposterior techniques. *American Academy of Orthopaedic Surgeons' Annual Meeting*. Washington, DC: American Academy of Orthopaedic Surgeons, 2005.

Matta J. Anterior approach for THA on the orthopaedic table in Barrack R (ed): *Hip Society Spring Meeting*. Washington DC: 2005.

McAndrew MP, Weinstein SL. A long-term follow-up of Legg-Calve-Perthes disease. *J Bone Joint Surg Am* 66:860–869, 1984.

Modig J, Hjelmstedt A, Sahlstedt, B, et al. Comparative influences of epidural and general anaesthesia on deep venous thrombosis and pulmonary embolism after total hip replacement. *Acta Chir Scand* 147:125–130, 1981.

Nolan D, Fitzgerald R, Beckenbaugh R, et al. Complications of total hip arthroplasty treated by reoperation. *J Bone Joint Surg Am* 57:977–981, 1975.

Ogden JA. Changing patterns of proximal femoral vascularity. *J Bone Joint Surg Am* 56:941–950, 1974.

Padgett DE, Holley KG, Cummings M, et al. The efficacy of 500 centigray radiation in the prevention of heterotopic ossification after total hip arthroplasty: A prospective, randomized, pilot study. *J Arthrop* 18:6677–686, 2003.

Pagnano M, Lewallen D, Hanssen A. Two-incision THA in 80 consecutive unselected patients: Prevalence of complications. *American Academy of Orthopaedic Surgeons Annual Meeting*. Washington, DC: American Academy of Orthopaedic Surgeons, 2005.

Pellicci PM, Bostrom M, Poss R. Posterior approach to total hip replacement using enhanced posterior soft tissue repair. *Clin Orthop Rel Res* 355:224–248, 1998.

Peterson HA, Winkelmann RK, Coventry MB. Nerve endings in the hip joint of the cat: Their morphology, distribution and density. *J Bone Joint Surg Am* 54:333–343, 1972.

Rao RR, Sharkey PF, Hozack WJ, et al. Immediate weightbearing after uncemented total hip arthroplasty. *Clin Orthop Rel Res* 349:156–162, 1998.

Ries M, Lynch F, Rauscher L, et al. Pulmonary function during and after total hip replacement. Findings in patients who have insertion of a femoral component with and without cement. *J Bone Joint Surg Am* 75:581–587, 1993.

Romano CL, Duci D, Romano D, et al. Celecoxib versus indomethacin in the prevention of heterotopic ossification after total hip arthroplasty. *J Arthrop* 19:14–18, 2004.

Rumi MN, Deol GS, Bergandi JA, et al. Optimal timing of preoperative radiation for prophylaxis against heterotopic ossification. A rabbit hip model. *J Bone Joint Surg Am* 87:366–373, 2005.

Schmalzried TP, Amstutz HC, Dorey FJ. Nerve palsy associated with total hip replacement. Risk factors and prognosis. *J Bone Joint Surg Am* 73:1074–1080, 1991.

Schwartz JT Jr, Mayer JG, Engh CA. Femoral fracture during non-cemented total hip arthroplasty. *J Bone Joint Surg Am* 71:1135–1142, 1989.

Sculco TP, Ranawat C. The use of spinal anesthesia for total hip-replacement arthroplasty. *J Bone Joint Surg Am* 57:173–177, 1975.

Sharrock NE, Cazan MG, Hargett MJ, et al. Changes in mortality after total hip and knee arthroplasty over a ten-year period. *Anesth Analg* 80:242–248, 1995.

Sharrock NE, Go G, Harpel PC, et al. The John Charnley Award. Thrombogenesis during total hip arthroplasty. *Clin Orthop Rel Res* 319:16–27, 1995.

Smith-Peterson M. Approach to and exposure of the hip joint for mold arthroplasty. *J Bone Joint Surg Am* 31:40, 1949.

Svensson O, Skold S, Blomgren G. Integrity of the gluteus medius after the transgluteal approach in total hip arthroplasty. *J Arthrop* 5:7–60, 1990.

Talbot NJ, Brown JH, Treble NJ. Early dislocation after total hip arthroplasty: Are postoperative restrictions necessary? *J Arthropl* 17:1006–1008, 2002.

Ulrich C, Burri C, Worsdorfer O, et al. Intraoperative transesophageal two-dimensional echocardiography in total hip replacement. Arch Orthop *Trauma Surg* 105:274–248, 1986.

von Knoch M, Berry DJ, Harmsen WS, et al. Late dislocation after total hip arthroplasty. *J Bone Joint Surg Am* 84-A:1949–1953, 2002.

Weber ER. Daube JR, Coventry MB. Peripheral neuropathies associated with total hip arthroplasty. *J Bone Joint Surg Am* 58:66–69, 1976.

Weeden SH, Paprosky WG, Bowling JW. The early dislocation rate in primary total hip arthroplasty following the posterior approach with posterior soft-tissue repair. *J Arthrop* 18:709–713, 2003.

Weinstein SL. Natural history of congenital hip dislocation (CDH) and hip dysplasia. *Clin Orthop Rel Res* 225:62–76, 1987.

Woolson ST, Adler NS. The effect of partial or full weight bearing ambulation after cementless total hip arthroplasty. *J Arthrop* 17:820–855, 2002.

Woolson ST, Mow CS, Syquia JF, et al. Comparison of primary total hip replacements performed with a standard incision or a mini-incision. *J Bone Joint Surg Am* 86-A:1353–1358, 2004.

Wright JM, Crockett HC, Delgado S, et al. Mini-incision for total hip arthroplasty; A prospective, controlled investigation with 5-year follow-up evaluation. *J Arthrop* 19:538–545, 2004.

CHAPTER 11

The Knee Joint

MICHAEL R. O'ROURKE/JOHN J. CALLAGHAN/ANDRÉ P. BOEZAART

▶ INTRODUCTION

This chapter excludes sport injuries to the knee; these are discussed in Chap. 17.

The goals of reconstructive surgery of the knee in adults are to maintain optimal function, minimize disability, and remove pain. All the joints of the lower extremity participate in locomotion. Pathologic conditions that affect the knee impair normal daily activities and the ability to walk. The broad spectrum of pathologic conditions affecting the knee includes soft tissue injuries to the ligamentous structures that provide stability, meniscal injuries, and arthritic conditions. This chapter focuses mainly on the degenerative arthritic conditions that affect the knee in adults. Ligamentous and meniscal injuries are discussed in the Chap. 17. The number of patients with pain and disability from arthritic conditions of the knees is increasing, as are the expectations of those who wish to maintain active lifestyles. Approximately 300,000 knee replacements are performed each year in the United States. The goal in treating these disorders is to optimize function and mobility while minimizing surgical risks.

▶ ANATOMIC CONSIDERATIONS

Developmental Anatomy

The knee forms between 5 and 7 weeks of gestation. The combined distal femoral and proximal tibial growth plates provide approximately 65 percent of the growth to the lower limb. The proximal tibial physis accounts for 60 percent of the tibial growth. The distal femoral physis contributes to 70 percent of the femoral growth. Limb growth is complete at approximately 13 to 15 years of age in females and 16 to 18 years of age in males.

Gross Anatomy

The knee has a rich anastomotic vascular network. The descending genicular artery branches from the femoral artery before it crosses the adductor hiatus and gives rise to the articular branch (crosses the vastus medialis muscle) and the saphenous branch (travels between the vastus medialis muscle and the sartorius muscle with the saphenous nerve). The superior medial genicular and superior lateral genicular arteries branch from the popliteal artery and pass around the distal femur superficial to the origins of the gastrocnemius muscle. The middle genicular artery branches from the popliteal artery and penetrates the posterior capsule to supply the cruciate ligaments. The inferior medial genicular artery branches from the popliteal artery and courses deep to the hamstring tendons and the medial collateral ligament approximately 2 cm distal to the joint line. The inferior lateral genicular artery travels immediately adjacent to the lateral joint line deep to the lateral collateral ligament. The genicular arteries passing anterior to the knee form a peripatellar anastomosis with additional contributions from the descending branch of the lateral femoral circumflex artery, anterior tibial recurrent artery, and circumflex fibular artery. During a standard medial parapatellar approach to the knee, the superior medial, inferior medial, and inferior lateral genicular arteries are compromised.

The knee has afferent fibers from the tibial nerve, common peroneal nerve, posterior branch of the obturator nerve, and femoral nerve. The posterior articular nerve branches from the tibial nerve, piercing the superior oblique ligament, with the middle genicular artery supplying the posterior capsule, meniscal structures, and cruciate ligament. The femoral nerve branches supply the quadriceps muscles and send branches to the superior articular capsule. The common peroneal nerve gives rise to the lateral articular nerve and recurrent peroneal nerve, which innervates the inferolateral capsule/lateral collateral and the anterolateral capsule, respectively. The infrapatellar branch of the saphenous nerve courses along the superior border of the pes anserine to supply the skin over the anteroinferior aspect of the knee. Anesthesia and paresthesia in the distribution of the infrapatellar branch are common after a standard medial parapatellar approach.

The synovial cavity extends approximately 6 to 8 cm above the superior pole of the patella. The collateral ligaments provide coronal plane stability. The medial collateral ligament consists of superficial and deep portions that extend from the medial upper condyle of the distal femur to the subperiosteum of the medial side of the proximal tibia. The semimembranosus contributes to the medial stabilizing complex, as do the tendon insertions of the sartorius, gracilis, and semitendinosus. The lateral-sided structures, provide stability in the coronal plane. The iliotibial band inserts onto Gerdes tubercle (lateral to the tibial tubercle) and provides stability in extension. The lateral collateral ligament provides stability in both flexion and extension, and the popliteus muscle contributes to stability, particularly in flexion. The posterolateral corner includes the capsular thickening (arcuate complex) and provides lateral stability, particularly in extension.

The anterior and posterior cruciate ligaments are intraarticular extrasynovial structures, which provide rotational and sagittal plane stability to the knee. The anterior cruciate ligament is the primary structure that resists anterior translation of the tibia and plays a secondary role in resisting external rotation of the tibia. The anterior cruciate ligament (ACL) has free nerve endings and mechanoreceptors that play a role in proprioception (derived from the posterior articular branch from the tibial nerve).

Meniscal structures have a fibrocartilaginous composition with a reasonably good peripheral blood supply, a "watershed" area, and a poor blood supply in the center. Afferent innervation mirrors the distribution of the vascular supply. The medial meniscus is attached to the deep medial collateral ligament and is semilunar in shape. The lateral meniscus is more circular and mobile, with an absence of direct connection with the lateral collateral ligament. The popliteal hiatus, located in the posterolateral aspect of the joint, coincides with an area of the lateral meniscus that has no attachment.

The proximal tibial plateau is relatively flat compared to the distal femur. The lateral tibial plateau is convex and the medial tibial plateau is concave. The meniscal structures act as an interposition between the relatively round femoral condyles and relatively flat tibial condyles to help distribute weight more evenly across the articulation. The mobility of the lateral meniscus accommodates the greater posterior translation of the contact point between the lateral femoral condyle and the lateral tibial plateau as the knee moves from an extended to a flexed position.

▶ BIOMECHANICS OF THE JOINT

The axis of motion is not a true hinge. The motion of the knee joint is a combination of rolling and gliding movements, which create an instant center of rotation that changes through a range of motions. The translation between the femur and the tibia is greatest in the lateral compartment compared to the medial compartment as the knee goes from an extended to a flexed position. This posterior translation ("rollback") of the femur relative to the tibia is important to obtain higher degrees of knee flexion. The posterior translation allows the distal femur to complete terminal flexion without impingement from the posterior tibia. In addition to the translation of the femur on the tibia, there is approximately 10 degrees of rotational change through the range of motion. As the knee goes from 10 to 30 degrees of flexion to full extension, there is an external rotation of the tibia of about 5 degrees. The cruciate ligaments assist in this guided motion. The ACL provides most of the restraint to anterior translation of the tibia with the knee at 30 degrees of flexion. The posterior cruciate ligament (PCL) provides resistance to posterior translation of the tibia in flexion. Normal knee motion is from 2 to 3 degrees of hyperextension to flexion of 140 degrees. During walking, the maximum flexion is usually less than 70 degrees; in climbing stairs, the maximum flexion is approximately 95 degrees.

▶ ETIOLOGY AND EPIDEMIOLOGY

Arthritis of the knee joint is defined by loss of the hyaline cartilage at the end of the femur and tibia, leading to contact between the subchondral bones. Arthritis can be primary or secondary. Primary osteoarthritis of the knees is more common in women than men and seems to be associated with obesity. There is a genetic predisposition to primary arthritis, and the typical age of presentation is in the sixth to eighth decades of life.

Secondary osteoarthritis may be due to traumatic conditions (tibial plateau fractures or ligamentous ruptures around the knee), meniscal injuries, previous surgical procedures, pigmented villonodular synovitis, and inflammatory conditions involving the knee (rheumatoid arthritis, lupus, psoriasis, gout, pseudogout). Chondrocalcinosis (calcium pyrophosphate deposition) leads to stiffening in the meniscal structures and hyaline cartilage, which predisposes them to higher contact stress and therefore earlier degenerative changes. Osteonecrosis of the knee occurs most commonly in the medial femoral condyle during the sixth and seventh decades of life and is more common in women.

▶ PATHOPHYSIOLOGY

The most common location of primary osteoarthritis of the knee is in the medial compartment. The wear tends to occur initially at the anteromedial aspect of the proximal tibia when the ACL is functioning. The wear pattern is generally posteromedial in patients with a deficient ACL. With the progressive varus deformity that results from loss of articular cartilage in the medial compartment, there is contact between the lateral femoral condyle and the tibial spines, leading to wear patterns in the central portion of the knee joint. This is often associated with changes in the articulation of the patellofemoral joint and subsequent patellofemoral osteoarthritis.

Primary osteoarthritis of the knee can also occur in the lateral compartment and is often associated with hypoplasia of the lateral femoral condyle. Valgus deformities are often associated with lateral tracking of the patella, increased femoral anteversion, and tibial torsion. In varus osteoarthritis, the ligamentous structures of the opposite compartment have normal tension and length; whereas in valgus osteoarthritis, the medial collateral ligament of the opposite medial compartment usually becomes lax as the deformity worsens. Laxity of the medial structures can be a source of pain preoperatively and makes the surgical treatment more difficult.

▶ SURGICAL PROCEDURE

Arthroplasty

Patient Selection/Indications
Arthroplasty of the knee includes procedures that resurface the distal femur and proximal tibia to prevent pain generated by bone-on-bone articulation. The options for resurfacing the knee joint include unicompartment knee arthroplasty and total knee arthroplasty. Total knee replacements retain the PCL, sacrifice the PCL, or replace it with an implant. All total knee replacements remove the ACL if it is still present.

The decision for knee arthroplasty should be made before the decision for a total or partial arthroplasty. Knee replacements are generally undertaken when the cartilage in at least one compartment is absent and the radiographs show bone-on-bone contact. When these criteria are met, decisions to proceed with surgical treatment are based on the patient's disability and pain. Great care must be taken in evaluating knee pain. Other sources of knee pain may be soft tissue instability, patellofemoral pain, hip pathology, lower back pathology, fibromyalgia, and other myofascial pain syndromes. If an arthroplasty is performed prematurely in the course of a disease or for an indication other than loss of articular cartilage, patients may be potentially worse off than before surgery. Some authors have described this condition as the "imperfect knee syndrome."

Unicondylar knee arthroplasties involve resurfacing the most involved compartment of the knee joint; this may be an option in a small subset of patients with isolated compartment arthritis without inflammatory disease. The ideal candidate for a unicompartment knee arthroplasty is generally a low-demand, older person of normal weight with single-compartment arthritic symptoms and an otherwise well-functioning knee with good range of motion and mild to moderate deformity. These operations can be performed for medial and lateral compartment disease, but they are more commonly performed for medial compartment disease owing to its higher frequency overall.

The advantages of a unicompartment knee arthroplasty are the retention of both cruciate ligaments, leaving a knee that functions with more normal kinematics. In addition, less invasive exposures are required during placement and the range of motion is generally higher after a unicompartment compared to a total knee replacement. Disadvantages are the potential for mechanical loosening and disease progression in the other compartments, leading to a less durable outcome than with total replacement.

Although controversial, mainstream indications include unicompartmental disease without contralateral tibiofemoral disease in a patient with good range of motion, focal symptoms in the involved compartment, and functioning cruciate ligaments. Relative contraindications to unicompartment knee arthroplasty are significant patellofemoral symptoms, ACL deficiency, knee flexion contracture of more than 5 degrees, subluxation, a highly active patient, and obesity.

There has been increased use of unicompartment knee arthroplasties for a subset of the population who are younger and more active. Many authors have doubts about the use of these devices in this patient population. The use of these arthroplasties in a younger patient population may be thought of as a bridge to delay a total knee replacement. High tibial osteotomy should be considered in younger patients with higher activity levels.

Early Treatment for Arthritis
Early treatments for knee arthritis include activity modification, orthotic devices to alter the mechanics of the

weight-bearing axis through the knee, anti-inflammatory medications, acetaminophen, and occasionally intraarticular injections. When these conservative treatments have been exhausted and the patient's disability and pain have increased, an arthroplasty procedure may be indicated.

Surgical Technique

Positioning and Tourniquet

The patient is usually positioned supine on the operating table. A tourniquet is commonly used during the procedure to minimize intraoperative blood loss, but some controversy exists as to the potential consequences, particularly in patients with risk for neuropathic pain, as in diabetes and vascular disease. Many surgeons choose to perform a knee arthroplasty without a tourniquet in patients with neuropathic pain or radiographic evidence of vascular calcifications. The duration and pressure of the tourniquet correlate with a potential for neurologic injury.

Exposure

Exposure of the knee for an arthroplasty is an anterior longitudinal incision over the knee exposing the extensor mechanism (Fig. 11-1). It is important to maintain the blood supply of the anterior skin flaps by minimizing dissection between the deep fascial plane and the overlying skin. Elevation of these flaps deep to the fascia will help maintain the viability of the skin flaps. This is particularly important when patients have had several previous knee operations. Every effort should be made to incorporate previous incisions so as to avoid skin necrosis.

The knee joint can be exposed through a quadriceps-splitting approach, the mid-vastus muscle-splitting approach, or a subvastus approach. Each of these exposures has advantages and disadvantages. The advantage of the quadriceps-splitting approach is a relatively atraumatic plane within the quadriceps tendon, allowing excellent exposure of the knee joint. This is historically the most commonly utilized knee exposure. There have been proponents of midvastus exposure, which extends from the medial side of the tibial tubercle along the medial side of the patella and veers in a medial superior direction through the midportion of the vastus medialis muscle. The potential advantage of this approach is to maintain the integrity of the quadriceps tendon. Disadvantages to this approach include muscle splitting and potential denervation of a portion of the vastus medialis muscle. A subvastus approach is one that elevates the entire quadriceps mechanism from the medial border of the vastus medialis muscle. The disadvantage of this approach is increased blood loss and limited exposure.

All of the medial exposures compromise the vascular supply to the patella from the superior medial geniculate and inferior geniculate arteries. Once the

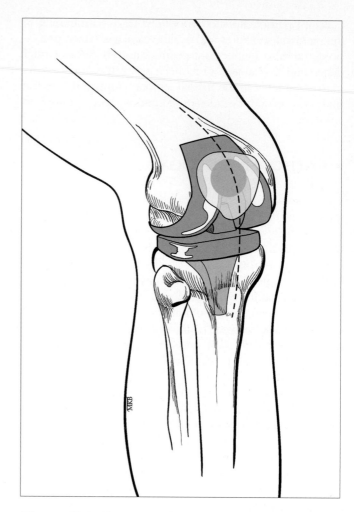

Figure 11-1. Exposure of the knee for an arthroplasty.

arthrotomy is performed through the medial side of the patella, the soft tissue structures on the medial proximal tibia are elevated in a subperiosteal plane to allow anterior translation and external rotation of the tibia relative to the femur, thus providing improved exposure. The medial release is larger in a varus knee than a valgus knee, which helps balance the tight medial structures at the completion of the arthroplasty. Traditionally, a portion of the infrapatellar fat pad is excised to allow adequate exposure of the knee joint. The patella may or may not be resurfaced (in the United States, the patella is most often resurfaced). The patella has traditionally been everted to provide access to the medial and lateral compartments of the tibiofemoral joint. Some surgeons have proposed avoiding a patellar eversion in order to minimize soft tissue tension within the extensor mechanism and thus improve short-term recovery.

A lateral parapatellar approach can be used for a valgus knee. The advantages of the lateral approach are that it minimizes release of the medial stabilizing structures and that it releases the lateral patellar retinaculum of the patella as part of the exposure. The disadvantages of the lateral approach are an inability to subluxate the tibia for exposure, difficulty closing the capsule following arthroplasty, the occasional need for a tibial tubercle osteotomy to improve exposure, and difficulty of a revision procedure through the same approach. Most surgeons choose a medial exposure for all joint replacements.

There has been a trend toward promotion of minimally invasive techniques and exposures for total knee replacement. Various authors have suggested that modifications of these traditional approaches are less intrusive in the suprapatellar cavity and less traumatic to the extensor mechanism.

Bone Preparation and Implantation

The sequence of bone cuts varies according to the surgeon's preferences. The goals of the surgery are to create a joint line that is parallel to the floor; thus, the tibia is cut parallel to the axis of the tibial shaft. This axis lies medial to the midpoint between the lateral and medial malleoli such that, on a radiograph, the axis passes through the center of the talus. The level of the resection of the proximal tibia is determined by the anticipated restoration of the composite tibial component. (For example, a composite tibial component of 10 mm would require a resection of the proximal tibia in the uninvolved compartment of approximately 10 mm.) The distal femur is resected such that the resection is perpendicular to the mechanical axis of the femur, which extends from the center of the femoral head rotation to the center of the distal femur. The combination of a tibial cut parallel to the floor and perpendicular to the mechanical axis of the femur results in a limb alignment that is mechanically neutral.

The alignment of these cutting jigs to the bones can be made with extramedullary or intramedullary alignment. The most common alignment for the femur is intramedullary and the most common alignment for the tibia is extramedullary. The advantage of intramedullary alignment on the femur is more accurate placement due to limitations in identifying landmarks intraoperatively. The disadvantages of intramedullary alignment relate to increased risk of fat embolism and its systemic effects. On the tibial side, extramedullary alignment is more easily achieved because these anatomic landmarks are readily palpable intraoperatively.

The remaining distal femoral cuts are based on the implant dimensions and the choice of sacrificing a retaining knee arthroplasty. Retention or substitution of the PCL is very controversial; excellent short- and long-term outcomes have been shown with both techniques. Those who support retention of the PCL argue that less bone is resected from the intercondylar notch, more normal movement is retained, and there is potential retention of afferent proprioception from the retained ligament. In general, a knee replacement that retains the PCL is less tolerant to changes in the level of the reconstructed joint line, and studies have shown paradoxical anterior translation of the femur relative to the tibia with flexion. Surgeons who remove the PCL believe that substitution for the function of the PCL with the implant is more predictable and minor changes in the joint line location are better tolerated.

Revision

The concepts in revision knee arthroplasty are similar to those in primary knee replacement. However, in the former, intramedullary stems are generally utilized as part of the reconstruction. Therefore both the femoral and tibial cuts are often based on intramedullary alignment. The goals of creating neutral mechanical alignment are the same in primary and revision operations. Most revision operations utilize metal augments to replace lost bone. The stem extensions into the metadiaphyseal regions of the tibia and femur may be cemented or uncemented.

Exposure for revision operations is more complex and often requires supplemental techniques to improve exposure when motion is limited and/or periarticular scars are excessive. Most of these exposure issues relate to management of the extensor mechanism. Options include extending the incision into the quadriceps tendon superior and lateral "quadriceps snip", extending the incision into the quadriceps tendon in a V-shaped fashion toward the lateral inferior aspect of the extensor mechanism ("quadriceps turndown"), or a tibial tubercle osteotomy. In revision operations, various degrees of ligamentous insufficiency may be encountered. To cope with this, there is a graduated level of constraints in implants based on different specifications by the manufacturers. These may vary from a semiconstrained to a fully constrained hinge implant.

Comorbidities

As with total hip arthroplasty, patients with end-stage osteoarthritis of the knee often have comorbidities that must be addressed in the perioperative period so as to reduce complications. Comorbidities include cardiopulmonary disease, diabetes, hypertension, and obesity (see Chap. 10). Many patients with arthritis have been treated with anti-inflammatory drugs and may have gastric or renal side effects because of this. Patients with inflammatory conditions, particularly rheumatoid arthritis, must be treated with particular care owing to involvement of other musculoskeletal areas. As with operations on any patient with rheumatoid arthritis, the cervical spine should be examined to ensure absence of significant instability or canal compromise (see Chap. 8).

Prophylaxis

Thromboprophylaxis

Thromboprophylaxis of some form is generally recommended for total knee replacements, just as they are with total hip replacements (see Chap. 4). The risk of fatal pulmonary embolism is lower in a total knee replacement than in a total hip replacement (see Chap. 10). The incidence of proximal thigh clots is lower with total knee replacements than with total hip replacements. Thromboprophylaxis protocols differ between surgeons and are based on experience and the level of concern. Early mobilization, compression stockings, venous compressive devices such as foot pumps, or sequential compression devices are often utilized. Some authors have recommended chemical prophylaxis with aspirin, warfarin, or low-molecular-weight heparin.

Antibiotic Prophylaxis

Antibiotic prophylaxis has been shown to be associated with decreased infection rates (see Chap. 3). When antibiotics are administered, it should be done 30 to 60 min before placing a tourniquet, so that the antibiotic concentrations in tissue at the surgical site are optimal.

► ANESTHETIC CONSIDERATIONS

Preoperative Measures

Patients presenting for knee arthroplasty often fall into the older age groups; therefore comorbidities associated with advanced age, rheumatoid arthritis, and obesity should be considered (see Chaps. 7, 8, and 12).

Surgical Requirements for Anesthesia

Optimal anesthetic techniques for lower extremity joint arthroplasty are those that provide analgesia of the operated extremity, adequate relaxation for retraction, the ability to monitor nerve function postoperatively, and avoidance of additional risks. The experience of the anesthesiologist and the hospital environment may dictate the safest and most effective anesthetic technique.

Techniques that minimize central "hangovers" are optimal for recovery and initiation of physical therapy. Preemptive pain control (oral narcotics and COX-II nonsteroidal anti-inflammatory agents) and antiemesis measures may be desirable.

Various forms of anesthesia are suitable for knee arthroplasty: general, regional, and neuraxial anesthesia. Most primary total knee replacements are performed in a timely manner, which makes them amenable to these techniques. Epidural and regional anesthetics have been shown to decrease the recovery period for these patients and to pose fewer risks than general anesthesia; they may also assist in postoperative analgesia.

Nerve Block

Unilateral nerve blocks for major proximal lower limb surgery are generally not optimal, since the nonoperated leg can become very uncomfortable for the patient—hence the patient may move it and thus distract the surgeon. Our choice for knee arthroplasty is to place a continuous femoral nerve block preoperatively (see Chap. 26), followed by a subarachnoid block (see Chap. 30) for the surgery. The femoral nerve block can also be done postoperatively, but not being able to observe patellar movements because of the bandaging may make this difficult. However, one can feel for contractions of the sartorius muscle (which originates from the superior anterior iliac spine). If there are clear anterior motor responses without sartorius contractions, it can only be the quadriceps muscles contracting. To place blocks postoperatively can be very painful for the patient, so it is advisable to place the block just before the spinal anesthesia loses all its effect or to make liberal use of potent analgesics, such as remifentanil. The catheters are left in place for 1 to 5 days, depending on the preference of the anesthesiologist and the surgeon; quadriceps function may be an important consideration. Low infusion rates and low concentrations of a drug such as ropivacaine usually preserve quadriceps muscle function. The patient can top this up by patient-controlled bolus injections whenever the quadriceps muscle function is not needed, as at night while the patient is sleeping (see Chap. 21).

Intraoperatively, the type and amount of sedation depends on the patient's requirements. Continuous infusion of propofol is often used at various infusion rates, although this sometimes disinhibits the patient; we prefer to use midazolam in varying dosages with or without small doses of meperidine, depending on the patient's requirements. We also provide patients with noise-cancellation headphones and music of their choice.

A common anesthetic technique is, however, still general anesthesia, although it is not optimal. Its use depends on the choice of the patient, the experience of the anesthesiologist, the choice of anticoagulation agent, and its timing (see Chaps. 4 and 30).

One of the disadvantages of femoral nerve catheters in the postoperative period is a slower return of quadriceps function. This may increase the risk of a fall while the patient is in the hospital; therefore measures to prevent this must be taken. Sciatic nerve blocks are a concern, particularly in valgus knee deformities, owing to the importance of early detection of sciatic and peroneal nerve palsies. These deficits can develop after the initial postoperative evaluation, within the first 24 h. They can be due to postoperative hematoma as well as positioning problems. Oral pain management is essential to provide optimal physical therapy in the recovery period following a total knee replacement. Multimodality pain control often allows the patient to optimize his or her pain control without the central effects of heavy narcotic use.

Because a tourniquet controls bleeding, the assistance of the anesthesiologist is not usually required. However, the use of tourniquets is becoming more and more controversial, and anesthesiologists may well in the near future be called on to help control bleeding in the surgical field. The principles are described in Chap. 10.

▶ POSTOPERATIVE PROTOCOL

The majority of total knee replacements in the United States are cemented arthroplasties (see Chap. 33). There are, however, proponents of uncemented femoral components, and there has been a resurgence of interest in uncemented tibial and femoral components. The postoperative protocol may vary based on the choice of an implant. With cemented total knee replacements, weight bearing is generally allowed as tolerated. Physical therapy is usually initiated on the day of surgery or first postoperative day. This therapy includes ambulation, generally with assistive devices, and exercises to restore early range of motion and quadriceps strength. Occasionally, knee immobilizers are used for a patient's safety in walking until quadriceps strength returns. During the recovery period, caution with extreme flexion is necessary to prevent extensor mechanism problems. Continuous passive motion is utilized to improve motion and may provide a psychological benefit to the patient in terms of visualization of a knee that moves as well as providing some early pain relief. Concerns about continuous passive range of motion are the possible contributions to limitation in terminal extension and potential compression of the peroneal nerve when the patient's mobility is decreased.

▶ POTENTIAL COMPLICATIONS

Postoperative complications include arthrofibrosis, nerve traction injuries, vascular insufficiency, extensor mechanism problems, or skin problems. Arthrofibrosis is related to many different factors including poor balancing, preoperative limited motion and scar formation from previous operations, aggressive scar formation during the recovery period, and insufficient or poor physical therapy during the postoperative period. Inadequate pain control may contribute to a patient's unwillingness to participate in physical therapy and range-of-motion exercises.

Peroneal Nerve Injury

Nerve injuries are rare. However, they are more common in a valgus knee with a flexion contracture than in varus knee deformities preoperatively. With the restoration of a normal mechanical axis, a valgus knee deformity tends to stretch the peroneal nerve as it crosses on the lateral

side of the knee just distal to the fibular head. In combination with a flexion deformity, this risk is increased, since the nerve passes posterior to the axis of the knee joint. Peroneal nerve injuries in the varus knee preoperatively are rare but can be related to tourniquet problems, postoperative pressure palsies from the patient's limited mobility, inadequate protection of the peroneal nerve, or excessively tight dressings. Postoperative hematomas can contribute to the development of postoperative nerve palsies. When a postoperative nerve injury is detected, the dressings should be removed and the possibility of an expanding hematoma examined. Compartment syndrome is rare but should be ruled out. Generally the knee is placed into flexion with no pressure on its lateral side to assist reversible changes in the peroneal nerve.

Extensor Mechanism

Extensor mechanism failure can occur intraoperatively or postoperatively with aggressive physical therapy and/or postoperative trauma due to quadriceps weakness. Extensor mechanism complications must be avoided and care taken to protect the patient during and after the operation. Education, aids for walking, and/or knee immobilizers can help to prevent these problems.

Skin Complications

Skin complications are devastating around total knee replacements, particularly at the inferior aspect of the wound, where there is minimal subcutaneous tissue over the proximal tibia. The blood supply to the anterior skin flaps is at risk if large undermining is performed. These flaps are at greater risk if previous incisions are not accounted for in planning surgical incisions. If a skin complication is encountered, aggressive soft tissue coverage should be instituted.

▶ KNEE ARTHRODESIS

Knee arthrodesis is rarely indicated before knee arthroplasty. Indications are septic arthritis or failure of an extensor mechanism due to neuromuscular disease. The most common indication for a knee arthrodesis is in patients with failed knee arthroplasty in the setting of an absent extensor mechanism or recurrent infection. Techniques for knee revision surgery include intramedullary nailing, plate fixation, and external fixation. An intramedullary nail tends to be the most desirable implant due to its load sharing capacity and immediate weight-bearing potential for the patient. The risks of intramedullary nailing are greatest in patients with sepsis, because of recurrent infection around the intramedullary nail. Other alternatives for knee fusion include external fixation, which is desirable in a complicated postinfectious case. However, the risk of nonunion is higher with external fixation than with intramedullary nailing. In addition, postoperative management is more complicated with external fixation than with intramedullary nailing.

SUGGESTED FURTHER READING

Archibeck MJ, White RE Jr. What's new in adult reconstructive knee surgery. *J Bone Joint Surg Am* 86(8):1839–1849, 2004.

Barrack RL, Bertot AJ, Wolfe MW, et al. Patellar resurfacing in total knee arthroplasty. A prospective, randomized, double-blind study with five to seven years of follow-up. *J Bone Joint Surg Am* 83-A(9):1376–1381, 2001.

Becker MW, Insall JN, Faris M. Bilateral total knee arthroplasty. One cruciate retaining and one cruciate substituting. *Clin Orthop Rel Res* (271):122–124, 1991.

Dennis D, Komistek R, Scuderi G, et al. In vivo three-dimensional determination of kinematics for subjects with a normal knee or a unicompartmental or total knee replacement. *J Bone Joint Surg Am* 83(90022):S104–S115, 2001.

Diduch DR, Insall JN, Scott WN, et al. Total knee replacement in young, active patients. Long-term follow-up and functional outcome. *J Bone Joint Surg Am* 79(4):575–582, 1997.

Fahmy NR, Chandler HP, Danylchuk K, et al. Blood-gas and circulatory changes during total knee replacement. Role of the intramedullary alignment rod. *J Bone Joint Surg Am* 72(1):19–26, 1990.

Iorio R, Healy WL. Unicompartmental arthritis of the knee. *J Bone Joint Surg Am* 85(7):1351–1364, 2003.

Laubenthal KN, Smidt GL, Kettelkamp DB. A quantitative analysis of knee motion during activities of daily living. *Phys Ther* 52(1):34–43, 1972.

Pagnano MW, Cushner FD, Scott WN. Role of the posterior cruciate ligament in total knee arthroplasty. *J Am Acad Orthop Surg* 6(3):176–187, 1998.

Rose HA, Hood RW, Otis JC, et al. Peroneal-nerve palsy following total knee arthroplasty. A review of The Hospital for Special Surgery experience. *J Bone Joint Surg Am* 64(3):347–351, 1982.

Sharrock N, Haas S, Hargett M, et al. Effects of epidural anesthesia on the incidence of deep-vein thrombosis after total knee arthroplasty. *J Bone Joint Surg Am* 73(4):502–506, 1991.

Swanik CB, Lephart SM, Rubash HE. Proprioception, kinesthesia, and balance after total knee arthroplasty with cruciate-retaining and posterior stabilized prostheses. *J Bone Joint Surg Am* 86(2):328–334, 2004.

CHAPTER 12

Foot and Ankle Surgery

MICHAEL L. SALAMON/CHARLES L. SALTZMAN/
VIJAYA GOTTUMUKKALA/ANDRÉ P. BOEZAART

▶ INTRODUCTION

This chapter deals with the foot and ankle as two entities. Common surgical procedures of the foot and ankle are discussed to give the orthopaedic anesthesiologist an insight into the intricacies of these conditions.

Foot pathology is very common. Most disorders can be successfully treated by nonoperative means, including the use of orthotics, physical therapy, anti-inflammatory medications, ambulatory aids, and shoe-wear modifications. When these measures fail to alleviate the symptoms, surgery is considered.

Although trauma victims form a significant subset of patients for these operative procedures in the acute setting, patients with rheumatoid arthritis, diabetes, degenerative disorders, congenital deformities of the foot, benign and malignant lesions of the foot, and those with neuromuscular disorders comprise the rest.

Surgery on the foot is often a large undertaking for both patient and family. The prolonged and confining convalescence period can be very difficult for them. Furthermore, pain in the first postoperative week can be substantial if it is not aggressively treated. Poorly managed postoperative pain may contribute to many detrimental consequences, including increased postoperative morbidity (pulmonary, cardiac, and thromboembolic), delayed convalescence, and even chronic pain. It is now known that a higher level of postoperative pain generally results in a lower quality of recovery. Although different analgesic techniques and regimens may be satisfactory (if analgesia is aggressively managed) from an outcome point of view, preliminary evidence suggests that regional analgesic techniques may allow for a superior quality of recovery as well as an increase in the quality of life and patient satisfaction.

Although there are many foot conditions that may require operative treatment, this chapter focuses on the most common circumstances in which surgery is necessary.

▶ PREOPERATIVE CONSIDERATIONS

Trauma victims comprise a significant group of patients for these procedures. After a thorough evaluation of other injuries, adequacy of fluid resuscitation and preexisting medical comorbidities need to be considered in planning the anesthetic management. Particular attention is necessary to airway issues and aspiration precautions. If the wound is open, minimizing time delay between the injury and surgery will significantly reduce the incidence of wound infection.

Rheumatoid arthritis patients with advanced rheumatoid arthritis pose a significant anesthetic challenge because of the multisystem involvement of the disease (see Chap. 8). Apart from the secondary involvement of the cardiopulmonary, hematologic, and renal systems, the challenges faced by the anesthesiologist pertain to airway management (cervical spine instability), vascular access, and positioning. These patients also have impaired immune systems, muscle wasting, and a hypermetabolic state, all of which contribute to an increased rate of postoperative infection and morbidity. It is therefore imperative for the anesthesiologist to thoroughly evaluate these patients for the severity of their disease and their pharmacologic history. Drug therapy in these patients is utilized to provide analgesia, control inflammation, and induce immunosuppression.

A well thought out anesthetic technique considering all of the above-mentioned concerns, with particular emphasis on aggressive management of postoperative pain, would contribute to a successful outcome.

Diabetes is a leading cause of both mortality and early disability. In the United States, it is the leading cause of nontraumatic limb amputations—in addition to other complications such as blindness and end-stage renal disease. Microvascular, neuropathic, and other concurrent diabetic complications lead to the development of the "diabetic foot" in patients at risk.

The principal goal in the anesthetic management of a diabetic patient is to evaluate him or her for any metabolic and infectious complications, end-organ dysfunction, and degree of glycemic control. Perioperative morbidity can be greatly reduced by paying particular attention to the tight control of hemodynamic parameters and blood sugar levels. Other anesthetic considerations in these patients are obesity, airway issues (stiff-joint syndrome), gastroparesis (risk of regurgitation and aspiration of gastric contents), vascular access (diabetic scleroderma), glucose and electrolyte abnormalities, hydration status, current medications, and being at risk for sudden death.

It is recommended that diabetic patients be scheduled for surgery early in the day so as to limit the duration of preoperative fasting. The diet-treated, well-controlled non-insulin-dependent diabetes mellitus (NIDDM) patient and patients with well controlled insulin-dependent diabetes mellitus (IDDM) undergoing brief outpatient procedures may not require any adjustment in their therapy, hospitalization, or any special treatment (including insulin) before or during surgery. Patients on oral hypoglycemic drugs have to be monitored closely, as these drugs can cause hypoglycemia for several hours after the last dose (chlorpropamide) or lactic acidosis (metformin). Whatever regimen of intravenous fluids and insulin therapy is chosen during the perioperative period, the goal is to avoid hypoglycemia, excessive hyperglycemia, ketoacidosis, and electrolyte disturbances. Preadmission is indicated only for patients with poorly controlled diabetes.

Neuromuscular Disorders

Charcot-Marie-Tooth (CMT) disease (peroneal muscular dystrophy) is the most common inherited cause of chronic motor and sensory peripheral neuropathy that results in foot deformities. Patients with CMT disease have a glove-and-stocking sensory loss along with distal muscle weakness and sensory ataxia, which leads to walking difficulties. There is a correlation between respiratory symptoms and proximal upper limb involvement. Therefore it is prudent to assess such patients for any upper limb weakness. Anesthetic considerations in these patients are related to their sensitivity to neuromuscular blocking drugs, positioning issues, and the possibility of postoperative

respiratory failure. Perioperative cardiac abnormalities have not been a consistent finding in these patients, and there is no evidence that patients with CMT1A are susceptible to malignant hyperthermia (MH) or a hyperkalemic response to succinylcholine. Preoperative workup in these patients is dependent on their age, clinical condition, and other comorbid conditions.

Benign and Malignant Lesions

Preoperative evaluation of patients with malignant lesions includes consideration of possible pathophysiologic side effects of the disease and the adverse effects of cancer chemotherapeutic drugs and radiation therapy. Correction of nutrient deficiencies, anemia, coagulopathy, and electrolyte disturbances might be needed. Patients with chronic pain might be on long-term opioid therapy; this must be taken into consideration during the perioperative period both for pain management and management of opioid withdrawal states. The presence of hepatic, cardiac, pulmonary, and renal involvement may influence the patient's workup and the anesthetic technique chosen. Attention to aseptic technique is important during the procedure for both surgical and anesthetic interventions, as immunosuppression occurs with chemotherapeutic agents. Immunosuppression produced by inhalational agents, surgical stress, and even blood transfusions during the perioperative period may have an undetermined effect.

▶ APPLIED ANATOMY OF THE FOOT AND ANKLE

To be proficient and successful with peripheral regional techniques, one must understand the gross anatomy of the foot and ankle, with particular emphasis on the nerve supply.

In order to provide complete anesthesia to the distal third of the leg, ankle joint, and the foot, blockade of the saphenous, common peroneal (superficial and deep peroneal), and tibial nerves (sural, medial and lateral plantar nerves) must be achieved (see Chap. 28). The chosen location of the blocks to be performed (classical ankle versus popliteal block of the sciatic nerve and saphenous) is primarily dependent on the location of surgery and other considerations, such as the site of tourniquet application.

Nerve Supply to the Lower Leg and Foot

Cutaneous

The saphenous nerve in the leg (purely cutaneous except for an articular twig to the inferior tibiofibular joint) runs down the medial border of the tibia immediately behind the great saphenous vein, crosses the vein in front of the medial malleolus, and reaches as far as the base of the great toe. This nerve supplies the cutaneous area over the medial side of the leg, ankle, and foot (see Chap. 28).

The superficial peroneal nerve supplies the front of the leg and the intermediate part of the dorsum of the foot. The superficial peroneal nerve pierces the fascia of the lateral leg compartment (peroneal muscles) to become superficial in the distal third of the leg, midway between the anterior tibia and the fibula. This nerve then branches into the medial and intermediate dorsal cutaneous nerves of the foot.

The sural nerve supplies the posterolateral part of the lower third of the leg as well as the lateral side of the foot and the little toe. The adjacent sides of the first and second toes are supplied by the medial division of the deep peroneal nerve, the lateral side of the little toe by the sural nerve, and all the remaining parts of the toes by the superficial peroneal nerve.

The skin on the dorsal surfaces of the terminal phalanges is supplied by the plantar nerves (branches of tibial nerve), the lateral plantar supplying the fifth and the lateral side of the fourth toes and the medial plantar supplying the remainder.

Medial calcaneal (terminal cutaneous branches of the tibial nerve) nerves supply the heel of the foot. The medial two-thirds and the lateral third of the sole are supplied by the corresponding plantar nerves.

Muscular Innervation

The muscular innervation of the leg and foot can be best understood by considering the individual compartments of the leg and the layers in the foot.

The muscles in the anterior compartment of the leg are innervated by the deep peroneal nerve (tibialis anterior by L4 and L5 and the rest by the L5 and S1 roots). The actions of the muscles in this compartment are mainly to dorsiflex the ankle and extend the toes. The tibialis anterior also produces inversion of the foot, and the peroneus tertius aids in the eversion of the foot.

The muscles in the posterior compartment of the leg are innervated by the tibial nerve (L4 and L5 and the S1, S2, and S3 roots). The muscles in this compartment of the leg are mainly involved with plantarflexion of the foot and flexion of the great toe and digits at all joints; they also help in walking by maintaining the longitudinal arches of the foot. The tibialis posterior is also involved with inversion of the foot.

The muscles in the lateral compartment of the leg are innervated by the superficial peroneal nerve (L5 and S1 and S2 roots). These two muscles, the peroneus longus and brevis, are involved in eversion and are also weak plantarflexors of the foot.

All three muscle layers in the foot are supplied by the medial and lateral plantar nerves (S2 and S3 roots), which are branches of the tibial nerve. The muscles of the foot are involved with abduction, adduction, and flexion movements of the digits and metatarsophalangeal (MTP) joints and maintenance of the transverse arch of the foot.

Articular Innervation of the Foot

Ankle Joint

The tibial nerve supplies the posterior part of the ankle joint. In addition, articular twigs are also received from the saphenous and deep peroneal nerves.

JOINTS IN THE FOOT

The deep peroneal nerve supplies the tarsometatarsal and MTP joints of the great toe. The medial plantar nerve supplies articular branches to the MTP and interphalangeal joints of the medial $3\frac{1}{2}$ toes. The lateral plantar nerve supplies articular branches to the MTP and interphalangeal joints of the lateral $1\frac{1}{2}$ toes. In addition, most of the intertarsal and tarsometatarsal joints are also innervated by the lateral plantar nerve.

Osteotomes of the distal third of the lower leg and foot are derived from the roots of L4 and L5 and from S1, S2, and S3.

► ANESTHETIC MANAGEMENT

In general, the choice of an anesthetic technique for surgical procedures of the foot depend on the particular requirements of the procedure, state of the patient's health, patient preference, duration of the procedure, and surgeon's preference (ability to perform neuromuscular examination in the postoperative period).

Most procedures on the foot can be done under regional anesthesia alone, regional anesthesia with sedation, or a combined continuous regional anesthesia with light general anesthesia. If general anesthesia is chosen as the primary anesthetic of choice, induction of anesthesia, airway management, and intraoperative maintenance including monitoring depend on the patient's existing comorbid conditions.

If regional anesthesia is desired, the choice is between a central neuraxial conduction blockade (seldom) and peripheral nerve blocks with sedation. The particular choice again is dictated by the patient's medical condition and choices. Patients on anticoagulant drugs or with any coagulation abnormalities are considered to represent an absolute contraindication for continuous central neuraxial conduction blockade. Peripheral nerve blocks have the advantage of ipsilateral anesthesia on the side of the surgery and lack the complications secondary to bilateral sympathetic blockade and the risk of spinal hematoma formation. *Continuous regional techniques* offer postoperative analgesia superior to that of conventional systemic opioid analgesia, thereby decreasing the side effects secondary to opioid use and decreasing postoperative morbidity while also enhancing passive rehabilitative measures and improving the quality of recovery. If single-injection peripheral nerve blockade is used as the anesthetic technique, it is important to prescribe adequate analgesic medications for postoperative pain management once the nerve block dissipates. Regional anesthesia should be the preferred technique whenever possible.

Position/Tourniquet

Most procedures on the foot can be done in the supine position. However, the prone position is commonly used for calcaneal osteotomy.

A tourniquet with a cuff pressure 100 mmHg higher than the systemic arterial pressure is used for most procedures so as to provide an optimal surgical field. During foot and ankle surgery, the surgeon often asks to have the foot-end of the operating table raised in order to minimize bleeding after release of the tourniquet. This is commonly done by placing the patient in the Trendelenburg position. Anesthesiologists should be cautioned against this practice, since the head-down position increases the intracranial pressure and may cause a decrease in cerebral blood flow and possibly cerebral edema. It may be a better practice to elevate both the feet and the head by flexing the patient into the "jackknife" position. This may especially apply to elderly patients. Patients with diabetes may continue to have some bleeding with the tourniquet inflated owing to their calcified vessels. Patients on chronic steroid medication should have appropriate padding placed under the tourniquet to minimize deleterious effects of pressure on the skin. Most procedures on the foot can be done with a tourniquet in the midcalf region. However, a thigh tourniquet is used for transtibial and Symes amputations and correction of flat foot and cavovarus abnormalities.

Intraoperative Anesthetic Management

Our preferred anesthetic technique for foot surgery, depending on the anticipated complexity of the surgery and the patient's medical condition, is general anesthesia. This is usually combined with an ankle block (see Chap. 28) or sciatic nerve block (see Chap. 27) placed before or after induction of general anesthesia. General anesthesia is typically induced and maintained with propofol, a laryngeal mask airway (LMA) with or without intermittent positive-pressure ventilation (IPPV), with air in oxygen. If a peripheral nerve block cannot be done for any reason, we use a remifentanil infusion for intraoperative analgesia. We typically place a peripheral nerve block (ankle, popliteal, or more proximal sciatic nerve block combined with a femoral nerve block or more distal saphenous nerve block), which provides excellent intra- and postoperative analgesia (see Chaps. 26, 27, and 28). The effects of an ankle or sciatic nerve block can last into the second day after surgery and a continuous nerve block is seldom indicated, although it is usually done for subtalar fusions and major ankle surgery. If a continuous nerve block is done, a continuous popliteal block is ideal for foot surgery, although a more proximal block is usually done for major foot and ankle surgery because of the positioning of the tourniquet around the thigh.

It is important to realize that the saphenous nerve, a branch of the femoral nerve, can provide sensory innervation all the way down to the big toe. The saphenous nerve also provides sensory innervation to the medial aspect of the ankle joint.

Because most or all foot and ankle surgery is done under tourniquet control of bleeding, the anesthesiologist does not have to be concerned about the control of the bleeding in the surgical field.

Postoperative Management

Most foot and ankle procedures are usually painful, with the possible exception of surgery for conditions related to diabetes mellitus. The effects of single-injection blocks, such as an ankle block or a popliteal block, can last up to 36 h and usually provide adequate postoperative analgesia (see Chaps. 27 and 28). However, especially in the case of major ankle surgery, pain usually outlasts the block and combined continuous sciatic and femoral blocks are commonly done to overcome this discomfort (see Chaps. 26 and 27).

If a peripheral nerve block cannot be done for some other reason, intravenous patient-controlled analgesia (PCA) with morphine sulfate or another suitable agent should be provided as a minimum.

► SURGICAL MANAGEMENT

Bunions/Hallux Valgus

Etiology/Epidemiology

Bunions are an affliction of a civilized shoe-wearing society. Epidemiologic evidence suggests that the incidence of bunions in unshod societies is approximately 3 percent, whereas among shod societies it is as high as 33 percent. Although there may be a genetic predisposition to bunions among some populations or families, the vast majority of bunions develop secondary to inappropriate shoe wear. In particular, shoes with elevated heel heights and narrow toe boxes are considered causal to the development of bunion deformities.

Surgical Techniques

There are over 150 different operations described to treat bunion deformities. The myriad of procedures indicates a lack of consensus and true understanding of optimal treatment approach. For mild deformities, it is common for surgeons to choose procedures that require less convalescence than for larger deformities. All of the procedures are done on the first ray (the first cuneiform, first metatarsal, and hallux). If an equinus contracture of the ankle exists, the surgeon may add a percutaneous tendoachilles lengthening or a gastrocnemius recession at the same time as the bunion operation to "unload" the forefoot. This is done because some surgeons believe that inability to dorsiflex the ankle past a neutral position contributes to the bunion deformity.

For major deformities, surgeons generally either fuse the first metatarsocuneiform joint or osteotomize and realign the first metatarsal. This is combined with soft tissue reconstruction of the first MTP joint and sometimes with other forefoot procedures involving the hallux and/or lesser toes. After osteotomy, internal fixation is usually used to hold the position of alignment. The soft tissue reconstruction is performed to allow the hallux to achieve better alignment.

Postoperative Protocol

After surgery, patients who have had less involved bunion operations are frequently allowed to bear weight as tolerated in a postoperative stiff-soled shoe. Patients who have more complex operations involving osteotomizing the metatarsal or fusion of the metatarsocuneiform joint are restricted from weight bearing on this part of the foot until the bones have healed. With osteotomies, this period is approximately 4 to 6 weeks. However, after an arthrodesis procedure, this period can be as long as 12 weeks. Immobilization ranges from use of a simple postoperative stiff-soled shoe to a short leg cast.

Common Complications

Complications of bunion surgeries include recurrence of deformity, nonunion of osteotomy, nerve injury or entrapment, avascular necrosis of the first metatarsal head, degenerative joint disease, stiffness of the MTP joint, deep venous thrombosis, and infection. Although immediate postoperative complications are relatively rare and bone healing usually occurs, nerve dysfunction with subtotal great toe numbness and recurrence of deformity are seen more commonly. Recurrence of deformity occurs secondary to the wearing of shoes that are too tight and is more common in both younger patients and those with generalized hypermobility of the soft tissues and joints.

Hammer Toes and Metatarsalgia

Etiology/Epidemiology

Hammer toes and metatarsalgia are common problems. Although hammer-toe deformities can occur from a neurologic cause, they are usually initiated by poorly fitting shoes. The second toe is most commonly affected, as it is the longest toe on most feet, and becomes deformed as it hits the end of the shoe. The third toe may become involved soon thereafter. A hallux valgus deformity may exacerbate or even cause a hammer-toe deformity. This occurs when the great toe moves into valgus and slides underneath the second and third toes. Subsequently, this causes decreased weight bearing by the toes, with more weight transferred proximally to the metatarsal heads. Metatarsalgia (or pain under the "ball" of the foot) may then ensue. If the hammer-toe deformity progresses, the natural history is that the plantar plate of the second MTP joint may be disrupted and the second toe will subluxate dorsally onto the second metatarsal head. Eventually the deformities of the joints may become fixed.

Surgical Indications/Contraindications

The indication for hammer-toe surgery is painful callus formation on the tip of the toes, on the dorsum of the phalanges, or along the plantar aspect of the metatarsal heads that is unresponsive to nonoperative treatment. The contraindications to the standard hammer-toe operation are insensitivity, recurrent infection, vascular insufficiency, and inflammatory arthritis.

Surgical Techniques

Fixed hammer toes require resection of bone. Typically this is combined with pin fixation. Flexible hammer toes can be treated with tendon lengthening or tendon transfers. Hammer-toe deformities with metatarsalgia may require a reconstruction of the MTP joint. The range of reconstruction includes soft tissue releases (extensor tendon lengthenings, dorsal capsular releases, collateral ligament releases), partial metatarsal head resections, or shortening procedures at the level of the metatarsal necks. When the metatarsals are shortened, surgeons try to maintain the normal cascade of relative length of the metatarsal heads. Therefore if the second metatarsal head is shortened proximal to the third, often the third will also need to be shortened so that the cascade is maintained.

Postoperative Protocol

Patients who undergo hammer-toe procedures are generally allowed to bear weight as tolerated on the heel and require a few days of extremity elevation. If metatarsal osteotomies are involved, weight bearing may be restricted for longer periods until bony healing is evident.

Percutaneous pins in the toes are usually left in place for 3 to 6 weeks and are easily removed in the clinic.

Common Complications

The most common complications of hammer-toe surgery include pin-tract infections, recurrence of deformity, continued pain at the level of the resected hammer toe, and stiffness of the toes. These complications are reduced by the use of early range-of-motion therapy and judicious pin care.

Forefoot Deformities and Rheumatoid Arthritis

Etiology/Epidemiology

Rheumatoid arthritis and the related inflammatory arthropathies affect approximately 5 percent of North Americans. The disease process includes both intra- and extraarticular pathology. The foot is the second most common site for initial inflammatory destructive changes, accounting for nearly 20 percent of first presentations. Early rheumatoid disease is often diagnosed by inflammation across the forefoot. The MTP joints have a strong predilection for inflammation. Inflammation of the MTP joints ultimately will result in subluxation or dislocation of these joints. The hallux typically goes into a valgus position. The lesser MTP joints usually dislocate dorsally and develop secondary hammer-toe deformities and metatarsalgia. Although nonrheumatoid operations are being done more commonly in the rheumatoid population, the standard treatment for a rheumatoid forefoot deformity is arthrodesis of the first MTP joint and resection arthroplasty of the lesser MTP joints, with or without hammer-toe correction. Therapeutic advances in cytokine molecular targeting medications appear to be slowing the progression of disease. This may change the way in which rheumatoid deformities are managed in the future.

Surgical Indications/Contraindications

The indication for rheumatoid forefoot reconstruction is the presence of painful deformities unresponsive to shoe modifications. Contraindications are chronic open ulcerations that have not been adequately treated nonoperatively, ongoing vasculitis, punctate hemorrhages of the nail fold suggesting inflammatory deposition vasculopathy, vascular insufficiency, and severe soft tissue atrophy secondary to chronic steroid use.

Surgical Techniques

Incisions on the forefoot are usually placed in a longitudinal fashion. These include incisions on the medial or dorsal aspect of the first MTP joint, between the second and third MTP joints, and between the fourth and fifth MTP joints. Through these incisions, the MTP joints are exposed. The first MTP joint is debrided of its articular surfaces and the second through fifth are generally treated with cascading metatarsal head resections. Hammer toes are either corrected operatively as described earlier or are corrected by simply realigning the toes via forceful manipulation. The toes are then held in position by percutaneously placed pins across the MTP joints for stabilization. The first MTP joint fusion is often the most difficult part of the procedure. Orientation of the first MTP arthrodesis in three dimensions is critical. Plates, screws, pins, or staples are used to hold the alignment of the fusion while it heals.

Postoperative Protocol

Patients who have forefoot fusions usually need to be restricted from weight bearing on the involved part of the foot until adequate bony healing has occurred. Rheumatoid patients are either placed in removable boots or short leg casts during the initial postoperative period. These patients generally have difficulty using standard crutches or walkers and require either modified platform crutches or walkers for ambulation in the postoperative period.

Common Complications

The most common complication of the rheumatoid forefoot operation is wound dehiscence. This problem is typically handled by local wound care but may require secondary procedures if infection becomes an issue. The second most common complication is nonunion at the fusion site, and this may require secondary procedures to obtain successful union. The shortened foot without the metatarsal heads functions well for most patients with rheumatoid arthritis, as these patients typically have low demands. Pain relief predictably occurs. However, for the higher-demand patient, resection of the metatarsal heads can be associated with the feeling of a functionally shortened foot, imbalance, and lack of terminal push off.

Diabetic Foot Problems

Etiology/Epidemiology

The Centers for Disease Control estimates that 16 million Americans are currently known to have diabetes mellitus and up to an equal number have undiagnosed diabetes mellitus or glucose intolerance. The epidemic of diabetes has been increasing exponentially over the past two decades. This has resulted in a large increase in the number of patients with end-stage problems. To varying degrees, the diabetic foot is characterized by chronic sensorimotor neuropathy, vascular disease, autonomic neuropathy, and impaired immune function. In the foot, the major cause of difficulties is directly related to the loss of protective sensation. Diabetic peripheral neuropathy involves the motor and sympathetic distributions and causes secondary toe clawing and decreased sweating. All together, the lack of sensation, toe clawing, and decreased sweating result in forefoot overload and secondary ulceration of the metatarsal heads or dorsum/tips of claw toes. Untreated ulcers frequently become secondarily infected, and this commonly leads to amputation. Surgery is occasionally performed for acute infections but is more commonly required to treat chronic infections of bone.

Surgical Indications/Contraindications

Indications for surgical treatment include abscess, necrotizing fasciitis, or the presence of chronic osteomyelitis. Antibiotics and appropriate wound management can generally treat acute osteomyelitis and cellulitis. The patient with a dysvascular limb needs to be revascularized before antibiotics will work. Partial forefoot amputations in dysvascular limbs are usually contraindicated.

Septic arthritis or abscesses in the deep spaces of the foot are relatively uncommon. When they do occur, surgical drainage is indicated. Drainage may be followed by use of closed suction drains or open packing. Acute abscesses and septic arthritis should be considered urgent surgical cases.

Chronic osteomyelitis is the most common indication for surgical management of the diabetic foot. Some parts of the foot are relatively expendable and others are essential. Decisions related to surgical amputation level reflect the functional use of each anatomic structure. The lesser toes can usually be amputated without cause for great concern. The great toe can also either be amputated in part or in full with minimal increased risk of causing pressure overload of the remaining foot that might lead to development of ulceration and osteomyelitis. Decision making regarding more proximal chronic infections is challenging, as the indications for performing a transmetatarsal-level amputation versus a ray resection are evolving. In general, either the first ray or the lateral one or two rays can be resected with preservation of relatively good foot function. Resection of a single, central ray (either the second, third, or fourth) can be performed. Infection of the first and second metatarsals, any two central metatarsals, or extensive involvement of the lateral two or more metatarsals requires an amputation at the transmetatarsal level. This is an excellent level for function, since the peroneus longus, peroneus brevis, and tibialis anterior tendons all still function. This means that the foot can still dorsiflex, plantarflex, invert, and evert. Moreover, postoperative orthotic management is quite simple. With a higher level of amputation, function of the aforementioned tendons is removed and the foot cannot be dorsiflexed or everted. In these circumstances, we tend to use a transtibial level of amputation. If the patient has calcaneal osteomyelitis in isolation and has a good vascular supply, we will consider a partial or complete calcanectomy.

In terms of major lower extremity amputations, we either perform a transtibial level amputation or a Symes amputation (ankle disarticulation). The transtibial amputation is performed on over 90 percent of patients. The indication for a Symes amputation is a patient who cannot afford a prosthetic leg or refuses to consider having a transtibial amputation. In general, amputees function much better with a transtibial amputation than a Symes amputation. The newest transtibial prostheses store and release energy efficiently in a single gait cycle. This results in better oxygen efficiency and is associated with a higher level of patient satisfaction.

Surgical Techniques

In general, antibiotics are held prior to surgery if the amputation is being done for reasons of infection. This allows the surgeon to obtain cultures from deep tissue, which is essential in guiding appropriate and effective antibiotic regimens. After cultures have been obtained, empiric antibiotic therapy can be started and later refined based on culture results. If an amputation is being done for reasons other than infection, perioperative antibiotics are appropriate. Wounds can be closed primarily if the amputation is at a level away from the infected tissue. If the incisions are near or through grossly contaminated tissues, the wounds should be left open and the incisions closed on a delayed basis, or they should be allowed to heal by secondary intention. In general, all visible nerves should be cut as proximally as possible and allowed to retract into the soft tissues, so that painful neuroma formation does not develop.

Amputations of the toes are relatively straightforward. Incisions are designed so that wound closure is easily achieved after bony resection. The amputations are usually done to a level where healthy tissue remains and are either transosseous amputations or disarticulations.

Ray resections can be a bit more challenging. Longitudinal incisions are used and must be planned so that wound closure is not under undue tension. Bony prominences should not remain in areas that bear weight and should ideally be well covered with soft tissue.

Transmetatarsal amputations are achieved by creating a longer plantar skin flap that is brought over the ends of the cut metatarsals and closed dorsally. This allows the thick plantar skin to protect the end of the residual foot and keeps the incision away from weight-bearing areas. The metatarsals are cut so that a smooth cascade is created.

The Symes amputation is an ankle disarticulation. The incision is planned so that when closure is complete, the tough heel pad is end-bearing. The incision usually ends up anterior to the ankle joint and is away from the end of the residual limb.

A below-knee or transtibial amputation is usually done approximately 13 to 15 cm distal to the tibial tubercle.

The major vessels are ligated and large nerves cut sharply and allowed to retract into the leg. A long posterior flap of skin and muscle is brought around the end of the cut tibia and fibula and closed just proximal to the ends of the bones. This produces a well-padded, durable residual limb that will be able to accept a prosthesis. Higher-level amputations are not discussed here.

Postoperative Protocol
Patients are typically admitted to the hospital for a few days postoperatively and receive intravenous antibiotics. If they have undergone partial resections of forefoot bones, we wait until the resected margins are evaluated by pathology for the presence of continued infection before switching to a home oral antibiotic regimen. If patients have evidence of continued infection, our practice is either to reoperate and resect more tissue or try a 4- to 6-week course of intravenous antibiotics. Otherwise, we proceed with oral antibiotics when the wound appears benign. An infectious disease specialist frequently guides antibiotic therapy.

Weight-bearing protocols depend on the level of the amputation and the patient's ability to cooperate. In general, we try to keep most patients off the operated limb for approximately 3 weeks, until the wounds are stable. Sutures are removed at about 3 weeks and the patient is fitted for appropriate shoes, orthotics, or prosthetics as needed.

Common Complications
The most serious complication during amputation of the foot is severe intraoperative blood loss. This occasionally occurs during attempts to control bleeding from calcified blood vessels. Such vessels may bleed profusely during a transtibial amputation despite use of a tourniquet. Since many of these patients have renal insufficiency and anemia, it is important to have blood available for transfusion.

Wound problems and recurrent infections are common in diabetic patients. These may require rehospitalization or reoperation. Patients who have recurrent plantar wound problems of the forefoot and an equinus contracture may require a tendoachilles lengthening or gastrocnemius recession to help unload these areas of high contact pressure.

Adult-Acquired Flatfoot Deformity

Etiology/Epidemiology
The prevalence of the acquired flatfoot deformity in adults appears to be increasing, along with our aging population. The deformity is associated with obesity and triceps surae tightness (equinus contracture). Surgeons classify these deformities as either fixed or flexible. Deformities are fixed if they are not passively correctable.

Flexible deformities can be reduced to a plantigrade position without forceful manipulation while the patient is awake in the clinic.

Surgical Indications/Contraindications
All flexible flatfoot deformities should be treated with physical therapy and orthotic management prior to consideration of surgery. Fixed deformities do not generally respond to orthotic management and rehabilitation and more often require surgery. The surgical treatments of adult-acquired flatfoot deformities are evolving. Fixed deformities are treated with fusion-type procedures. In general, older or obese patients are also treated with fusion procedures. The flexible deformities are treated with extraarticular osteotomies and tendon transfers. Fusions of intrinsically unstable joints can also be included if needed.

Contraindications to surgery include patients who are unwilling to comply with prolonged non-weight-bearing protocols, patients with bilateral disease who cannot avoid weight bearing, those with vascular insufficiency, and patients whose neurologic complications preclude operative management.

Surgical Techniques
For fixed deformities, the surgical technique involves an arthrodesis of the subtalar (talocalcaneal) joint and often the calcaneocuboid and talonavicular joints. The subtalar joint arthrodesis is performed through a lateral approach. The subtalar joint is fixed with screws. If there is any residual varus deformity after the subtalar arthrodesis is performed, the talonavicular and calcaneocuboid joints must be included in the arthrodesis. Fixation is achieved by using screws, staples, or long pins. Bone grafts may need to be used, especially if the talonavicular joint is to be fused. Autogenous bone graft can be harvested from the iliac crest or the proximal tibia distal to the lateral joint line of the knee. The use of allograft in place of autograft is becoming more popular, although its efficacy is unclear.

For a flexible deformity, the typical operation involves realignment of the calcaneal tuberosity through a lateral hindfoot approach. This incision is placed below the sural nerve along the lateral aspect of the calcaneus; the calcaneus is then osteotomized and displaced medially approximately 1 cm. Fixation is achieved using one or two screws. The second part of the procedure involves a transfer of the flexor digitorum longus (FDL) tendon to the insertion of the posterior tibial tendon. The loss of toe flexor function is not noticed by patients after the FDL transfer. In some patients, a midfoot fusion must be performed at the same time because of residual instability of the metatarsal cuneiform or naviculocuneiform joints. If this is the case, the surgeon will have to remove the joint's articular surfaces and stabilize it, usually with two screws. Tendoachilles lengthening and gastrocnemius recession are often required to obtain good alignment for the fixed deformities and can be used in addition to the operations for the flexible deformities.

Postoperative Protocol

The postoperative protocol for both types of operations is similar. Patients are maintained non-weight-bearing for approximately 6 weeks in a short leg cast. The position of the foot is gradually reduced from an inverted/plantarflexed position for the flexible deformities. The position of the foot for the fixed deformities is set at the time of surgery and does not follow cast changes. At 6 weeks, radiographs are taken, and if bone healing is progressing satisfactorily, the patient is put in either a walking boot or walking cast. For the flexible deformities, orthotics can be used up to a year after surgery to maintain the position of soft tissues. In general, orthotics are not needed after fusion procedures of the hindfoot.

Common Complications

Complications of these operations include nerve entrapment or transection of either a branch of the superficial peroneal nerve or the sural nerve. Other complications include nonunion, recurrence of deformity, continued pain, and the need for reoperation. Deep venous thromboses are rare in this population and anticoagulation is generally not used except in patients who have a family history of hypercoagulability.

The Cavovarus Foot

Etiology/Epidemiology

The prevalence of cavovarus (high arches/inverted heel) feet in the general population is relatively low. A cavovarus foot deformity is most commonly secondary to a progressive neuromuscular disorder such as Charcot-Marie-Tooth (CMT) disease (hereditary sensorimotor neuropathy). Of the progressive neuromuscular diseases, CMT disease is the most prevalent in North America. Progressive demyelination of nerves to specific muscle groups occurs in a characteristic fashion. Typically, the intrinsic muscles are affected first, followed by larger extrinsic muscles such as the tibialis anterior and peroneus brevis. Other muscles in the anterior compartment, the posterior compartment, and the peroneus longus may be affected later in the process. From a hereditary standpoint, CMT disease is characterized by variable penetrance and variable mixed phenotypic expression within families and even between a single patient's two limbs. Because of this, it is very difficult to predict the final outcome of the disease process. Surgical procedures to treat deformity are static interventions along a continuum of progressive neurologic dysfunction. The primary goal of surgery for these patients is to create a stable, plantigrade foot that can be braced.

The other general class comprising patients with cavovarus feet is the "idiopathic" group, as these patients do not have neuromuscular dysfunction. Most procedures done for these patients can result in long-standing static improvement of deformities.

Patients with a unilateral cavovarus foot need careful assessment. Most have a history of leg trauma and have sustained some form of leg or foot compartment syndrome. However, some patients have spinal cord abnormalities such as tumor or syringomyelia that need to be investigated prior to surgical reconstruction.

Surgical Indications/Contraindications

The indications for cavovarus foot reconstruction include unbraceable feet with recurrent instability or focal plantar pressure problems. Contraindications include patients who have unrealistic expectations regarding their ultimate functional outcome (especially patients with progressive neuromuscular disease), vascular insufficiency, and ongoing infection.

Surgical Techniques

The surgical technique depends on the deformity. Like the flatfoot, fixed deformities are treated with hindfoot fusion procedures. Flexible deformities are treated with aggressive realignment and tendon transfer procedures.

The mainstay of the realignment procedures is to elevate the first ray with a dorsiflexion closing wedge first metatarsal osteotomy and then slide the heel into a more valgus position through a lateral closing wedge calcaneal osteotomy. Except in children, where fixation of the first metatarsal may not be needed, both of these are stabilized with hardware. Tendon transfers are done to balance the foot. The standard transfers include centralizing the tibialis anterior (if still functioning) to the central midfoot, resulting in a more lateral pull, and transfer of the peroneus longus to the peroneus brevis to augment hindfoot eversion and reduce declination of the first ray. An open tendoachilles lengthening is also often used. To augment ankle dorsiflexion in patients with profound tibialis anterior weakness, the posterior tibial tendon can be transferred to the dorsum of the foot, passing it through the interosseous membrane. With severe deformity of the great toe, the hallux interphalangeal joint is often fused and the extensor hallucis longus is transferred proximally to the neck of the first metatarsal. The common claw-toe deformities can be treated in a variety of ways. The surgical options for treating claw toes include flexor tenotomies with pinning versus intrinsic substitution tendon transfers. The plantar fascia of the foot is released to decrease the cavus deformity.

Postoperative Protocol

The feet are usually casted for a minimum of 6 weeks. Patients remain non-weight-bearing for the first 4 to 6 weeks and then are allowed to bear weight once radiographs show evidence of osseous healing.

Common Complications

Because of the lack of sensation, patients with neuromuscular disease are prone to cast-related complications. Wound problems are not uncommon. Nerve dysfunction in focal areas of the foot is also common, although it does not seem to bother most patients with CMT disease. Such problems are not as well tolerated by patients with idiopathic cavovarus feet. Progressive weakness and deformity among patients with CMT disease is a common problem after reconstructive procedures. Patients need to understand before surgery that their surgical intervention is a static one in a continuum of a progressive disease. Bracing may be required throughout the patient's life.

▶ THE ANKLE JOINT

Ankle surgery involves certain unique considerations. The soft tissue around the ankle is limited, with little or no muscle coverage. Therefore, to maintain optimal blood flow and healing, direct approaches are preferable to the dissection of large flaps. The use of tourniquets should be limited to as little time as possible, generally less than 90 min. Incisions are generally made with a view to avoid nerves so as to prevent postoperative scarring and pain. Elevation of the ankle is desired during and after surgery to minimize swelling. Postoperative immobilization is common, but it must be done in neutral ankle position to avoid pain and plantarflexion contracture secondary to gravity.

▶ ANATOMIC CONSIDERATIONS

Developmental Anatomy

The lower limb bud begins to develop at 27 to 28 days of gestation. The nerves of the lumbosacral plexus grow into the limb bud from the fifth through seventh embryonic weeks, innervating muscle and cutaneous tissues. The continued growth and rotation of the limb results in the adult dermatomal pattern. Each dermatome represents the sensory fibers of one dorsal root, with some overlapping and individual variability. Joints, such as the ankle joint, are formed from the interzonal mesenchyme between developing bones, giving rise to the capsule and ligaments, the joint cavity, and the synovial membrane.

Surgical Anatomy

The ankle (talocrural) joint is a hinge-type synovial joint located between the distal tibia and fibula and the talus. The talus articulates in the mortise of the ankle, which is formed by the medial malleolus, the distal tibial articular surface, and the lateral malleolus of the fibula. The joint is uniaxial, with dorsiflexion-plantarflexion movement. A fibrous capsule and the medial and lateral collateral ligament complex support the joint. The deltoid ligament (medial) is composed of the tibionavicular, anterior tibiotalar, posterior tibiotalar, and tibiocalcaneal ligaments. The lateral ligaments are the anterior talofibular, posterior talofibular, and calcaneofibular ligaments.

The blood supply to the ankle joint is derived from the malleolar branches of the peroneal, anterior tibial, and posterior tibial arteries. The innervation of the ankle joint derived from the tibial and deep peroneal nerves and the saphenous nerve medially. The skin around the ankle is innervated by the medial cutaneous branch of the saphenous nerve (medial), sural nerve (posterolateral), and superficial peroneal nerve (anterolateral).

The anterior tibial artery, along with the deep peroneal nerve, crosses under the extensor hallucis longus muscle from medial to lateral at the level of the ankle joint, becoming the dorsalis pedis artery. The medial branch of the deep peroneal nerve goes on to innervate the first web space. Thus, in the distal leg, this neurovascular bundle lies between the tibialis anterior tendon and the extensor hallucis longus tendon; in the foot, it lies between the extensor hallucis longus and the extensor hallucis brevis. The posterior tibial artery and nerve pass posterior to the medial malleolus between the flexor digitorum longus and flexor hallucis longus and deep to the flexor retinaculum. (Please refer to "Applied Anatomy of the Foot and Ankle," above, for details on the cutaneous nerve supply.)

▶ ANKLE ARTHROPLASTY

Total ankle arthroplasty is usually indicated for ankle pain due to (noninfectious) arthritis that has not responded to nonoperative treatment. These patients have typically endured long-standing, debilitating ankle pain.

An extensive anterior incision is made over the ankle (Fig. 12-1). The deep peroneal nerve, branches of the superficial peroneal nerve, and dorsalis pedis artery are protected as the joint is approached lateral to the tibialis anterior tendon. After adequate exposure is obtained, jigs and/or cutting blocks are used to guide the saw cuts that remove the articular surfaces. The talar and tibial surfaces are prepared and appropriate components implanted. Fluoroscopy is used to evaluate the saw cuts as well as the positioning of the components. The wound is meticulously closed in layers.

Depending on implant design, the distal tibia-fibula joint may be fused and fixed with screws during the procedure. An Achilles' tendon lengthening may be needed to achieve the needed dorsiflexion of the ankle.

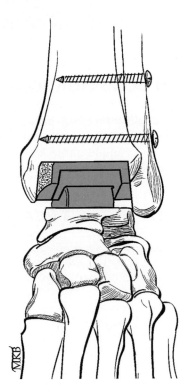

Figure 12-1. Anterior projection of an implanted Agility Ankle Replacement (Depuy, Inc., Warsaw, IN). This implant requires a tibiofibular syndesmosis fusion for proper function. All other ankle replacements do not involve screw fixation of the syndesmosis.

▶ ANKLE ARTHRODESIS

Arthrodesis or fusion of the ankle joint is indicated for pain in patients with arthrosis, deformities that are being corrected, or chronic instability in whom nonoperative treatments have failed. These patients have typically suffered from long-standing debilitating ankle problems. The patients who need arthrodesis are generally younger, more active, more demanding, and heavier than those who need ankle arthroplasty.

The ankle joint may be approached laterally, anteriorly, by a two-incision technique (minimally invasive with small anteromedial and anterolateral incisions), or arthroscopically assisted. The lateral common approach is made with an incision along the distal fibula curving to the base of the fourth metatarsal between the sural and superficial peroneal nerves. The soft tissues are dissected to expose the sinus tarsi and ankle joint. The fibula is osteotomized 2 cm proximal to the ankle joint. The remainder of the ankle joint is exposed with the removal of the distal fibula. The articular cartilage of the ankle is removed from the distal tibia and talus using a sagittal saw, osteotomes, and/or curettes to give broad, flat cancellous surfaces. A second incision can then be made if needed over the anterior medial aspect of the medial malleolus to expose the medial ankle joint. The articular surfaces of the lateral medial malleolus and lateral talus are then prepared in a similar manner. The appropriate position is then obtained and the joint is fixed with interfragmentary screws between the talus and tibia.

Note that numerous techniques have been described for ankle arthrodesis and fixation. Screw placement is variable. Some surgeons use a portion of the removed fibula as a strut graft on the lateral side of the fusion with screw fixation. The joint surfaces may be prepared for fusion arthroscopically if little deformity exists, and screw fixation can be obtained percutaneously. External fixation may be used in cases of revision or infection. In the case of deformity or revision surgery, an iliac crest bone graft may be required.

▶ EXTERNAL FIXATION

External fixators can be used around the ankle joint for a variety of indications. These include temporizing or definitive fracture treatment, ankle arthrodesis (primary or revision), deformity or malalignment near the ankle, and distraction of an arthritic ankle joint. Patient profiles are also variable. These individuals may have experienced acute trauma or chronic pain with possible failed prior procedures. They may suffer from diabetes, vascular disease, infection, or poor soft tissues around the ankle that may preclude other methods of treatment.

Preassembled or modular Ilizarov external fixator frames can be used around the ankle. Two circular rings are fixed to the tibia in the lower midshaft and supramalleolar area using wires or half pins for each ring. The wires or pins are placed into the bone through small incisions in the skin. The wires are tensioned and the pins and wires are fixed to the rings. Half rings are fixed to the calcaneus (two wires), talus (one wire if needed), and metatarsals (two wires) in a similar manner. If not preassembled, the foot half rings are attached to the tibial rings with threaded bar linkages and distraction or compression is applied across the ankle joint as required. Pins and wires are placed so as to optimize mechanical stability and avoid neurovascular structures.

Many different external fixation frames are available that may use a combination of pins or wires to fix the bones to the frame. The locations of pin placement and the number of pins will vary among the different fixator types.

Postoperatively, the patient may be kept from weight bearing or may bear partial weight. Complications vary owing to the multiple indications for external fixators, but they include pin-site infection, neurovascular injury, and tendon injury.

▶ SUPRAMALLEOLAR OSTEOTOMY

Osteotomy near the ankle joint can be used to treat congenital or acquired mechanical malalignment of the distal tibia. The patient population is variable, including children, adolescents, and adults.

A medial incision is made, centered at the level of the planned osteotomy. A small lateral incision at the same level may be needed if a fibular osteotomy is also required. An osteotomy is made parallel to the ankle joint at the appropriate level (usually at the level of the deformity). In the case of an open-wedge osteotomy for varus correction, the osteotomy is wedged open and a structural bone graft placed. In the case of a closing wedge osteotomy for valgus correction, a second osteotomy at the appropriate angle to the first bone cut is made and the defects are closed together. In either case, the osteotomy is fixed with a plate and screws. A specialized external fixator frame may be employed to perform gradual correction in cases of complex deformity.

▶ ANESTHETIC CONSIDERATIONS

Anesthetic considerations are similar to those involved in major foot surgery. Ankle block is inappropriate; continuous sciatic and femoral blocks are usually done for operative and postoperative analgesia in the major ankle surgery discussed above (see Chaps. 26 and 27).

Associated comorbidities and medications are similar to those discussed earlier in connection with surgery of the foot.

▶ PATIENT POSITIONING

The patient is positioned supine with the foot at the end of the operating table; a thigh tourniquet is usually used. Bumps may be used under the affected hip to rotate the ankle and foot medially, as may be surgically indicated.

▶ POSTOPERATIVE PROTOCOL

Postoperatively, the patient is immobilized in a splint and kept from bearing weight. Generally the dressing is changed on day 1 and day 14 and physical therapy begun at 6 weeks.

▶ COMMON COMPLICATIONS

Complications of ankle arthroplasty include neurovascular injury, tendon injury, infection, and wound-healing problems. Complications of ankle arthrodesis and osteotomy include the above plus nonunion and malunion.

SUGGESTED FURTHER READING

Antognini JF. Anesthesia for Charcot-Marie-Tooth disease: A review of 86 cases. *Can J Anesth* 39:398–400, 1992.

Canale ST, Campbell WC. *Campbell's Operative Orthopaedics,* 10th ed. 2004.

Crosby ET, Lui A. The adult cervical spine: Implications for airway management: *Can J Anesth* 37:77–93, 1990.

Firestein GS. Rheumatoid arthritis. *Sci Am Med* 3:1–15, 2002.

Goldman L, Ausiello D. *Cecil Textbook of Medicine,* 22d ed. Vol 2. 2004:1425–1452.

Kehlet H, Dahl JB. Anesthesia, surgery and challenges in postoperative recovery. *Lancet* 362:1921–1928, 2003.

Lam SL, Hodgson AR. A comparison of foot forms among the non-shoe and shoe wearing Chinese population. *J Bone Joint Surg* 40:1058, 1958.

Lupski JR, Chance PF, Garcia CD, et al. Inherited primary peripheral neuropathies. *JAMA* 270:2326–2330, 1993.

Macarthur A, Kleiman S. Rheumatoid cervical joint disease: A challenge to the anesthetist. *Can J Anesth* 40:154, 1993.

Mann RA, Coughlin MJ. *Surgery of the Foot and Ankle,* 7th ed., 1999.

Nathanson BN, Yu DG, et al. Respiratory muscle weakness in Charcot-Marie-Tooth disease. *Arch Intern Med* 1149:1389–1391, 1989.

Pellici PM, Ranawat CS, Tsairis P, et al. A prospective study of the progression of rheumatoid arthritis of the cervical spine. *J Bone Joint Surg Am* 63:342, 1981.

Perkins FM, Kehlet H. Chronic pain as an outcome of surgery: A review of predictive factors. *Anesthesiology* 93:1123–1133, 2000.

Romanes GJ. *Cunningham's Manual of Practical Anatomy,* 13th ed. Oxford, UK: Oxford University Press, 1966.

Wu CL, Fleisher LA. Outcomes research in regional anesthesia and analgesia. *Anesth Analg* 91:1232–1242, 2000.

Wu CL, Richman JM. Postoperative pain and quality of recovery. *Curr Opin Anesthesiol* 17:455–460, 2004.

CHAPTER 13

The Pediatric Spine

JOSEPH D. TOBIAS/DANIEL G. HOERNSCHEMEYER

▶ INTRODUCTION

Spinal surgery is one of the most common of the major orthopaedic operations in children. Spinal deformities that require surgery may be caused by congenital, acquired, or traumatic conditions. They may be due to primary defects of the vertebral column (hemivertebrae), neuromuscular disease (muscular dystrophy, cerebral palsy), or related to cancer, infections, or therapy. In spinal surgery, irrespective of the cause of the deformity that is being corrected, there are several surgical factors that may result in morbidity or death, including underlying disease, positioning of the patient, blood loss, and neurologic damage. To limit such problems, these patients should be approached in a standardized manner. This includes (1) a preoperative evaluation to identify comorbid features; (2) the anesthetic plan with attention to monitoring, patient positioning, maintenance of normothermia, techniques to limit the need for homologous transfusion, and control of coagulation function during large-volume transfusions; and (3) the postoperative regimen to maintain hemodynamic and respiratory parameters and to provide analgesia.

Spinal surgery in children may involve any level of the vertebral column through an anterior approach or a posterior approach or, in the case of thoracic and lumbar spine procedures, a combined anteroposterior (AP) procedure. However, the vast majority of the operations performed in pediatric patients involve long-segment surgery on the thoracic and lumbar spine. This chapter reviews the developmental and gross anatomy of the spine and gives an outline of the specific surgical procedures; preoperative assessment; anesthetic care, including methods to limit the need for homologous blood transfusion and spinal cord monitoring; and postoperative care, including pain management.

▶ DEVELOPMENTAL AND GROSS ANATOMY OF THE SPINE

Overview

The spine can be divided into four regions corresponding to four natural spinal curves: cervical, thoracic, lumbar, and sacral. The "normal" spine shows thoracic and sacral kyphosis and cervical and lumbar lordosis. The lordosis curvature of the cervical neck and of the lumbar spine develops in a response to weight bearing. As the posterior neck muscles of an infant gain strength, the spine develops lordotically to support the heavy head. At about 12 months of age, the lumbar spine develops a lordotic curve as a result of walking. Cervical and lumbar lordoses are considered secondary curves due to weight bearing. Their purpose is to keep the spine balanced and reduce the workload on the posterior spinal musculature. Thoracic and sacral kyphoses are considered to be primary curves. Normal cervical lordosis typically ranges from 20 to 40 degrees, while lumbar lordosis ranges between 30 and 50 degrees. An acceptable thoracic kyphosis curvature is 20 to 50 degrees. Medically, there is a broad range of acceptable sacral curvature, since S1–S5 are fused in a kyphotic angle.

Abnormal curvatures of the spine are scoliosis and kyphosis. Scoliosis is a complex three-dimensional deformity that involves changes in the coronal, sagittal, and axial alignment of the spine. The structural changes include wedging of the vertebral body, rotation of the vertebral body to the convex side of the curve, and deformities of the posterior elements. These changes are greatest at the apex of the curve. At this point, one will find the pedicle shortened and thickened, the lamina heavier, and the spinous process deviated toward the concave aspect of the curve. The vertebral body becomes wedge-shaped and thicker on the concave aspect of the curve owing to compression during spinal growth, while the vertebral body becomes thinner on the convex side, since it is expanded. The transverse processes approach the sagittal plane on the convex side and are positioned more toward the concave side in the frontal plane. Additionally, rib prominence is often noticed on the convex side of the curve owing to the rotation of the thoracic vertebrae. These structural abnormalities cause an asymmetrical thoracic cavity that may compromise respiratory function.

Scoliosis can have many causes. Congenital scoliosis represents a failure of formation or failure of segmentation of the vertebrae. Neuromuscular scoliosis may be caused by cerebral palsy, muscular dystrophy, myelomeningocele, poliomyelitis, or other diseases that affect the muscles or nervous system. Syndromes associated with a scoliotic spine include Marfan's syndrome, neurofibromatosis, and bone dysphasia. Idiopathic scoliosis is by far the most common of all scolioses and is classified according to age of development.

Abnormal kyphosis is usually classified as postural kyphosis, congenital kyphosis, or Scheuermann's kyphosis. Postural kyphosis, often referred to as round-back deformity, is a flexible spinal deformity that responds well to nonoperative treatments. Less common but more serious is congenital kyphosis. Surgery is usually recommended for this condition because of its rapid rate of progression, at 5 to 7 degrees per year, and the potential for neurologic damage. Congenital kyphosis, like congenital scoliosis, is known to be caused by a failure of part or all of the vertebral body to form or a failure of segmentation of part or all of the vertebral body.

Scheuermann's kyphosis presents in the thoracic, thoracolumbar, and/or lumbar spine. The etiology of both thoracic and thoracolumbar disease is unknown, although many researchers have suggested hormonal, nutritional, traumatic, vascular, and genetic factors as possible causes. Trauma is medically accepted to be the cause of lumbar Scheuermann's kyphosis. Clinically, all three variations of Scheuermann's kyphosis show rigidity in the affected area. Radiographically, more than 5 degrees of wedging of at least three adjacent vertebrae in a lateral view is necessary for the diagnosis. Radiographs will also show that the vertebral endplates are irregular and the disk plates narrowed. Schmorl nodes, thought to be the result of a herniated disk protruding through the weakened endplate, are often visible on x-ray films. Treatment includes nonoperative methods and surgery, depending on the symptoms and the degree of curvature. A curve of more than 75 to 80 degrees warrants surgery.

The Spinal Cord and Spinal Nerves

There are 31 pairs of spinal nerves: 8 cervical, 12 thoracic, 5 lumbar, 5 sacral, and 1 coccygeal. The first cervical root exits between the skull and C1, while the root of the eighth cervical nerve exits between C7 and T1. Thereafter, all nerve roots exit at the same level as their corresponding vertebrae. However, one should realize that the nerve roots branch off the spinal cord at a higher level than their actual exit through the intervertebral foramen. Specifically, the spinal nerve usually travels caudad adjacent to the spinal cord before exiting through the vertebral foramen. The development of these nerves is complex. The neural tube, which is crucial in embryonic development, becomes the central nervous system, and the neural crest forms the majority of the peripheral nervous system. As the neural tube closes, the neural crest cells migrate between the neural tube and the somite to form the peripheral nervous system, Schwann cells, and melanocytes. The neural tube becomes the spinal cord, the brain, and the peripheral afferent nerves and preganglionic fibers of the autonomic nervous system. When the neural tube closes, the dorsal region separates into two halves, the alar and basal laminae, referred to as the roof and floor plates. The alar plate becomes the sensory pathways, or dorsal columns, while the basal plates develop into the motor pathways. The motor pathways or the ventral horn neurons develop axons that form the ventral roots. The axons of the ganglion cells form central processes, which become the dorsal roots and peripheral processes that end in sensory organelles. Motor neurons become functional before sensory nerves. Autonomic nerve function is established last.

Dissection shows that the motor fibers are located on the anterior side of the spinal cord and the sensory fibers on the posterior side. A group of motor fibers is referred to as a ventral root (anterior root), while a collection of sensory fibers form a dorsal root (posterior root). The sensory nerves have groups of cell bodies outside of the spinal cord known as the dorsal root ganglia, which contain the nuclei of the sensory nerves. Directly lateral to the ganglia, the anterior and posterior (ventral and dorsal) nerve roots join to form a common spinal nerve surrounded by a dural sheath. This is the point where the peripheral nerve begins. Immediately after formation, the peripheral nerve divides into a small dorsal (posterior) ramus and a much larger ventral (anterior) primary ramus. The posterior primary rami innervate the paraspinous muscles on either side of the vertebral column and a narrow strip of overlying skin. All of the other muscles and skin are innervated by the anterior primary rami, which form the cervical, brachial, lumbar, and sacral nerve plexuses and the intercostal nerves.

Further dissection reveals the layers (meninges) that protect the spinal cord: the dura mater, arachnoid layer, and pia mater. The dura mater, the most external layer, is composed of connective tissue, is gray in color, and is easily identified. A narrow subdural space separates the dura mater from the next layer, the arachnoid. This middle layer provides much of the vascular supply. Between the arachnoid layer and the deepest layer, the pia mater, lies the subarachnoid space, which contains the cerebrospinal fluid; it protects the nerve pathways by acting as a shock absorber. The pia mater is closely adherent to the spinal cord and the individual nerve roots. It is highly vascularized to provide the blood supply to the underlying neural structures.

The spinal cord extends from the foramen magnum to L1–L4, depending on the age of the patient. The caudal end of the cord moves from its initial position of L3–L4 in infancy to its adult position at L1. The spinal cord terminates as the conus medullaris; below this, the thick flexible dural sac contains the spinal nerves collectively known as the cauda equina. Within the cauda equina, is the filum terminale, which extends from the conus medullaris to the coccyx and acts as an anchor to keep the lower spinal cord in its normal shape.

Vascular Components

The blood supply to the spinal cord involves several arteries and arteriolar branches. The anterior arterial trunk and the two posterior lateral trunks, which arise from the vertebral arteries, are important aspects of the blood supply to the cervical, thoracic, and lumbar cord. To assist these longitudinal arterial pathways, there are up to 17 radicular arteries anteriorly and as many as 25 posteriorly. The thoracic and lumbar radicular arteries are supplied by the aorta, while the vertebral arteries supply the majority of the radicular arteries in the cervical spine. In addition, the artery of Adamkiewicz, which is usually located on the left at T9–T11, feeds the lumbar section. It is the largest of the radicular arteries supplying the spinal cord by anastomosing with the anterior (longitudinal) spinal artery. Injury to the artery of Adamkiewicz can cause devastating ischemia of the lower spinal cord and paraplegia. Additionally, the blood supply of the thoracic spine is more tenuous than that of the cervical or lumbar spine, especially at the T4–T9 watershed area, which is more prone to ischemic injury.

A pair of segmental arteries, arising from the aorta, is present at every vertebral level to provide blood to the extra- and intraspinal structures. The segmental arteries divide into many branches at the intervertebral foramen. A second network of segmental arteries lies within the spinal canal in the loose connective tissue of the extradural space. This second network provides an alternative pathway of blood flow that ensures adequate spinal cord circulation after ligation of the segmental arteries during surgery.

Body Components

The outer layer of the vertebrae consists of dense, solid cortical bone made of compact Haversian systems. On the inside is cancellous or trabecular bone; a porous, loosely connected bone. This bone is weaker and more susceptible to disease and loss of density than cortical bone. The outer cortical bone extends above and below the superior and inferior ends of the vertebrae to form rims. The pedicles, consisting of dense cortical bone surrounding the medullary canal, are two short, rounded processes that extend posteriorly from the lateral margin of the dorsal surface of the vertebral body. The anterior third of the pedicle and the vertebral body together are referred to as an anterior arch.

The posterior arch, which attaches laterally to the anterior arch, includes the laminae, processes (spinous process, transverse process, superior particular process), and posterior two-thirds of the pedicles. The laminae are two flat plates of bone extending medially from the pedicles to form the posterior wall of the vertebral foramen. The part of the lamina located between the superior and inferior articular processes is called the pars interarticularis. Spondylolysis is a defect in the pars interarticularis, most commonly at the L5 level.

There are three spinal processes or projections of bony tissue that are attachment sites for tendons and ligaments. Two inferior and two superior articular processes extend from the junction of the pedicles and laminae. The inferior and superior articular processes meet to form facet joints. The facet joints are surrounded by a capsular membrane containing synovial fluid that, together with the intervertebral disk, provide mobility of the spine. Two transverse processes (one on each side of the pedicles) extend laterally and provide an attachment point for ligaments and tendons. A single spinous process, which rises posteriorly from the junction of the two laminae, also provides an attachment point for ligaments and tendons and serves as a lever for motion of the vertebrae.

Other bony components include the endplate and apophyseal ring. Endplates are located superiorly and inferiorly within the rim of each vertebral body. Each endplate consists of a cartilaginous external layer and a bony internal layer and provides vascular nutrition to the avascular intervertebral disk. These endplates also serve as growth rings, predominately in height, for the vertebral bodies. The endplates are closed by 17 to 18 years of age. The apophyseal ring of cortical bone surrounds the vertebral body below portions of the endplate. During surgical procedures, it is important to leave as much as possible of this bony endplate intact so as to prevent an implanted device from penetrating into the soft cancellous bone. The endplate is well vascularized, offering an excellent site for a fusion graft. The apophyseal ring is an ideal site for interbody fusion devices.

Surgical Procedures on the Pediatric Spine

Scoliosis is a lateral and rotational deformity of the vertebral column and it is most commonly idiopathic (60 to 70 percent), although it may also result from neuromuscular or congenital bony deformities. It is three to four times more common in females than males. Surgery is indicated when the Cobb angle is greater than 40 degrees in the lumbar spine or 50 degrees in the thoracic spine. The goals of surgery are to stop further progression of the deformity and in many cases to partially correct it. Progressive curvature invariably leads to restrictive lung disease, respiratory insufficiency, chronic hypoxemia and hypercarbia, and death from cor pulmonale in the third to fifth decades of life.

The surgical treatment of pediatric spinal deformity can be divided into anterior and posterior procedures. The surgeon's decision to use one or both of these approaches depends on the age of the patient, the underlying cause of the spinal deformity, and the severity of the curve. A patient with neuromuscular scoliosis can usually be treated surgically by using a posterior procedure but may require an anterior spinal release and fusion to aid correction, depending on the severity of the deformity. Procedures for the treatment of idiopathic scoliosis include anterior spinal release and fusion when a posterior procedure is involved, anterior spinal fusion with instrumentation for certain thoracic and thoracolumbar curves, and more recently thoracoscopic procedures to minimize dissection and decrease the morbidity of anterior spinal surgery.

Posterior procedures are effective in treating a wide variety of spinal deformities in children. Again, the underlying cause, degree of curvature, and patient's age will determine the type of procedure. For the juvenile patient with idiopathic scoliosis, nonsegmental posterior spinal instrumentation without fusion is used. This is also known as a growing rod. Posterior spinal fusion with segmental instrumentation is the "gold standard" for treating the adolescent patient with idiopathic scoliosis. Patients with neuromuscular scoliosis will often require fixation to the pelvis in addition to the posterior spinal fusion to control their pelvic obliquity, which can affect their sitting balance. Posterior procedures for the treatment of congenital scoliosis are often performed in combination with anterior procedures. This includes a convex hemiepiphysiodesis or an in situ fusion to stop further progression of the curve. Posterior spinal fusion alone with instrumentation can be used to treat the older adolescent with congenital scoliosis.

Anterior Surgery for Scoliosis

Anterior approaches typically result in successful correction of the curvature while limiting the extent of the fusion. For all anterior approaches, the patient is placed in the lateral decubitus position and the operating table in a flexed position. For right thoracic curves, the patient is placed in a left lateral decubitus position. The opposite is true for a left lumbar curve. The upper arm is moved forward and rotated away from the posterior portion of the spine. To minimize pressure on the brachial plexus, an axillary roll should be placed between the table and the patient's shoulder. Keeping all areas well padded is important to preventing nerve damage.

The surgeon will access the spine through the bed of the convex fifth rib for visualization of T5–T12 or via the bed of the tenth rib for access to the thoracolumbar spine. The initial incision extends anteriorly to the lateral border of the rectus sheath. The length of the incision will depend on the exposure required. As a general rule, the rib to be excised corresponds to the most superior vertebral body requiring exposure. For example, with a T6–T12 anterior fusion, the fifth rib would be excised. The rib below the level of incision is removed. The surgeon will split the costal cartilage anteriorly, which can later serve as a landmark for closure. When access to vertebral levels below T12 is necessary, the diaphragm must be divided. With fine dissection and gentle retraction, the peritoneum is separated off the diaphragm and the psoas muscle. Once the spine is exposed, retractors are positioned to protect the lung tissue and peritoneum. The surgeon can now access the vertebral disk or vertebral body, remembering that segmental vessels will be encountered at each level. Vascular compromise of the spinal cord after ligation of many segmental vessels is uncommon.

Video-Assisted Thoracoscopic Surgery

Video-assisted thoracoscopic technique is a new method for the surgical treatment of scoliosis. Specialized monitoring equipment is necessary for these surgical procedures, including the scope, light sources, cameras, flexible portals, monitors, and specific instrumentation. The anesthesiologist should be familiar with the use of double-lumen tubes with one-lung ventilation (see below). Contraindications to this method include a patient's inability to tolerate single-lung ventilation, severe respiratory insufficiency, or high airway pressures with positive-pressure ventilation and previous thoracotomy. After general anesthesia is induced, the patient is turned into the lateral decubitus position, as previously mentioned for the anterior approach, and one-lung ventilation instituted. The upper arm is placed on a stand with the shoulder abducted and flexed. An axillary roll is positioned between the patient's shoulder and the operating table. The surgeon identifies and outlines the scapular borders, 12th rib, and iliac crest. The first portal is usually placed at or near the T6–T7 interspace in the posterior axillary line. The surgeon makes an incision, continues with electrocautery through the intercostal muscle to enter the chest cavity, and ensures that the lung is deflated. Flexible portals are inserted in the intercostal spaces with a trocar. Using a blunt-tipped needle, a roentgenogram is completed to confirm the disk spaces.

The parietal pleura is completely resected with care not to ligate any segmental vessels. The surgeon then removes the disks and endplates. After the necessary diskectomies are completed, rib grafts are harvested through the portal sites. Before closure, a chest tube is placed through the most posterior inferior portal. The pleura may be closed or left open. The chest tube is connected to water seal and the anesthesiologist tests for an air leak in the reinflated lung.

Perioperative problems include bleeding, damage to the lung tissue, dural tears, lymphatic injury, and sympathetic nerve changes on the operative side. If hemostasis cannot be obtained and visualization remains poor, conversion to an open anterior approach may be required. Postoperatively, pulmonary problems can occur within the deflated lung. Often, mucous plugs form in this lung, requiring consistent, thorough suction, breathing treatments, and breathing exercises.

Posterior Surgery for Scoliosis

Because of recent advancements with segmental posterior spinal instrumentation, correction of both sagittal and coronal plane spinal deformities is felt to be superior to older systems such as the Harrington rods (Fig. 13-1). For this reason, the posterior approach to the spine has become increasingly popular. The posterior instrumentation method takes advantage of the spinous processes, pedicles, facets, and laminae to control the alignment of the vertebral bodies with the use of laminar hooks, pedicle hooks, pedicle screws, facet screws, and wires. The patient is placed prone on an appropriate spinal frame so that the inferior vena cava is less compressed and the abdomen hangs free. Traditionally a Hall frame or more recently a Jackson table is used to support the patient without increasing intraabdominal pressure. The patient's face should be well padded to avoid any pressure on the eyes. The patient's back is completely draped, with the entire spine and the iliac crest (for graft harvest) exposed.

The surgeon makes a midline incision over the spinous processes, splitting the apophysis and using subperiosteal dissection to expose the transverse processes laterally. The appropriate vertebrae are then identified using fluoroscopy or a plain radiograph. After a facetectomy and wide posterior release at each level, instrumentation is performed. Pedicle hooks, pedicle screws, laminar hooks, and sublaminar wires are inserted at the appropriate levels to obtain adequate correction. The first rod is placed on the concave side of the curve and subsequently rotated to correct the spinal deformity. Changes in spinal cord function, seen with neuromonitoring, usually occur during this phase of the surgery. While correction is maintained with the first rod, the second rod is placed. Cross-links are added to increase the torsional stiffness of the rod.

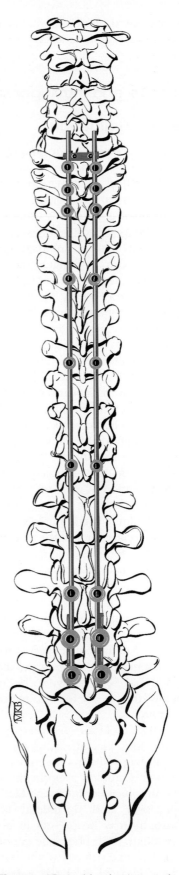

Figure 13-1. Harrington rods.

Decortication of the posterior elements prepares the spine for fusion. Bone grafts and layered closure complete the operation.

▶ Preoperative and Intraoperative Care

Preoperative Evaluation

The first step in the anesthetic care of these patients is a thorough preoperative evaluation to identify comorbid features that may affect their perioperative care. The effect of the disease on airway management is of primary importance. Patients presenting for surgery of the cervical spine should be assumed to have an unstable cervical spine or the potential for subluxation during neck movement, which can endanger the spinal cord. Problems of the cervical spine may be due to trauma or a congenital syndrome (Trisomy 21, achondroplasia, or rarer craniofacial syndromes such as Pfeiffer's, Apert's, or Crouzon's syndromes). Subluxation and upper cervical intervertebral fusions have been reported in 30 percent of patients with Pfeiffer's syndrome, while odontoid hypoplasia and the risk of C1–C2 subluxation have been reported in patients with Crouzon's syndrome and the mucopolysaccharidoses (see Chap. 6). Even in the absence of such problems, scoliosis or kyphosis may limit normal movement of the cervical spine and make endotracheal intubation difficult. Preoperative evaluation of spinal abnormalities, including a physical examination with an evaluation of neck movement, should be supplemented as needed with radiographic examination (flexion/extension films) or computed tomography (CT) scanning. An additional abnormality that may affect airway management is foramen magnum stenosis, which has been reported in patients with achondroplastic dwarfism. It results from hypertrophy of the bony margins of the foramen magnum, which can cause narrowing of the cervical spinal canal and compression of the cervical spinal cord or medulla. In children with achondroplasia who show neurologic or respiratory symptoms related to foramen magnum stenosis, the diameter of the foramen magnum has been shown to be three standard deviations below the mean for age-matched controls with normal stature.

Patients with craniofacial syndromes may also have midface abnormalities that affect airway management, including difficult bag-valve-mask ventilation and endotracheal intubation. Common abnormalities of the craniofacial syndromes include micrognathia, microstoma, midface hypoplasia, and lip/palatal abnormalities. Glossal hypertrophy may be present in neuromuscular conditions (see Chap. 6). If fiberoptic endotracheal intubation is anticipated, the patency of the nares should be assessed because choanal atresia is a feature of these syndromes. The equipment required for management of a difficult airway, as outlined by Vener and Lerman, should be readily available, including fiberoptic bronchoscopes and various sizes of laryngeal mask airways. During airway manipulation, excessive cervical spinal movement is prevented by manual in-line stabilization. In older, cooperative children and adolescents, awake intubation techniques commonly used in adults (intravenous sedation with glossopharyngeal nerve and superior laryngeal nerve blockade) followed by direct laryngoscopy or fiberoptic bronchoscopy may be feasible for endotracheal intubation.

After the airway examination, organ systems should be examined in sequence. Nervous system problems may be frequent comorbid features in children presenting for spinal surgery. Children with scoliosis presenting for posterior spinal fusion may have cerebral palsy and static encephalopathy, which may sometimes be complicated by mental retardation and seizure disorders. The preoperative evaluation should document therapeutic anticonvulsant concentrations in the serum. Anticonvulsant medication should be administered preoperatively to maintain therapeutic levels and should be started again during the postoperative period. The induction of hepatic enzymes by certain anticonvulsants may increase the metabolism of several drugs, including neuromuscular blocking agents (NMBAs) and some anesthetic induction agents. Increased intraoperative doses of these drugs may therefore be necessary for children treated with anticonvulsants. Mental retardation and visual and hearing disturbances may obviously make assessment of the patient difficult. Some degree of intellectual impairment is noted in 30 to 50 percent of patients with Duchenne's muscular dystrophy. These effects may also complicate the postoperative course by making pain assessment difficult.

Depending on the degree of scoliosis and the associated conditions, respiratory function may be compromised due to restrictive lung disease. Patients with scoliosis have decreased vital capacity, total lung capacity, and forced expiratory volume, while the residual volume remains normal. The decrease is greater in patients with congenital or infantile scoliosis than in those with adolescent scoliosis. The severity of the impairment is related to the angle of the scoliosis, the number of vertebral levels involved, the cephalad level of the scoliosis, and the loss of normal thoracic kyphosis. Muirhead and Conner found that 14 of 41 children with either infantile or congenital scoliosis had a moderate or severe ventilation defect (40 to 59 percent predicted for age) compared to only 4 of the 51 children with adolescent scoliosis. They also found that no child whose vital capacity was greater than 40 percent of that predicted for age required postoperative respiratory support. The effect of surgery on lung function depends on the surgical approach and the type of surgery. Surgical procedures that involve the thorax (anterior spinal fusion) reduce lung function for 3 months, with a return to preoperative values by 2 years. However, a pure posterior approach improves respiratory function at both 3 months and 2 years.

Controversy also exists about the degree of respiratory compromise that may contraindicate scoliosis surgery. In adults it has been suggested that a reduction of the forced vital capacity (FVC) or the forced expiratory volume in 1 s (FEV_1) to less than 40 to 60 percent of the predicted value may indicate a higher risk of postoperative complications and the need for postoperative mechanical ventilation. However, the criteria used to predict postoperative respiratory function in adults cannot necessarily be applied to children, because there are generally fewer comorbid features such as cardiac disease in children. The fact that preoperative tests of pulmonary function in children have little predictive value has been demonstrated by Tobias et al. Although the authors noted a consistent decrement in predicted-for-age values after 32 thoracotomies in 19 pediatric oncology patients, with a decrease in the FVC (percent predicted for age) from 68 ± 3.6 to 60 ± 2.4 percent ($p < 0.01$) and the FEV_1 from 69 ± 4.2 to 60 ± 3.8 percent ($p < 0.01$), no permanent morbidity was noted in the small cohort of patients with severe restrictive lung disease. Five of the patients had severe preoperative decreases in pulmonary function (less than 40 percent predicted for age). In this group the incidence of morbidity, defined as a postoperative need for ventilation and supplemental oxygen for more than 12 h or persistent air leak, was 3 of 5 versus 3 of 20 in patients with mild or moderate lung disease (60 to 80 percent predicted for age). There was, however, no postoperative mortality and no need for prolonged mechanical ventilation. Respiratory function may be further threatened by conditions that predispose to chronic upper respiratory tract infections or recurrent bouts of aspiration due to chronic gastroesophageal reflux. Any of the neuromuscular disorders (e.g., Duchenne's muscular dystrophy) may significantly affect respiratory function by adding chronic lung disease to the restricted function associated with the scoliosis. In all patients with severe restrictive lung disease, the decision to operate must therefore be based on an assessment of the potential for long-term postoperative ventilation versus the potential of benefits of surgery.

Cardiovascular abnormalities in patients with scoliosis may be due to the primary disease process or less commonly due to cor pulmonale and chronic hypoxemia from restrictive lung disease. The latter is uncommon because scoliosis is frequently treated before cardiovascular effects develop. Various neuromuscular conditions, such as the muscular dystrophies or myotonic dystrophies, may lead to changes in myocardial contractile function or conduction abnormalities. Of these conditions, Duchenne's muscular dystrophy is the most common disorder, with an incidence of 1 in 3300 male births. It is inherited as an X-linked disorder, which presents as weakness during the fourth to eighth years of life. The diagnosis is confirmed by muscle biopsy. The genetic defect results in a deficiency of the protein dystrophin in skeletal, cardiac, and smooth muscle. As these patients enter their second decade of life and definitely by the third decade, the myocardium is progressively affected by depressed contractility, conduction disturbances, and arrhythmias. Several reports in the literature have described a significantly increased risk of morbidity and even mortality during anesthetic care in patients with Duchenne's muscular dystrophy. Sethna et al. reported intraoperative cardiac arrest and death in 2 of 25 patients. In patients with associated myopathic conditions, the preoperative evaluation should include echocardiography and a 12-lead electrocardiogram (ECG).

The preoperative evaluation and preparation of the patient are essential to limit the use of allogeneic blood products. This may include arrangements for preoperative autologous donation with or without the use of erythropoietin (see below for a discussion of intraoperative techniques to limit the need for homologous transfusion). Patients presenting for major orthopaedic surgery may have chronic medical or nutritional conditions that affect blood coagulation. Chronic treatment with anticonvulsants, including phenytoin and carbamazepine, may adversely affect coagulation function. Poor nutritional status and poor intake of vitamin K may predispose to chronically low levels of vitamin K–dependent coagulation factors, resulting in preoperative coagulation dysfunction. Preoperative screening of coagulation function and simple measures such as the administration of vitamin K (oral or intramuscular) may prevent these problems. Patients with chronic orthopaedic problems and pain frequently use NSAIDs. Although acetylsalicylic acid irreversibly inhibits cyclooxygenase and platelet function for the life of the platelet, NSAIDs cause reversible inhibition of platelet function, which depends on the plasma concentration and half-life of the NSAID. Discontinuation of most NSAIDs for 2 to 5 days before surgery will result in the return of normal platelet function.

Premedication, Anesthetic Induction, Monitoring and Positioning

Premedication may include (1) high-flow nebulization of albuterol and an anticholinergic agent such as ipratropium in patients with airway reactivity; (2) gastrointestinal prophylaxis with H_2 antagonists (e.g., ranitidine), oral nonparticulate antacids and motility agents for patients at risk for aspiration; (3) dexamethasone for patients with airway reactivity as well as to decrease postoperative nausea and vomiting; (4) an anticholinergic agent such as glycopyrrolate or atropine to dry secretions, especially if fiberoptic intubation technique is planned, to blunt airway reactivity and to prevent bradycardia during laryngoscopy and endotracheal intubation; and (5) an anxiolytic. Premedication for anxiolysis follows the standard practice in pediatric anesthesia, including oral midazolam in patients without intravenous access or intravenous midazolam in those with such access.

After premedication, the patient is transported to the operating room and routine American Society of Anesthesiology (ASA) monitors are attached. In the operating room, normothermia should be maintained. This is particularly important in patients with little body fat. Normothermia is generally easily maintained by (1) keeping the operating room warmed until the patient is positioned and covered; (2) warming intravenous fluids, blood and blood products; and (3) the use of forced-air warming devices. Normothermia affects coagulation and makes its maintenance one of many essential steps to control blood loss.

The technique of anesthetic induction is guided by the patient's medical conditions, an assessment of the ease of intubation, and the patient's preference when appropriate. For anterior or posterior spine surgery, a reinforced endotracheal tube may be used to prevent inadvertent airway occlusion during surgical dissection and neck flexion. When neck flexion is prolonged, a nonreinforced endotracheal tube may become bent and occluded. In the patients with stable cardiovascular function, there are several options for the induction and maintenance of anesthesia. These include either inhalation techniques that utilize sevoflurane or halothane in oxygen or intravenous anesthesia. In patients with existing intravenous lines, several of the commonly used intravenous induction agents are suitable. If it is intended to perform endotracheal extubation in the operating room or immediately postoperatively, propofol may provide a more rapid awakening and a better recovery profile during the immediate postoperative period than barbiturates, while etomidate is an appropriate choice in patients with diminished myocardial function.

When adequate bag-mask ventilation has been achieved, inhalation or intravenous induction can be followed by the administration of a nondepolarizing neuromuscular blocking agent (NMBA). Succinylcholine is contraindicated in patients with various neurologic and myopathic conditions, given the potential for rhabdomyolysis, hyperkalemia, and cardiac arrest. Similar problems with succinylcholine may occur in patients after a spinal cord injury. Therefore our practice includes the use of intermediate-acting (vecuronium, rocuronium, cis-atracurium, atracurium) or short-acting (mivacurium) nondepolarizing NMBAs. The doses of these agents should be adjusted by using train-of-four (TOF) monitoring, especially in patients with myopathies, in whom the response to these agents can vary. In patients with underlying neuromuscular disease, a single dose of an intermediate-acting agent may cause prolonged neuromuscular blockade. We have found similar variability even when using mivacurium in these patients. We have also noted that the response to neuromuscular blocking (onset and duration of action) did not correlate with the patient's preoperative muscle strength.

After the airway is secured, adequate intravenous access and invasive cardiovascular monitoring are obtained.

Several factors may cause hemodynamic changes during spinal surgery in children, including the patient's associated medical conditions, positioning on the operating table, blood loss, and the administration of vasoactive agents to induce controlled hypotension. Arterial monitoring is routine in the majority of cases of pediatric spinal surgery. Adequate vascular access for the administration of blood, intravenous fluids, and medications is mandatory. This generally includes two large-bore (16- or 14-gauge) peripheral intravenous cannulas. The need for more invasive hemodynamic measurements remains controversial. Our practice has been to monitor central venous pressure (CVP) in patients with underlying conditions that may affect their myocardial function or in those in whom a protracted postoperative course is expected and prolonged venous access may be needed, such as patients with severe cerebral palsy and mental retardation. However, the correlation of CVP with myocardial function becomes less reliable in the prone position. Supkis et al. demonstrated that CVP increased from 8.7 ± 1.3 to 17.7 ± 2.5 mmHg when patients were turned from the supine to the prone position. At the same time the left ventricular end-diastolic pressure measured by transesophageal echocardiography decreased from 37.1 ± 2.9 to 33.2 ± 3.0 mmHg, thereby demonstrating a decrease in ventricular filling despite the increased CVP. The accuracy and utility of CVP measurements in the prone position are therefore questionable in such patients. Other monitoring procedures follow the routine recommended by the ASA, including electrocardiography, precordial or esophageal stethoscopy, observation of end-tidal carbon dioxide and temperature plus placement of a urinary catheter.

When appropriate vascular access and monitoring have been established, the patient is positioned on the operating table. The position will depend on the specific type of surgery but is generally prone or lateral. For cervical spinal and upper thoracic surgery, the head may have to be in a neutral position, supported in a ring device with the face directed toward the floor. Alternatively, for posterior spinal fusion that does not involve the lower cervical or high thoracic area or isolated lumbar surgery, the patient can be positioned prone and the head turned 90 degrees, thereby limiting the potential for pressure points on the eyes and face. Regardless of the positioning, careful padding of pressure points is necessary, since these surgical procedures may last up to 8 to 12 h.

The patient is positioned to minimize venous pressure at the surgical site in order to reduce bleeding. This is done by placing rolls under the chest and pelvis to keep the abdomen free and by reverse Trendelenburg positioning. The latter also helps to limit the development of dependent edema in the face, tongue, and upper airway and may also limit the increase in intraocular pressure (IOP), which may occur with prone positioning. Increased IOP due to prone positioning has been proposed as a possible cause of the rare but devastating complication of blindness following these surgical procedures. Keeping the abdomen free also facilitates mechanical ventilation by preventing restriction of diaphragmatic movement. Alternatively, specialized frames (e.g., the Wilson frame) can be used to position the patient so that venous pressure and surgical bleeding are decreased. For anterior procedures, the patient is positioned in the lateral position and a thoracotomy is performed to gain access to the vertebral column. There is also increasing experience with thoracoscopic approaches for such procedures. Regardless of whether open thoracotomy or thoracoscopy is performed, one-lung ventilation (OLV), as described below, will be required.

One-Lung Ventilation for Anterior Approaches

There are three basic options for OLV: (1) a double-lumen endotracheal tube (DLT), (2) a bronchial blocker, and (3) selective mainstem intubation. The smallest commercially available double-lumen endotracheal tube is 26 Fr, which precludes its use in patients less than 8 to 10 years of age. When the patient's size permits, a DLT may be preferable because it provides several advantages over other techniques of lung separation, including (1) rapid and easy separation of the lungs, (2) access for suctioning of both lungs, (3) a rapid switch to two-lung ventilation if needed, and (4) the feasibility of providing continuous positive airway pressure (CPAP) or oxygen insufflation to the operative lung should it become necessary.

In patients in whom a DLT cannot be used, the bronchus on the operative side can be occluded with a balloon-tipped catheter placed under fiberoptic bronchoscopic guidance. Several different devices can be used as bronchial blockers, including a Fogarty embolectomy catheter, atrioseptostomy catheter, pulmonary artery catheter, the Arndt endobronchial blocker (Cook Critical Care, Birmingham, IN), and the Univent endotracheal tube (Fuji Systems, Tokyo, Japan). Devices with a small central channel allow some suctioning, but not enough to clear the lung of secretions. Instead, it is used to deflate the operative lung and improve surgical visualization or for the insufflation of oxygen and the application of CPAP. Without the central channel, air or gas cannot escape from the lung once the balloon is inflated. The lung may therefore not deflate completely and may obscure surgical visualization. If there is no separate central channel, the lung can be manually compressed by the surgeon during a brief period of apnea and the balloon then inflated prior to the provision of positive-pressure ventilation.

Regardless of which catheter and technique of placement are chosen, there is a risk that the bronchial blocker may be displaced during the surgical procedure or repositioning of the patient. If this occurs, the bronchial blocker may occlude the tracheal lumen just beyond the ETT, resulting in inadequate ventilation. Continuous auscultation of breath sounds on the nonoperative side and monitoring of inflating pressures and respiratory compliance should help to identify this problem rapidly. Clinical experience indicates that inflating the balloon of the bronchial blocker with saline instead of air may limit its movement and dislodgment. With any change in the patient's position, the correct position of the bronchial blocker should be confirmed with fiberoptic bronchoscopy or auscultation.

The third method of OLV is selective endobronchial intubation. The major disadvantage of mainstem intubation is that it is not possible to change quickly to two-lung ventilation or vice versa. Furthermore movement of the ETT may cause extubation, which can be particularly troublesome when the patient is in the lateral decubitus position. Intubation of the right mainstem bronchus can generally be performed blindly, but intubation of the left bronchus requires bronchoscopic guidance because of anatomic differences in orientation of the bronchi.

When OLV is being utilized, general anesthesia is maintained with a combination of intravenous and inhalational agents. Because hypoxic pulmonary vasoconstriction (HPV) restricts blood flow to the nonventilated lung to limit hypoxemia, any nonspecific vasodilator (terbutaline, albuterol, isoproterenol, dobutamine, nicardipine, nitroglycerin, sodium nitroprusside, or an inhalational anesthetic agent) can impair oxygenation. Isoflurane has been shown to affect hypoxic vasoconstriction less than halothane or enflurane. However, no difference in oxygenation has been noted with isoflurane, sevoflurane, or desflurane at concentrations of 1 MAC. Anesthesia is supplemented as needed with intravenous agents including opioids, ketamine, benzodiazepines, propofol, and barbiturates, which have no clinically significant effect on vasoconstriction. Ventilation is maintained with tidal volumes of 8 to 10 mL/kg, the rate being adjusted as needed to maintain normocarbia. Hypocarbia is avoided because it may interfere with hypoxic pulmonary vasoconstriction (HPV). If adequate oxygenation cannot be maintained with 100% oxygen to the nonoperative side, CPAP of 4 to 5 cmH$_2$O can be applied to the operative lung provided that a DLT, Univent, or bronchial blocker with a central channel is used. Although this will improve oxygenation, it may also distend the operative lung to some degree and impair surgical visualization. Another option to improve oxygenation is to apply positive end-expiratory pressure (PEEP) to the nonoperative side. Applying excessive PEEP to the down or nonoperative side may impair oxygenation by increasing HPV in the nonoperative lung and shunting blood to the nonventilated, operative side. If the above measures fail, it may be necessary to ventilate both lungs intermittently.

Techniques to Limit Homologous Transfusion

There is increasing recognition of the potential adverse effects associated with the administration of allogeneic blood products, including the transmission of infectious diseases, immunosuppression, acute lung injury, transfusion reactions, and graft-versus-host disease. Techniques to limit the need for homologous blood products include (1) general methods such as preoperative optimization of coagulation function, anesthetic technique, proper patient positioning, and maintenance of normothermia (see above); (2) autologous transfusion, including preoperative donation with the use of erythropoietin and intraoperative collection using acute normovolemic hemodilution (ANH); (3) intraoperative and postoperative blood salvage; (4) pharmacologic manipulation of the coagulation cascade with epsilon-aminocaproic acid (EACA), tranexamic acid, aprotinin, desmopressin (DDAVP), and recombinant factor VIIa (rFVIIa); and (5) controlled hypotension (see Chap. 14). Surgery without the use of allogeneic blood products is best accomplished by combining several of these techniques.

The choice of intraoperative fluid administration may affect coagulation function and blood loss. During ANH (see below), blood is removed and replaced with crystalloids and/or colloids. Due to the dilution of anticoagulatory factors such as antithrombin III, hemodilution increases coagulation function. Albumin and gelatins have been found to have no effect or may actually improve coagulation function. Medium- or high-molecular-weight hydroxyethyl starches, because of their effects on von Willebrand factor (vWF), adversely affect coagulation function, (particularly platelet function) when used in doses exceeding 10 to 15 mL/kg.

Preoperative Donation

Although preoperative donation of autologous blood was first suggested by Fantus in 1937, when he founded the first blood bank in the United States, the technique did not became popular until the 1980s. Advantages of the technique include reduced exposure to allogeneic blood, the availability of blood for patients with rare phenotypes, reduction of blood shortages, avoidance of transfusion-induced immunosuppression, and the availability of blood to some patients who refuse transfusions based on religious beliefs. There are no limitations in regard to a patient's weight or age. Patients who weigh 50 kg or more donate a standard unit of blood (450 mL), while those who weigh less than 50 kg donate proportionately smaller volumes. The hematocrit should be ≥33 percent prior to each donation. Red blood cell production can be augmented by iron supplementation and the administration of erythropoietin (see below). Donations may be made every 3 days, but the usual practice is to donate one unit per week. The last unit should be donated at least 5 to 7 days before surgery to allow plasma proteins to normalize and to restore intravascular volume.

Acute Normovolemic Hemodilution

Acute normovolemic hemodilution (ANH) involves the removal of blood on the day of surgery (generally after the induction of anesthesia) and its replacement with crystalloid or colloid solution. Blood is removed by means of a large-bore intravenous cannula or a central line and is replaced with an equal volume of colloid or crystalloid in a ratio of 1 to 3. The blood is collected in standard CPD-A blood-bank bags and weighed to ensure that the appropriate amount is removed. The blood is kept in the operating room at room temperature for up to 4 h. A significant advantage of ANH over stored autologous blood is that the coagulation factors and platelets are still active. Intraoperatively, the blood is then infused in the opposite order to that in which it was withdrawn so that the units with the highest hematocrit value are saved until the end of the procedure, when bleeding is the least. The amount to be removed, is determined by the following formula:

$$\text{Estimated blood volume} \times (\text{initial hematocrit} - \text{target hematocrit})/\text{starting hematocrit}$$

Mechanisms that maintain oxygen delivery despite decreased hematocrit values include a decrease in blood viscosity (which increases venous return), peripheral vasodilation, increased cardiac output, and rightward shift of the oxyhemoglobin dissociation curve. Additionally, as oxygen delivery declines, oxygen extraction at the tissue level can increase to maintain adequate oxygenation. Fontana et al. evaluated the effects of ANH in 8 adolescents undergoing posterior spinal fusion for idiopathic scoliosis. Hemodilution decreased the hemoglobin from 10.0 ± 1.6 gm/dL to 3.0 ± 0.8 gm/dL. Oxygen delivery decreased from 532.1 ± 138.1 to 262 ± 57.1 mL/min/M^2, oxygen extraction ratio increased from 17.3 ± 6.2 to 44.4 ± 5.9 percent, and cardiac output increased without a change in the heart rate. Mixed venous oxygen saturation decreased from a baseline level of 90.8 ± 5.4 to 72.3 ± 7.8 percent after ANH.

Intraoperative Blood Salvage

There are three techniques to salvage blood intraoperatively. Semicontinuous flow devices were the first to be introduced and, although they are the most complex, are still the type used most commonly. The disposable equipment consists of an aspiration and anticoagulation assembly, a reservoir (various sizes are available), a centrifuge bowl, a waste bag, and tubing. A double-line aspiration set includes an anticoagulation line that permits heparin or citrate to combine with the aspirated blood at a controlled rate. The anticoagulated blood is collected in a disposable reservoir containing a filter. The filtered blood is then pumped into a bowl, centrifuged, washed with saline, and pumped into a reinfusion bag. Most of the white blood cells, platelets, clotting factors, free plasma hemoglobin, and anticoagulant are removed in the washing process and disposed of in the waste bag. The process takes approximately 5 to 10 min and yields a blood cell suspension with a hematocrit value of 45 to 60 percent.

The second type of intraoperative salvage, otherwise known as the canister collection technique, uses a rigid canister with a sterile, disposable liner. Blood is aspirated from the wound and anticoagulant added in a manner similar to that of semicontinuous flow devices. The blood can be washed before infusion or reinfused without washing. Functioning platelets and coagulation factors are present in the unwashed blood, but it poses an increased risk of adverse effects due to cellular debris, free hemoglobin, and fragmented blood components. This type is rarely used in the perioperative setting.

The third type of collection uses a single-use, self-contained rigid plastic reservoir with an anticoagulant (citrate) placed in it before use. This apparatus is most commonly used for postoperative blood collection and reinfusion. The surgical drains are connected to the canister, which is replaced and the blood reinfused every 4 h. Coagulation factors and platelets are present in this blood, but adverse effects may occur as a result of cell fragmentation and the release of free hemoglobin.

Suggested indications for intraoperative blood salvage include an anticipated blood loss exceeding 20 percent of the patient's blood volume or a procedure during which more than 10 percent of patients require transfusion. Contraindications include situations in which there may be contamination of the collected blood with infectious or noninfectious agents (infected wounds, amniotic fluid, hemostatic agents, or protamine). Potential complications include air and fat embolism, hemolysis, pulmonary dysfunction, renal dysfunction, coagulopathy, hypocalcemia, and sepsis. Coagulopathy may be related to the initiation of disseminated intravascular coagulation (DIC) by improper technique and the infusion of blood cell fragments or the infusion of residual anticoagulant after washing. Hemolysis may occur if the suction level is too high or if the aspiration method causes excessive mixing of air with blood. Free hemoglobin may be released during salvage and washing because of erythrocyte damage. Free hemoglobin levels exceeding 100 to 150 mg/dL may lead to hemoglobinuria and acute renal failure, as the binding capacity of haptoglobin is saturated and free hemoglobin is filtered in the renal tubules. Metabolic consequences of cell salvage may also be seen, including a metabolic acidosis and alterations in electrolytes such as magnesium, calcium, and potassium. These alterations may be lessened by using a balanced electrolyte solution instead of saline for washing the cells before reinfusion. Regardless of the technique, periodic measurement of electrolytes and acid-base status is suggested during blood salvage.

Pharmacological Manipulation of the Coagulation Cascade

Various agents have been used prophylactically to decrease blood loss, even in patients with normal baseline coagulation function. Although these agents have been studied in well-designed, prospective trials, the results of the studies are conflicting. A theoretical issue with any of these agents is the potential to cause a prothrombotic state with venous or arterial thrombotic complications.

Desmopressin (DDAVP) is a synthetic analog of vasopressin initially used in the treatment of diabetes insipidus. It affects hemostasis by promoting the release of factor VIII and vWF from endothelial cells. Factor VIII, a glycoprotein, accelerates the activation of factor X by factor IX. The hemostatic functions of vWF include increasing platelet adherence to vascular subendothelium, formation of molecular bridges between platelets to increase aggregation, protection of factor VIII in plasma from proteolytic enzymes, and stimulation of factor VIII synthesis. Prospective trials have failed to show an effect of DDAVP on blood loss during spinal surgery in pediatric patients.

Epsilon-aminocaproic acid (EACA) and tranexamic acid (TA) are γ-amino carboxylic acid analogs of lysine that inhibit fibrinolysis by preventing the conversion of plasminogen to plasmin. Plasminogen is activated by tissue plasminogen activator to form plasmin, which cleaves fibrin, thereby preventing the formation of the fibrin mesh. This fibrinolytic system is a basic defense mechanism that prevents the excessive deposition of fibrin following the activation of the coagulation cascade. Plasmin can also hydrolyze activated factors V and VIII. EACA and TA bind to the lysine group, which binds plasminogen and plasmin to fibrinogen, thus displacing these molecules from the fibrinogen surface and inhibiting fibrinolysis. EACA is administered at an intravenous loading dose of 100 to 150 mg/kg followed by an infusion of 10 to 15 mg/kg/h. Ninety percent is excreted in the urine within 4 to 6 h of administration. TA is 7 to 10 times as potent as EACA and may be used at lower doses (loading dose of 10 mg/kg followed by an infusion of 1 mg/kg/h). Ninety percent is present in the urine after approximately 24 h. Adverse effects of EACA or TA may be related to the effect on coagulation function and the route of excretion. Since these agents are cleared by the kidneys, thrombosis of the kidneys, ureters, or lower urinary tract may occur if urologic bleeding is present. Both EACA and TA may be associated with hypotension during rapid intravenous administration. Florentino-Pineda et al. evaluated the efficacy of EACA (100 mg/kg followed by 10 mg/kg/h) in 28 adolescents undergoing posterior spinal fusion. Patients who received EACA had decreased intraoperative blood loss (988 ± 411 mL versus 1405 ± 670 mL, $p = 0.024$) and decreased transfusion requirements (1.2 ± 1.1 U versus 2.2 ± 1.3 U, $p = 0.003$).

Aprotinin is a naturally occurring serine protease inhibitor first isolated from bovine lung in 1930. Aprotinin's effects on coagulation function are twofold: (1) inhibition of fibrinolysis through the inactivation of several serine proteases, including trypsin and plasma kallikrein, which convert plasminogen to plasmin, and (2) preservation of platelet adhesion by protecting membrane-bound glycoprotein receptors (vWF receptor) from degradation by plasmin. Aprotinin is administered intravenously and undergoes rapid redistribution into the extracellular fluid, followed by accumulation in renal tubular epithelium with subsequent lysosomal degradation. The dose is expressed as kallikrein-inhibitory units (KIU). To date, most of the experience with aprotinin has involved patients undergoing cardiovascular surgery, although its efficacy has also been demonstrated in adult patients undergoing orthopaedic surgery procedures. Potential adverse effects of aprotinin include allergic reactions and renal toxicity. Anaphylactic reactions have been reported and are more frequent in patients previously exposed to aprotinin. However, even in these cases, the incidence of anaphylaxis is less than 0.1 percent. Reports of aprotinin's effect on renal function have been controversial. Renal toxicity is postulated to result from aprotinin's strong affinity for renal tissue and subsequent accumulation in proximal tubular epithelial cells or its inhibition of serine proteases (kallikrein-kinin system). With high doses, obstructed proximal convoluted tubules and swollen tubular epithelial cells have been observed microscopically. These effects have been shown to be reversible in experiments on dogs. Additional adverse effects include decreases in renal plasma flow, glomerular filtration rate, and electrolyte excretion, which result from the inhibition of intrarenal kallikrein activation and decreased prostaglandin synthesis.

Controlled Hypotension

Controlled hypotension (also referred to as deliberate or induced hypotension) may be defined as a reduction of systolic blood pressure to 80 to 90 mmHg and a reduction of mean arterial pressure (MAP) to 50 to 65 mmHg, or a 30 percent reduction of baseline MAP (see Chap. 14). The latter is relevant for children whose baseline MAP may already be within the range of 50 to 65 mmHg. Although the main purpose of controlled hypotension is to limit intraoperative blood loss, an additional benefit may be improved visibility of the surgical field. As explained fully in Chap. 14, reduction of arterial blood pressure will not necessarily decrease bleeding which is mainly venous in origin. Depressing cardiac output with beta-adrenergic blocking agents may decrease cardiac output, increase venous pressure and increase bleeding. Drugs that decrease venous pressure, such as trinitroglycerin (TNG), are ideal.

Advances in drug therapy have provided several drugs for controlled hypotension in children. The available agents for controlled hypotension can be divided into those used alone (primary agents) and adjunctive or secondary agents used to limit the doses and adverse effects of primary agents. Primary agents include regional anesthetic techniques, the inhalational anesthetic agents (halothane, isoflurane, sevoflurane), the nitrovasodilators (sodium nitroprusside and nitroglycerin), trimethaphan, prostaglandin E_1 (PGE_1), and adenosine. The calcium channel blockers and beta-adrenergic antagonists have been used as primary agents and as adjuncts to other agents. The drugs primarily used as adjuncts include the angiotensin-converting enzyme inhibitors and alpha-adrenergic agonists such as clonidine. If neurologic monitoring is used (see below), the potential impact of the agent used for controlled hypotension must be considered.

Sodium nitroprusside (SNP) is one of the most commonly used agents for controlled hypotension. It is a direct-acting nonselective peripheral vasodilator that primarily dilates resistance vessels, leading to venous pooling and decreased systemic vascular resistance. It has a rapid onset of action (approximately 30 s), a peak hypotensive effect within 2 min, and a return of blood pressure to baseline values within 3 min of its discontinuation. Sodium nitroprusside releases nitric oxide (formerly termed endothelial-derived relaxant factor), which in turn activates guanylate cyclase, leading to an increase in the intracellular concentration of cyclic guanosine monophosphate (cGMP). Cyclic GMP decreases the availability of intracellular calcium through one of two mechanisms: decreased release from the sarcoplasmic reticulum or increased uptake by the sarcoplasmic reticulum. The net result is decreased free cytosolic calcium and vascular smooth muscle relaxation. Adverse effects include rebound hypertension, coronary steal, increased intracranial pressure, increased intrapulmonary shunt with ablation of HPV, platelet dysfunction, and cyanide/thiocyanate toxicity. Direct peripheral vasodilation also results in baroreceptor-mediated sympathetic responses with tachycardia and increased myocardial contractility in normovolemic patients. The renin-angiotensin system and sympathetic nervous system are also activated. The result is increased cardiac output, which may offset the initial drop in MAP. Plasma catecholamine and renin activity may remain elevated after discontinuation of SNP, resulting in rebound hypertension.

Nicardipine is a calcium channel blocker of the dihydropyridine class that dilates the systemic, cerebral, and coronary vasculature, with limited effects on myocardial contractility and stroke volume. Nicardipine does have some intrinsic negative chronotropic effects, which may limit the rebound tachycardia. Like other direct-acting vasodilators, nicardipine and the other calcium channel antagonists may increase intracranial pressure. Studies comparing SNP with nicardipine have demonstrated several potential advantages of nicardipine, including fewer episodes of excessive hypotension, less rebound tachycardia, less activation of the renin-angiotensin and sympathetic nervous systems, and in some studies, decreased blood loss. One disadvantage of nicardipine is that its effect is somewhat prolonged (20 to 30 min) following discontinuation of the infusion. The references listed at the end of this chapter provide a more comprehensive review of the agents available for controlled hypotension.

Spinal Cord Monitoring

The incidence of neurologic deficits following surgical procedures on the vertebral column when spinal cord monitoring is not used has been estimated at 3.7 to 6.9 percent. This can be decreased to less than 1 percent with appropriate monitoring. The American Academy of Neurology in its guidelines on intraoperative monitoring concluded that "considerable evidence favors the use of monitoring as a safe and efficacious tool in clinical situations where this is a significant nervous system risk, provided its limitations are appreciated." An important limitation, shown by animal studies, is that within less than 10 min of changes noted in monitoring, permanent damage is done.

There are four techniques of intraoperative monitoring: (1) the ankle clonus test, (2) the wakeup test, (3) somatosensory evoked potentials (SSEPs), and (4) motor evoked potentials (MEPs).

The *ankle clonus test* was the first to be used to assess spinal cord integrity intraoperatively. During the normal awake state, descending inhibitory fibers prevent clonus in response to an ankle stretch. The reflex is also inhibited during deep levels of anesthesia. However, during emergence from anesthesia, inhibition of the central descending pathways allows ankle clonus to be elicited following dorsiflexion of the foot/ankle. If there has been damage to the spinal cord, flaccid paralysis will be present and therefore no spinal reflexes can be elicited. To elicit ankle clonus, neuromuscular blockade must be reversed or absent and the patient is allowed to emerge from general anesthesia as is done with a wakeup test (see below). In most circumstances, the ankle clonus test can be elicited before the patient regains consciousness and therefore is usable at a deeper level of anesthesia than a true wakeup test. The test is extremely sensitive and specific; however, it does not provide a continuous monitor of spinal cord function.

The *wakeup test* was originally reported in the 1970s as a means of monitoring spinal cord integrity. Use of the technique requires a preoperative explanation to the patient about the test, its purpose and timing during the procedure, and the fact that there may be some intraoperative recall of its performance. At the appropriate time, neuromuscular blockade is reversed and the plane of anesthesia decreased. The speed with which a patient will awaken and respond to verbal stimuli has been facilitated by the use of short-acting anesthetic agents (desflurane, propofol, and remifentanil). With the use of these agents, a successful wakeup test can generally be accomplished within 3 to 10 min of the surgeon's request. Alternatively, reversal agents can be used to antagonize the effects of benzodiazepines and opioids. The depth of anesthesia and the patient's awakening can also be judged by the use of neurophysiological monitors such as the BIS monitor (Aspect Medical, Newton, MA). When the patient reaches a light plane of anesthesia, a voluntary movement in the motor groups above the level of surgery (e.g., squeezing one's hand) is requested initially followed by a request to move the lower extremities. Once a positive response is achieved in the lower extremities, anesthesia is deepened by the administration of propofol or thiopental. Although easy to perform, the test does entail certain risks, including having an awake patient in the prone position on the operating table. Inadvertent or sudden movements may injure the patient or cause dislodgement of venous cannulas, arterial cannulas, or the endotracheal tube or may lead to hypertension with increased bleeding. Like the ankle clonus test, it provides only a single assessment of spinal cord integrity. In most centers, the wakeup test is used only when there are questionable findings on electrophysiologic monitoring (see below).

Electrophysiologic monitoring includes somatosensory evoked potentials (SSEPs) and MEPs (see Chap. 14). The first are monitored by stimulation of a distal nerve, generally in the leg (posterior tibial) and measuring the response at the cervical level and the central nervous system via standard electroencephalographic electrodes. The pathways involved include the peripheral nerve, the dorsomedial columns (fasciculus gracilis and fasciculus cuneatus) of the spinal cord, and the cerebral cortex. SSEPs do not monitor anterior cord (motor) function. Given the close proximity of the motor and sensory tracts the spinal cord, damage to the motor tracts generally results in damage to the sensory tracts, making SSEPs a fairly reliable measure of motor function. However, since the dorsomedial tracts and the anterior aspect of the spinal cord do not share the same arterial supply, isolated damage to the motor tract has been reported while the SSEP was normal.

Since SSEPs can be affected by anesthetic agents, baseline recordings are performed after an appropriate level of anesthesia has been achieved. The variables measured include both the height of the response (amplitude) and the time it takes the response to travel from the periphery to the central nervous system (latency). Significant changes include a reduction in the amplitude of ≥50 percent or an increase in the latency of

≥10 percent. Both the inhalational anesthetic agents and nitrous oxide cause a decrease in the amplitude and an increase in the latency of SSEPs; however, acceptable monitoring can be achieved with 0.5 MAC of isoflurane or desflurane in 50 to 60 percent nitrous oxide. Intravenous anesthetic agents have been shown to have less of an effect on SSEPs, making total intravenous anesthesia with propofol or midazolam combined with an opioid an effective technique. Neuromuscular blocking agents have no effect on SSEPs.

More recently, owing to the concern that there can be isolated motor damage with normal SSEPs, many centers have started to monitor MEPs along with SSEPs. Like SSEPs, MEPs are affected by the type of anesthetic agent used. Various techniques have been recommended and there remains variation from center to center. With MEP monitoring, the level of neuromuscular blockade must be kept stable, with maintenance of one to two twitches of the train-of-four or elimination of the use of an NMBA. We prefer to use neuromuscular blockade with a short-acting agent only for endotracheal intubation and no NMBAs during the operation. Anesthesia is provided by continuous infusion of a combination of intravenous agents (propofol and remifentanil). We have also found that these agents can be effectively titrated to provide controlled hypotension with a limited need for antihypertensive agents.

▶ Postoperative Care Including Pain Management

One of the keys to the successful care of children after spinal surgery is to provide a smooth transition from the operating room to the intensive care unit (ICU). This process begins with the preoperative preparation and instruction of the patient preferably with a tour of the ICU. The patient should also be instructed regarding the correct use of incentive spirometry and patient-controlled analgesia if the use of these devices is planned. In some institutions and with specific patients (idiopathic scoliosis with no underlying medical conditions), direct postoperative admission to the ward and not the PICU may be feasible. In such instances, a 2- to 4-h stay in the postanesthesia care unit is used to ensure cardiorespiratory stability.

At the completion of the procedures, it may be desirable to have an appropriate level of responsiveness so that a neurologic examination can be performed to evaluate adequate upper and lower extremity function. The continuation of mechanical ventilation into the postoperative period is decided on an individual basis. When there is any possibility that postoperative mechanical ventilation may be needed, this should be discussed preoperatively with the parents and the patient. Mechanical

ventilation may be needed owing to neuromuscular disorder, preoperative pulmonary dysfunction, or the surgical procedure (blood loss of more than one blood volume). In specific cases, the best option may be to provide 2 to 4 h of postoperative mechanical ventilation to ensure cardiorespiratory stability, normal coagulation function, and correction of metabolic variables. Once this is accomplished, the trachea can be extubated in the ICU.

Owing to the length of the surgical incision and extensive bony and soft tissue dissection in spinal surgery, there will be significant postoperative pain. Effective analgesia is therefore essential to provide a stable postoperative course. Effective analgesia is generally best provided by using analgesic agents, anxiolytic agents, and medications to control muscle spasms. Muscle spasms may be particularly troublesome in patients with underlying cerebral palsy. Options for the provision of analgesia include intravenous administration and/or regional anesthesia. For intravenous administration, we prefer the use of patient-controlled analgesia (PCA), or, when the patient may not be able to activate the device, we use nurse-controlled analgesia. By using the device in this manner, the bedside nurse has ready access to a supply of opioid to provide an immediate dose to a patient who is in pain. Before starting PCA, an appropriate level of analgesia must be achieved by the careful titration of opioid. This is generally done in the operating room at the completion of the surgical procedure. When the remifentanil infusion is discontinued, we titrate in additional doses of morphine (0.02 mg/kg) or hydromorphone (3 to 4 μg/kg) based on the patient's respiratory rate and complaints of pain. Once adequate analgesia is achieved, the PCA device is started to maintain analgesia. Given the significant interpatient variability, it is necessary to use age-appropriate pain scores and adjust the PCA according to the patient's response.

To limit the total dose of opioid, adjunctive agents can be used. The potential adverse effects of nonsteroidal anti-inflammatory drugs (NSAIDs) on bone formation is still controversial. Given these concerns, many centers do not to use these agents after spinal surgery in children. We prefer to administer acetaminophen (10 mg/kg either by mouth or per rectum) every 4 to 6 hours around the clock. Because many of these patients tend to develop muscle spasms or require anxiolysis, benzodiazepines such as diazepam may be added to the postoperative regimen as needed or at fixed intervals. Alternatively, α_2-adrenergic agonists may be used to relieve anxiety and muscle spasms. Dexmedetomidine is a novel α_2-adrenergic agonist which currently has FDA approval for the sedation of adult patients in the ICU for 24 h. Unlike clonidine, it has a half-life of 2 to 3 h, thereby allowing its titration by continuous infusion. Given its limited effects on respiratory function and its ability to potentiate opioid-induced analgesia, it may also help to provide anxiolysis following major surgical procedures. In our experience a continuous infusion of dexmedetomidine (0.25 to 0.5 µg/kg/h) may be efficacious in these patients. Adverse effects of analgesia, including respiratory depression may occur especially in patients with comorbid features. Close monitoring of respiratory function with continuous pulse oximetry may therefore be necessary.

Given its success in other surgical procedures, there is much interest in the possible use of regional anesthesia to control pain after spinal surgery in children. Published reports on regional anesthesia after spinal surgery have included several variations: (1) the dose of the medications used; (2) the route of delivery (intrathecal or epidural); (3) the mode of delivery (single dose, intermittent bolus dosing, or continuous infusion); (4) the number of catheters used (one versus two); (5) the medications infused (opioids or local anesthetics or both); (6) the opioid used (morphine, fentanyl, hydromorphone); (7) analgesic regimen of the control group if present (intermittent "as needed" morphine or PCA); (8) the type of surgery (short-segment lumbar fusion, short-segment laminectomy for dorsal rhizotomy, posterior spinal fusion, and anterior spinal fusion); and (9) the surgical approach (open versus thoracoscopic). A review of the reports on regional anesthetic techniques after spinal surgery in children is outlined in Tables 13-1 through 13-4. The evaluation of regional anesthetic techniques is clouded by the variation in these techniques. Future trials are needed to determine the optimal postoperative analgesic regimens for these procedures.

▶ **TABLE 13-1.** INTRATHECAL MORPHINE FOLLOWING ANTERIOR OR POSTERIOR SPINAL FUSION

Authors and References	Type of Surgery	Analgesic Technique	Outcome
Dalens B, Tanguy A. *Spine* 13:494–498, 1988.	Anterior spinal fusion (n = 5) Posterior spinal fusion (n = 12)	Open label trial with no comparison or control group. Lumbar intrathecal morphine: 0.02 mg/kg.	No patient required supplemental analgesia during the initial 36 postoperative h.
Blackman RG et al. *Orthopedics* 14:555–557, 1991.	Posterior spinal fusion (n = 33)	Open label trial, no control group. Lumbar intrathecal morphine mean dose: 0.01 mg/kg; range: 0.007–0.019 mg/kg) in 10 mL of normal saline.	Duration of postoperative analgesia (mean: 18.8 h; range: 0–40 h). Early respiratory depression (n = 3), late respiratory depression (n = 4). Authors postulate this was related to large volume of fluid used for intrathecal injection.
Goodarzi M. *Paediatr Anaesth* 8:131–134, 1998.	Posterior spinal fusion (n = 80)	Prospective, randomized trial. Lumbar intrathecal morphine (0.02 mg/kg) plus intrathecal sufentanil (50 mcg) compared to inhalational agent plus intravenous sufentanil.	Decreased intraoperative blood loss in the intrathecal group and longer duration of analgesia. Mean duration of postoperative analgesia: 14.5 h, range 0–36 h with intrathecal morphine versus immediate need for analgesia in the intravenous sufentanil group.
Gall O et al. *Anesthesiology* 94:447–452, 2001.	Posterior spinal fusion (n = 30)	Prospective, randomized trial. Lumbar intrathecal morphine: 0.2 or 5 mcg/kg.	Decreased intraoperative blood loss with 5 mcg/kg. Decreased postoperative intravenous morphine use and lower pain scores at 2, 4, and 14 h in 2 and 5 mcg/kg group. No difference in adverse effect profile.

▶ **TABLE 13-2.** SINGLE EPIDURAL CATHETER WITH INTERMITTENT DOSING FOLLOWING POSTERIOR SPINAL FUSION OR DORSAL RHIZOTOMY

Authors and References	Type of Surgery	Analgesic Technique	Outcome
Amaranth L et al. *Clin Orthop Rel Res* 249:223–226, 1989.	Posterior spinal fusion (n = 35)	Epidural catheter at L_{1-2} versus intermittent intravenous or intramuscular morphine. Epidural morphine (30–50 mcg/kg) every 12–24 h.	Epidural patients had decreased requirements for postoperative IV/IM morphine.
Adu-Gyamfi Y et al. *J Internat Med Res* 23:211–217, 1995.	Posterior spinal fusion (n = 22)	Open label trial with no control group. Epidural catheter at T_{8-9} and dosed with 2 mg morphine plus 4 mL of 0.25% bupivacaine.	Complete analgesia in 18 of 22 patients. Mean pain score: 0.6 ± 0.1 in the other 4 patients. Epidural doses per day: 5.5 ± 1.9. Days catheters left in place: 4.1 ± 0.7 days.
Sparkes ML et al. *Pediatr Neurosci* 15:229–232, 1989.	Dorsal rhizotomy (n = 28)	Open label trial with no control group. Intermittent, epidural morphine (0.05 mg/kg). Sixteen of 28 patients also received bupivacaine.	Adequate analgesia in all patients without intravenous opioids. Days catheters left in place: 3. Duration of analgesia following epidural morphine: 11.44 ± 3.1 h; range: 6.5 to 18 h.
Lawhorn D et al. *Pediatr Neurosurg* 20:198–202, 1994.	Dorsal rhizotomy (n = 14)	Prospective, randomized trial. Epidural morphine (80 mcg/kg) or epidural morphine (80 mcg/kg) plus butorphanol 40 mcg/kg).	Adequate analgesia in both groups. Decreased incidence of nausea/vomiting, pruritus, and oxygen desaturation in the epidural morphine plus butorphanol group.

▶ **TABLE 13-3.** SINGLE EPIDURAL CATHETER WITH A CONTINUOUS INFUSION FOLLOWING POSTERIOR OR ANTERIOR SPINAL FUSION

Authors and References	Type of Surgery	Analgesic Technique	Outcome
Arms DM et al. *Orthopedics* 21:539–544, 1998.	Posterior spinal fusion (n = 12)	Open label trial. Morphine (30–50 mcg/kg) plus 5–10 mL of 0.25% bupivacaine followed by 4–10 mL/h of 0.0625–0.125% bupivacaine plus morphine 5–10 mcg/kg.	Satisfactory postoperative analgesia in all patients.
Shaw BA et al. *J Pediatr Ortho* 16:374–377, 1996.	Posterior spinal fusion (n = 50), anterior spinal fusion (n = 5), anterior–posterior fusion (n = 16)	Retrospective (n = 30) and prospective, open label evaluation (n = 41). Continuous infusions of 0.0625–0.125% bupivacaine plus hydromorphone (n = 61) or morphine/fentanyl (n = 10).	Successful analgesia in 64 patients (arousable yet denying pain). Of the remaining 7, there were 5 failures and 2 that could not be assessed.

(Continued)

▶ **TABLE 13-3.** SINGLE EPIDURAL CATHETER WITH A CONTINUOUS INFUSION FOLLOWING POSTERIOR OR ANTERIOR SPINAL FUSION (*Continued*)

Authors and References	Type of Surgery	Analgesic technique	Outcome
Cassady JF Jr et al. *Reg Anesth Pain Med* 25:246–253, 2000.	Posterior spinal fusion (n = 33)	Prospective, randomized trial of epidural bupivacaine plus fentanyl versus morphine (patient-controlled analgesia).	No difference in analgesic efficacy. Epidural group had a faster return of bowel sounds.
Turner et al. *Anaesthesia* 55:367–390, 2000.	Posterior spinal fusion (n = 14)	Open label trial with no control group. Epidural fentanyl + bupivacaine	Used dye injection of demonstrate location of catheter. No analgesia obtained if dye was not seen in epidural or paravertebral space.
Lowry KJ et al. *Spine* 26:1290–1293, 2001.	Anterior spinal fusion (n = 10)	Open label trial. Intraoperative placement of epidural catheter via anterior approach. Bolus dose of hydromorphone + fentanyl followed by continuous infusion of hydromorphone + 0.1% ropivacaine.	Adequate analgesia obtained in all patients without adverse effects.

▶ **TABLE 13-4.** DUAL EPIDURAL CATHETER WITH CONTINUOUS INFUSION FOLLOWING SPINAL FUSION

Authors and References	Type of Surgery	Analgesic Technique	Outcome
Tobias JD et al. *Paediatr Anaesth* 11:199–203, 2001.	Posterior spinal fusion (n = 14)	Dual epidural catheter. Tip of upper catheter at T_{1-4} and lower L_{1-4}. Bolus: hydromorphone (5 mcg/kg) + fentanyl (1 mcg/kg) diluted in 0.3 mL/kg of normal saline with 0.1 mL/kg into upper catheter and 0.2 mL/kg into lower catheter. Continuous infusion: 0.1% ropivacaine + hydromorphone (10 mcg/mL) at 0.2 mL/kg/h into lower catheter and 0.1 mL/kg/h into upper catheter.	Adequate analgesia as assessed using pain scores.
Ekatodramis G et al. *Reg Anesth Pain Med* 49:173–177, 2002.	Posterior spinal fusion (n = 23)	Dual epidural catheter technique. Tip of upper catheter at T_{4-6} and lower catheter at $T_{12}-L_1$. Initial bolus: 0.0625% bupivacaine after normal postoperative neurologic examination followed by a continuous infusion of 0.0625% bupivacaine + fentanyl 2 mcg/mL + clonidine 3 mcg/mL at 10 mL/h.	Complete analgesia at rest in all patients. Adequate analgesia with mobilization and respiratory physiotherapy in 19 of 23 patients. The other 4 required supplemental intravenous morphine for pain scores greater than 30 (maximum score = 100).

► SUMMARY

Many challenges face the anesthesiologist during spinal surgery in children. As with any surgical procedure, the care of these patients begins with a thorough preoperative evaluation to identify comorbid features, which are present in many of these patients. Idiopathic scoliosis is a common disease, and many of these patients will have associated neurologic or myopathic conditions that affect anesthetic care. Intraoperative issues include techniques for airway management, vascular access, blood conservation, patient positioning, intraoperative neurologic monitoring, the administration of blood and blood products, and the maintenance of fluid and electrolyte homeostasis. There is also a need for a smooth transition to the postoperative period, with ongoing monitoring to ensure stable cardiorespiratory function and an aggressive approach for the provision of effective postoperative analgesia.

SUGGESTED FURTHER READING

Beschetti GD, Moore JS, Smith JG, et al. Techniques for exposure of the anterior thoracic and lumbar spine. *Spine: State of the Art Reviews* 12:599, 1999.

Bunnell WP. The natural history of idiopathic scoliosis. *Clin Orthop* 120:229, 1988.

Butler MG, Hayes BG, Hathaway MM, et al. Specific genetic diseases at risk for sedation/anesthesia complications. *Anesth Analg* 91:837–855, 2000.

DePalma L, Luban NLC. Autologous blood transfusion in pediatrics. *Pediatrics* 85:125–128, 1990.

Diaz JH, Belani KG. Perioperative management of children with mucopolysaccharidoses. *Anesth Analg* 77:1261–1270, 1993.

Florentino-Pineda I, Blakemore LC, Thompson GH, et al. The effect of epsilon aminocaproic acid on perioperative blood loss in patients with idiopathic scoliosis undergoing posterior spinal fusion. *Spine* 26:1147–1151, 2001.

Fontana JL, Welborn L, Mongan PD, et al. Oxygen consumption and cardiovascular function in children during profound intraoperative normovolemic hemodilution. *Anesth Analg* 80:219–225, 1995.

Goodnough LT, Rudnick S, Price TH, et al. Increased preoperative collection of autologous blood with recombinant human erythropoietin therapy. *N Engl J Med* 321:1163–1168, 1989.

Hamill CL, Lenke LG, Bridwell KH. Use of pedicle screw fixation to improve correction in the lumbar spine in patients with idiopathic scoliosis: Is it warranted? *Spine* 121:1241, 1996.

Hersey SL, O'Dell NE, Lowe S, et al. Nicardipine versus nitroprusside for controlled hypotension during spinal surgery in adolescents. *Anesth Analg* 84:1239–1244, 1997.

King HA. Selection of fusion levels for posterior instrumentation and fusion in idiopathic scoliosis. *Orthop Clin North Am* 19:247, 1988.

Kurz A, Sessler DI, Lenhardt R, for the Study of Wound Infection and Temperature Control Group. Perioperative normothermia to reduce the incidence of surgical-wound associated infection and shorten hospitalization. *N Engl J Med* 334:1209–1215, 1996.

Laupacis A, Fergusson D, for the International Study of Perioperative Transfusions (ISPOT) Investigators. Drugs to minimize perioperative blood loss in cardiac surgery: Meta-analyses using perioperative blood transfusion as the outcome. *Anesth Analg* 85:1258–1267, 1997.

Muirhead A, Conner AN. The assessment of lung function in children with scoliosis. *J Bone Joint Surg* 67:699–702, 1985.

Regan JJ, Mack MJ, Picetti GD III. A technical report on video-assisted thoracoscopy in thoracic spinal surgery: Preliminary description. *Spine* 20:831–837, 1995.

Ruttmann TG, James MF, Viljoen JF. Haemodilution induces a hypercoagulable state. *Br J Anaesth* 76:412–414, 1996.

Ruttmann TG, James MFM, Aronson I. In vivo investigation into the effects of haemodilution with hydroxyethyl starch (200/0.5) and normal saline on coagulation. *Br J Anaesth* 80:612–616, 1998.

Schmied H, Kurz A, Sessler D, et al. Mild hypothermia increases blood loss and transfusion requirements during total hip arthroplasty. *Lancet* 347:289–292, 1996.

Sethna NF, Rockoff MA, Worthen HM, et al. Anesthesia-related complications in children with Duchenne muscular dystrophy. *Anesthesiology* 68:462–465, 1988.

Sloan TB. Anesthetic effects on electrophysiologic recordings. *J Clin Neurophysiol* 15:217–226, 1988.

Taylor RT, Manganaro L, O'Brien J, et al. Impact of allogeneic packed red blood cell transfusion on nosocomial infection rates in the critically ill patient. *Crit Care Med* 30:2249–2254, 2000.

Testa LD, Tobias JD. Techniques of blood conservation. Part 1: Isovolemic hemodilution. *Am J Anesthesiol* 23:20–28, 1996.

Theroux MC, Corddry DH, Tietz AE, et al. A study of desmopressin and blood loss during spinal fusion for neuromuscular scoliosis: A randomized, controlled, double-blinded study. *Anesthesiology* 87:260–267, 1997.

Tobias JD. A review of intrathecal and epidural analgesia after spinal surgery in children. *Anesth Analg* 98:956–965, 2004.

Tobias JD. Airway management in the pediatric trauma patient. *J Intens Care Med* 13:1–14, 1998.

Tobias JD. Anesthetic implications of thoracoscopic surgery. *Paediatr Anaesth* 9:103–110, 1999.

Tobias JD, Atwood R. Mivacurium in children with Duchenne muscular dystrophy. *Paediatr Anaesth* 4:57–60, 1994.

Tobias JD, Bozeman PM, Mackert PW, et al. Postoperative outcome following thoracotomy in the pediatric oncology patient with diminished pulmonary function. *J Surg Oncol* 52:105–109, 1993.

Vedantam R, Lenke LG, Bridwell KH, et al. A prospective evaluation of pulmonary function in patients with adolescent idiopathic scoliosis relative to the surgical approach used for spinal arthrodesis. *Spine* 25:82–90, 2000.

Vener DF, Lerman J. The pediatric airway and associated syndromes. *Anesth Clin North Am* 13:585–614, 1995.

Weinstein JN, Rydevik BL, Rauschnig W, et al. Anatomic and technical considerations of pedicle screw fixation. *Clin Orthop* 284:34, 1992.

CHAPTER 14

The Adult Spine

SERGIO MENDOZA-LATTES/ANDRÉ P. BOEZAART

▶ THE CERVICAL SPINE

Special Anatomic Considerations

The surgical anatomy of the cervical spine is divided into that of the craniocervical junction and the subaxial cervical spine (Fig. 14-1). The first includes the occiput (C0), atlas (C1) and axis (C2) vertebrae. The atlas vertebra has the form of a ring, with two lateral articular masses that articulate with the occipital condyles cephalad and with the superior facets of the axis caudad. The atlas and axis provide 40 percent of the total rotation of the cervical spine. This occurs around the odontoid process (dens). The stability between C1 and C2 depends on the lateral-mass facet-joint capsules and on the transverse ligament of the atlas, which prevents anteroposterior (AP) translation of the dens. Pathology that can potentially damage this ligament includes trauma and inflammatory pannus, as that from rheumatoid arthritis (Fig. 14-2). Instability of C1–C2 may be repaired by a C1–C2 fusion. Advanced arthritis may also erode the articular surfaces of C0–C1 and C1–C2. As a consequence, the axis migrates closer to the foramen magnum and the dens may intrude into the cranium. If this basilar invagination is reducible with traction, the patient is operated under skeletal traction and the occiput is fixed or fused in the reduced position to the cervical spine (craniocervical fusion). Nevertheless, if the dens cannot be reduced or there are other conditions that occupy the anterior spinal canal and displace the brainstem, this may be decompressed anteriorly via transoral exposure.

The subaxial cervical spine consists of five vertebrae linked by five joints at each level: the intervertebral disk (a symphysis), two facet joints, and two uncinate processes. These joints provide significant range of motion and also protect the neural elements. This area may be approached for fusion and/or decompression from both the anterior and posterior aspects of the neck.

Anterior decompression includes anterior diskectomy or corpectomy and fusion. Posterior decompression may be by laminectomy or laminoplasty. In general, posterior decompression is preferred for multilevel disease with a lordotic cervical spine. The anterior approach to the subaxial cervical spine is a standard, widely used procedure. The approach takes advantage of the anatomic planes of the neck and requires only minimal soft tissue disruption.

Patient Profile

A wide array of patients may present, including young and healthy patients who have suffered an injury as well as elderly patients with long-standing spinal cord dysfunction secondary to myelopathy. A spine affected by rheumatoid arthritis requires special attention and is discussed later (see also Chap. 8). Multiple other comorbidities may be present in the elderly group. Finally, there are also those who have suffered spinal cord injury, whose management deserves special consideration.

Common Comorbidities

Comorbidities and, therefore, the indications for the procedure may vary significantly. Most frequently, patients who require fusion for injuries or for cervical disk disease are young and present without comorbidities. Patients with cervical spondylotic myelopathy, on the other hand, are frequently in their sixth or seventh decade of life and present with one or more comorbidities as well as long-term spinal cord dysfunction. Patients suffering from rheumatoid arthritis and subsequent atlantoaxial instability frequently

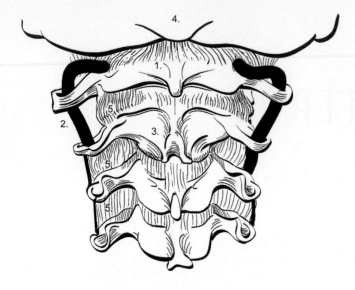

1. Posterior arch of C1 (atlas)
2. Vertebral artery
3. Posterior arch of C2 (axis)
4. External occiptal protuberance
5. Facet joint capsules

Figure 14-1. Posterior surgical anatomy of the cervical spine.

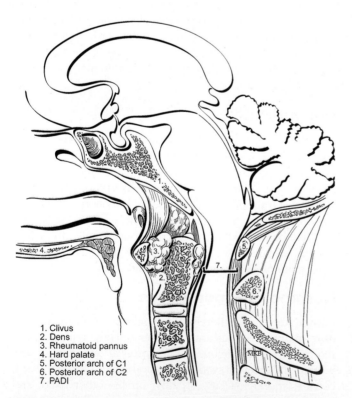

1. Clivus
2. Dens
3. Rheumatoid pannus
4. Hard palate
5. Posterior arch of C1
6. Posterior arch of C2
7. PADI

Figure 14-2. Sagittal view of the pathologic anatomy of the upper cervical spine in inflammatory arthritis. There is atlantoaxial subluxation and the posterior atlanto-dens interval (PADI) is reduced.

present with multiple medical problems, including those associated with chronic steroid therapy.

Spinal Cord Injury

The loss of sympathetic tone produces generalized vasodilatation below the level of the injury. The intravascular volume is expanded, which leads to hypotension. Additionally, there is an increase in vagal tone due to sympatholysis, resulting in bradycardia, which reduces cardiac output and further adds to the reduction of systemic blood pressure. Fluid management is therefore crucial. Too aggressive attempts to treat neurogenic shock solely by the administration of fluids may cause fluid overload and pulmonary edema. Furthermore, some patients may have concomitantly suffered pulmonary contusion. The resultant hypoxia not only worsens the effects of oligemia but may also contribute to the progression of secondary injury of the spinal cord. Optimal oxygenation is mandatory, and anticholinergic drugs such as atropine may be used to counteract bradycardia. Careful administration of vasopressors is indicated to control vasomotor disturbances, and great care must be taken to identify and treat other associated injuries, such as liver and spleen lacerations, which may be masked by the spinal cord injury. If the injury is above the level of C4, respiratory function may be compromised owing to involvement of the phrenic nerve, and assisted ventilation may be required after surgery. Additionally, gastroparesis and immobility increase the risk of aspiration pneumonia. Nasogastric tubes are therefore essential.

Positioning on the Operating Table

Positioning may directly influence surgical exposure and fusion alignment. Correct positioning is also necessitated to preserve neurologic function. Once the patient is anesthetized, there are no warning signs of maneuvers that might be damaging to the cervical spinal cord. This is especially important in cases of instability and cervical canal stenosis. General precautions include moving the patient in a rigid cervical orthosis at all times and head-to-trunk immobilization during transfers.

Positioning for Anterior Surgical Exposure

For anterior cervical exposure, the neck should lie in a neutral or slightly extended position. This is achieved by placing a roll under the scapulae. Care must be taken in positioning an elderly patient with a stenotic spinal canal. Gardner-Wells tongs may be used to assist in positioning and also to help in immobilizing the head and neck. The shoulders may be taped down distally to facilitate fluoroscopic visualization of the cervicothoracic junction. The arms are carefully padded and wrapped to the sides. If autologous bone is required for grafting, the anterior iliac crest may be prepared. A horseshoe or Mayfield head rest is padded with a soft roll, adapted, and secured. After the anesthesiologist has secured the airway, the surgeon should hold the patient's head and gently extend the neck slightly. Most of this extension should involve the occipitocervical junction. Once adequate positioning has been obtained, the head rest is secured and, if necessary, a head halter or tong traction applied. Finally, the head of the bed is slightly elevated to decrease venous bleeding. The knees can be raised to prevent the patient from sliding down during the operation and to protect the sciatic nerve from traction injury.

Positioning for Posterior Cervical Exposure

For posterior cervical exposure, the neck must be aligned close to neutral, with some degree of forward thrust of the head. If instability is caused by flexion, care must be taken not to increase traumatic deformity. When occipitocervical and/or atlantoaxial fixation is planned, flexion of the head creates space for exposure and instrumentation by maximizing the distance between the occiput and the posterior arches of the atlas and axis. A horseshoe or Mayfield head rest is recommended. In occipitocervical fixation the head should be aligned in a functional position at the time the implants are fixed.

For both anterior and posterior procedures, the arms are carefully positioned next to the body, with elbows, wrists, and hands well padded. Wrist straps may be used for traction, especially for lower cervical or cervicothoracic fusions. In this situation, lateral fluoroscopy may be very difficult because the shoulders may obstruct the x-rays; therefore downward traction of the shoulders may be needed.

Potential complications due to positioning include nerve trauma at the ulnar tunnel, at the carpal tunnel, or in the axillae. In the lower extremities, the most common nerve compression syndromes associated with positioning include femorocutaneous and peroneal nerve palsies. The orbits should also be free of any external compression.

Authors' Surgical Technique

Anterior Cervical Decompression and Fusion (ACDF)

The anterior exposure to the cervical spine has been widely used since its original description in 1958. As described, this approach is useful for single- or multiple-level diskectomy and cervical corpectomy. The removal of a vertebral body is useful in trauma where the thecal sac is invaded by a fragmented vertebral body or as an alternative to multiple-level diskectomy and interbody fusions, where the pseudoarthrosis (nonunion) rate increases in proportion to the number of levels of attempted fusion.

Magnification is recommended, and the skin is incised horizontally, starting from the midline and extending laterally. The surface landmarks for the incision are the hyoid at C3, the thyroid cartilage at C4–C5,

and the cricoid cartilage at C6. A longitudinal incision following the anteromedial border of the sternocleidomastoid muscle is indicated for the treatment of multilevel surgery, as for two or more vertebrae. With a properly placed horizontal incision, up to three diskectomies may be performed. If multiple corpectomies are planned, a longitudinal incision is preferred.

Following incision, the platysma muscle is divided longitudinally, strap and sternocleidomastoid muscles are identified, and the superficial layer of fascia is divided (Fig. 14-3). The pretracheal fascia is exposed, and the strap muscles are divided longitudinally to identify the medial border of the carotid sheath. The omohyoid muscle may be transected if more extensive exposure is required. The strap muscles, trachea, and esophagus are retracted medially, and the prevertebral fascia is exposed. A needle is used to mark the appropriate disk space, and AP and lateral fluoroscopy is used to confirm the appropriate level, and the midline.

Once the appropriate disk space is confirmed, the prevertebral fascia and longi colli muscles are dissected and Cloward-type retractor blades are placed with the distal lips lying deep in these muscles. All static retractors cause pressure on the soft tissues, including the airway, carotid artery, and internal jugular vein; this pressure should therefore be relieved at regular intervals. It may be advantageous to reduce the endotracheal cuff pressure to avoid mucosal ischemia.

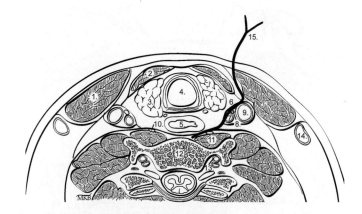

1. Sternocleidomastoid muscle
2. Strap muscles
3. Thyroid
4. Trachea
5. Esophagus
6. Carotid sheath
7. Common carotid artery
8. Vagus nerve
9. Internal jugular vein
10. Phrenic nerve
11. Longus colli muscle
12. Body of C4 vertebra
13. Vertebral artery
14. External jugular vein
15. Plane of approach to the anterior cervical spine

Figure 14-3. Cross section through the neck demonstrating the intermuscular approach to the anterior cervical spine.

The disk is then removed, as are anterior osteophytes. To visualize the posterior annulus and spinal canal, the vertebrae are distracted with a Cloward distractor or Caspar spreader. Microsurgical curettes, Kerrison rongeurs, and a nerve hook are used to complete the diskectomy and examine the spinal canal for evidence of any compressing elements. If disk material is suspected to be lying posterior to the posterior longitudinal ligament (PLL), this is removed, avoiding pressure on the dura. Free disk fragments are removed with a pituitary rongeur.

After decompression, arthrodesis is done by positioning a graft between the endplates. The distractor system is removed, and fluoroscopy is used to confirm correct placement. A low-profile titanium plate may also be added for increased stability (Fig. 14-4).

If two adjacent disks have been removed, a Leksell rongeur is used to create a trough in the vertebral body. The remainder of the vertebral body is then burred down to the posterior cortex, which is finally removed with curettes and a Kerrison rongeur. The lateral margins of the corpectomy must always be limited to the projection of the uncovertebral processes in order to protect the vertebral arteries.

The muscles are repositioned and the platysma and subcutaneous tissue layer and skin sutured. The patient's neck is stabilized with a cervical orthosis.

Posterior Cervical Decompression and Fusion

After prone positioning of the patient and surgical preparation, a vertical incision is made from the superior occipital protuberance to the prominent spinous process of C7. Epinephrine (1:500,000) may be used to help with hemostasis. After dissection of the subcutaneous tissue layer, the trapezius fascia and paraspinal muscles are dissected from the tip of the spinous processes, extending laterally to the lateral aspect of the articular processes. Dissection beyond the facet joints or articular processes may result in denervation of the muscles and may also threaten the vertebral artery. Intraoperative x-rays or fluoroscopy are used to confirm the correct anatomic site. Decompression procedures—including foraminotomy, laminectomy, and laminoplasty—are carried out through this exposure (Fig. 14-5). In laminoplasty, the posterior arch is hinged open to increase the AP diameter of the spinal canal, thus maintaining the integrity of the posterior tension band. Laminectomy also allows decompression of the thecal sac, but this may compromise the stability of the spine. Foraminotomy allows access to decompress a single nerve root without compromising spinal stability.

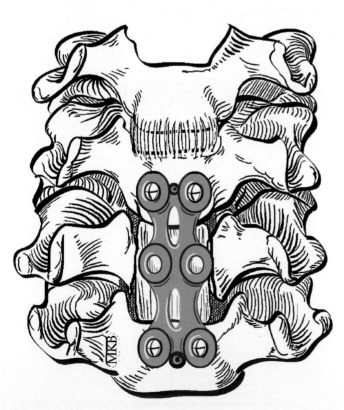

Figure 14-4. View of the anterior exposure of the cervical spine. A corpectomy has been replaced by interbody strut graft and anterior plate reconstruction.

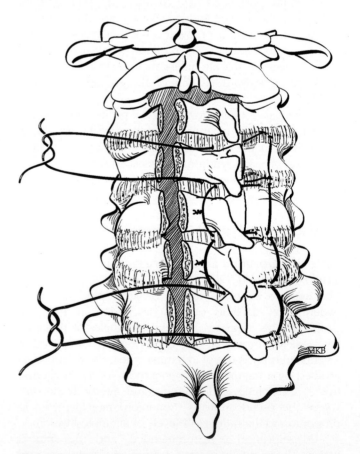

Figure 14-5. Posterior approach to the cervical spine with a laminoplasty. Note that the laminae have been hinged open, the so-called open door.

Screws may be placed into the lateral articular processes. The technique described by Magerl is the most popular owing to its many biomechanical advantages and because it protects the neurovascular structures, though not completely. This is so especially during drilling, which is targeted cranially from 30 to 40 degrees, following the direction of the superior articular surface and laterally 25 to 30 degrees to avoid the vertebral artery. The screws are connected to plates or rods, providing rigid fixation of the segments with disordered motion.

The articular surfaces and the lateral processes are prepared for arthrodesis with a high-speed burr so as to provide decorticated bone for bone graft only. Finally, the wound is closed in three layers and a cervical orthosis applied.

Occipitocervical Fusion

With the patient in the prone position, a midline incision is made from the caudal aspect of the occiput to the C3 spinous process. The deep dissection is kept as close to the midline as possible, although the median raphe or ligamentum nuchae may follow a tortuous course, making it difficult to remain in an avascular plane for the dissection. The ligamentous attachments of the C2 spinous process are identified and subperiosteally elevated. The exposure extends no further than the medial one-third of the facet joint between C2 and C3. The midline of the occiput is exposed subperiosteally. The posterior tubercle of C1 is palpated and subperiosteal dissection performed. Excessive pressure on the posterior arch of C1 can cause accidental penetration of the atlantooccipital membrane, which may injure underlying structures. The dura can be especially vulnerable in cases of C1–C2 instability. The vertebral artery and vein are vulnerable beyond a point 15 mm from the midline as the artery courses from a slightly posterior foramen transversarium of C1 in a posteromedial direction to enter the foramen magnum, just cephalad of the ring of C1. If the atlantooccipital membrane is accidentally penetrated proximally to the superior border of the ring of C1, the vertebral artery lies more medial, where it may be vulnerable. Arterial bleeding in this location may have disastrous consequences. Additional care must be taken when these structures are being dissected in rotatory dislocations of C1–C2, because the vertebral artery is stretched across the joint where C1 is dislocated anteriorly.

After dissection, instrumentation is started by inserting 4.5- to 5.25-mm screws into each side of the occiput, avoiding penetration of the skull. Cerebrospinal fluid (CSF) may leak, but this stops once the screw is placed. Ideally, three screws per side are placed.

Transarticular C1–C2 screws are then placed starting at the midline of the caudal aspect of the inferior facet of C2, aiming toward the lateral mass of C1 through the C1–C2 joint. This procedure is fluoroscopically guided and provides reliable fixation of this joint. Additionally, a sublaminar wire loop is passed under the posterior arch of C1 and anchored under the spinous process of C2. The free ends are used to hold an H-shaped bicortical autograft from the base of the occiput to the posterior arch of C2. The wires are tied, firmly fixing the graft, and the transarticular screws are connected through a rod to the occipital screws. The wound is then closed in three layers and a cervicothoracic orthosis (CTO) is applied.

Anesthetic Considerations

Spinal Cord Monitoring

Spinal cord monitoring is widely used during cervical and thoracic spinal procedures. Intraoperative neurophysiologic monitoring of the spinal cord has proven beneficial in minimizing the risks of neural injury during surgery.

The Wakeup Test

Traditionally, the wakeup test (WUT) has been considered the "gold standard" that provides a "snapshot" of the neurologic situation. This test is performed after instrumentation, decompression, and correction of the deformity have been completed. It consists of decreasing the anesthesia, typically by administering an infusion of remifentanil or alfentanil with propofol or inhalational anesthesia to the point where the patient is able to follow verbal commands. The patient must be fully reversed from any neuromuscular blocking agents and is first asked to squeeze the anesthesiologist's hand to indicate his or her ability to respond and then to move the feet and toes. If hand movement occurs but foot movement does not, the surgeon will undo corrective procedures or remove implants invading the spinal canal in order to reassess the situation. Removal or modification of instrumentation within 3 h after the onset of a neurologic deficit may significantly decrease permanent damage. Spinal cord perfusion and oxygenation must be optimized. High doses of steroids can be used to prevent the progression of secondary injury to the spinal cord, but this is controversial.

Because inhalational anesthetics make timing of the wakeup test very difficult, opioids like remifentanil with nitrous oxide and propofol or ketamine are anesthetic agents of choice. Risks involved with the wakeup test include accidental extubation, dislodgment of instrumentation, injury, bronchospasm, recall of intraoperative events, and psychological trauma, air embolism, and cardiac ischemia. Success and safety are therefore very dependent on informing the patient properly beforehand. Midazolam is also helpful in causing anterograde amnesia.

Somatosensory Evoked Potentials

Somatosensory evoked potentials (SSEPs) allow for continuous assessment of spinal cord function, primarily the function of the sensory system. The negative predictive value of SSEPs is reported to be 99.93 percent, and this assessment is started immediately after the induction of anesthesia. A peripheral nerve, usually the posterior tibial nerve at the ankle, is stimulated, and cortical potentials are recorded with surface electrodes. Early positive potentials after stimulation are recorded at 31 ms (P31), followed by a small negative potential at 35 ms (N35) and subsequent sizable positive potentials at 40 ms (P40). The P31 potential arises from the brainstem and is more consistent and resistant to anesthetic agents than P40, which is a cortical response. An increase in latency and decrease in amplitude may be observed at clinically used concentrations of inhalation anesthetic agents. This decreases the specificity and sensitivity of the monitoring. This false-positive response is dose-dependent. It has been determined that 0.5 MAC of halothane or 1.0 MAC of isoflurane, sevoflurane, or enflurane combined with 50% nitrous oxide will provide adequate sensitivity and specificity of the monitoring. Data for desflurane are not available. Additionally, stable spinal cord blood flow and oxygenation provide more consistent responses. This requires normal temperature and blood pressure as well as optimal oxygenation, hematocrit, and glucose.

Motor Evoked Potentials

Motor evoked potentials (MEPs) are motor responses of the limb muscles obtained by transcranial electrical stimulation or by magnetic pulse stimulation of the motor cortex. A brief muscle response is recorded in the lower extremities. This tests the pathways of the motor neurons. Transcranial electrical stimulation requires the application of high voltage and may be painful to the conscious patient. Magnetic stimulation is not painful but requires a sizable coil and cable that is extremely sensitive to positional changes, making its use during surgery impractical. Electrical stimulation thus seems more practical for intraoperative monitoring. MEPs are also very sensitive to anesthetic agents. Halogenated inhalational agents must be avoided. Nitrous oxide also interferes with MEP recordings and may be used as an adjunct to propofol anesthesia with a concentration below 50%. Neuromuscular blockade makes this type of monitoring of spinal cord function impossible, but neuromuscular blockade to one to two twitches of the train-of-four nerve stimulator monitor may be permissible. It is important to discuss the problem with neurophysiologists before neuromuscular blocking agents are used.

Postoperative Analgesia

Anterior cervical exposure requires little dissection; tissue disruption and postoperative pain are therefore limited and little analgesia is required. Most commonly, the pharynx and larynx are edematous and inflamed, causing dysphagia. This requires alimentation with cool fluids as well as mashed and semisolid foods until symptoms subside. If bone was removed from the iliac crest for grafting, this commonly becomes the main source of pain.

Pain following posterior cervical exposure requires more analgesia because tissue disruption is greater than with anterior exposure. The patient with spinal cord injury also suffers from pain at the operative site and may also have other complex regional pain or neuropathic pain syndromes that necessitate intensive management.

Associated Medication

Antibiotic prophylaxis is similar to that in other musculoskeletal procedures where implants are used. Modern guidelines for using prophylactic antibiotics are outlined in Chap. 4.

A further consideration is the use of steroids. A patient admitted with a spinal cord injury will have received high-dose steroid therapy. This usually includes 30 mg/kg of methylprednisolone (Solu-Medrol) as a bolus diluted in normal saline and infused over 30 min. Thirty minutes after this bolus has been completed, a continuous infusion of methylprednisolone at 5.4 mg/kg/h is initiated for 24 or 48 h. Although this protocol is currently considered the standard of care in most emergency department settings, its use remains a matter of controversy. Not only has its usefulness been questioned but it has also been pointed out that high-dose steroids may increase perioperative morbidity, particularly surgical-site infection, pneumonia, and gastrointestinal hemorrhage. Finally, existing studies lack control for surgical interventions, stratification of the patient population, and the use of summed motor scores and functional assessment of improvement in motor function. Mortality after hospitalization for spinal cord injury currently reaches approximately 7 percent in the first year; this is attributed mainly to multiple trauma and respiratory and infectious complications. Mortality is directly proportional to the level of injury and the patient's age. Although not proved by evidence in the clinical literature, the timing of surgical intervention may be a key factor determining neurologic outcome. There is wide support for early surgical intervention and early rehabilitation. Improved nursing care and attempts to reduce systemic complications seem to be among the most important factors that reduce mortality and improve neurologic outcome.

Physical Therapy Goals and Requirements in the Postoperative Period

Reconstruction procedures of the cervical spine often provide enough stability to allow the patient to begin rehabilitation. If there is doubt about stability or bone quality, a cervical orthosis must be used to protect the bone-implant interface. Upper extremity loading is restricted until fusion is achieved. Exposure to potential trauma is also avoided, including participating in sport—especially contact sport, use of all-terrain vehicles, horseback riding, etc.

For patients with anterior cervical decompression and fusion, out-of-bed activities are encouraged on the day of surgery, and patients are usually discharged from the hospital after 1 or 2 days. Generally one or two visits by the physical therapist and occupational therapist are sufficient to provide instructions on care and independence in daily activities. Patients subject to more extensive posterior procedures may require an additional day of hospitalization for pain control.

In cases of spinal cord injury, the reconstruction of the spine should be stable enough to allow for all rehabilitation procedures, including pulmonary rehabilitation, orthostatic rehabilitation, the acquisition of transfer skills, and self-care.

Special Intra- and Postoperative Surgical Requirements

The Unstable Cervical Spine

There is currently no consensus on the definition of clinical instability of the spine. It has been defined as the loss of the capacity of the spine to support physiologic loads while still maintaining a harmonious relationship between the vertebrae in such a way that there is neither initial nor subsequent damage to the spinal cord or the development of incapacitating deformity or pain. A checklist that facilitates its clinical application has also accompanied this definition. The checklist also includes images that reveal destruction of the bony architecture, the presence of neural deficit, anticipated dangerous loading, spinal canal narrowing, and static/dynamic (flexion-extension) radiographic signs (>3.5 mm of subluxation or more than 11 degrees of focal kyphosis). For the patient who undergoes general anesthesia, the most important predictor of paralysis is the space available for the cord (SAC). The SAC is the distance between the posterior cortex of the vertebral body and the spinolaminar line. In a cohort of 49 patients with rheumatoid arthritis who underwent joint arthroplasty, almost 50 percent presented criteria for instability with subaxial subluxation of the cervical spine >3 mm; nevertheless, only 8 percent presented with SAC ≤13 mm.

At the level of the atlantoaxial complex, the SAC is significantly greater than that in the subaxial cervical spine. The "rule of thirds" describes the relationship between the dens and the spinal cord inside the ring of the atlas. The dens and the thecal sac occupy one-third each, leaving a safety margin of a third of the anteroposterior diameter of the spinal canal. The relationship between C1 and C2 is maintained by its lateral masses

and by the transverse ligament of the atlas. If the distance between the anterior margin of the dens and the posterior margin of the ring of the atlas (atlanto-dens interval) exceeds 4 mm, then most likely the transverse ligament is incompetent. Nevertheless, a SAC ≤13 mm is a major clinical predictor of spinal cord injury. The posterior atlanto-dens interval (PADI) represents the SAC at the level of the atlas and has a negative predictive value of 94 percent for the development of paralysis if the measurement is greater than 14 mm. The PADI is especially useful in determining risks for chronic atlantoaxial instability, such as rheumatoid arthritis and Down's syndrome. Other conditions include the presence of a hypoplastic dens, os odontoideum, rheumatoid arthritis, or a pseudoarthrosis of the dens.

In cases of cervical instability, the unconscious patient is at particular risk. Fiberoptic endoscopically assisted intubation of the patient is preferable. The patient is turned and transferred to the operating table with a rigid cervical orthosis in position. Sometimes surgeons prefer to place the patient in the prone position before general anesthesia is induced. This allows for neurologic assessment after positioning. Common causes of cervical instability include trauma and destructive lesions caused by infection or malignant tumor growth.

Cervical Stenosis

The patient with a narrowed cervical spinal canal may be at particular risk of developing central cord syndrome if the neck is extended. The normal sagittal diameter of the spinal canal in the subaxial cervical spine is approximately 17 to 18 mm in healthy people, and the spinal cord diameter is approximately 10 mm in this same region. Cervical stenosis is defined as an anteroposterior spinal canal diameter ≤13 mm by a Torg (Pavlov) ratio of less than 0.8. This ratio is the size of the spinal canal relative to the anteroposterior dimensions of the vertebral body. A Torg ratio of less than 80 percent represents a risk factor for the development of myelopathy in patients with cervical spondylosis.

The dimensions of the spinal canal change with flexion-extension movements. When the neck is extended, the spinal cord may be compressed between the posterior vertebral bodies' osteophytes projecting from the posterior lip of the inferior endplate and the superior border of the lamina of the vertebra immediately below, resulting in a central cord syndrome. Flexion, on the other hand, results in tension forces on the spinal cord, and concomitant compression of the ventral spinal cord against endplate osteophytes and disk material. Furthermore, during extension, the cervical cord shortens and its cross-sectional area increases. Simultaneously, the ligamentum flavum bulges inward to further reduce the SAC and compress the spinal cord. Neck extension poses the greatest risk of cord injury because the SAC is narrowed with simultaneous expansion of the cervical cord. Neutral alignment of the neck must thus be maintained at all times, since that position provides the largest SAC.

Patients with a significant risk of spinal cord compression and ischemia, due either to traumatic instability or stenosis, should be stabilized before anesthesia induction. This is possible only for anterior cervical exposure with the patient supine. Fiberoptic assisted intubation in awake patients is mandatory to prevent manipulation of the neck. When awake, the patient is able to provide feedback, and continuous neurologic assessment is possible. If anesthesia must be induced before positioning the patient, as for posterior cervical exposure, it is important to position the patient with a rigid cervical orthosis constantly in place.

Complications

Neurologic Injury

Injury to the spinal cord is probably the most feared complication associated with spinal procedures. The Cervical Spine Research Society has surveyed 5356 cases and has reported an incidence of 1.04 percent neurologic complications, with 0.2 to 0.4 percent of these being spinal cord injuries. The figure was lower for anterior procedures than for posterior procedures. Intraoperative management as well as the principles of prevention have been described earlier.

Vascular Complications

Although ACDF involves minimal blood loss, the approach involves displacing the carotid sheath and all its contents. Although injury to the carotid artery is extremely rare, bradycardia may result from a vasovagal response caused by retraction of the carotid sheath. Other structures that may bleed during and after surgery are the thyroid vessels as well as the superficial jugular vein.

Vertebral artery laceration is rare, with a reported incidence of 0.5 percent. These injuries usually occur during cervical corpectomy. Anatomic variants of the trajectory of this artery and excessive lateral resection of the vertebral body are the key factors. The vertebral artery is approximately 5 mm from where a decompression is performed at the C6 level and is situated in the posterior quarter of the vertebral body, allowing a very narrow margin of safety when the lateral nerve roots are being decompressed.

Control of bleeding from vertebral artery laceration is difficult. Ligation may result in cerebellar infarction with cranial nerve palsies, transient dysphagia and dysarthria, persistent posterior fossa circulatory insufficiency, vocal cord paralysis, and quadriplegia. A report on 100 patients with vertebral artery ligation gave a mortality of 12 percent, secondary to brainstem ischemia.

Postoperative Visual Loss

This devastating complication of spinal surgery has frequently been reported in the literature on anesthesia in orthopedics and neurosurgery with an incidence of approximately 0.2 percent. In an attempt to identify risk factors and preventive measures, the American Society of Anesthesiologists developed the "postoperative visual loss (POVL) registry" in June 1999 and had registered 79 cases by the end of summer 2003. Although this does not represent the true occurrence of this problem, this registry revealed some interesting facts. First, ischemic optic neuropathy (ION) was by far the most common cause of visual loss. Second, the most common procedures associated with POVL were spine surgery (54 percent) followed by cardiac surgery (10 percent). Third, most of the spinal cases involved prolonged prone positioning (median 8 h) and large blood losses (median 2.3 L). Age does not seem to matter. Some cases occurred in young, healthy patients with 3 h prone time and minimal blood loss. Nevertheless, the incidence does seem to increase dramatically for prone times ≥5 h. Venous congestion may be important, in association with hypotension and anemia.

Finally, of the spine surgery cases in the prone position that developed POVL, 77 percent had their heads positioned with a foam support and 18 percent with Mayfield tongs.

Other Complications

Horner's syndrome may occur because of an injury to the cervical sympathetic plexus. This plexus lies within the longi colli muscles and can be injured by dissection or excessive pressure from a retractor blade. The syndrome may be temporary or permanent.

The recurrent laryngeal nerve may be damaged, causing hoarseness and vocal cord paralysis. The hoarseness is usually temporary, but cases have been reported in which the vocal cords were permanently paralyzed. Care must be taken when considering a second procedure with contralateral exposure. Visual inspection of the vocal cords is recommended before surgical intervention.

Laceration of the dura is uncommon during cervical spinal surgery. If it does occur, repair should be attempted. Possible complications include dural-cutaneous fistula, secondary Arnold-Chiari phenomenon, and cranial nerve dysfunction. The thecal sac may be lacerated as a result of a traumatic injury or may be damaged during ossification of posterior longitudinal ligament (OPLL) surgery.

Postoperative dysphagia is a common yet underreported problem, which may last up to a year. This complication has been reported in up to 50 percent of patients 1 month after surgery and in 12 percent of patients after 1 year. The dysphagia is commonly mechanical but may also be accompanied by odynophagia, breathing difficulties in 18 percent, and pneumonia during the early postoperative period. Patients with gastroesophageal reflux disorder are more likely to experience breathing difficulties in the postoperative period. The etiology of dysphagia is not completely understood.

During the procedure, inadvertent perforation of the esophagus may occur. This is a very serious complication, including the development of osteomyelitis, abscess formation, and mediastinitis. The incidence of this complication has been reported to be between 0.2 and 0.9 percent of all anterior cervical exposures, and one-third of these injuries occur during surgery. Protruding graft, hardware, or cement, which may erode the esophagus in the postoperative period, accounts for the other two-thirds. Early recognition and immediate management are vitally important.

In the postoperative period, the most urgent complication is acute respiratory distress due to cervical hematoma. Careful intraoperative hemostasis as well as a postoperative drain deep to the aponeurosis help to prevent this problem. Immediate treatment includes orotracheal intubation. A cricothyroidotomy may be lifesaving, along with immediate drainage of the hematoma. If the patient has been subjected to prolonged surgery, especially in the prone position, edema may develop around the neck and compromise the upper airway. Steroid therapy may be useful in coping with this complication.

Finally, although extremely uncommon, a hematoma of the spinal canal may develop. This will lead to progressive neurologic deterioration. This situation also requires immediate exploration. The diagnosis is confirmed by magnetic resonance imaging (MRI) or computed tomography (CT) myelography.

▶ THE THORACIC SPINE

Indications and Special Anatomic Considerations

The thoracic spine provides structural support, limited motion, and protection of the neural elements. The stability and rigidity of this part of the spine partially depends on its relationship with the rib cage through the costovertebral and costotransverse joints. Injury to the heads of the ribs is an indirect sign of significant torsional stress on the spine and must not be overlooked. In addition, the close relationship with the mediastinum and lungs must warn of potential injuries to these structures, especially when there is evidence of translational or shearing forces that have acted on the thoracic spine.

Posterior surgery to the thoracic spine includes that for the correction of deformities, stabilization after trauma or tumor resection, and decompression of the thoracic spinal cord. Anterior surgery is most commonly undertaken for decompression of the thoracic spinal cord from trauma, tumor, infection, or degenerative pathology such as thoracic disk herniation. Anterior surgery also plays an increasing role in the correction of deformities, alone or combined with a posterior procedure. More detail on the correction of deformities in the pediatric population is given in Chap. 14.

Patient Profile

The patient profile ranges from the healthy young adult with a deformity or a herniated disk to the chronically ill patient with an infection or tumor.

It must be always kept in mind that the enormous energy required to injure the thoracic spine may have damaged other organs or systems. With lung contusions, prone positioning of the patient may potentially disrupt pulmonary blood flow and cause ventilation/perfusion mismatch.

Similar considerations apply to patients with spinal cord injury, such as those described in the discussion of the cervical spine, above. In thoracolumbar trauma, the patient with paralysis is even more likely to have occult abdominal or thoracic trauma, which must be thoroughly evaluated.

Common Comorbidities

For the anterior exposure to the thoracic or thoracolumbar spine, a thoracotomy is required. This exposure significantly decreases the values of pulmonary function tests (PFTs) for up to 2 years. Patients with previous lung disease must be carefully evaluated, and planning for the postoperative period is mandatory. Ventilatory assistance may be required after surgery. In patients with injuries to the thoracolumbar spine, pulmonary contusion may be relevant in deciding on the timing and laterality of the surgical exposure. Spinal instability will not allow adequate mobilization of the patient, and it may be impossible to achieve adequate pulmonary function. Gas exchange can be further compromised by single-lung ventilation during spinal surgery, and the surgical team must decide whether the patient will be able to tolerate one-lung ventilation for several hours.

Positioning on the Operating Table

Posterior Approach to the Thoracic Spine

This exposure requires prone positioning. Most surgeons prefer to use a four- or five-post frame. The face is positioned on contoured foam, taking care to prevent pressure and congestion around the eyes. Some devices with a mirror allow continuous observation of endotracheal tube placement. Care should also be taken to avoid compression of the abdomen, since this increases venous congestion and intraoperative bleeding from venous epidural sinuses. Decompression of the abdomen and inferior vena cava reduces epidural blood flow, which allows better visualization of structures in the spinal canal. If the fusion is carried into the lumbar spine, preservation of the sagittal alignment is essential. This is further discussed below, under positioning for lumbosacral fusion exposures.

The superior posts should be positioned under the patient's rib cage, while the inferior posts should be positioned underneath the anterior iliac spine. For heavier patients, a transverse post across the superior chest, two posts on the inferior rib cage, and two posts on the iliac crests are used. The legs are supported with pillows. Care should be taken to prevent excessive pressure on the breasts in female patients.

The arms are positioned with 90 degrees or more of flexion of the elbows and 90 degrees or less abduction of the shoulders. The arms rest on well-padded boards, and special care is taken to avoid pressure on the ulnar grooves and the wrists. The axillae must also be protected against compression.

Prone positioning checklist:

No pressure on eyes to ensure normal retinal blood flow

Endotracheal tube unobstructed

Head not lower than heart to prevent cerebral congestion and decreased cerebral blood flow

Neck not extended but neutral

Abdomen free to prevent venous congestion, increased bleeding, and epidural venous congestion

Breasts not compressed

Male genitals free and not compressed

Urinary catheter free and not compressed or obstructed

Legs supported; femoral nerves free from compression

Shoulders abducted 90 degrees or less

Elbows flexed 90 degrees or less

Ulnar nerves free and not compressed

Median nerves at wrists free of compression; wrists neutral

Ventilation bilateral and normal

Intravenous and arterial lines free and unobstructed

Anterolateral Approach to the Thoracic Spine

This exposure requires lateral positioning, usually on the patient's right side. The left-sided exposure is the most convenient, especially for the lower thoracic spine and thoracolumbar junction. Retracting the right hemidiaphragm may be difficult. The spleen is smaller and therefore easier to retract than the liver. In addition, the vena cava (on the right side) can be lacerated more easily than the aorta. Because of its pulsation, the aorta is easier to locate on the left side (Fig. 14-6). This is especially important when resection includes soft tissue mass extension from tumor or infection. Nevertheless, there are conditions when a left-sided exposure will not be convenient, as in

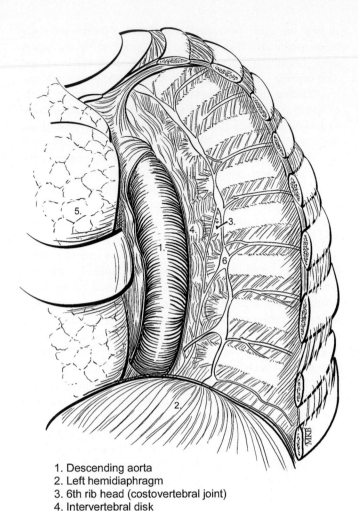

1. Descending aorta
2. Left hemidiaphragm
3. 6th rib head (costovertebral joint)
4. Intervertebral disk
5. Left lung lower lobe
6. Sympathetic chain

Figure 14-6. Left-sided thoracotomy exposure. The lung has been retracted anteriorly, and the dome of the left hemidiaphragm is observed.

the correction of scoliosis with a right-sided curve. If the operation involves the upper thoracic spine (T1–T4), it is convenient to approach the spine from the right side so as to avoid the aortic arch. If the vertebral bodies are small, as in small people, spinal implants may be relatively prominent and the aortic wall may be eroded by the pulsations of the artery against them. The right arm is abducted and flexed as far cephalad as possible to allow mobilization of the scapula anteriorly and superiorly. Since left-sided exposures are more frequent, the following description considers the patient lying on his or her right side.

The patient is transferred to the operating table in a supine position. After anesthesia has been induced and the endotracheal tube (usually a double-lumen tube to facilitate one-lung ventilation) is inserted, the patient is turned to a lateral decubitus position and a roll is placed underneath the axilla to prevent circulatory disturbance to the right arm (Fig. 14-7). Most surgeons prefer silicone

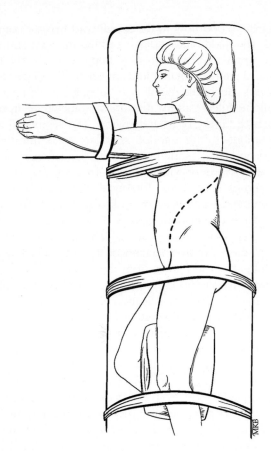

Figure 14-7. Positioning and skin incision for left-sided thoracoabdominal exposure.

padding. Foam padding is also placed underneath the right leg from the hip down to the foot. The head is supported with pillows or foam, maintaining neutral alignment of the neck. The trunk is supported on the sternum and the back by padded supporting attachments or by a beanbag. The pelvis is supported by adhesive tape or straps over the left greater trochanter, which is always protected by foam padding. In procedures involving decompression of the spinal canal or instrumentation of the spine, stable positioning is important for surgical orientation and intraoperative imaging. The right arm is supported by a foam-padded arm board with the shoulder at 90 degrees of extension and the left is extended on top of this, separated by pillows or other soft padding. Special supporting devices for the upper arm are available. Some surgeons prefer to flex the table at the patient's waist in order to increase the space between the ribs. Tilting the table into a reverse Trendelenburg position facilitates retraction of the hemidiaphragm by displacing the abdominal viscera caudally. This position also facilitates venous drainage and decreases surgical bleeding from the epidural venous sinuses or obstruction of vision by them.

Authors' Surgical Technique

Posterior Spinal Fusion and Instrumentation

After a standard midline incision of the skin and subcutaneous tissues, the thoracic fascia and paraspinal musculature are dissected in a subperiosteal manner with a bovie cautery and a Cobb elevator. After the skin incision, 1:500,000 epinephrine may be used to provide hemostasis. Stripping of the muscles subperiosteally prevents muscle tearing and excessive bleeding. Self-retaining retractors are inserted, and tissue ischemia is avoided by intermittently decreasing the pressure. The facet joint capsules are stripped and the cartilage removed with the use of a high-speed burr and curettes. Care is taken to avoid injury to the facet joints that are not to be included in the fusion. Intraoperative x-ray or fluoroscopy is convenient at this point to confirm the levels to be operated on. To prepare the spine for fusion, the transverse processes and laminae are also decorticated with the use of a high-speed burr.

Instrumentation consists of sublaminar hooks, pedicle screws, and rods. Hooks are placed either facing in a caudal direction and anchored over the superior border of the lamina or facing in a cephalad direction and anchored under the inferior border of the lamina. To place each hook, the ligamentum flavum is removed from its attachment with a curette; once the spinal canal is visualized, a Kerrison rongeur is used to square off the anchoring point on the lamina. Hooks of different sizes and angulations are available and are determined by the orientation and dimensions of the lamina and spinal canal. The hooks will occupy a portion of the posterior spinal canal. The number of hooks and the pattern of placement are planned before surgery and depend on the corrective maneuvers that are deemed necessary. Once all hooks have been positioned, they are connected with rods, and compression or distraction forces are applied as appropriate. These forces may significantly modify the contours and dimensions of the spinal canal.

The bone graft is placed laterally, over the decorticated transverse process and along the lateral aspect of the lamina and decorticated pars interarticularis region as well as on the facet joints. Finally, the wound is closed in three layers.

Thoracoabdominal Approach for Corpectomy and Reconstruction

Injuries to the thoracolumbar spine frequently occur at the thoracolumbar junction (T10–L2). Corpectomies of these transitional segments or instrumentation for deformity correction requires thoracoabdominal exposure. This starts with a skin incision placed over the 10th rib (Fig. 14-7). If the approach involves higher levels, the rib chosen is at the level of the affected vertebral body or one level higher. For the upper thoracic spine (T1–T4), the arm is placed as far cephalad as possible so as to mobilize the scapula anteriorly and superiorly.

The musculature is divided in line with the rib and includes the latissimus dorsi and external oblique (Fig. 14-8). The rib is dissected subperiosteally and is cut from the costochondral junction anteriorly and as far posterior as possible. After removal of the rib, the abdominal muscles are transected with a bovie cautery, in line with the skin incision. The posterior aspect of the approach should not reach the midline. The costochondral cartilage is divided longitudinally, exposing the retroperitoneal space. The peritoneum is dissected bluntly from the abdominal wall and from the undersurface of the diaphragm and forced distally toward the side opposing the approach. The chest cavity is opened along the rib bed by longitudinal division of the parietal pleura. Wet laparotomy sponges are placed on the borders of the thoracotomy, and a rib spreader is placed to allow for better visualization. The lung is retracted with a sponge-covered malleable (Fig. 14-6). At this point, the spine is identified and the posterior parietal pleura are incised in line with the midline of the vertebral bodies. Dissection is started over the intervertebral disks because they are easy to identify. Next, the segmental vessels are identified in the midline of the vertebral bodies. These vessels are elevated with a dissector and ligated or clipped and successively cut. If these vessels are cut too near the aorta, there is a risk of bleeding from an orifice in the aorta. On the other hand, if they are cut too near the

foraminae, blood flow to the spinal cord may be compromised. The midthoracic spinal cord has the least abundant blood supply and the narrowest bony confines. The anterior spinal artery is smaller in diameter and in 85 percent of the cases depends mainly on a single accompanying radiculomedullary artery that arises somewhere from T9 through L2 (artery of Adamkiewicz). The segmental arteries contribute to the anterior medullary artery through the anterior radicular branch. Collateral circulation is usually present in close proximity to the foramen and includes anastomoses at the same foraminal level distal to the ligated segmental artery or by radicular arteries originating from adjacent segmental vessels. This critical zone of the spinal cord may predispose the patient to an ischemic insult to the cord after ligation of the segmental vessels, especially if cut too short from these anastomoses. Some surgeons favor temporary ligation and evaluation of the SSEPs. In our experience, ligation of the segmental vessels in the midportion of the vertebral body has proven to be a safe procedure. After ligation, the mediastinal structures are easily displaced and a malleable retractor is placed for protection during the procedure.

The diaphragm can be circumferentially transected approximately 2 cm from the chest wall insertion. If it is sectioned too peripherally, reconstruction may be very difficult; if too medially, hemostasis may be difficult and the phrenic innervation may be compromised. Different or alternate colored marking sutures are placed, which will enable appropriate reconstruction at the end of the procedure. If the dissection continues distally into the upper lumbar spine, the psoas muscle should be cautiously dissected off the anterior surface of the lumbar vertebral bodies, or the lumbar plexus may be injured.

For the upper thoracic spine, the skin incision surrounds the inferior and medial aspects of the scapular wing. The trapezius muscle is dissected along the skin incision, and latissimus dorsi muscles are dissected as far caudally as possible. When the rib cage is encountered, the dissection continues as described above.

When the exposure has been completed, the intervertebral disks are excised, starting with an incision in the annulus fibrosus. The nucleus pulposus is removed with curettes and pituitary rongeurs. If anterior release is necessary for mobilization of the spine, the annulus and the anterior longitudinal ligament must be circumferentially excised. Angled curettes and Kerrison rongeurs are used for this purpose. The surgeon's fingertips should be able to circumferentially palpate the disk, including the contralateral side of the exposure. A small portion of the posterior annulus and posterior longitudinal ligament are left intact. After the diskectomy has been completed, endplates are freed of all cartilage with ring curettes to prepare them for fusion.

If the purpose of diskectomy is that of spinal canal decompression, the rib head is removed by the use of

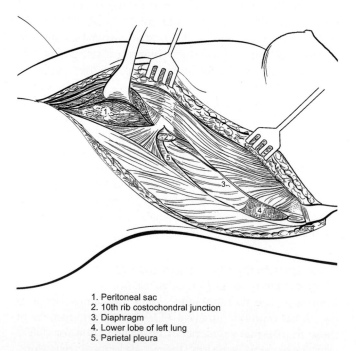

1. Peritoneal sac
2. 10th rib costochondral junction
3. Diaphragm
4. Lower lobe of left lung
5. Parietal pleura

Figure 14-8. Thoracoabdominal exposure. The 10th rib has been resected and the parietal pleura opened. The lung and diaphragm are visible and the retroperitoneal space is visible underneath the diaphragm.

osteotomes and a Kerrison rongeur, allowing access to and view of the spinal canal. Extruded disk material may be removed by this route. If the purpose of the surgery is a corpectomy to decompress the spinal canal from bone fragments, the ipsilateral pedicle may also be removed, with great caution to protect the emerging segmental nerve. The vertebral body, including the ipsilateral cortex, is excised with osteotomes, a high-speed burr, curettes, and pituitary rongeurs. The anterior and contralateral cortices are preserved for protection of the mediastinal structures. When the vertebral body has been cavitated, the retropulsed bone is removed in a posteroanterior direction, away from the thecal sac. The procedure is completed when the dura is free of all compressing elements.

Finally, for the reconstruction of the spine, an interbody strut graft is measured and placed between the adjacent endplates. A wide variety of materials may be used, including autograft, allograft fibula or humerus, titanium-mesh or carbon-fiber cages, according to the surgeon's preference. After reconstruction, a titanium plate is secured to the adjacent vertebral bodies with bicortical screws, which are placed under fluoroscopic guidance.

When the decompression and reconstruction of the spine have been completed, the diaphragm is reconstructed with a running, nonabsorbable suture. Incomplete reconstruction of the diaphragm may lead to the development of a hernia. The pleura may be closed with running suture. Many times, due to the presence of the implants, this is not possible. Revision procedures show evidence of complete epithelial coverage 2 weeks after a

pleural defect occurs. Some surgeons feel that insistence on sealing a pleural defect may actually carry the mediastinal structures closer to the metallic implants. The chest is thoroughly lavaged and the lungs are allowed to reexpand. Careful inspection for air leakage or injuries to the visceral pleura is carried out. One or two chest tubes are left in the chest cavity, and the chest is closed. First, the ribs are approximated with a nonabsorbable threaded interrupted suture. The intercostal muscles and the parietal pleura are then closed with a running suture and similarly the latissimus dorsi on a separate plane.

Costotransversectomy Approach

This is a posterior extrapleural approach that allows access to the lateral aspect of the vertebral bodies (Fig. 14-9). The positioning of the patient is similar to that for posterior spinal fusion. The incision may be in the midline or just lateral to the midline over the costotransverse junction. After dissection of the skin and subcutaneous tissues, the costotransverse joint is approached through the erector spinae muscles. The base of the rib and the transverse process are removed. Great care is taken to avoid disrupting the parietal pleura. If this were likely to occur, the patient would have to be warned that a chest tube might be required in the postoperative period. The spinal canal and the dura are approached by laminectomy and by removal of the ipsilateral pedicle. Great care is taken with the neurovascular bundle exiting caudal to the pedicle. The spinal cord is safely decompressed, with optimal visualization. Compressing elements on the midline, such as a central disk protrusion or OPLL, may not be accessible by this approach. This approach is not suitable for placement of a

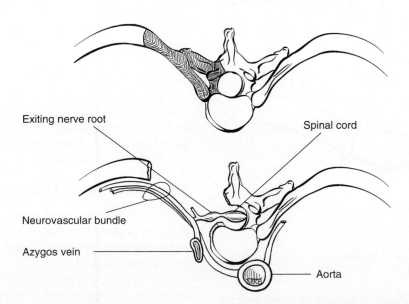

Figure 14-9. Costotransversectomy approach. After resection of the ipsilateral pedicle, the spinal cord may be decompressed through a posterior approach to the thoracic spine.

structural interbody graft. The anterolateral approach is preferred for these cases (Fig. 14-10).

Anesthetic Considerations

Spinal cord monitoring is preferred for most operations on the thoracic spine. Anesthetic recommendations are similar to those described for cervical spinal procedures.

Measures to prevent iatrogenic spinal cord injury are similar to those described for cervical spinal procedures. In particular, hypotensive anesthesia is to be avoided, especially when the anatomy of the spinal canal is significantly altered or when the thecal sac is manipulated. Similar considerations apply to anterior procedures when the segmental vessels are ligated.

Blood Loss and the Quality of the Surgical Field

Bleeding due to surgery to the spine is mainly from venous epidural sinuses. Arterial or capillary bleeding

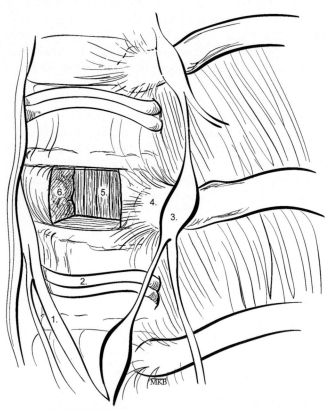

1. Splanchnic nerve
2. Segmental vessels
3. Sympathetic trunk
4. Rib head
5. Posterior longitudinal ligament
6. Intervertebral disk

Figure 14-10. View through a left-sided thoracotomy exposure. The intervertebral disk has been partially removed. The segmental vessels are on the midportion of the adjacent vertebral bodies.

plays no role or a very small role during spinal surgery. It is therefore important to keep the venous pressure as low as possible while still maintaining cardiac filling and cardiac output. It is of no value to decrease the arterial pressure. Furthermore, measures that decrease the cardiac output, and therefore increase the central venous pressure, should be avoided. This includes the popular yet senseless practice of reducing the arterial blood pressure with beta-blocking agents. This will only serve to increase the bleeding from venous sinuses and worsen the surgical field.

Apart from keeping the blood volume optimal and adequately positioning the patient, keeping pressure off the abdomen, venous dilators like trinitroglycerin will further help to decrease bleeding. If the central venous pressure is abnormally high, it may even be necessary to administer small doses of furosemide. A central venous pressure lower than that of the surgical field will cause air to be sucked into the venous system, with resulting air embolism. Although this is rare, it may be the cause of an otherwise inexplicable state of hemodynamic instability. It is therefore essential to monitor the central venous pressure and keep it approximately at the same level as the main surgical activity.

Analgesia

When anterior exposure to the thoracic spine is used, intercostal block with 0.25% bupivacaine at the time of closure is recommended. Epidural block above and below the level of surgery provides excellent analgesia, and so does thoracic paravertebral block. These two procedures provide short-term analgesia and help with pulmonary rehabilitation and ventilation. Recovery of ventilatory mechanics is fundamental for functional recovery and in avoiding pulmonary complications. Pain management must be optimized, and we insist on the frequent use of an incentive spirometer.

Patients who do not receive epidural or paravertebral block usually require intravenous morphine or hydromorphone patient-controlled analgesia (PCA) for the first 24 to 36 h. Thereafter they are managed with oral opioids such as oxycodone.

Associated Medication

Patients with spinal cord injury may be receiving high doses of steroids. Steroids may also be given when monitoring indicates possible damage to the spinal cord during the operation.

Treatment with prophylactic antibiotics is started 1 h before the operation and repeated every 6 h during the procedure. Thereafter, antibiotics are continued until all indwelling catheters have been removed, including chest tubes and the urinary catheter.

Physical Therapy Goals and Requirements in the Postoperative Period

Patients undergoing surgery for deformity usually have very stable constructs and require very little if any external immobilization. Out-of-bed activities are encouraged, with assistance, on the first day after surgery. These patients can walk or sit on a recliner as tolerated. Age obviously has an enormous influence on the speed of recovery. If there has been any anterior surgery, respiratory therapy is started immediately. This includes use of an incentive spirometer. Upright posture is encouraged because of its benefits for pulmonary toilette. Chest tubes are removed on the second to third days after surgery, and patients with either anterior and/or posterior fusions are discharged within 5 to 7 days. Physical therapy goals include independent walking (may be aided by a walker), transfers, personal hygiene, and some stair steps. If these goals are not met within the first week, patients are transferred to a rehabilitation facility for 2 to 4 weeks, especially elderly patients.

The reconstruction of the spine should be stable enough to allow all necessary rehabilitation procedures, including pulmonary rehabilitation, and the acquisition of transfer skills and self-care.

Special Intra- and Postoperative Surgical Requirements

Lung retraction is probably one of the most important considerations during anterior surgery to the thoracic spine. In open thoracotomy, handheld malleable retractors may collapse the lung sufficiently. Nevertheless, we are increasingly performing anterior operations on the thoracic spine through video-assisted thoracoscopic spinal surgery (VATSS). The exposure is minimal, requiring three or four 15- to 20-mm portals to perform a corpectomy. The success of this procedure depends largely on adequate lung deflation. This is obtained either by use of a double-lumen endotracheal tube or a bronchial blocker. The double-lumen tube tends to be obstructed by mucous plugs due to its smaller diameter. The patient may develop inadequate gas exchange during the procedure, requiring reexpansion of the lung and fiberoptic inspection and lavage of the lumens of the tube. The bronchial blocker also provides adequate lung collapse, but it may require repositioning during the procedure.

Common Problems (Pre-, Intra- and Postoperative)

Vascular Injuries

The proximity of the greater vessels obviously makes a vascular injury possible. In the thoracic spine, most intraoperative problems may be caused by inappropriate handling and ligation of the segmental vessels. Careful dissection and respect for anatomic landmarks is the best way to prevent damage to these vessels.

Spinal Cord Injury

Although it is very uncommon, spinal cord injury is among the most devastating complications of spinal surgery. In a large single-center case series, including adult and pediatric deformity cases, a 0.37 percent incidence of major neurologic complications was reported. All these patients underwent combined anterior and posterior exposure, they all had ligation of segmental vessels, and they were all subject to intraoperative controlled hypotension.

Although most surgeons now prefer to use spinal cord monitoring, some surgeons have described false-negative results. The mechanisms of injury are multifactorial and include those related to the anatomic configuration of the spinal canal, the placement of spinal instrumentation, and adequate perfusion of the spinal cord. The first of these mechanisms is most commonly associated with the correction of deformity and realignment of the spinal canal, while the second may have to do with the space occupied by instrumentation, including laminar hooks or misplaced pedicle screws.

Spinal cord injury may also occur in the immediate postoperative period because of the development of an expanding epidural hematoma. This problem must be addressed immediately and includes surgical evacuation of the hematoma and management of coagulopathies. Patients who have received multiple transfusions and suffer from dilutional decrease in coagulation factors may benefit from transfusion of fresh frozen plasma and platelets. In spite of all immediate efforts, damage may be permanent.

Dural Laceration

This complication may occur as a result of trauma or secondary to aggressive decompression of the thecal sac. In particular, patients with OPLL may have an ossified dura, which may leave a dural defect at the time of removal. In the chest, this creates a particular problem due to the negative intrathoracic pressure. A dural-pleural fistula creates a strong gradient for the leakage of spinal fluid. This gradient may force the spinal cord into the defect and may even produce a herniation of the cord. The patient will then develop further signs and symptoms of myelopathy. The consequences of spinal fluid leakage are discussed in the section on the lumbar spine, below.

Pulmonary Complications

Atelectasis is very common, but aggressive respiratory therapy in the early postoperative period is effective in preventing it. If this is not aggressively done, atelectasis may lead to pneumonia. Other complications include hemothorax, pneumothorax, and chylothorax.

Diaphragmatic rupture and the formation of a hernia are extremely rare complications and may be avoided by proper reconstruction of the divided diaphragm.

▶ THE LUMBAR SPINE

Indications and Special Anatomic Considerations

In contrast to the rigid thoracic spine, the lumbar spine makes motion of the trunk possible while also providing structural support to approximately 60 percent of the body weight as well as protection to the neural structures. The conus medullaris lies somewhere between the T12–L1 and the L1–L2 disk spaces. The cauda equina floats within the spinal fluid contained by a thecal sac.

The vast majority of degenerative conditions—including disk herniation, spondylosis, and osteoarthritis—occur in the last two or three disk spaces.

Patient Profile

An increasing number of elderly people seek surgical care for symptoms of spinal stenosis. This is explained by increase in life expectancy and increased functional demands. Advanced age is accompanied not only by comorbid conditions but also by a decreased physiologic reserve. Attention to detail is important for patient safety and early recovery. Fluid volume management, oxygen transport, perfusion, and metabolic control constitute the most important elements. Continuous evaluation of hemoglobin, gas exchange, and lactic acid are recommended during prolonged surgery.

Common Comorbidities

Multiple comorbidities are frequently seen in elderly patients who undergo lumbar decompression with or without fusion. Diabetes, high blood pressure, coronary artery disease, and chronic obstructive pulmonary disease (COPD) are common in this age group.

Positioning on the Operating Table

Posterior Approach to the Lumbar Spine
The posterior approach requires prone positioning. Patients who do not need fusion, such as microdiscectomy or laminectomy for decompression of a stenotic spine, may be positioned in the semigenupectoral ("90/90," or knee-chest) position with the use of an Andrews frame or with the double bend of a Maquet table. The patient's back should be parallel to the floor; knees and hips are flexed slightly past 90 degrees. Many surgeons prefer the prone position on a flat table with a Wilson frame. Care must be taken to avoid compression of the abdomen. Decompression of the abdomen and inferior vena cava helps to reduce epidural blood flow, allowing better visualization (see "Blood Loss and the Quality of the Surgical Field," above). Additionally, if the spine remains in lordosis, the interlaminar space is closed down and an unnecessary amount of laminectomy will be required to expose the disk.

For lumbar fusion procedures, the most important function of positioning is to preserve the sagittal contours of the lumbosacral spine. A radiolucent fourposter frame or similar device is recommended, and padding should be added to maintain the hips fully extended. This position preserves normal lordosis, thus avoiding flat-back deformity. The superior posters should be positioned under the patient's rib cage and the inferior ones under the anterior iliac spine.

The arms are positioned with 90 degrees of flexion at the elbows and less than 90 degrees of abduction at the shoulders. The arms rest on well-padded arm boards and care is taken to avoid pressure on the ulnar grooves and wrists. Care is also taken at the superior posts, which must not exert pressure on the axillae. In women, pressure on the breasts must be minimized. In heavier patients, we prefer a five- or six-post configuration instead of four to allow better distribution of the weight. The male genitals should also be free of pressure. (See "Prone positioning checklist" on page 164.)

Anterolateral Retroperitoneal Exposure of the Lumbar Spine
These approaches require lateral positioning. The positioning is similar to that required for the anterior exposure of the thoracic spine and is adequate for anterolateral retroperitoneal exposure of the lumbar spine as well as for transpleural retroperitoneal (thoracoabdominal) exposure of the thoracolumbar junction. The patient is placed in a lateral decubitus position with the side to be operated on facing up. Since left-sided exposures are more frequent, the following description considers the patient to be lying on his or her right side.

The patient is transferred from the preanesthesia cart to the operating table in a supine position and then turned 90 degrees. An axillary roll is placed to prevent circulatory obstruction to the right arm. Our preference is for silicone padding. Foam padding is also placed underneath the right leg from the hip down to the foot. Pressure on the peroneal nerve on the right side must be avoided. The head is supported with pillows or foam, taking care to maintain the alignment of the neck. The chest cage is supported on the sternum and the back by pads and adhesive tape or by a beanbag. The pelvis is supported by adhesive tape over the greater trochanter, which is always protected by foam padding. In procedures involving decompression of the spinal canal or instrumentation of the spine, stable positioning is essential for surgical orientation and intraoperative imaging. Finally, the right arm is supported by a foam-padded arm board with the shoulder at 90 degree extension and the left is extended on top of this, separated by pillows or other soft padding. Some surgeons prefer to break the table at the patient's waist in order to increase the space between the inferior rib border and the ilium. This is particularly beneficial for the lower lumbar spine.

Anterior Trans- or Retroperitoneal Exposure of the Lumbar Spine

The exposure to the two or three lower lumbar segments requires supine positioning with hyperextension of the lumbosacral junction. This is obtained by placing foam padding underneath the lumbar region. The table is then tilted into the Trendelenburg position. This helps to displace the abdominal contents cephalad, facilitating the exposure. Owing to the necessary mobilization of the iliac vessels, some authors recommend pulse oximeters in both the upper and lower extremities.

Authors' Surgical Technique

Lumbar Microdiskectomy

The level of the disk to be removed is confirmed with fluoroscopy. A 1-in. midline skin incision is then made (Fig. 14-11). After dissection of the skin and subcutaneous tissues, the dorsal lumbar fascia and paraspinal musculature are dissected in a subperiosteal manner from the tip of the spinous process all the way lateral to the corresponding facet joint. A Taylor retractor is placed lateral to this joint, and the ligamentum flavum is released with a small

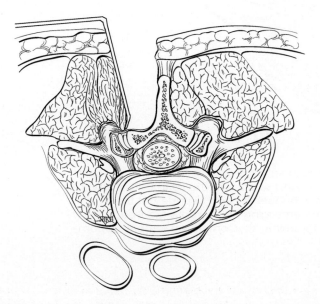

Figure 14-11. Midline posterior approach to the lumbar spine. The paravertebral muscles have been dissected subperiosteally.

angled curette from the inferior and superior borders of the adjacent laminae as well as from the medial edge of the superior facet. A Kerrison rongeur is used to remove several millimeters of the cephalad lamina and 2 to 3 mm of the medial border of the inferior facet. The ligamentum flavum is then removed in a piecemeal manner. The medial border of the superior facet is visualized and removed with a Kerrison rongeur. A nerve root retractor is used to displace the dural sac and the emerging nerve root toward the midline of the spinal canal. Epidural veins are usually encountered, and these are coagulated with a bipolar cautery. This allows optimal visualization of the disk and the herniation. The extruded disk fragments are now removed with a pituitary rongeur. If the extrusion is subligamentous, the posterior longitudinal ligament is incised with a knife in a horizontal manner. Following this, the spinal canal is thoroughly explored with a 4-mm Murphy ball-tipped probe to determine whether there are any residual disk fragments or any other compressing elements on the dural sac or emerging nerve root.

This procedure may be carried out under microscopic or loupe magnification. There are certainly advantages to the use of a microscope, but their consideration is beyond the scope of this chapter.

When the procedure is complete, 40 mg of Depo-Medrol is deposited on the interlaminar space and the wound is closed in three layers. After closure, the skin is injected with 0.25% bupivacaine.

Lumbar Decompression

Laminectomy has become the standard procedure for surgical decompression in lumbar spinal stenosis. A midline skin incision is made. After dissection of the subcutaneous tissues, the dorsal lumbar fascia and paraspinal musculature are dissected in a subperiosteal manner, from the tip of the spinous processes all the way lateral to the corresponding facet joints (or transverse processes if fusion is going to be done). After thorough hemostasis, the inferior half of the superior spinous process as well as the superior half of the inferior spinous process and all intermediate spinous processes are removed with a rongeur. The laminae are thinned down with a Leksell rongeur or a high-speed burr. A Kerrison rongeur is then used to remove the remainder of the laminae and ligamentum flavum in a caudad-to-cephalad direction (Fig. 14-12*A*). The dural sac is now centrally decompressed and can be manipulated to allow access to the lateral recesses or subarticular areas of the spinal canal. A partial medial facetectomy is performed by undercutting with a 45-degree Kerrison rongeur all the way lateral to the medial wall of the pedicles (Fig. 14-12*B*). The nerve roots are identified and followed into the corresponding foramina with an overlying Kerrison rongeur removing all overlying spurs (Fig. 14-12*C*). A 4-mm Murphy ball-tip probe is used

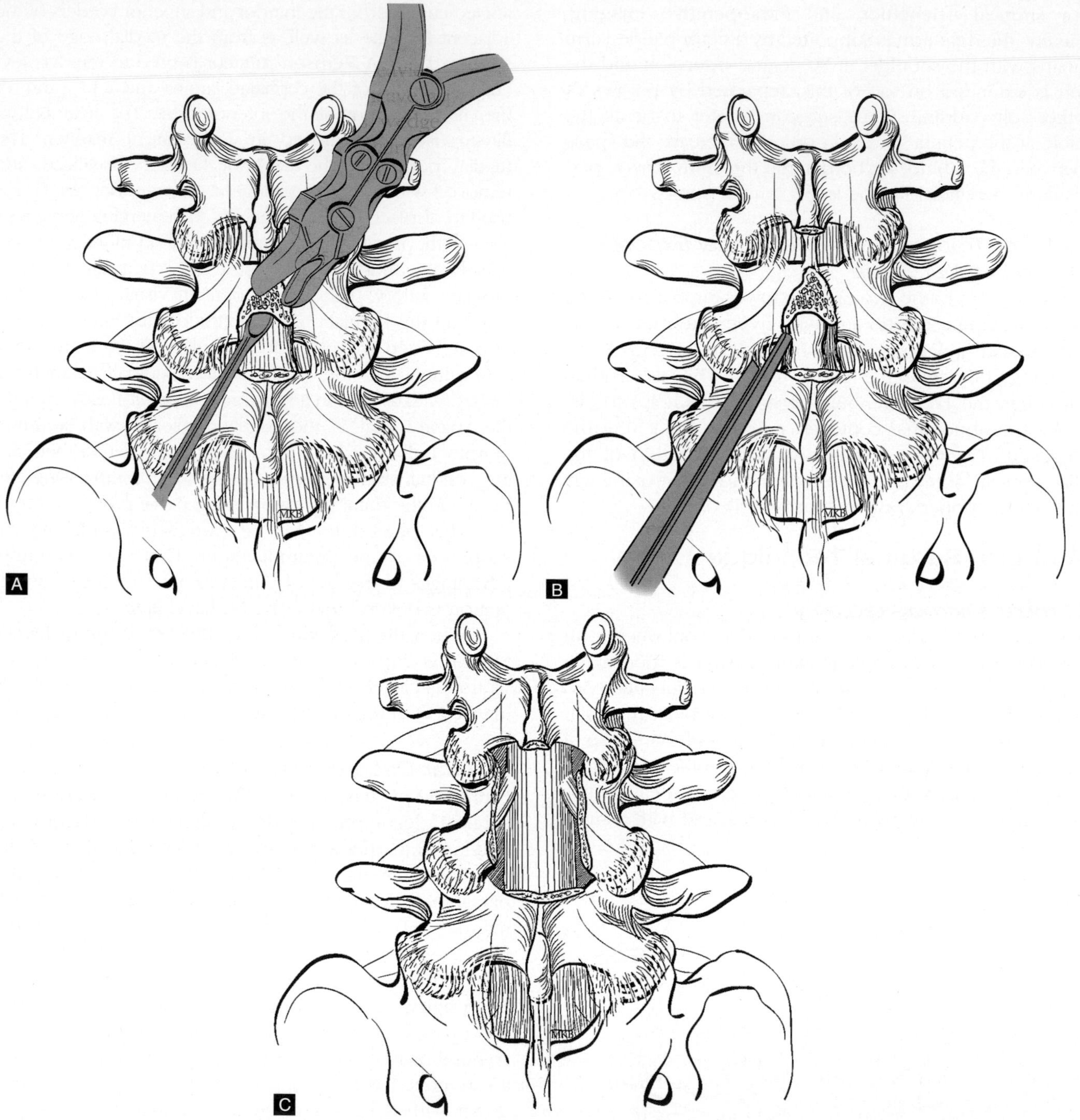

Figure 14-12. Lumbar decompression. After posterior exposure of the spine, the spinous process is cut and a curette or small Cobb is used to dissect the ligamentum flavum from the undersurface of the lamina. *A.* A Kerrison ronguer is used to undercut the hypertrophic facet joints and ligamentum flavum. *B.* The emerging nerve roots are freed of any compressing elements all the way toward the foramina. *C.* Completed lumbar decompression.

to determine whether decompression is adequate. Closure is similar to that for microdiskectomy.

Anterior Lumbar Interbody Fusion

This procedure is indicated mainly for the caudal lumbar disks, namely L5–S1, L4–L5, and/or L3–L4. The approach to this area of the lumbar spine must allow the surgeon to see the disks facing the midline, and it requires either a retro- or transperitoneal exposure. The first choice should be retroperitoneal exposure, especially in male patients. Our second choice is the transperitoneal exposure, but we prefer it for obese patients, revision exposures, and for patients in whom the abdominal retroperitoneum or pelvis have been exposed previously.

An infraumbilical vertical incision is extended proximally to the pubis. The rectus fascia is opened longitudinally with the incision; the rectus abdominis muscle is then retracted laterally, exposing the posterior rectus fascia. This is done to avoid damage to the segmental (T6–T12) innervation of the rectus. The arcuate line is identified. The preperitoneal space is encountered, and the peritoneum is dissected away from the posterior rectus sheath before incising the sheath. Great care is taken to avoid injury to the inferior epigastric vessels. The exposure continues by dissection of the retroperitoneal space. The peritoneum is mobilized from medial to lateral by gentle digital dissection. Once the psoas muscles are reached, the peritoneal sac is protected with wet laparotomy sponges and retractors are placed. Care must be taken with the ureter on the side of the dissection.

In the transperitoneal approach, the peritoneum is incised in line with the rectus sheath. The bowels are packed cephalad to expose the posterior peritoneum, which is also incised in a longitudinal manner, exposing the great vessels and the lumbar spine.

The next part of the dissection consists of mobilizing the greater vessels to allow for the orthopaedic procedure (Fig. 14-13). The aorta and vena cava usually bifurcate at the height of the L4–L5 intervertebral disk, but higher or lower bifurcations are not infrequent. We recommend a thorough preoperative assessment of the vascular anatomy with MR angiography (MRA) as well as planning the direction in which the greater vessels are to be mobilized. The parasympathetic plexus (hypogastric) is distributed as a diffuse plexus that courses around the aorta and head distal from the bifurcation in the presacral area. Great care is taken in protecting this plexus, so as to avoid the complication of retrograde ejaculation. The middle sacral artery and/or lower segmental vessels and ascending lumbar vein are ligated at the level and side of mobilization. The psoas muscles mark the lateral limits of the dissection. The ureters may occasionally be visible and must be retracted with the peritoneum.

The lower lumbar disks should be directly visible at this point. Retractor blades are then placed on a table-

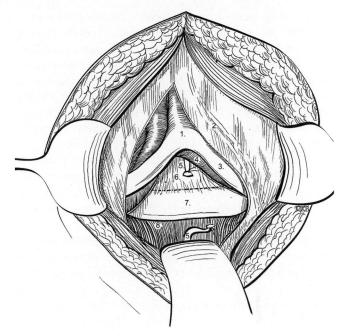

1. Aorta
2. Iliolumbar vessels
3. Left common iliac artery
4. Left common iliac vein
5. Middle sacral artery
6. L5 vertebral body
7. L5–S1 intervertebral disk
8. S1 vertebral body (sacrum)

Figure 14-13. Anterior retroperitoneal exposure of the L5–S1 intervertebral disk. This disk conforms to the apex of the promontorium and is distal to the bifurcation of the greater vessels. The middle sacral artery and vein and hypogastric plexus are in the midline.

mounted retractor system, including vascular retractors. Some systems anchor with pins into the vertebral bodies. The orthopaedic procedure consists of removal of the anterior annulus and anterior longitudinal ligament, complete removal of the nucleus pulposus, and preparation of the endplates with curettes and osteotomes. Fusion is achieved by implanting a femoral ring allograft or cage with bone graft. This approach is also optimal for total disk replacement or disk arthroplasty.

Instrumented Posterior Lumbar Fusion

After a standard midline dissection of the skin and subcutaneous tissues, the lumbar fascia is dissected in a subperiosteal manner with a bovie cautery and a Cobb elevator. After the skin incision, 1:500,000 epinephrine may be used for hemostasis. This dissection is advanced from the tip of the spinous process all the way lateral to the tip of the transverse processes. Stripping the muscles subperiosteally prevents tearing of the muscles and excessive bleeding. The superior and inferior segments are sequentially stripped, depending on the levels to be fused. Self-retaining retractors are then placed, but prolonged pressure on the paravertebral musculature is avoided by freeing the pressure intermittently to prevent necrosis. The intervening facet joint capsules are stripped and the cartilage is removed with a high-speed burr and curettes. Great care is taken to avoid damage to the facet joints that will not be fused. Some bleeding may occur, especially during the dissection of the pars interarticularis, where the superior articular artery may be damaged. Bipolar cautery is recommended to avoid injury to the exiting nerve root.

To prepare the spine for fusion, the facet joints are stripped of their capsules and articular cartilage and the transverse processes and laminae are decorticated with the use of a high-speed burr. The ala of the sacrum is also decorticated if needed (Fig. 14-14).

Instrumentation consists of pedicle screws and rods. Landmarks for placing pedicle screws in the lumbar spine include the midline of the transverse process and the lateral cortex of the pars interarticularis. A Leksell rongeur or a high-speed burr is used to decorticate the entry position. A pedicle opener or "gearshift" is then used to perforate the pedicle, and a ball-tipped pedicle probe is used to palpate the inner walls of the trajectory of the screw hole. An appropriately sized tap is next used, and finally the screw is inserted. The structures at risk during the insertion of pedicle screws include the dural sac medially, the exiting nerve root medial and caudal to the pedicle, and the greater vessels anteriorly.

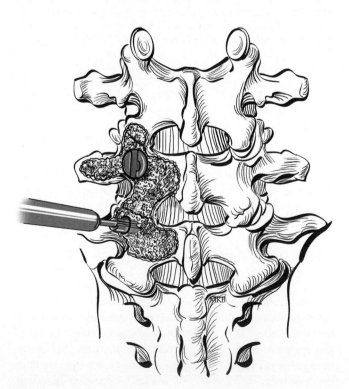

Figure 14-14. Preparation for pedicle screws. The transverse process, lamina, and facets have been decorticated.

These vessels lie anterior to the vertebral bodies above L3 or L4 and caudal to L4; the bifurcating common iliac arteries and veins take a more lateral position, directly anterior to the pedicles. For the placement of sacral (S1) pedicle screws, bicortical purchase is strongly recommended. The internal and external iliac artery and vein lie laterally along the sacral ala, and any penetration of the anterior cortex must be done with extreme caution. In the anterior midline of the sacrum, the middle sacral artery may also be injured.

The bone graft is placed laterally, over the decorticated transverse process and along the lateral aspect of the lamina and decorticated pars interarticularis region as well as the facet joint.

In longer surgical incisions, we use a medium-sized drain between the fascia and the skin. The wound is closed in three layers.

TRANSFORAMINAL LUMBAR INTERBODY FUSION (TLIF)

As an additional step in posterior lumbar fusion, an interbody device or cage may also be placed. The major reasons for doing this are to restore sagittal contours, strengthen the load-bearing characteristics of the construct, and increase the chances of obtaining a successful fusion. The inferior articular process is removed with an osteotome and the superior articular process is then removed in a piecemeal manner with a Kerrison rongeur. This allows access to the intervertebral disk. The dural sac lies medially, underneath the ligamentum flavum, and the exiting nerve root is on the superolateral aspect of the foraminotomy. Both the thecal sac and emerging nerve root are protected with retractors. Annulotomy is performed with a knife blade, and the disk is completely removed with disk shavers, pituitary rongeurs, and sharp curettes. The cartilage endplates are removed as well to prepare the adjacent vertebrae for interbody fusion. The anterior interbody space (posterior to the anterior annulus) is packed with bone graft; an interbody device is placed between both endplates and filled with bone graft as well. Fluoroscopy is used to assess correct placement of the cage.

Posterior Iliac Crest Bone Graft

Morcellized corticocancellous autograft may be obtained by the same skin incision used for a lumbopelvic fixation or by a separate incision. If the spinal fusion extends into the sacrum, the subcutaneous tissue layer is undermined and the posterior iliac crest approached through a separate fascial incision that stretches approximately 4 cm from the posterior superior iliac spine (PSIS), in an anterior direction. The gluteal musculature is dissected in a subperiosteal manner and a Taylor retractor is placed in the depth of the wound under direct vision. Great care is taken not to use any sharp instruments in the sciatic notch. The Taylor retractor or a sharp Cobb may not only injure the sciatic nerve but also lacerate the superior gluteal artery, in which case bleeding will be very difficult to control. Alternatively, a vertical incision may be made 4 cm lateral to the PSIS. After dissection of the skin and subcutaneous tissues, the procedure is as described above.

The graft is obtained by removing the lateral cortex of the ilium with the use of osteotomes. The cancellous bone is then obtained by exposing the cortex of the ilium with gouges and curettes. Care is taken to avoid penetrating the inner cortex of the ilium and potentially damaging the sacroiliac joint or ilioinguinal nerve (Fig. 14-15). When sufficient bone graft has been removed, surface bleeding of the bone is controlled by bone wax and Gelfoam. The aponeurosis is then closed with a running suture. Wound drains are usually not necessary.

Anesthetic Considerations

Microdiskectomy is usually performed under general anesthesia, but it may also be performed under epidural or local anesthesia. Advantages of epidural anesthesia include shorter recovery room time, faster return of alertness, absence of postoperative nausea and vomiting, and superior postoperative pain management. Additionally, there can be

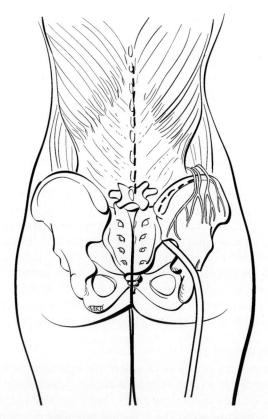

Figure 14-15. Incisions for posterior lumbar exposure and posterior iliac crest bone harvesting. Note the relationship with the clunial nerves and the sciatic notch.

less intraoperative bleeding due to decreased venous pressure (see "Blood Loss and the Quality of the Surgical Field," above). Disadvantages of epidural anesthesia include hypotension, difficulty in obtaining an airway in case of an adverse intraoperative emergency and the fact that the patient may move the upper body during the procedure. The patient may also be uncomfortable during the surgery. Furthermore, the volume of the anesthetic may further compromise severely diminished canal dimensions due to a large disk extrusion. Epidural anesthetics may also increase urinary retention, requiring an overnight hospital stay. Laminectomy for decompression and posterior spinal fusion requires general anesthesia, mostly due to the length of the procedure. For these procedures, as in thoracic spinal fusion, control of the surgical field and reduction of intraoperative bleeding are important anesthetic considerations (see the discussion of thoracic spinal fusion, above).

Analgesia

After microdiskectomy, patients may be discharged on the same day or after a 23-h hospitalization regimen. They are mobilized within a few hours and may require only mild enteral analgesics, since this surgery is generally not painful. More extensive procedures, including laminectomy or lumbar fusion, require longer hospital stays and more intensive pain control. It is recommended that the patient become mobile on the day after surgery. Intrathecal morphine (0.004 mg/kg, or 0.3 mg for the average patient, injected by the surgeon before closing the wound) or epidural analgesia (the catheter placed by the surgeon prior to closure of the wound) have been shown to be very effective analgesic measures.

Associated Medication

Most elderly patients with degenerative conditions of the lumbar spine also have one or more comorbid conditions that require specific management.

Prophylactic antibiotics are used for all spinal procedures. Because the intervertebral disk is poorly vascularized, it is more vulnerable to a disk-space infection (diskitis). In general, this occurs with an incidence of 1 percent for lumbar diskectomy; but this figure doubles in diabetic patients. For all implant procedures, antibiotics are continued until all indwelling catheters have been removed. (See Chap. 3 for antimicrobial prophylaxis and Chap. 4 for thromboprophylaxis.)

Physical Therapy Goals and Requirements in the Postoperative Period

Patients who underwent microdiskectomy are encouraged to resume their activities in a short time. Ambulation and physical therapy are initiated on the same afternoon after surgery. A corset is used, mostly for comfort, after discharge from the hospital. Patients are encouraged to increase their activities progressively but to avoid bending, stooping, or lifting heavy objects during the first 2 weeks. Return to work is within 2 weeks for occupations that are not physically challenging; otherwise, patients may return to work in 4 to 6 weeks after an intensive course of physical therapy. Similar guidelines are observed for laminectomy. Nevertheless, this operation is indicated mostly for elderly patients; the surgery is longer, and the resulting physiologic impact greater. Hospital stays are therefore longer, but this must be decided individually.

In the case of fusions, patients begin with out-of-bed activities on the first day after surgery. Especially in the elderly, transfer to a recliner may be sufficient. Ambulation is increased slowly throughout the following days. Hospital goals for discharge include independent transfers, independent gait (may include the use of a walker), and stair climbing. Occupational therapy consultation is provided to help patients resume daily activities. If these goals are not achieved within the first 5 to 7 days, we recommend transfer to a rehabilitation facility for 2 to 4 weeks until these goals are met. Otherwise, patients are discharged with recommendations for a progressive walking program, with strict instructions against bending, stooping, or lifting. Especially in the case of instrumented fusions in the osteoporotic spine, a rigid brace is recommended for all out-of-bed activities.

Special Intra- and Postoperative Surgical Requirements

Neuromuscular blockade is helpful for surgery to the lower lumbar spine, especially in obese or very muscular patients; it may be very difficult to obtain adequate access to this area. Completely paralyzed paravertebral musculature is easier to retract laterally and allows for better visualization. Nevertheless, thereafter, complete recovery of neuromuscular function in order to monitor electromyographic (EMG) activity should be achieved for spontaneous as well as for stimulus-evoked modalities. This is discussed further in the next section.

Common Problems (Pre-, Intra- and Postoperative)

Complications of Iliac Bone Graft Harvesting

Donor-site problems have a reported incidence of 8 to 39 percent and range from minor wound problems to severe, persistent donor-site pain, neurovascular injury, and even loss of pelvic stability. The most common problem is that of pain, which can be severe within the first 6 months but tends to diminish thereafter. Other complications that may have direct intraoperative implications include herniation through the ilium, lateral femoral cutaneous nerve injury

(meralgia paresthetica), and injury to the superior cluneal nerves or ilioinguinal nerve.

The superior gluteal artery may be injured by dissection with a sharp instrument or by retraction over the sciatic notch. Bleeding is extremely difficult to control, and owing to its anatomic location, repair or ligation is not only difficult but may cause other complications, including sciatic nerve injury and injury to the ureter or iliac vessels. In our opinion, the best way to deal with this problem includes tamponade by direct pressure and endovascular repair or selective embolization.

The stability of the sacroiliac joint may be damaged by removing excessive amounts of the inner cortex of the posterior ilium as well as by damage to the sacroiliac ligaments. Pelvic instability and pain are the long-term consequences of such damage. In patients with persistent sacroiliac joint pain after graft harvesting, there is a high prevalence of inner cortical disruption of the ilium.

Problems with Pedicle Screw Placement

As previously mentioned, soft tissue structures may be harmed by misplaced pedicle screws. A review of the literature reveals that in cadaver studies, experienced surgeons breech the cortex of the pedicle 5.5 to 31.3 percent of the time; in clinical studies, between 28.1 and 39.9 percent of pedicle screws are misplaced. Nevertheless, only 1.6 to 5 percent of clinical series present with irritation or injury to the adjacent nerve roots. Current methods to avoid this problem include pedicle probing, visualization of axial landmarks by fluoroscopy, image-guided navigation systems, neuromonitoring with stimulus-evoked EMGs, and sensory evoked potentials. The latter have had limited success because they are not sensitive enough to detect individual nerve root dysfunction. Evoked EMG has become an increasingly popular technique to confirm correct pedicle screw placement in the lumbar and sacral spine. The intact pedicle cortex insulates the adjacent nerve root from the stimulating current, and relatively high levels of energy are required to stimulate it, while the stimulation threshold is lower after a cortical breach in the pedicle. Electrodes are placed in muscle groups whose nerve roots are at risk from misplaced screws. Because EMG monitoring is strongly influenced by paralysis from pharmacologic agents and chronic nerve compression, neuromuscular blockade is reversed after exposure is completed.

Vascular Injury

A serious complication of anterior spinal surgery is laceration of the greater vessels, with significant blood loss. These injuries occur very rarely, but they do have disastrous consequences. The reported mortality of operative injury to a major vessel has ranged up to 50 percent. If the patient survives, blood supply to the spinal cord may also be affected. Although the incidence of these injuries is extremely low, it could be underestimated, because the clinical manifestations may be extremely variable. Sometimes the effects are readily apparent early on, but they may also manifest in the long term, as is the case of arteriovenous fistulas or pseudoaneurysm in the retroperitoneal space.

During anterior exposure of the lower lumbar spine, direct pressure on the iliac artery may promote arterial occlusion, especially in patients with risk factors for thrombosis (obesity, smoking, hypotensive anesthesia, prolonged retraction time, and history of thrombosis). Great care is taken with patients who have demonstrated atheromatous plaques.

Deep Venous Thrombosis and Pulmonary Embolism

The incidence of deep venous thrombosis as revealed by ultrasound has been reported in 0.6 to 2 percent and by venographic studies in 10.8 to 17.7 percent of patients subjected to spinal surgery (see Chap. 4). The occurrence is higher for lumbar spinal surgery (26.5 percent) than for cervical spinal surgery (5.6 percent), and the prevalence of proximal deep venous thrombosis is 0.9 percent. Fatal pulmonary embolisms have been described in many case reports, but the exact incidence is not yet clear. Risks factors include lengthy procedures, prone positioning, prolonged recumbence after surgery, and motor paralysis of the lower extremities, as is the case for patients with spinal cord injuries. One particular reason that may explain a higher incidence in lumbar surgery may be the use of Hall-Reston type frames with direct pressure on the inguinal region, thus increasing venous stasis in the lower legs. The same holds true for prolonged retraction of the iliac vessels during anterior exposure to the lower lumbar spine.

Several methods to prevent these complications have been attempted; nevertheless, there is no clear consensus on the optimal regimen. Both pharmacologic and mechanical methods have been shown to reduce this risk. Pharmacologic prophylaxis is not a well-accepted method for reducing this risk, because it may increase the risk of formation of an epidural hematoma with potentially catastrophic neurologic damage. For this reason, most surgeons prefer mechanical prophylaxis. Venographic studies show that most of the thrombi are in the calves, and they may occur proximally only occasionally. The effects of mechanical methods to prevent thrombosis have not been clearly demonstrated in spinal surgery (see Chap. 4).

Dural Lacerations

In spite of meticulous surgical technique, dural lacerations sometimes cannot be prevented during lumbar spinal surgery, particularly in cases of spinal stenosis and previous laminectomies. The reported incidence is 4.6

percent in patients subjected to laminectomy for lumbar stenosis, 9.8 percent if the surgery is revision, and 1.8 percent in disk surgery. Some authors have reported even higher numbers for patients with lumbar stenosis, possibly as a consequence of an atrophic dura. It is noteworthy that accidental durotomy constitutes the second most frequent cause for malpractice claims in lumbar spinal surgery.

The manifestations of intracranial hypotension may be quite dramatic, with cranial nerve dysfunction, tonsillar herniation, cerebellar hemorrhage, brainstem compression, and respiratory arrest. More commonly, patients present with orthostatically induced headaches, vertigo, or a subarachnoid-cutaneous fistula. This may potentially cause and signal meningitis. Repair is warranted. The etiology of cerebellar hemorrhage has been ascribed to reduced intracranial CSF pressure, which increases the difference between intravascular pressure and CSF pressure. Alternatively, extensive CSF loss causes downward displacement of the cerebellum and stretching of the superior vermian veins. Other nontraumatic risk factors include hypertension, coagulation disorders including anticoagulant therapy, and vascular malformations.

When dural laceration is diagnosed, it must be repaired. The exposed nerve roots are protected with a cottonoid, the laminectomy is made adequate, and the dura is sutured with running monofilament, nonabsorbable 5–0 suture. Care is taken to avoid catching the nerve roots into the suture. The repair is then tested for leakage by applying a Valsalva maneuver. Fibrin glue is used to cover the repair at the end of the procedure. The patient is left in flat bed rest for the subsequent days, which lowers the intrathecal pressure and thus promotes healing of the dura.

If CSF drainage continues after surgery, Trendelenburg positioning or a blood patch may be attempted. The placement of an intrathecal lumbar drain may also facilitate healing. Prophylactic antibiotics are used, and the height of the drain receptacle is adjusted to obtain 50 to 100 mL of CSF per 8-h shift over 4 days. Alternatively, the patient may be returned to the operating room for repair.

▶ APPENDIX

Common Surgical Procedures

Fusion: Surgical arthrodesis allowing permanent immobilization of a joint by inducing bone growth across the joint space. For example, in the subaxial cervical spine, two adjacent vertebral bodies have five joints, allowing for motion between them. This includes the intervertebral disk, the facet joints (one on each side) and the uncovertebral processes. In an anterior procedure, an interbody structural load-bearing bone graft is placed between the vertebral endplates to allow bone growth between the vertebral bodies. In a posterior procedure, the facet joint surfaces are partially destroyed, and the lateral masses are bridged together by morcellized cancellous bone graft.

Anterior cervical decompression and fusion (ACDF): Anterior approach to the cervical spine, removal of the intervertebral disk and interbody fusion.

Corpectomy: Surgical excision of the vertebral body, including the two adjacent intervertebral disks. This procedure is intended for decompression of the spinal canal and for reconstructive purposes. The spine is then reconstructed with a structural bone graft and plate instrumentation.

Anterior instrumentation: Placement of anterior plate to increase stability and to promote fusion.

Laminectomy: Removal of the laminae and spinous process to increase the AP dimensions of the spinal canal, thus relieving pressure on the thecal sac.

Laminoplasty: This procedure is intended to increase the AP diameter of the spinal canal while preserving the posterior tension band, thus avoiding iatrogenic deformity (kyphosis). There are several different techniques, but the posterior arch is interrupted on one side of the spine and hinged on the opposite side, producing an open-door effect. As the laminae are splayed, the cord migrates posteriorly and the pressure is reduced.

Posterior cervical lateral-mass instrumentation: Screws are positioned in the articular processes and are subsequently interconnected by plates or rods.

Posterior wire fixation: Multiple techniques include the passage of wires or titanium cables through the spinous processes or facets so as to reproduce stability on motion segments that have become unstable.

Craniocervical fusion: Surgical arthrodesis between the occiput and the cervical spine. This is achieved by inserting a structural bone graft, which spans the base of the occiput, posterior to the opisthion, and down to the posterior arch of C1 and C2. Several techniques have been described, but probably the most widely used includes occipital plates anchored with screws connected through rods to the lateral processes of the subaxial cervical spine and the pars interarticularis of C2.

Transarticular C1–C2 screws: Screws are driven from the inferior articular process of the axis through the C1–C2 joint into the lateral mass of the atlas, as described by Magerl. This allows for C1–C2 fusion procedures.

Gallie or Brooks wiring technique: These techniques for C1–C2 arthrodesis consist of sublaminar wires that are passed anterior to the posterior arch of C1 and C2 (Brooks) and then over a structural bicortical graft that is used to provide fusion. This requires both posterior arches to be intact.

Dens screws: Anterior exposure is required at the height of the C4 vertebral body so as to obtain adequate angulation for the insertion of screws through the anteroinferior corner of the body of the axis and into the dens. This procedure is indicated for dens fractures with a risk factor for nonunion.

Transoral decompression: This approach allows for removal of ventrally situated bony abnormalities causing cervicomedullary compression from the base of the clivus to the body of the axis. The approach is through the soft palate and posterior wall of the pharynx. After excision of the anterior arch of the atlas, the dens is fully viewed and may be completely removed.

Anterior release: The thoracic or thoracolumbar spine is approached anteriorly to removing the intervertebral disks. This allows for increased flexibility of the spine and provides enhanced deformity correction. The endplates are curetted free of cartilage and bone graft is packed in between in order to obtain interbody fusion.

Posterior Thoracospinal fusion: A fusion is a surgical arthrodesis that allows permanent immobilization of a joint by inducing bone healing across the joint space. Through a posterior approach to the thoracic or thoracolumbar spine, the transverse processes are decorticated and a morcellized bone graft is laid in the inter-transverse-process area to allow bone to bridge between the vertebral segments. This may be combined with posterior instrumentation, including hook, screw, and rod constructs.

Thoracolumbar corpectomy: Complete or subtotal removal of a vertebral body in the thoracic spine, including the two adjacent disks, with the purpose of decompressing the spinal cord and/or reconstructing the anterior column. The void is filled with a structural bone graft or a cage device packed with morcellized bone.

Anterior instrumentation: Placement of anterior plate or rod-screw construct to obtain increased stability and promote fusion. In scoliosis surgery, anterior instrumentation may be used to correct the curvature, avoiding a posterior procedure after anterior release.

VATSS (video-assisted thoracoscopic spinal surgery): Endoscopic or mini-open thoracotomy allows access to the anterior thoracic spine for most standard procedures, including anterior release, corpectomy, spinal cord decompression, and anterior instrumentation.

Costotransversectomy: A posterior extrapleural approach to the anterior and middle column of the spine, including the vertebral body and ipsilateral pedicle. This allows for adequate decompression of the spinal canal. It also allows for partial reconstruction of the anterior column.

Microdiskectomy: The spinal canal is approached through the interlaminar space, with a very small laminotomy (hemi-, semilaminectomy), with the purpose of removing an extruded disk fragment.

Lumbar decompression: This procedure is intended for the treatment of lumbar spinal stenosis. The spinal canal is approached through wide laminectomies, with the purpose of removing osteophytes, and other hypertrophic structures that produce pressure over the thecal sac.

Posterior lumbar fusion: Surgical arthrodesis is obtained by decorticating the intervening facet joint as well as the transverse processes. Morcellized bone is placed in the intertransverse process area, providing a scaffold for vascular ingrowth and bone formation.

Anterior lumbar interbody fusion (ALIF): Surgical arthrodesis is obtained by placing a structural graft or device between the vertebral bodies through an anterior exposure. The endplates are prepared by curetting them free of cartilage. If a cage is used, it is filled with bone graft to allow for the formation of a bone bridge.

Posterior lumbar interbody fusion (PLIF) and transforaminal lumbar interbody fusion (TLIF): Surgical arthrodesis is obtained by placing a structural graft or device between the vertebral bodies through a posterior exposure. If the approach to the disk includes a laminectomy and displacement of the thecal sac, this is defined as a PLIF. If the approach is through a foraminotomy, this is defined as a TLIF.

Circumferential spinal fusion ("360-degree fusion"): Surgical arthrodesis including both posterior intertransverse process fusion and anterior lumbar interbody fusion.

"270" fusion: An anterior lumbar fusion is complemented by the implantation of posterior instrumentation without posterior arthrodesis. This has become increasingly popular with the advent of percutaneous posterior spinal instrumentation.

SUGGESTED FURTHER READING

Apel DM, Marrero G, King J, et al. Avoiding paraplegia during anterior spinal surgery: The role of somatosensory evoked potential monitoring with temporary occlusion of segmental spinal arteries. *Spine* 16(Suppl 8):S365–S370, 1991.

Bazaz R, Lee MJ, Yoo JU. Incidence of dysphagia after anterior cervical spine surgery: A prospective study. *Spine* 27(22):2453–2458, 2002.

Bohlman H, Emery S, Goodfellow D, Jones P. Robinson anterior cervical diskectomy and arthrodesis for cervical radiculopathy: A long-term follow-up of one hundred and twenty-two patients. *J Bone Joint Surg* 75(A):1298, 1993.

Büttner-Janz K. Surgical approach, in Büttner-Janz K, Hochschuler S, McAfee P (eds): *The Artificial Disc*. Berlin: Springer-Verlag, 2003.

Cammisa FP, Girardi FP, Sangani PK, et al. Incidental durotomy in spine surgery. *Spine* 25(20):2663–2667, 2000.

Clements D, Morledge D, Martin W, Betz R. Evoked and spontaneous electromyography to evaluate lumbosacral pedicle screw placement. *Spine* 21:600–604, 1996.

Found EM, Weinstein JN. Surgical approaches to the lumbar spine, in Frymoyer JW (ed): *The Adult Spine: Principles and Practice*. New York: Raven Press, 1991.

Graham JJ. Complications of cervical spine surgery: A five-year report on a survey of the membership of the Cervical Spine Research Society by the Morbidity and Mortality Committee. *Spine* 14:1046–1050, 1989.

Grauer JN, Tingstad EM, Rand N, et al. Predictors of paralysis in the rheumatoid cervical spine in patients undergoing total joint arthroplasty. *J Bone Joint Surg* 86(A):1420–1424, 2004.

Hurlbert RJ. Methylprednisolone for acute spinal cord injury: An inappropriate standard of care. *J Neurosurg* 93:1–7, 2000.

Jellinek D, Platt M, Jewkers D, et al. Effects of nitrous oxide on motor evoked potentials recorded from skeletal muscle in patients under total anesthesia with intravenously administered propofol. *Neurosurgery* 29:558–567, 1991.

Lee LA. ASA postoperative visual loss registry: Preliminary analysis of factors associated with spine operations. *ASA News* 67(6):7–8, 2003.

Machida M, Yamada T. Spinal cord monitoring, in Weinstein SL (ed): *Pediatric Spine Surgery*. Philadelphia: Lippincott Williams & Wilkins, 2001.

Menezes AH. Surgical approaches to the craniocervical junction, in Weinstein SL (ed): *Pediatric Spine Surgery*. Philadelphia: Lippincott Williams & Wilkins, 2001.

Montesano PX, Magerl F. Lower cervical spine arthrodesis: Lateral mass plating, in Clark CR and The Cervical Spine Research Society Editorial Committee (eds): *The Cervical Spine*, 3d ed. Philadelphia: Lippincott-Raven, 1998.

Morpeth JF, Williams MF. Vocal cord paresis after anterior cervical discectomy and fusion. *Laryngoscope* 110:43–46, 2000.

Oda T, Fuji T, Kato Y, et al. Deep venous thrombosis after posterior spinal surgery. *Spine* 25(22):2962–2967, 2000.

Panjabi M, White A. Biomechanics of non-acute cervical spinal cord trauma. *Spine* 13:838–842, 1988.

Patel CK, Fischgrund JS. Complications of anterior cervical spine surgery. *AAOS Instr Course Lect* 52:465–469, 2003.

Pathak KS, Annadio BS, Kalamchi MD, et al. Effect of halothane, enflurane and isoflurane on somatosensory evoked potentials during nitrous oxide anesthesia. *Anesthesiology* 66:753–754, 1987.

Ravishankar V, Lenke LG, Bridwell KH, et al. A Prospective evaluation of pulmonary function in patients with adolescent idiopathic scoliosis relative to the surgical approach used for spinal arthrodesis. *Spine* 25(1):82–90, 2000.

Riew KD, McCulloch J. Microdiscectomy: Technique and utility in lumbar disc disease. *Semin Spine Surg* 11(2):119–137, 1999.

Rosner M. Medical management of spinal cord injury, in Pitts LH, Wagner FC (eds): *Craniospinal Trauma*. New York: Thieme, 1990:213–225.

Sullivan JA. Bone grafting, in Weinstein SL (ed): *Pediatric Spine Surgery*. Philadelphia: Lippincott Williams & Wilkins, 2001.

Tetzlaff JE, Yoon HJ, O'Hara J. Influence of anesthetic technique on the incidence of deep venous thrombosis after elective lumbar spine surgery. *Reg Anesth* 19(Suppl):28, 1994.

Truumees E, Herkowitz HN. Lumbar spinal stenosis: Treatment options. *Instr Course Lect* 50:153–161, 2001.

Zindrick MR, Ibrahim KI. Pedicle screw instrumentation, in Weinstein SL (ed): *Pediatric Spine Surgery*, 2d ed. Philadelphia: Lippincott Williams & Wilkins, 2001.

CHAPTER 15

Hand Surgery

CURTIS STEYERS/ANDRÉ P. BOEZAART

▶ INTRODUCTION

Regional anesthesia is the mainstay of anesthesia for the hand; ineffective anesthesia or partially failed blocks prevent the surgeon from accomplishing the intended goals and will likely compromise the results of the surgery. Except in children, where regional anesthesia is handy for the prevention of operative and postoperative pain, nerve blocks are often used as the sole anesthetic.

For all the surgical procedures discussed in this chapter, it is assumed that regional anesthesia is used, which includes axillary block (see Chap. 25), infraclavicular block (see Chap. 24), or supraclavicular block (see Chap. 23). Intravenous regional anesthesia (Bier block) is also used, but it is losing popularity. For completeness sake, it is discussed briefly further on.

▶ LIGAMENT RECONSTRUCTION AND TENDON INTERPOSITION (LRTI) ARTHROPLASTY FOR THE THUMB

Carpometacarpal Joint (LRTI Procedure)

Indications and Anatomic Considerations
Ligament reconstruction and tendon interposition (LRTI procedure) arthroplasty for the thumb's carpometacarpal joint is most commonly indicated for symptomatic osteoarthritis of the carpometacarpal joint (CMCJ) of the thumb. Patients with posttraumatic arthritis and inflammatory disorders are occasionally also candidates for this procedure.

Specific activities that are difficult in this condition include any maneuver that requires strong key pinch,

such as holding a heavy book, or strong span grasp, such as turning a tight jar lid.

Inspection of the hand frequently reveals no apparent abnormalities, but in the latter stages of this disorder, the thumb metacarpal begins to collapse into the hand as its proximal end subluxates dorsally from its articulation with the trapezium. This occurs as the articular cartilage thins and erodes and the volar beak ligament, which holds the thumb metacarpal to the trapezium, attenuates. Initial treatment for this condition includes some modification of activity when feasible, anti-inflammatory medications, splints, and intraarticular corticosteroid injections. Those patients in whom conservative treatment fails and who continue to complain of pain, causing significant functional impairment, are candidates for surgical reconstruction of the CMCJ.

Several anatomic features are especially important to any surgical procedure near the basilar thumb region of the hand. Incisions in this region unavoidably risk injury to the cutaneous innervation of the area. The terminal divisions of the superficial radial nerve, the palmar cutaneous branch of the median nerve, and the terminal fibers of the lateral antebrachial cutaneous nerve may be encountered during any dissection in this region. The number, location, and distribution of these nerve branches are somewhat variable, and they are easily injured. The dorsal branch of the radial artery crosses the dorsum of the scaphotrapezial joint as it passes through the floor of the anatomic snuffbox and is also at risk during this procedure. It must be identified, gently mobilized, and its articular branches cauterized to avoid postoperative wound hematoma or hand ischemia.

Patient Profile
A typical patient is a 55- to 70-year-old woman who complains of the insidious onset of aching pain near the

basilar region of her thumb, which is related to activity. Although this condition is frequently bilateral, the dominant hand is usually the most troublesome.

Positioning on the Operating Table

The patient is placed in the supine position and her arm is placed on a hand table attached to the surgical bed. The shoulder should not be abducted more than 90 degrees or externally rotated excessively in order to avoid inadvertent injury to the shoulder joint and rotator cuff. A tourniquet cuff is placed about the proximal arm over cotton padding. All bony prominences are padded and care is taken to assure that the legs remain uncrossed.

Surgical Technique

The limb is exsanguinated with an elastic wrap and the tourniquet inflated to a pressure of 250 mmHg. A variety of incisions may be used to expose the CMCJ of the thumb. They all include a dorsal component over the CMCJ and snuffbox region and some also include a palmar extension in the region of the distal palmar crease. Cutaneous nerves are identified and carefully mobilized. The radial artery is mobilized and gently retracted with soft vessel loops. The surgeon then incises the scaphotrapezial and CMCJ capsule to expose these joints. Capsular flaps are sharply dissected from the surface of the trapezium, which is then removed. Care is taken to avoid injury to the flexor carpi radialis (FCR) tendon in the base of the wound. A channel is created in the base of the thumb metacarpal starting from the dorsal cortex and ending at the volar base. A distally based flap of FCR tendon is then harvested through one or more small incisions in the volar forearm and delivered into the cavity formerly occupied by the trapezium. This tendon is then delivered through the channel in the metacarpal base from volar to dorsal using a loop of fine wire. The tendon flap will function as a stabilizing ligament to hold the thumb metacarpal in place.

The thumb metacarpal is then pinned in a position of wide abduction and extension. The tendon flap is pulled taut and sutured into place. The remaining tendon is packed into the cavity formerly occupied by the trapezium to function as a biological spacer. The joint capsule is sutured closed over the tendon interposition and the tourniquet deflated. Bleeding is controlled with compression and electrocautery. When satisfactory hemostasis is achieved, the vessel loop is removed and the wounds are closed with fine nonabsorbable sutures. A soft dressing is applied, followed by a plaster splint that holds the wrist in slight dorsiflexion and encircles the thumb.

Anesthetic Considerations

General anesthesia is very seldom used for this operation. Any one of the single-injection periclavicular blocks (supra- or infraclavicular; see Chaps. 23 and 24) or the axillary block (see Chap. 25) is ideal for this surgery.

We typically place an infraclavicular block plus a block of the intercostobrachial nerve. Intraoperatively, we achieve high patient satisfaction with light sedation with meperidine and/or midazolam combined with music of the patient's choice by noise-cancellation earphones.

Analgesia

The single-injection block is generally sufficient to provide optimal postoperative analgesia; continuous nerve blocks are not indicated. The patient, however, must be instructed to protect the vulnerable nerves of the arm (radial, ulnar, and to a lesser extent median nerves) from accidental trauma or pressure during the postoperative period while the arm is blocked (see Chap. 32).

Depending on the agent used for the block (see Chap. 18), one can expect the block to be effective for 4 to 8 h postoperatively; the patient should start taking oral analgesic agents before sensation returns to the hand.

Associated Medication

Patients may be elderly or suffer from rheumatoid arthritis and take medication associated with these conditions (see Chaps. 7 and 8). One dose of prophylactic antibiotics is usually given intravenously before the tourniquet is inflated (see Chap. 3).

Postoperative Care

The sutures are removed approximately 10 to 14 days after surgery. Postoperative pain is most notable for the first 2 or 3 days and is usually controlled with prescription oral narcotics. The pin is removed 3 to 4 weeks later and the patient is fitted for a hand-based opponens splint. Hand therapy begins at this time to restore thumb motion and pinch strength. Splinting is routinely discontinued at 6 weeks.

▶ OTHER COMMON HAND PROCEDURES

Palmar and Digital Fasciectomy

Indications and Anatomic Considerations

Palmar and digital fasciectomy is indicated for patients with Dupuytren's disease who develop finger flexion deformities that severely impair hand function.

Patient Profile

A typical patient is a 60- to 70-year-old man with painless flexion deformities of his fingers. These patients often have several significant comorbidities, including a history of alcohol abuse and associated liver dysfunction.

Positioning on the Operating Table

Standard patient and limb positioning is used, and the surgical procedure must be completed under tourniquet control.

Surgical Technique

The diseased fascia commonly displaces the digital nerves. The surgeon must clearly identify each nerve in order to avoid injury to these structures. This must be done with confidence and cannot be done without a completely bloodless operative field. A variety of incisions may be used to expose the diseased fascia. A common technique includes a transverse palmar incision at the level of the distal palmar crease, which is then left open at the conclusion of the procedure ("open-palm technique"). Regardless of the design of the skin incisions, the diseased fascia is next exposed by reflecting the skin flaps. Beginning proximally, the common and proper digital neurovascular bundles are identified and protected as the diseased tissue is resected. After the removal of all abnormal palmar and digital fascia, the tourniquet is deflated and hemostasis established. The incisions are then closed. When appropriate, Z plasties are designed, cut, and transposed at digital flexion creases. The transverse palmar incision is not closed but rather covered with the postoperative soft dressing.

Anesthetic Considerations

Palmar fasciectomy is very seldom done with general anesthesia. Any of the periclavicular brachial plexus blocks (supraclavicular (see Chap. 23) or an infraclavicular (see Chap. 34) or axillary block is appropriate for this surgery.

Intraoperatively we normally use very little or no sedation but provide soothing music of the patient's choice through noise-cancellation headphones. This approach seems very satisfactory.

Analgesia

Postoperative pain is generally minimal; a single-injection brachial plexus block is usually sufficient to deal with it. Oral analgesics can be used if required.

Associated Medication

Elderly patients may be receiving various drugs to treat comorbid conditions. A single intravenous dose of a prophylactic antibiotic agent may be used 3 min before the tourniquet is inflated (see Chap. 3).

Postoperative Care

Gentle finger range-of-motion exercises begin immediately. The dressing is usually changed 3 to 5 days postoperatively, at which time more aggressive exercise begins and the patient is encouraged to start using the hand more actively. Sutures are removed 2 weeks postoperatively.

The open palmar wound heals by secondary intention within 6 weeks.

Carpal Tunnel Release

Indications

Surgery for carpal tunnel release is indicated for patients with carpal tunnel syndrome who fail to respond to conservative care or in whom evaluation reveals objective deficits in the sensory or motor function of the median nerve.

Patient Profile

Patients presenting with carpal tunnel syndrome fall into all adult age groups, but the typical patient is a middle-aged woman.

Positioning on the Operating Table

Positioning on the operating table follows the routine for hand surgery (see above).

Surgical Technique

After exsanguination of the limb, the tourniquet is inflated and a short longitudinal incision made in the interthenar interval. Subcutaneous tissues are retracted and the palmar fascia is incised to expose the transverse carpal ligament. The ligament is then divided under direct vision to open and expose the contents of the carpal tunnel. The skin is closed, a low-profile soft dressing applied, and the tourniquet deflated.

This surgery is sometimes performed endoscopically.

Anesthetic Considerations

This procedure is typically completed under local anesthesia with sedation, which is especially helpful to alleviate anxiety and reduce the likelihood of unanticipated patient movement during the procedure. Local anesthetic is first infiltrated slowly into the subcutaneous plane, just proximal to the flexion crease of the wrist, across the width of the distal forearm. A mixture of lidocaine and bupivacaine is commonly used, but epinephrine is always avoided. This effectively blocks the palmar cutaneous branches of the median and ulnar nerves. A second injection is begun by inserting the needle through the anesthetized distal forearm skin just ulnar to the palmaris longus tendon at the flexion crease of the wrist. Local anesthetic is infiltrated distally into the subcutaneous tissues by advancing the needle distally in line with the third web space. No attempt is made to infiltrate anesthetic agent into the carpal tunnel or to complete a formal median nerve block.

Some surgeons perform this surgery under Bier block, but in the hands of a skilled surgeon, this procedure generally takes less than 10 to 15 min, while the tourniquet has to be inflated for a minimum of 30 min after a Bier block (see above). Apart from the fact that a Bier block provides no postoperative analgesia, it generally slows down operating room turnover, although some surgeons and anesthesiologists are very proficient and happy with this technique.

Analgesia

Minimal postoperative analgesia, at most oral analgesics, is required if the surgery is performed with a field block as described above.

Postoperative Care

Sutures are removed 10 to 14 days later and the patient gradually resumes normal activity. Postoperative pain is usually minimal and easily controlled with mild analgesics.

Trigger Finger Release

Indications

Trigger finger release is indicated for patients who fail to experience satisfactory improvement following corticosteroid injection into the flexor tendon sheath of the involved finger or thumb. Patients with this condition complain of painful locking or snapping as they flex and extend the affected finger. The ring finger and thumb are most frequently affected and the most common comorbidity is diabetes mellitus.

Patient Profile

This condition occurs in any age group from infancy to old age but is commonly associated with diabetes mellitus (see Chap. 12).

Surgical Technique

The limb is exsanguinated and the tourniquet inflated. An incision is made through the anesthetized skin and the subcutaneous tissues are separated to expose the first annular pulley. The surgeon must be especially careful to avoid injury to the adjacent digital nerves, especially in the thumb, where these nerves are found just a few millimeters below the dermis and where they can be lacerated with an overly aggressive skin incision. The first annular pulley is then incised and the patient asked to flex and extend the finger to ensure that full and unrestricted motion has been restored. The wound is closed, a small soft dressing applied, and the tourniquet deflated.

Anesthetic Considerations

The procedure begins with infiltration of local anesthetic into the subcutaneous tissues at the level of the distal palmar crease in the axis of the affected finger. For the thumb, infiltration is completed in the flexion crease of the metacarpophalangeal joint.

Analgesia

Minimal postoperative analgesia, at most oral analgesics, is required if the surgery is performed with a field block as described above.

Postoperative Care

The patient begins active range-of-motion exercise immediately and sutures are removed 10 to 14 days later. Postoperative pain is easily managed with over-the-counter analgesics.

▶ PEDIATRIC CONDITIONS

Syndactyly Reconstruction

Indications

Syndactyly occurs when adjacent digits fail to separate completely during fetal development. It is a condition characterized by variable degrees of fusion of the soft tissue and skeletal elements of adjacent digits. Any digits may be affected, but the long and ring fingers are most commonly involved. Separation of the digits and reconstruction of the interdigital web are indicated in nearly all cases; typically surgery is completed between the ages of 6 and 18 months.

Patient Profile

Patients are typically infants between 6 and 18 months of age. Other congenital conditions are common; specifically, cardiac abnormalities and malignant hyperpyrexia may be complicating factors (see Chap. 6).

Positioning on the Operating Table

A tourniquet is applied about the proximal arm and the entire arm and one or both groins are prepped and draped free for harvest of a full-thickness skin graft.

Surgical Technique

The procedure begins by designing skin incisions that will provide a dorsal skin flap to resurface the interdigital web and that avoid creating longitudinal scars along the surfaces of the newly separated digits (Fig. 15-1*A* and *B*). Skin flaps are developed and defatted to expose the interdigital space. Fascial bands are divided and any fusions of tendon or skeletal elements separated. Not infrequently, the common digital nerve bifurcates distally between the conjoined fingers instead of in the distal palm. In this situation the two proper digital nerves are separated from one another by sharp dissection in order to place the dorsal skin flap in an appropriate position. The common digital artery may also bifurcate distally, in which case one or the other of the proper digital arteries must be sacrificed to allow proper separation of the fingers. After complete separation, the dorsal flap is sutured into place with fine absorbable suture. The other interdigitating skin flaps are then sutured to one another (Fig. 15-1). All remaining skin defects are then resurfaced with full-thickness

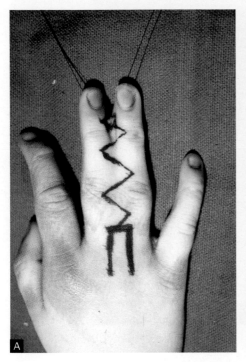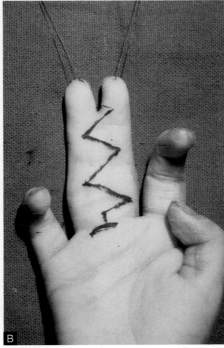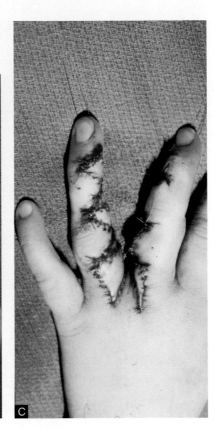

Figure 15-1. Syndactyly.

skin graft harvested from the groin or lower abdomen. A snugly fitting postoperative dressing is then applied to ensure skin graft survival.

Anesthetic Considerations

Syndactyly reconstruction is completed under general anesthesia and routine pediatric anesthetic principles apply (see Chap. 6). Peripheral nerve block may be appropriate to provide intraoperative analgesia (see Chap. 31); airway management may be with a laryngeal-mask airway or endotracheal tube, as appropriate.

Analgesia

Analgesic requirements in the postoperative period are low and, if a peripheral nerve block was done, this is usually all that is required. We typically use a nerve block and acetaminophen suppositories, which provides excellent analgesia.

Postoperative Care

A long arm cast must also be applied to protect the dressing for approximately 2 weeks. The cast and dressing are then removed and appropriate wound care provided.

▶ OTHER COMMON PEDIATRIC CONDITIONS

Other common pediatric conditions include thumb hypoplasia (Fig. 15-2A and B), thumb duplication (Fig. 15-3A and B), and absent fingers from conditions including amniotic disruption sequence (constriction ring syndrome), symbrachydactyly, and transverse terminal absence (Fig. 15-4). Thumb hypoplasia varies in severity from very subtle deficiencies to complete absence of the thumb and is often associated with other disorders. These include cardiac anomalies (Holt-Oram' syndrome), blood dyscrasias (Fanconi's anemia and thrombocytopenia–absent radius syndrome), and a collection of anomalies known as the VACTERL (vertebral anomalies, anal atresia, cardiac abnormalities, tracheoesophageal fistula, esophageal atresia, renal anomalies, radial defects, and lower limb anomalies) association. Treatment varies from reconstruction of the existing thumb to ablation of the thumb and pollicization of the index finger.

Thumb duplication is not associated with the same risk of associated problems as is thumb hypoplasia. Surgical treatment is nearly always indicated and is directed at reconstruction of a single, stable, well-aligned

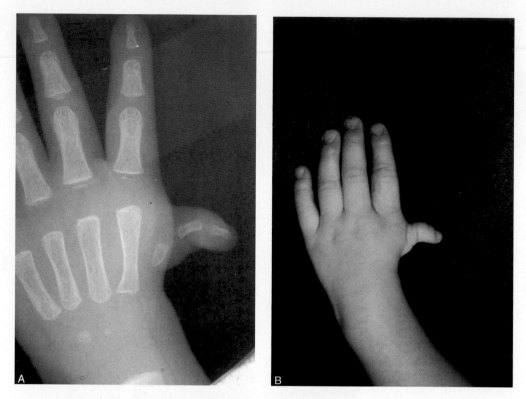

Figure 15-2. Thumb hypoplasia.

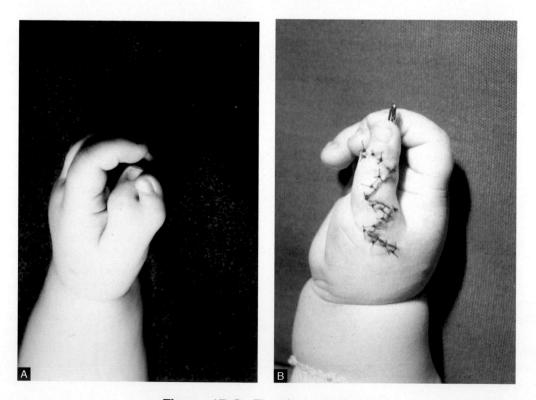

Figure 15-3. Thumb duplication.

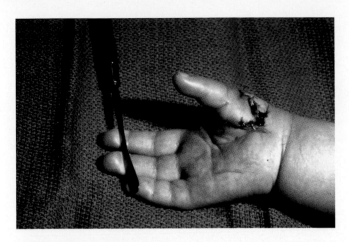

Figure 15-4. Pollicization.

thumb with a functional range of motion using the existing components of the two available thumbs. Treatment for patients with missing or hypoplastic digits includes augmentation of existing parts or replacement of missing parts by transfer of tissues from other sources.

▶ INTRAVENOUS REGIONAL ANESTHESIA (BIER BLOCK)

There are many variations of the Bier block. In short, the Bier block is defined by the use of a double tourniquet. It is useful for short procedures but offers no analgesia in the postoperative period. This—together with the fact that the peripheral nerve blocks are so effective, fast in onset, safe, and provide excellent postoperative analgesia—has caused the Bier block to be used by fewer surgeons and anesthesiologists.

In the Bier block, an intravenous cannula is inserted in the arm to be operated. The arm is then elevated and "exsanguinated" by an Esmarch bandage. The proximal tourniquet inflated to 250 to 300 mmHg (or 100 mmHg above the systolic blood pressure) and 30 to 60 mL of 0.5% lidocaine is injected through the intravenous cannula. This tourniquet is kept inflated for a minimum of 30 min. The proximal tourniquet is first inflated and kept inflated until it becomes uncomfortable, at which time the distal tourniquet is inflated to the same pressure and the proximal tourniquet is deflated.

After 30 min, the tourniquet can be deflated. Some experts recommend cycling the two tourniquets as a means of limiting the systemic uptake of lidocaine, although this is controversial.

Complications include systemic toxic effects such as cardiac arrhythmia, loss of consciousness, convulsions, vertigo, and nystagmus. Most surgeons prefer to operate under conditions of peripheral nerve block.

SUGGESTED FURTHER READING

Blair EF, Steyers CM (eds). *Techniques in Hand Surgery.* Baltimore: Williams & Wilkins, 1996.

Burton RI, Pellegrini VD Jr. Surgical management of basal joint arthritis of the thumb: Part II. Ligament reconstruction with tendon interposition arthroplasty. *J Hand Surg* 11A:324–332, 1986.

Green DP, Hotchkiss RN, Pederson WC, Wolfe SW (eds): *Green's Operative Hand Surgery.* Philadelphia: Elsevier Churchill Livingstone, 2005.

Katz JN, Simmons BP. Clinical practice: Carpal tunnel syndrome. *N Engl J Med* 346:1807–1812, 2002.

Keret D, Ger E. Evaluation of a uniform operative technique to treat syndactyly. *J Hand Surg* 12A:727–729, 1987.

Light TR. Treatment of preaxial polydactyly. *Hand Clin* 8:161–175, 1992.

Lister GD. Reconstruction of the hypoplastic thumb. *Clin Orthop* 195:52–65, 1985.

Lubahn JD, Lister GD, Wolf T. Fasciectomy and Dupuytren's disease: A comparison between the open palm technique and wound closure. *J Hand Surg* 9A:53–58, 1984.

McCash CR. The open palm technique in Dupuytren's contracture. *Br J Plast Surg* 17:271–280, 1964.

Rhoades C, Gelberman H, Manjarris JF. Stenosing tenosynovitis of the fingers and thumbs. *Clin Orthop Rel Res* 190:236–238, 1984.

CHAPTER 16

Common Fractures

TODD MCKINLEY/ANDRÉ P. BOEZAART

► INTRODUCTION

Fractures are among the most common disorders treated by orthopaedic surgeons. They encompass a wide variety of injuries, from nondisplaced fractures of a digit to an open crushed pelvis. However, all fractures have one thing in common: pain. Therefore adequate pain control plays a pivotal role in the successful treatment of fractures.

The goal of fracture treatment is to restore the function of the injured extremity as well as possible. Treatment principles are to reduce the fracture into acceptable alignment and maintain the reduction with some type of stabilization. Reductions can often be performed using closed techniques; however, a substantial number of them require surgery. Fractures too can frequently be stabilized with closed techniques, such as bracing or casting. However, many are better treated with internal or external fixation. In any event, most fractures require some type of intervention to be treated successfully.

Successful reduction and stabilization are usually prohibitively difficult without adequate pain control; anesthesia is therefore a vital part of fracture treatment. This chapter describes common fractures of the upper and lower extremity. Fractures of the spine, hand, and foot are addressed in other chapters. Open fractures, crush injuries, and compartment syndromes are also discussed. The treatment principles for each fracture, with particular attention to anesthetic considerations, are discussed.

► UPPER EXTREMITY FRACTURES

Proximal Humeral Fractures

Fractures of the proximal humerus are common injuries and most often occur in elderly patients who have suffered a fall (Fig. 16-1). Most of these fractures are treated non-operatively with short-term immobilization followed by rehabilitation. However, higher-energy injuries in younger patients frequently require surgical reduction and fixation.

Patient Profile
Most of the patients with these injuries are elderly. However, younger patients often sustain higher-energy injuries, including proximal humeral fractures in motor vehicle accidents or falls. They can also be hurt by sports injuries and often have associated dislocations of the shoulder.

Fracture Classification
Most orthopaedic surgeons adhere to the Neer classification of proximal humeral fractures. Neer described four parts of the proximal humerus, including the head and anatomic neck, the greater tuberosity, the lesser tuberosity, and the humeral shaft. He described a part as displaced if it had translated more than 1 cm or angled more than 45 degrees from its normal position. Most lower-energy fractures in older patients are two-part fractures of the surgical neck. This is a fracture of the shaft off the humeral head inferior to the tuberosities. It is distinguished from an anatomic neck fracture, which fractures through the base of the articular surface within the joint. Three- and four-part fractures involve a displaced fracture of the shaft and displaced fractures of one or both of the tuberosities. In younger patients, these are usually high-energy injuries.

Treatment
The vast majority of lower-energy fractures in older patients are treated closed. They are immobilized for a short period followed by shoulder rehabilitation. In elderly

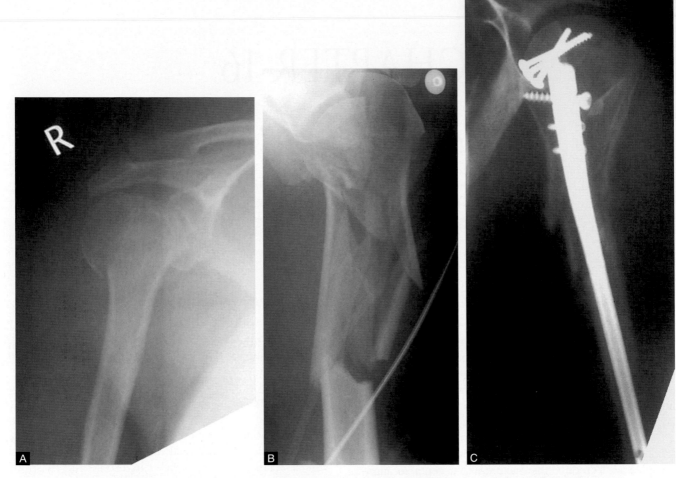

Figure 16-1. Fractures of the proximal humerus are typically due to low-energy falls in elderly patients (Fig. 16-1*A*) and are treated conservatively. In younger patients, the fractures are higher-energy injuries, such as this four-part fracture sustained by a 48-year-old woman in an automobile accident (Fig. 16-1*B*). In younger patients, displaced fractures are typically treated with open reduction and internal fixation (Fig. 16-1*C*).

patients with grossly displaced three- and four- part fractures, the most common treatment is humeral head replacement. Surgery is delayed until the patient is medically stabilized, usually several days after the injury, and it is done through an anterior approach, usually through the deltopectoral interval, and the prosthesis is cemented into the proximal humerus.

In younger patients with displaced fractures, open reduction with internal fixation is the mainstay of treatment. More extensive fractures are usually reduced and stabilized through an open approach, either directly from the lateral deltoid or through the deltopectoral interval. The patients are usually placed supine or in a beach chair type of position. Internal fixation usually involves some type of plate-and-screw construct. In patients with certain two- and three-part fractures (surgical neck fractures, greater tuberosity fractures, anatomic

neck fractures), closed reduction with percutaneous fixation has been shown to be a successful treatment option. The goal of surgery is adequate realignment of the displaced fracture fragments with stable internal fixation to afford early motion and function once the humeral head is healed. Postoperatively, the patients are given antibiotics and are usually allowed a very limited motion regime for the first several weeks after surgery. Once early healing is established, increases in the range of motion and activity are permitted.

Anesthetic Considerations

Communication between the surgeon and anesthesiologist is important to position the patient properly to allow surgical and fluoroscopic access without jeopardizing the patient's airway. The anesthesiologist must be informed that forceful manipulation of the fracture is likely and the airway should be reinforced as necessary. Muscular paralysis greatly aids in manipulation and reduction of these fractures. Postoperative pain management with an indwelling catheter has also helped patients substantially (see Chaps. 20, 21, and 23).

Patients suffering high-energy humeral fractures often have associated lung injury; this should be evaluated and treated appropriately.

Humeral Shaft Fractures

Humeral shaft fractures are relatively common injuries. The vast majority of these fractures have excellent outcomes when treated closed. However, a small subset of these fractures require surgical treatment, including open fractures, unstable and grossly deformed fractures, and injuries of the floating elbow type (a humeral fracture and ipsilateral forearm fracture).

Patient Profile

Fractures of the humeral shaft occur in a wide variety of patients, including older patients, who often sustain them by falling, or younger patients, who sustain them in higher-energy injuries due to motor vehicle accidents or falls. They can also be sustained through sports injuries, in which a large torsional force is applied to the humerus, as in wrestling or arm wrestling.

Treatment

The humerus is circumferentially encased in muscle. Therefore most fractures have excellent inherent hydraulic stability from swelling, fracture hematoma, and circumferential muscle. The circumferential muscle sleeve is also an outstanding conduit to the supply of blood. Because of this, most humeral fractures are maintained in excellent alignment with closed methods and predictably heal well. The arm is initially placed in a splint, which is eventually followed by a functional fracture brace. Activity is progressively allowed as the fracture heals.

Because the humerus achieves normal function even when substantially deformed, most fractures do not require operative reduction and fixation. However, in fractures with greater than 30 to 40 degrees of angulation after closed reduction or in open fractures, operative treatment can improve patient outcomes. The mainstay of treatment of humeral shaft fractures is open reduction and internal fixation using a plate-and-screw construct. Some surgeons advocate intermedullary fixation for these fractures. However, many studies have showed no improvement in arm strength in patients treated with intramedullary nails compared to open techniques. There is also a substantial incidence of shoulder pain in patients treated with intramedullary fixation.

Patients can be placed in a supine position for an anterolateral approach or in the prone position for a posterior approach on a radiolucent table. The fracture is aligned and compressed with a large plate and screws. Postoperatively patients are allowed to move the shoulder and elbow but have limited use of the limb for several months until healing takes place; then their activity is increased accordingly.

Anesthetic Considerations

Humeral shaft fractures are sometimes sustained in high-energy injuries; therefore the principles of treating a multiply injured patient apply (see Chap. 2). These fractures do not need to be fixed to mobilize a patient in an intensive care unit, and treatment should be delayed until the patient is completely stable. Complete muscular paralysis greatly facilitates reduction. Because the radial nerve is intimately associated with the humeral shaft, there is a substantial incidence radial nerve palsy due to the initial injury. There is also a substantial incidence of iatrogenic radial nerve palsies following surgery to fix these fractures, especially with posterior approaches. Because of this, nerve blocks should be done with caution or even avoided during and after the surgery.

Intraarticular Fractures of the Elbow

Intraarticular fractures of the elbow include those of the distal humerus, proximal ulna, and radial head (Fig. 16-2). These fractures occur in a wide variety of patients and can result from falls or from high-energy impacts, as in motor vehicle collisions. Some of the most comminuted fractures can occur from lower-energy mechanisms. There is often gross displacement of the articular surface. Therefore a substantial number of intraarticular elbow fractures are treated with open reduction and internal fixation.

Classification

There is no widely accepted classification of distal humeral fractures or proximal ulnar fractures. Frequently more than one bone is fractured. Therefore these injuries are best described by first identifying which bones are fractured. Second, the amount of comminution and displacement, with particular attention to the amount of articular comminution, further describes the fracture. It is particularly important to determine whether there is an associated elbow dislocation. Fracture-dislocations of the elbow usually indicate that a severe soft tissue injury has also occurred.

Fractures of the radial head are frequently described by the Mason classification. This indicates the number of bone fragments, the size of the fragments, and the amount of comminution. Severely comminuted Mason type III radial head fractures are particularly difficult to treat with surgery, in contrast to Mason type II injuries, which involve two pieces or less of the radial head and can be treated with open reduction and internal fixation.

► LOWER EXTREMITY FRACTURES

Pelvic Ring Fractures

Pelvic ring fractures are typically high-energy injuries (Fig. 16-3). Widely displaced pelvic fractures are usually associated with massive hemorrhage and can result in death (see Chap. 2). The massive forces required to break the pelvis also damages the pelvic viscera and vasculature, which can cause life-threatening hemorrhage. Because of these potentially lethal injuries, pelvic fractures are often treated on an emergency basis.

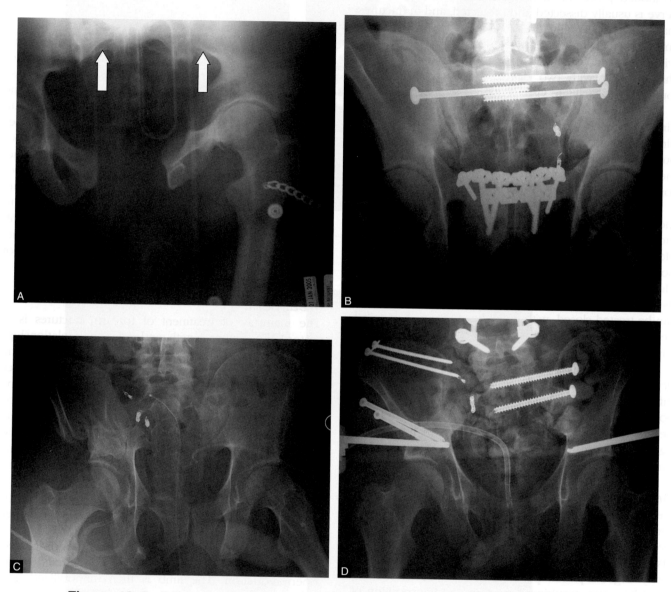

Figure 16-3. Pelvic ring injuries can be life-threatening due to severe hemorrhage. Fig. 16-3A is an AP x-ray view of the pelvis a 52-year-old male pedestrian struck by a pickup truck. The patient has wide diastases at the symphysis pubis anteriorly and widened sacroiliac joints posteriorly. This is an AP compression injury, which is particularly prone to bleed heavily. The patient was treated with application of an immediate pelvic binder. Several days later, after 28 U of blood had been administered, he had percutaneous fixation of the posterior pelvic ring and open reduction with internal fixation of his symphysis (Fig. 16-3B). Figure 16-3C is an AP x-ray of the pelvis of a 28-year-old man who was involved in a side-on collision ("T-boned") while driving his car, resulting in a lateral compression– type of pelvic ring injury. The patient had percutaneous fixation of the posterior pelvic ring and application of a low-profile external fixator to control the anterior pelvic ring (Fig. 16-3D).

Classification

There are several classifications for pelvic fractures. The classification of Young and Burgess is particularly useful, as it correlates the mechanism of injury with the resulting pelvic deformity. Such a deformity has been shown to be predictive of blood loss and associated injuries. The Young and Burgess classification separates pelvic ring injuries caused by lateral compression, anteroposterior (AP) compression, vertical shear of the pelvis, and combined mechanical injury. Lateral compression injuries decrease the pelvic volume at the time of impact and therefore cause less tensile and shear injury to the pelvic vasculature. Hemorrhage is therefore usually less than with AP types of injuries, but it can still be substantial. Typically, the pelvis is struck from the side and folded in on itself. These are often stable injuries, but higher-energy impacts can result in pelvic instability. A substantial incidence of closed head and chest injuries occur concomitantly with lateral compression pelvic fractures.

AP compression-type injuries usually result from a massive anterior-to-posterior force, which opens the pelvis at impact. The pelvic viscera and vascular structures are thus subjected to large stretching and shearing forces at impact that can cause massive pelvic hemorrhage. Intraabdominal injuries and massive blood loss within the first 24 to 48 h are frequent in patients with AP pelvic fractures. Mortality is decreased dramatically if immediate pelvic stabilization is performed.

Vertical shear injuries usually result from a fall. The classic sign is that the affected hemipelvis is displaced proximally compared to the opposite side. The pelvic vasculature is not subjected to as much stretch and shear stress and less blood is typically needed than in AP compression-type injuries.

Treatment

Severe pelvic fractures are life-threatening injuries (see Chap. 2). Hypotensive patients with unstable pelvic ring fractures should have immediate stabilization of the pelvis done during resuscitation. Pelvic binders are effective devices that provide immediate pelvic stability while allowing other diagnostic and therapeutic measures to proceed. Patients who remain hypotensive after application of a pelvic binder and adequate fluid resuscitation require immediate further intervention. Patients with suspected exsanguinating intraabdominal or intrathoracic injuries should proceed to surgery to control hemorrhage. Patients without exsanguinating injuries should undergo pelvic angiography. Definitive treatment of unstable, displaced pelvic fractures is delayed until the patient is adequately resuscitated.

Pelvic ring injuries that are unstable are definitively reduced and stabilized with internal or external fixation or a combination of both techniques. Stabilization involves techniques that stabilize the anterior and posterior pelvic ring. Open or closed reduction techniques can be used for both anterior and posterior pelvic injuries.

Pelvic fractures with posterior instability can be stabilized with the patient in the supine or prone position. Most of these injuries are reduced and stabilized with percutaneous techniques in the supine position. Reduction is achieved with traction and percutaneous insertion of pins into the iliac wing. Reduction is confirmed on AP, inlet, outlet, and lateral x-rays of the articulation between the pelvis and the sacrum. The posterior pelvic ring is stabilized with percutaneous placement of iliosacral screws under fluoroscopic guidance. This is a technically demanding operation with little margin of error for screw placement. Typically a lateral view of the sacrum combined with inlet and outlet views of the pelvis is used to ensure proper insertion of the screws. Screws are typically inserted from the pelvic wing into the S1 body of the sacrum.

Open techniques are infrequently used for stabilization of the posterior hemipelvis. For fractures with substantial vertical migration or displaced fractures treated on a delayed basis, open posterior techniques are commonly used. Patients are positioned prone. Iliosacral screws, plates, and fixation to the lower lumbar spine are reported stabilization techniques. Open techniques have a substantial incidence of wound complications. Common complications of posterior pelvic internal fixation include nerve root injury due to misplaced screws.

The anterior pelvic ring can be reduced closed and stabilized with percutaneous external fixation pins. Reduction can be facilitated by traction and manipulation through percutaneous pins placed into the anterior pelvic ring. The pins are incorporated into an external fixator to hold the reduction. External fixators provide minimal stability for the posterior pelvic ring and are used strictly in acutely hypotensive patients for resuscitation or to control the anterior pelvic ring. Therefore they are used independently for fractures with anterior rotational instability with intact posterior vertical stability or as adjunctive anterior fixation in fractures with anterior rotational and posterior vertical instability. The pins can be inserted either through the top of the iliac crest, aiming toward the acetabulum, or just above the acetabulum, aiming toward the sciatic notch. Open techniques of anterior pelvic reduction and stabilization usually involve an anterior approach to the pelvic ring. This is done through a transverse lower abdominal incision with the patient in a supine position. Reduction can be done with skeletal clamps, and the anterior pelvic ring is typically stabilized with a plate placed on top of the superior ramus. Open reduction is used for more widely displaced and rotated disruptions of the anterior pelvic ring.

Anesthetic Considerations

The immediate concern in patients with pelvic ring injuries is life-threatening bleeding (see Chap. 2). Patients with severe AP injuries required on average 35 U of blood during their first 48 h of hospitalization. Severe lateral compression and vertical shear injuries required 7 to 9 U of blood during the same period. Associated thoracic and abdominal injuries are common. Aggressive resuscitation in these severely injured patients cannot be overemphasized. Patients who are adequately resuscitated initially need careful observation to detect recurrent hemodynamic instability. It is the responsibility of the surgical and anesthetic team to monitor the patient closely and intervene rapidly when necessary.

Percutaneous stabilization techniques are technically demanding and depend on good fluoroscopic visualization. Nitrous oxide increases bowel gas, which makes it more difficult to visualize reduction; it should therefore not be used as part of an anesthetic during these cases. Neuromuscular paralysis eliminates the large muscular forces that resist reduction and is therefore helpful in realigning the pelvis. Principles of dealing with severely traumatized patients as described in Chap. 2 are followed.

Acetabular Fractures

Acetabular fractures are challenging orthopaedic injuries that require a team approach to optimize treatment (Fig. 16-4). These fractures can occur as isolated injuries due to relatively low forces or they can be one of many high-energy injuries in a single patient. Displaced fractures are often treated with open reduction and internal fixation (Fig. 16-5). Surgical treatment of these fractures can be among the most challenging in orthopaedic surgery. The prolonged surgery and substantial blood loss make preoperative communication between the surgeon and anesthesiologist absolutely necessary.

Patient Profile

Acetabular fractures occur in a wide variety of patients. They can result from high-energy trauma such as motor vehicle accidents or from simple falls, usually in older osteopenic patients. As with most fractures, they are more common in males. Preoperative comorbidities parallel the age of the patient and the force that caused the injury.

Fracture Classification

The most widely used classification of acetabular fractures is that of Letournel and Judet. It divides these fractures into simple and associated types. The pelvis encompassing the acetabulum is divided into the anterior and posterior columns. Simple types include isolated fractures of the anterior or posterior column, isolated fractures of the anterior or posterior wall, and transverse fractures across both columns. The associated types are more complex fractures representing column fractures with concomitant wall fractures, fractures that separate the anterior and posterior columns from each other, and fractures that completely separate the acetabulum from the rest of the pelvis. The Letournel and Judet classification has been shown to aid in choosing surgical approaches and is modestly helpful in predicting outcomes.

Treatment Options

Several authorities have demonstrated that outcomes are closely correlated with the quality of reduction of the articular surface. Therefore, displaced fractures in patients who are able to tolerate surgery and remain reasonably physically active are treated with open reduction and internal fixation. Patients who cannot tolerate a larger operation or those who have a severe fracture pattern that predicts a poor outcome (e.g., severe comminution that is irreparable, severe injury to the femoral head, or severe preexisting arthritis) should be treated without surgery.

Fractures are approached directly depending on the fracture type and location. Posterior fractures are exposed through a Kocher-Langenbach approach, which is similar to a posterior approach for a total hip replacement. This is done through approximately a 20-cm incision that involves releasing the gluteal sling and external rotators of the hip after splitting the gluteus maximus muscle. Care must be taken to avoid injury to the sciatic nerve or excessive traction on it because this operation is associated with a substantial incidence of nerve palsy, especially to the peroneal division of the sciatic nerve. This approach is a common one for posterior column injuries, posterior wall fractures, and transverse fractures. Patients can be positioned either prone or in the lateral decubitus position.

Most complex associated injuries and anterior injuries are approached anteriorly through an ilioinguinal or iliofemoral approach. The ilioinguinal approach is a complex one, which involves cutting through the lower abdominal wall proximal to the inguinal ligament from the midline of the abdomen, coursing laterally to the pelvis. This approach isolates the femoral artery, vein, and nerve. These are large vessels with a potential for massive blood loss if iatrogenic injury occurs. The iliofemoral approach is more lateral than the ilioinguinal approach. Although it does not violate the abdominal wall and allows the surgeon to inspect the joint, it limits access to the inside of the pelvis and the superior ramus. The iliofemoral or ilioinguinal approaches are both performed with the patient in the supine position.

For more complex fractures or fractures treated on a delayed basis, more extensive approaches to the acetabulum are used. These include the extended iliofemoral approach and the modified extended iliofemoral approach. Both approaches expose the inside and outside of the pelvis. They are usually reserved for the most

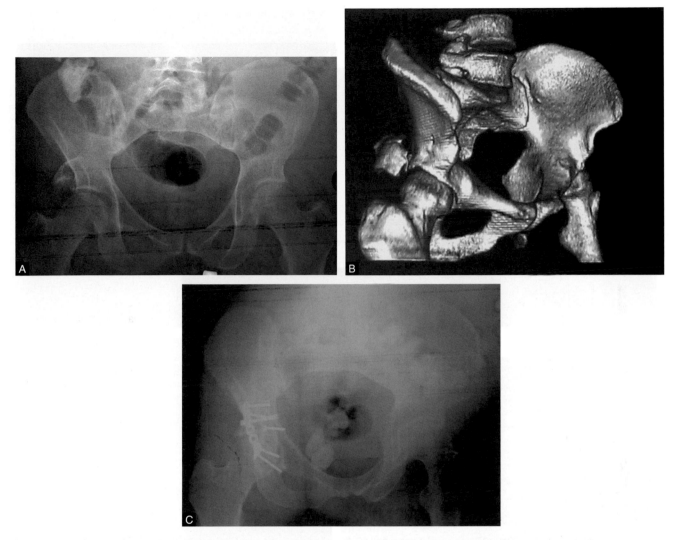

Figure 16-4. This is an AP pelvic x-ray of a 41-year-old man who struck his knee against the dashboard of his car in an automobile accident (Fig. 16-4*A*). The patient sustained a posterior wall acetabular fracture, best visualized on an obturator oblique three-dimensional reconstructed CT image (Fig. 16-4*B*). This fracture is best treated through an open posterior approach and secured with a plate-and-screw internal fixation configuration (Fig. 16-4*C*).

difficult fracture patterns in younger patients, which involve both the front and back of the acetabulum, or fractures treated on a delayed basis. These approaches are associated with substantial blood loss and involve prolonged surgery.

As with any large orthopaedic operation, substantial complications occur. The incidence of iatrogenic nerve injuries has been reported to be as high as 30 percent, but in experienced hands is usually less than 10 percent. Most surgeons who treat fractures avoid regional anesthesia due to the suspicion that they increase nerve palsies. Infection rates vary between 1 and 5 percent and are more common in multiply injured patients. There have been reports of catastrophic complications from femoral artery thrombosis with ilioinguinal approaches,

but these are rare. However, such cases must be monitored closely postoperatively. Deep venous thromboses occur, but when patients are treated with anticoagulants, symptomatic pulmonary emboli are rare.

Anesthetic Considerations

There are several technical considerations that need to be discussed between the orthopaedic surgeon and anesthesiologist. The reduction of acetabular fractures is visualized with fluoroscopy. Pelvic fluoroscopy gives poor results when there is contrast material in the bladder or colon or with excessive bowel gas. The use of nitrous oxide as part of the anesthetic causes a substantial amount of bowel gas, which compromises fluoroscopic visualization of fracture reduction and hardware placement.

full weight bearing. These patients are mobilized as soon as possible to avoid the complications of recumbency, including deep venous thrombosis, skin ulcers, and pneumonia. They are usually anticoagulated unless they have a medical contraindication.

Anesthetic Considerations

The main anesthetic considerations are dictated by the patient's medical comorbidities. Hip fracture surgery is not typically associated with prolonged surgical times or substantial blood loss, but patients usually have multiple medical problems. Eiskjaer et al. demonstrated improved outcomes in patients who had optimization of medical comorbidities preoperatively, usually under the direction of an internist (Eiskjaer 1991). Communication among the surgeon, internist, and anesthesiologist is of utmost importance in these cases. Hip fracture surgery can be successfully accomplished under regional anesthesia. Attention must be paid to pulmonary function under several circumstances. Intramedullary fixation for intertrochanteric fractures has been theorized to produce fat emboli during reaming and insertion of the intramedullary nail. Likewise, fat emboli occur during pressurization of the bone cement used during hemiarthroplasty.

One anesthetic technique that has proven satisfactory is to do a continuous femoral nerve block (with tunneling of the catheter toward the abdomen so as not to interfere with the surgical site) as soon as possible. This provides analgesia for most of the femur and the patient can then be transported comfortably to and from the radiology department, onto x-ray tables, and so on and prepared for surgery. In the operating room, after placement of monitoring, the patient can be positioned in the lateral decubitus position with the side of the fracture down (which does not cause pain because the nerve supply to the femur has been blocked) and a unilateral subarachnoid block can be done using 1 mL of 0.75% "heavy" bupivacaine (see Chap. 30). The patient is kept in the lateral decubitus position for 10 to 20 min to allow the unilateral spinal subarachnoid block to fix. This technique has no or very few hemodynamic implications and almost any patient, regardless of physical condition, can be operated on with this anesthetic technique. Appropriate sedation should be used intraoperatively and the continuous femoral nerve block can be used postoperatively, depending on the patient's coagulation status and the timing of thromboprophylactic drugs (see Chap. 4).

Femoral Fractures

Femoral fractures usually result from high-energy injuries, but they also occur as isolated fractures due to lower-energy forces (Fig. 16-8). They most frequently result from motor vehicle collisions or falls from heights and frequently cause multiple injuries (see Chap. 2). Because of the great forces involved, the patient's overall physiologic status often plays a substantial role in the management of the fracture.

Classification

Femoral fractures are best classified based on their longitudinal location. Fractures from the lesser trochanter to approximately 6 cm distal to it are subtrochanteric fractures. Extraarticular fractures from the diaphyseal-metaphyseal junction and distal to this point are distal femoral fractures. Fractures between these two points are diaphyseal fractures. Although the great majority of femoral fractures are treated with intramedullary nailing, surgical technique is affected by the longitudinal location of the fracture.

Treatment

Operative stabilization is the treatment of choice for nearly all femoral fractures. Because of the high incidence of associated fat embolism, femoral fractures should be fixed as early as possible (see Chap. 5). The vast majority of subtrochanteric fractures, diaphyseal femoral fractures, and distal femoral fractures are stabilized with intramedullary fixation. Intramedullary fixation nails can be inserted antegrade through the proximal femur or retrograde through the knee.

Antegrade nailing can be done utilizing different types of patient positioning. The patients are often placed on a fracture table with skeletal traction, usually applied through a proximal tibial traction pin. They are placed supine or in the lateral decubitus position. The majority of orthopaedic surgeons choose the supine position because of its familiarity; however, lateral decubitus positioning offers advantages, particularly with subtrochanteric fractures and in obese patients. Anterograde nailing is the treatment of choice for subtrochanteric fractures and is also excellent treatment for diaphyseal fractures and distal femoral fractures. Closed reduction is performed using the fracture table prior to skin preparation and confirmed fluoroscopically. When the nail is in the proper position, crosslock screws are secured through the bone and nailed to prevent any twisting deformities of the leg postoperatively.

Retrograde nailing has gained popularity over the past decade, with increasing evidence that it causes minimal clinical problems in the knee. The distal femur is opened through the knee joint, either by an arthrotomy or small incision through the patellar tendon, and the nail is inserted from distal to proximal. Patients are positioned supine on a radiolucent table and are not placed in skeletal traction. This positioning makes retrograde nailing particularly appropriate in patients who have multiple orthopaedic injuries that are being operated on simultaneously. Retrograde nailing is also indicated in patients with ipsilateral pelvic trauma and is frequently technically easier in obese patients.

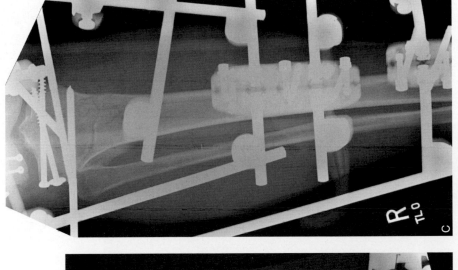

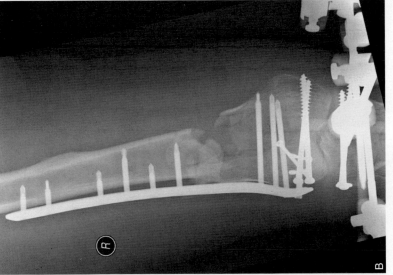

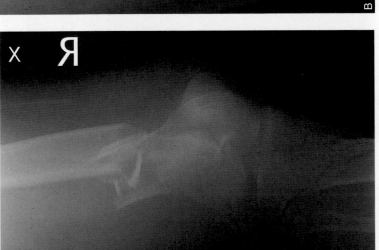

Figure 16-8. Intraarticular fractures of the knee are usually treated with open reduction and internal fixation. This 19-year-old man was involved in a motorcycle accident, sustaining an intraarticular fracture of his distal femur and proximal tibia (Fig. 16–8A). He had compartment syndromes of both his thigh and leg and was initially treated with fasciotomies and spanning external fixation. He returned to the operating room and underwent internal fixation of the distal femoral fracture and both internal and external fixation of the tibial plateau fracture (Figs. 16-8B and C). Four months later, both fractures had healed, but the patient has a substantial defect in his distal femur (arrow)(Figs. 16-8D and E).

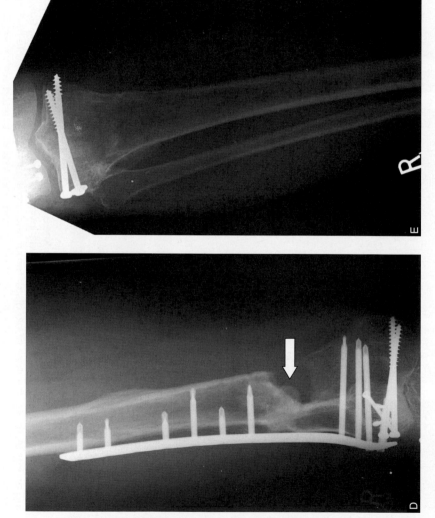

Figure 16-8. (*Continued*)

Most patients with intramedullary fixation can be mobilized with full weight bearing. Multiply injured patients will be given some form of prophylaxis for venous thrombosis, but it is debatable whether patients with isolated femoral fractures who start moving soon after surgery need antithrombotic prophylaxis.

Anesthetic Considerations

Patients who have sustained femoral fractures frequently have multiple injuries; in such cases a team is necessary to treat the patient properly. Particular care must be taken with chest-injured patients. These patients benefit from early stabilization of their fracture (within 24 h), but a small number may develop severe pulmonary complications and multiple organ failure when immediate intramedullary stabilization is done. A number of patients also have associated fat embolism; the earliest sign of this may be petechiae in the axilla and inner upper arm. This should warn the anesthesiologist of early fat embolism and an unstable intraoperative course (see Chap. 5).

The concept of damage-control orthopaedics has been proposed for multiply injured patients with femoral fractures. The fractures in these patients are initially stabilized with external fixation, which is exchanged for intramedullary fixation 5 to 7 days later. It has been hypothesized that fat emboli produced during canal reaming and nail insertion cause pulmonary complications. The anesthesiologist must pay particular attention to the patient during these parts of the procedure. In chest-injured patients, a lateral decubitus position can be potentially hazardous if an injured lung is in the dependent position. This creates substantial ventilation/perfusion mismatches, and chest-injured patients are therefore placed in the supine position when a fracture is fixed with nailing.

The reduction of femoral fractures, especially without skeletal traction, can be particularly difficult. Full neuromuscular paralysis greatly facilitates reduction. Because reduction maneuvers can be sudden and sometimes "violent," a secure airway should be ensured before reduction is undertaken.

Intraarticular Fractures about the Knee

Intraarticular fractures about the knee are common injuries and are usually caused by high-impact motor vehicle accidents or falls (Fig. 16-8). These fractures include intraarticular distal femoral fractures and tibial plateau fractures and have a bimodal distribution. High-energy comminuted fractures result from vehicular trauma or falls from substantial heights. Low-energy fractures occur mostly in older patients, usually due to falls.

Classification

The most widely accepted classification of intraarticular fractures of the distal femur is that proposed by the Orthopaedic Trauma Association. Type B fractures are unicondylar and type C fractures affect both condyles. However, these fractures are better described by the amount of articular surface comminution, articular surface displacement, and metaphyseal comminution above the articular surface. These anatomic features are important in deciding on surgical technique.

Tibial plateau fractures are commonly classified by the system of Schatzker. However, their anatomic features describe these fractures better. It is important to determine whether the fracture is limited to the medial or lateral plateau, or involves both sides of the proximal tibia. The amount of articular surface comminution, articular surface displacement, and comminution between the articular segments and the proximal tibia are also important features that guide treatment. The most common tibial plateau fracture is a low-energy fracture of the lateral plateau resulting from a fall in an elderly patient. However, high-energy, bicondylar fractures are also common and among the most difficult to treat.

Treatment

Intraarticular fractures of the knee invariably present with pain and swelling. It is important to determine the mechanism of injury. Knee injuries resulting from small forces (falls) are usually isolated, in contrast to those resulting from vehicular trauma, which are frequently accompanied by other injuries. The extremity must be thoroughly inspected for any breaks in the skin, which likely represent an open fracture. It is also important to address the vascular status, especially in high-energy injuries.

Proximal tibial fractures are particularly prone to develop compartment syndromes. This is particularly true in patients who sustain "bumper injuries" from being struck by a car. The hallmark signs of compartment syndrome—including a tense leg, progressive pain, and pain with passive stretch of the compartment—must be thoroughly investigated in these patients.

The majority of intraarticular distal femoral fractures are treated with operative reduction and fixation. Surgery is usually aimed toward securing an anatomic reduction of the articular surface and stabilizing the articular segment to the shaft of the femur in proper alignment. With recent improvements in technique and fluoroscopy, the majority of these fractures are treated through limited approaches. Patients are placed supine on a radiolucent table, and a limited approach to the articular portion of the fracture is made through an anterior or anterolateral incision. This articular reduction is usually secured with screws. The articular segment is then realigned with the distal femoral shaft and secured with internal fixation, using either a plate or intramedullary nail. There is usually an 8- to 12-week period of limited weight bearing; however, patients are encouraged to begin knee motion immediately.

Fractures of the tibial plateau are frequently treated with operative reduction and fixation (Fig. 16-8). In selected elderly patients with well-aligned stable joints, nonoperative treatment is very successful. In younger patients, patients with gross deformity of the articular surface, or those with knee instability, operative reduction and fixation are the preferred treatment. In fractures with modest articular comminution and displacement, open reduction and internal fixation are the most common treatment. Patients are placed supine on a radiolucent operating table and the fracture is approached through a single anterior incision or an incision directly over the fracture. Some bicondylar tibial plateau fractures are approached by a two-incision technique. Reduced articular fragments are secured with screws and the articular segment is stabilized to the tibial shaft, usually with some type of plate fixation.

As techniques have improved, limited approaches have become more effective in treating tibial plateau fractures. The articular surface is reduced and secured through percutaneous incisions, and the articular segment is stabilized to the tibial shaft with percutaneously placed plates or external fixation. There is usually an 8- to 12-week period of limited weight bearing; however, patients are encouraged to begin knee motion immediately.

Anesthetic Considerations

As with any fracture, the forces required to reduce intraarticular fractures around the knee are substantial. This is particularly true in femoral fractures. Full muscular paralysis is a tremendous benefit for patients in these operations. Postoperative pain is severe, and a regional pain catheter is beneficial for patients with distal femoral fractures. However, compartment syndromes occur in fractures of the tibial plateau. Therefore regional anesthesia may be contraindicated during the postoperative period in these patients to avoid masking the progressive pain associated with a compartment syndrome, which serves as an indicator of is development.

Tibial Fractures

Tibial fractures are among the most common fractures in orthopaedic surgery. They result from both low- and high-energy mechanisms. High-energy open tibial fractures are among the most difficult orthopaedic injuries to treat successfully. Higher-energy tibial fractures are often encountered in multiply injured patients, and a team approach utilizing general surgery, orthopaedic surgery, and anesthesiology is important in managing these patients successfully.

Classification

There is no effective classification of tibial fractures. These are individual injuries with individual characteristics that

must be respected; the type of bone and soft tissue injury better describes them. The bone injury is described by the location of the fracture in the bone, whether it is segmental, the amount of comminution, and the degree of deformity. The soft tissue injury describes whether the fracture is open or closed, involves crushing, or is prohibitively swollen. Compartment syndromes are common sequelae of tibial fractures and require immediate fasciotomy to avoid muscle necrosis and consequently the need for amputation.

Treatment

Tibial fractures can frequently be successfully treated by closed reduction and casts provided that adequate limb length and alignment can be maintained in a long leg cast. For closed fractures with unacceptable deformity, the mainstay of treatment is intramedullary nailing. This is usually performed on a radiolucent operating table with the patient in the supine position. Alternatively, patients can be placed supine on a fracture table with traction exerted with a traction pin through the calcaneus. Intramedullary fixation nails are uniformly inserted through a small incision around the knee.

Open tibial fractures are treated with surgical debridement followed by stabilization. Lower-grade open fractures without substantial contamination can be treated definitively with intramedullary fixation at the time of injury. Higher-grade and grossly contaminated fractures are aggressively debrided and stabilized with an external fixator. Serial debridements are done until the wound can be safely closed. Closure is achieved primarily or with muscle flaps to cover the fracture in more severe open fractures. Rotational flaps of the gastrocnemius or soleus muscles are usually used to cover proximal and midshaft fractures. Distal fractures, requiring soft tissue coverage, are covered by free muscle transfer, usually by a latissimus dorsi or serratus anterior muscle flap. At the time of wound closure, definitive fixation is performed. Some of these fractures are treated definitively with an external fixator, but the majority are treated by removing the external fixator and performing intramedullary nailing.

Anesthetic Considerations

High-energy tibial fractures are frequently part of multiple injuries (see Chap. 2). Physicians must be aware of the patient's hemodynamic status, because severe open tibial fractures can cause severe intraoperative blood loss. Patients with crush injuries can develop high serum potassium and creatinine kinase levels and must be monitored for cardiac disturbances.

Compartment syndromes occur frequently in patients with tibial fractures. They are most common in high-energy closed proximal tibial fractures but can occur in any tibial fracture, including open fractures. Patients should not have regional anesthesia because it masks the severe pain that is the most characteristic symptom of a developing compartment syndrome. This applies to patients both before and after surgery, because a substantial number of compartment syndromes occur after surgery.

Ankle Fractures

Ankle fractures are among the most common injuries treated by orthopaedic surgeons (Fig. 16-9). They encompass a wide population, from young, active people to geriatric patients. Ankle fracture surgery is designed to restore a properly aligned and stable articulation between the talus and the distal tibia. This is achieved by reconstituting the proper length and rotation of the fibula and continuity of the medial structures that support the ankle.

Classification

There are several common classifications for ankle fractures. Most orthopaedic surgeons generally categorize them into fractures that involve the lateral malleolus, the medial malleolus, or both. The Weber classification divides injuries according to the level of the fibular fracture into three categories: A, B, and C. Weber A fractures are fibular fractures below the ankle joint. They are generally stable and do not require operative treatment. Weber type B

fractures extend from the level of the ankle joint to several centimeters proximal to the ankle. Displaced Weber B injuries usually benefit from fibular reduction and fixation. Weber C fibular fractures are 4 cm or more above the ankle joint. These injuries predictably disrupt the articulation between the distal fibula and tibia; therefore fixation between these two bones will often be required.

Another common classification of ankle fractures was proposed by Lauge-Hansen. Their description takes into account fracture mechanism and foot position at the time of injury. Fracture patterns described by this system include injuries called supination–external rotation injuries, supination adduction injuries, pronation–external rotation injuries, and pronation-abduction injuries.

Treatment

The goal in treating any ankle fracture is to reduce the talus securely into its proper relation with the distal tibia to provide stable articulation. In patients with minimally displaced fibular fractures without a shift of the talus, this can be done with closed treatment and casting.

In patients with displaced fractures and subluxation of the talus, open reduction with internal fixation is usually the treatment of choice. Fixation of the medial

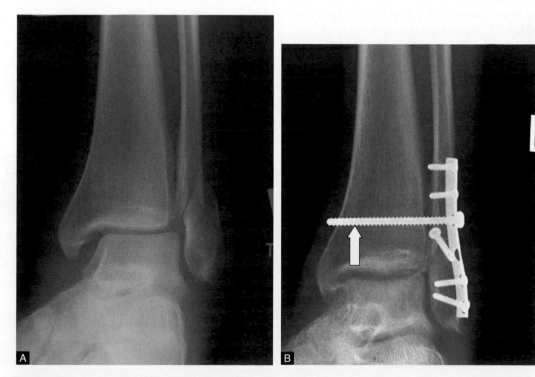

Figure 16-9. Rotational ankle fractures result in displacement of the talus from its normal alignment with the distal tibia (Fig. 16-9*A*). These fractures are best treated by open reduction and internal fixation to restore the normal relationship between the talus and the distal tibia (Fig. 16-9*B*). If the supporting syndesmotic ligaments that bind the distal tibia and fibula together are disrupted, the two bones are secured with a screw (arrow).

or lateral malleolus is most commonly achieved with direct approaches to the fracture site and internal fixation. The distal fibula is frequently secured with a small plate and screws, while the medial malleolus is often internally fixed with screws alone. After adequate fixation of the fractures is achieved, the stability of the articulation between the distal fibula and tibia is assessed. Normally, the two bones are held tightly together at the ankle joint by multiple ligaments called the ankle syndesmosis. Disruption of the syndesmosis creates an unstable articulation between the talus and the distal tibia, which has been shown to create abnormal stresses across the ankle joint and predictably will cause ankle arthritis. In syndesmotic injury, therefore, the tibia and fibula at the ankle joint are reduced back into their proper articulation and secured to each other with one or two screws.

Patients are typically splinted or casted soon after surgery. After a modest period of protected weight bearing, patients are allowed to progress in their weight bearing while also working on range-of-motion and rehabilitation exercises.

Anesthetic Considerations

The force required to reduce bone displacements is substantially decreased by muscular paralysis. Complete muscle paralysis therefore aids in restoring the length of a fractured fibula; this is particularly helpful in fractures that are several weeks old. Ankle fractures are frequently too swollen for immediate surgery, which will be postponed from 2 to 4 weeks. Complications such as compartment syndrome and nerve injury are rarely associated with ankle fractures; regional anesthetics are therefore good options in these patients.

Open Fractures

Open fractures comprise any injury in which a fractured bone is exposed by a wound or by piercing of the skin. These fractures encompass a wide magnitude of injuries and in general are orthopaedic emergencies. Prompt treatment is important to avoid infections or amputations and to ensure the best outcome.

Classification

The most widely used system to classify open fractures is that of Gustillo and Anderson. Their classification evolved from retrospective and prospective studies of over 1000 open fractures. They classified open fractures into types I, II, and III injuries. Type III injuries were further divided based on injury severity and vascular status.

Type I open fractures result from lower-energy injuries and present as small wounds that are not grossly contaminated. These are typically "inside-out" types of injuries where an indirect force that caused the fracture also forced the bone through the skin. By definition, the laceration is 1 cm or less in length.

Type II open fractures are typically low- to moderate-energy injuries. These wounds are less than 10 cm long and are not grossly contaminated or crushed. Type II open fractures are related more closely to type I wounds than to type III wounds. They are best thought of as low- to moderate-energy injuries in which the laceration is simply more extensive than in those with type I small puncture wounds.

Type III open fractures result from high-energy injuries that cause larger, grossly contaminated open wounds, moderate to severe bone comminution, and crushed limbs (Fig. 16-10). These are immediate limb-threatening injuries. Open fractures that are grossly

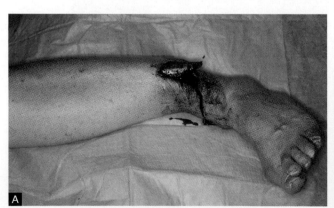
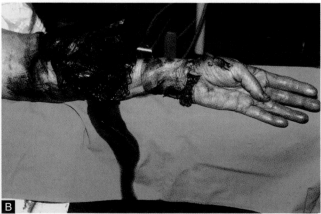

Figure 16-10. Open fractures come in different shapes and sizes. Types I and II are often inside-out wounds, as in this 23-year-old woman who was injured in an automobile accident (Fig. 16-10A). In contrast, type III open fractures are usually high-energy direct blows that can crush tissue, as depicted in this 75-year-old woman who was injured in a tornado (Fig. 16-10B).

contaminated are also considered type III open fractures regardless of wound size, comminution, or crushing. These may result from injuries in a farmyard or during submersion under water. Type III open fractures are further subdivided into IIIA, IIIB, and IIIC injuries. Type IIIA open fractures represent high-energy injuries that do not require rotational muscle flaps or free soft tissue transfer to cover the fracture. Type IIIB open fractures are more extensive than type IIIA open fractures, and these injuries cause tissue loss requiring some type of rotational muscle flap or free tissue transfer to cover the wound. Type IIIC open fractures comprise any type of open fracture in which the limb has been rendered dysvascular by an arterial disruption. Complications such as infection and amputation increase dramatically with type IIIB and IIIC open fractures.

Treatment

The treatment of open fractures includes aggressive debridement of crushed, nonviable, or grossly contaminated tissue, fracture stabilization, and prophylactic antibiotics. Many patients have sustained high-energy injuries and associated intraabdominal, intracranial, or intrathoracic injuries.

Antibiotics should be started immediately on presentation to the emergency department, and all patients should receive antitetanus injections. All patients with open fractures should be given a first-generation cephalosporin. Patients with type III open fractures with crushed tissue should have an aminoglycoside added to the antibiotic regimen to cover against gram-negative infection. Patients with grossly contaminated wounds should also have coverage against anaerobic organisms, therefore receiving triple antibiotics. Gross contamination should be crudely debrided and irrigated in the emergency room. All fractures should be splinted or placed in traction with povidone-iodine (Betadine)–soaked dressings.

Surgical debridement and stabilization should then proceed on an emergency basis. Patients should be taken to the operating room as soon as it is physiologically safe to proceed with surgery. The hallmark of surgical treatment is complete debridement of the entire zone of injury. Type I and II open injuries can often be treated definitively and safely in the first operation. After thorough debridement, definitive internal fixation such as intramedullary nailing or plate-and-screw fixation can proceed immediately, with predictably good results. Type III open fractures, especially those with crushed or grossly contaminated tissue, usually requires serial debridements. These fractures are usually stabilized with some sort of external fixation at the initial debridement. External fixation can be definitive, but it is frequently exchanged for internal fixation when the surgeon has decided that it is safe to close the wound.

Anesthetic Considerations

Open fractures frequently accompany immediately life-threatening injuries, which obviously require treatment before the fracture does. Decisive communication among the general surgeon, orthopaedic surgeon, and anesthesiologist is mandatory to optimize the treatment of these patients. These patients have frequently lost much blood, and the surgical team must be prepared to administer large blood transfusions (see Chap. 2). The physicians must also be prepared to treat the consequences of massive blood loss, massive blood transfusions, and crushed tissue (see Chap. 2). Blood potassium levels can increase rapidly, disturbing cardiac rhythm and increasing creatinine kinase levels, which can cause acute renal failure. Patients can also quickly develop a hypocoagulopathy.

Patients with type III injuries will require frequent dressing changes after the operation, especially in cases of contaminated wounds and type IIIB wounds. Because dressing changes are frequent and painful, pain control becomes very important. Indwelling regional catheters can greatly decrease pain in these patients, particularly during dressing changes (see Chaps. 20 and 21). These patients usually make multiple trips to the operating room. Communication between the surgeon and the anesthesia team can minimize the number of anesthetics that patients are subjected to during this acute injury phase.

Compartment Syndrome

Compartment syndromes occur when excessive pressure develops within a closed fascial compartment, rendering the tissue within the affected compartment ischemic. Orthopaedic compartment syndromes occur in the upper extremities, lower extremities, and the gluteal region. These syndromes have multiple causes, but they are most commonly due to trauma and fractures. Aggressive emergency treatment is essential to prevent the loss of a limb.

Etiology

The most common cause of compartment syndromes is a fracture. They are often caused by higher-energy closed fractures but can also occur with lower-energy forces and in open fractures. There is often a history of direct blunt injury to the limb, as when a tibia is struck by the bumper of a car. They occur most commonly with closed tibial fractures and are particularly common in proximal tibia fractures.

Vascular injuries can also lead to compartment syndromes. Arterial bleeding within a closed compartment can rapidly cause excessive intracompartmental pressure. Alternatively, reperfusion after prolonged ischemia can cause excessive swelling, leading to a compartment syndrome. This typically occurs after a revascularization procedure. Compartment syndromes can also result from external causes, such as casts, constrictive dressings, or "antishock" lower extremity garments. They have also been reported in patients subjected to prolonged lithotomy positioning in obstetric and urologic reconstructive operations.

Pathophysiology

The final common physiologic mechanism is excessive intracompartmental pressure, which compromises perfusion and causes microcirculatory failure in the tissues of the compartment. As the intracompartmental pressure rises, it eventually exceeds the arteriolar pressure, causing a rapid failure of the local capillary anastomoses and loss of blood flow to the tissues. Excessive pressure also inhibits venous return, further blocking blood flow within the compartment.

Tissue damage depends on the duration of the compartment syndrome. Muscle tissue can usually survive 4 h of ischemia, but more than 8 h of ischemia causes irreversible damage. Peripheral nerves will continue to conduct normally for up to 1 h of complete ischemia and will survive without injury when subjected to 4 h of ischemia; however, they will be irreversibly damaged after 8 h.

Diagnosis

The characteristic symptom of compartment syndrome is progressive, unrelenting pain. These patients frequently report severe increases of pain with a fairly rapid onset. This is mainly a clinical diagnosis, especially in patients at risk. The leg is firm and often shiny. The earliest and most reliable physical sign is severe exacerbation of tenderness of the affected compartment by manual compression of the compartment or passive stretching of the muscles within the compartment. A gentle squeeze of the calf or passive flexing of the toes or ankle is excruciatingly painful to these patients.

Because compartment syndrome is a microcirculatory failure, the peripheral pulses are usually intact. This is in direct contrast to an acute arterial thrombosis. The misconception that the legs of patients with compartment syndrome are pulseless needs to be corrected. The pulses are often bounding, and only very late in a compartment syndrome, when pressures are dramatically elevated, does the affected extremity become pulseless. Owing to increased perfusion to the subcutaneous tissues surrounding the compartment, the leg is pink and shiny, in contrast to a mottled, pale extremity seen in cases of arterial thrombosis. Early in a compartment syndrome, the peripheral nerves function normally. It is not until the compartment syndrome has advanced that patients complain of tingling and numbness. Finally, in advanced cases, the limb becomes paralyzed.

In an alert patient with a firm, painful leg that becomes more painful with gentle passive stretching, the diagnosis should be made immediately and emergency fasciotomies be performed. In less obvious cases, compartment pressures can be measured. There are several commercial pressure transducers that measure intracompartmental pressure; an arterial line pressure transducer works just as well. There is debate as to what pressure constitutes a compartment syndrome. Several authors have advocated fasciotomy when intracompartmental pressure is greater than 30 mmHg. Others have recommended a threshold of 45 mmHg, with close monitoring of patients with pressures between 30 and 45 mmHg. In a prospective study of 116 patients, those with intracompartmental pressures below 45 mmHg and a differential pressure greater than 30 mmHg (diastolic pressure minus compartment pressure) all had excellent outcomes without fasciotomies.

One note of caution should be emphasized. Commercially available catheters and arterial pressure transducers are very sensitive to technique. Readings often drift substantially after the transducer is inserted into the compartment, making it difficult to determine the true intracompartmental pressure. Precise history and close, serial physical examinations of patients who are at risk are therefore essential. Particular attention must be paid to multiply injured patients or any patient who cannot communicate.

The hallmark symptom of this syndrome is unrelenting pain; it is therefore important to lower the threshold pressure that indicates the necessity for fasciotomy when patients cannot express their pain.

Treatment

Once the diagnosis of compartment syndrome is established, the affected compartments should be decompressed immediately. Delay is unacceptable because a devastating necrosis of the muscles and permanent damage to the nerves will ensue if 8 h or more elapse after the onset of the syndrome. Most nerve blocks last 8 h or longer and will mask this important symptom. Nerve blocks are therefore absolutely contraindicated if there is any risk of compartment syndrome.

Fasciotomies within 4 h of the development of a compartment syndrome usually have excellent outcomes (Fig. 16-11). A problem arises when a compartment syndrome is suspected to have been missed. Delayed fasciotomies may open a compartment full of necrotic muscle tissue and result in infection, often necessitating amputation. Although there are some disagreements, the general consensus is that limbs with missed compartment syndromes should not be opened.

The most common compartment syndromes are those in the leg and forearm. The patients are placed supine on an operating table. Regional anesthetics or peripheral nerve blocks must be avoided in these patients. Pressure in the four compartments of the leg—including the anterior, lateral, superficial posterior, and deep posterior parts—must be released along their entire length. Leg compartment syndrome pressures can be released through one or two incisions. Limited incision fasciotomies are dangerous, because failure to release the skin fails to manage the underlying problem

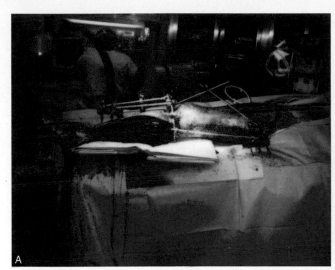

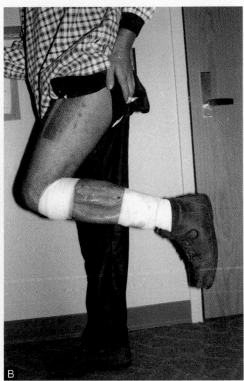

Figure 16-11. Compartment syndromes are immediate limb-threatening injuries. They require emergent fasciotomies to avoid limb amputation (Fig. 16-11A). The fractures are often temporarily spanned with external fixation (Fig. 16-11A) and definitively fixed on a delayed basis. Prompt treatment can enable these patients to maintain excellent function (Fig. 16-11B).

and places the sural and superficial peroneal nerves at undue risk of surgical laceration. Pressure in forearm compartment syndromes is released with an extensive anterior approach to the forearm, which includes release of the volar fascia from the carpel tunnel distally to across the elbow proximally. Again, the incision should extend the full length to release the skin and the fascia should be opened under direct visualization. The opened tissues are irrigated and packed with moist dressings. Patients usually return to the operating room 3 to 5 days later for skin grafting or closure of the wounds.

Crush Injuries

Orthopaedic crush injuries are often associated with other life-threatening injuries (Fig. 16-12). They are usually the result of high-energy forces such as those that occur in motor vehicle collisions or the result of large structures falling onto and trapping people. The fractures are usually open and limb-threatening, but they can also occur as closed injuries. These injuries are frequently also life-threatening, and their prompt treatment may avoid death or amputation.

Diagnosis

The diagnosis of a crush injury is often obvious and is obtained by history and examination. Frequently, these patients are trapped in vehicles or by large objects that have fallen onto them. People trapped with an arm or leg held by a heavy weight are likely to have crush injuries. Although the superficial extent of a crush injury can easily be seen, the full and deeper extent of such an injury is not obvious. Cranial, thoracic, and abdominal injuries must be thoroughly investigated. Systemic manifestations of massive rhabdomyolysis, such as acute renal failure, should be anticipated (see Chap. 2).

The diagnosis of a closed crush injury in a limb is more difficult. It is important to know whether limbs have been trapped or caught under large heavy objects. It is also important to recognize that direct massive blows in and around the pelvic and gluteal region can cause internal crushing or degloving-type injuries. Such injuries frequently occur in motor vehicle accidents or when people fall from heights with severe direct blows to the pelvis or gluteal region. Patients with closed crushing injuries usually present with an insensate limb with massive tense swelling, which develops rapidly after the injury. It is important to distinguish this from a compartment syndrome,

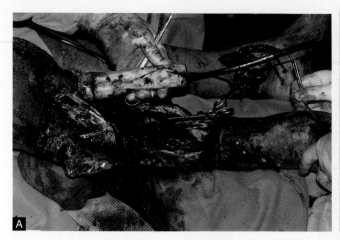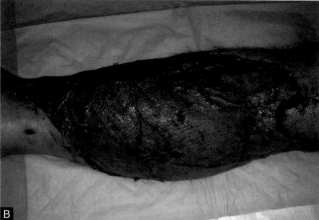

Figure 16-12. Crush injuries are limb-threatening (Fig. 16-12*A*). There is not only severe soft tissue injury but the bone is often also comminuted or missing. Frequently, these limbs are best treated with immediate amputation, but some may be salvaged. Limbs usually require soft tissue procedures for bone coverage, which often calls for transfer of a free muscle (Fig. 16-12*B*).

because myonecrosis has usually already occurred in crushing injuries and fasciotomies in such cases almost invariably lead to infections and amputations.

Treatment

Crushed limbs with open fractures require emergency treatment to try to save function in the limb and avoid amputation. Life-threatening injuries of the head, chest, or abdomen must be promptly addressed. However, a crushed open limb is itself a life-threatening injury that also needs to be treated immediately, especially in patients who are bleeding to death. Immediate amputation should be performed in life-threatening crush injuries with uncontrolled bleeding when the limb cannot be saved. Immediate amputation is also indicated when bone and soft tissue reconstruction cannot restore adequate function. This is especially true in cases of lower extremity injuries that include devastating injuries of the foot, in which a below-knee amputation can save part of the leg. Early amputation of a crushed upper extremity is much less desirable, because it is usually better to save any potential function of the hand than to resort to a prosthesis.

If the aim is to save a limb, the initial surgery is aimed at adequate debridement of all the tissue that is crushed and appears nonviable followed by skeletal stabilization. This is frequently accomplished by external fixation, often of adjacent joints. These operations are usually associated with a large blood loss. Patients are typically placed supine on a radiolucent operating table with widely prepped fields. The surgeon must be careful to expose the entire zone of injury completely, because crushing injuries often extend far beyond the externally visible zone of injury. Patients should be started on antibiotics to cover not only gram-positive bacteria but also gram-negative and anaerobic bacteria. Usually a first generation cephalosporin, an aminoglycoside, and antibiotics such as penicillin or clindamycin are given immediately (see Chap. 3). However, caution must be used in administering an aminoglycoside due to its nephrotoxicity. These patients often have massive rhabdomyolysis, which can cause kidney failure and in turn can be severely exacerbated by an aminoglycoside antibiotic.

Patients usually require multiple debridements and dressing changes. Analgesia with indwelling epidural or peripheral nerve block catheters can be extremely beneficial in these patients, not only to provide anesthesia and analgesia but also to improve blood flow by the resultant sympathectomy. Patients will return to surgery at 24- to 48-h intervals until all crushed tissue has been removed and the extremity has a clean bed of tissue with the ability to heal. The next step in their treatment is wound coverage. Depending on the extent of tissue loss, this is achieved by the simplest measures possible. In some cases, skin grafts are adequate. However, rotational muscle flaps or free tissue transfer is often necessary. Definitive skeletal stabilization is done concurrently with or before definitive wound coverage. Depending on the severity of the injury and the fracture characteristics, definitive stabilization can be external or internal fixation. Wound coverage must be done before or concurrently with internal fixation so as to avoid infection.

SUGGESTED FURTHER READING

Bone LB, Johnson KD, Weigelt J, et al. Early versus delayed stabilization of femoral fractures. A prospective randomized study. *J Bone Joint Surg Am* 71:336–340, 1989.

Burgess AR, Eastridge BJ, Young JW, et al. Pelvic ring disruptions: Effective classification system and treatment protocols. *J Trauma* 30:848–856, 1990.

Dalal SA, Burgess AR, Siegel JH, et al. Pelvic fracture in multiple trauma: Classification by mechanism is key to pattern of organ injury, resuscitative requirements, and outcome. *J Trauma* 29:981–1000; discussion 1000–1002, 1989.

Eiskjaer S, Ostgard SE. Risk factors influencing mortality after bipolar hemiarthroplasty in the treatment of fracture of the femoral neck. *Clin Orthop Rel Res* 270:295–300, 1991.

Garden RS. Malreduction and avascular necrosis in subcapital fractures of the femur. *J Bone Joint Surg Br* 53:183–197, 1971.

Gustilo RB, Anderson JT. Prevention of infection in the treatment of one thousand and twenty-five open fractures of long bones: Retrospective and prospective analyses. *J Bone Joint Surg Am* 58:453–458, 1976.

Lauge-Hansen N. Fractures of the ankle II: Combined experimental-surgical and experimental-roentgenologic investigation. *Arch Surg* 60:957, 1950.

Letournel E. Acetabulum fractures: Classification and management. *Clin Orthop Rel Res* 151:81–106, 1980.

Mason M. Some observations on fractures of the head of the radius with review of one hundred cases. *Br J Surg* 42:123–132, 1954.

Matta JM. Fractures of the acetabulum: Accuracy of reduction and clinical results in patients managed operatively within three weeks after the injury. *J Bone Joint Surg Am* 78:1632–1645, 1996.

McQueen MM, Court-Brown CM. Compartment monitoring in tibial fractures. The pressure threshold for decompression. *J Bone Joint Surg Br* 78:99–104, 1996.

Neer CS. Displaced proximal humeral fractures. I. Classification and evaluation. *J Bone Joint Surg Am* 52:1077–1089, 1970.

Pape HC, Auf'm'Kolk M, Paffrath T, et al. Primary intramedullary femur fixation in multiple trauma patients with associated lung contusion—A cause of posttraumatic ARDS? *J Trauma* 34:540–547; discussion 547–548, 1993.

Pape HC, Hildebrand F, Pertschy S, et al. Changes in the management of femoral shaft fractures in polytrauma patients: From early total care to damage control orthopedic surgery. *J Trauma* 53:452–461; discussion 461–462, 2002.

Young JW, Burgess AR, Brumback RJ, et al. Pelvic fractures: Value of plain radiography in early assessment and management. *Radiology* 160:445–451, 1986.

Zuckerman JD, Skovron ML, Koval KJ, et al. Postoperative complications and mortality associated with operative delay in older patients who have a fracture of the hip. *J Bone Joint Surg Am* 77:1551–1556, 1995.

CHAPTER 17

Sports Injuries to the Shoulder, Knee, and Ankle

MORGAN H. JONES/BRIAN R. WOLF/ANNUNZIATO (NED) AMENDOLA/
G. MICHAEL BLANCHARD, JR./ANDRÉ P. BOEZAART

▶ INTRODUCTION

In this chapter common sports injuries to the shoulder, knee, and ankle are discussed. Other joints are also affected by sports injuries, but these three joints are especially affected, and each joint is discussed separately. Injuries and conditions of these joints not related to sports are dealt with separately; the reader is encouraged to refer to these chapters as well (Chaps. 7, 11, and 12).

▶ SPORTS INJURIES TO THE SHOULDER JOINT

Biomechanics

The shoulder is a unique joint owing to its tremendous range of motion. Most shoulder problems can be subdivided into three categories: instability problems, rotator cuff disease, and arthritis. The glenohumeral joint has minimal bony constraint because of the relatively small and shallow nature of the glenoid in relation to the humeral head. This minimal bony constraint allows a wide arc of movement but also makes the shoulder susceptible to instability problems, which may be traumatic or atraumatic in nature. Shoulder instability is most frequently encountered in younger patients. Stability to the shoulder is provided by static restraints such as the labrum, capsule, and glenohumeral ligaments. The primary glenohumeral ligaments are thickenings of the capsule as opposed to clearly discrete structures. Dynamic

stability is provided to the shoulder by the rotator cuff, long head of the biceps tendon, and periscapular muscles. Shoulder instability can be anterior, inferior, posterior, or in multiple directions.

Pathophysiology of Shoulder Instability

The most common shoulder instability problem is anterior or anteroinferior shoulder instability resulting from a traumatic dislocation. During this traumatic event the anterior capsule and inferior glenohumeral ligament (IGHL) undergo stretch injury. The anteroinferior capsulolabral attachment to the glenoid can also be disrupted. This is called a Bankart or Perthes lesion (Fig. 17-1). The IGHL attaches to the glenoid in the region of this Bankart lesion. A substantial percentage of patients will suffer recurrent subluxation and dislocation of the shoulder following this initial event due to residual laxity in the capsule and the Bankart lesion. Posterior shoulder dislocation is less common. A reverse Bankart lesion can be present, with detachment of the posterior or posteroinferior capsulolabral complex. Surgical management in these patients is focused on direct repair of damaged structures and possibly some reduction in capsular volume.

A subset of patients suffer shoulder laxity that is intrinsic in nature and not secondary to overt trauma. This is often referred to as multidirectional instability. It is most frequently seen in patients in their second and third decades and can be aggravated by overhead arm movements or sports. This problem is secondary to an overall excessive capsular volume in the shoulder as

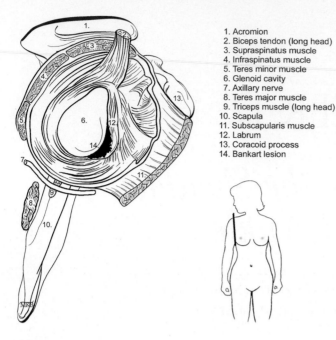

1. Acromion
2. Biceps tendon (long head)
3. Supraspinatus muscle
4. Infraspinatus muscle
5. Teres minor muscle
6. Glenoid cavity
7. Axillary nerve
8. Teres major muscle
9. Triceps muscle (long head)
10. Scapula
11. Subscapularis muscle
12. Labrum
13. Coracoid process
14. Bankart lesion

Figure 17-1. Bankart lesion.

opposed to a discrete tear or detachment. Surgical management in this subset of patients is not taken lightly and focuses on shifting the capsule to decrease the overall volume of the glenohumeral joint.

▶ OPERATIONS OF THE SHOULDER JOINT

Diagnostic Arthroscopy

Indications and Special Anatomic Considerations

Diagnostic arthroscopy of the shoulder is indicated for the symptomatic shoulder in which—after the history, physical examination, and appropriate imaging studies—the diagnosis is not clear, and when the symptoms do not respond to conservative treatment. In addition, arthroscopic treatment of shoulder disorders should always begin with a diagnostic arthroscopy. With all shoulder surgeries that involve arthroscopy, the bony landmarks of the shoulder are indicated with a surgical marker. This can be more difficult in very muscular or obese patients. The bony landmarks include the palpable acromion, acromioclavicular joint, distal clavicle, and coracoid process.

Patient Profile

Diagnostic shoulder arthroscopy is considered for patients of any age with persistent pain or disability of the shoulder. Patients presenting with sports injuries of the shoulder are usually young, healthy adults.

Positioning on the Operating Table

The patient may either be positioned in the "beach chair" position, or in the lateral decubitus position. During shoulder arthroscopy in the beach chair position, a mechanical arm holder, a Mayo stand table, or an assistant holds the arm to aid in positioning the shoulder. In the lateral decubitus position, the arm is subjected to approximately 15 lb of traction to maintain distraction of the joint, shoulder abduction, and slight forward flexion. During beach chair positioning, the head and airway can be at risk as traction is applied to the arm. Extreme care must be taken to secure the head and neck to prevent injury. This is less of a problem during lateral decubitus positioning because the arm is in a constant position.

Surgical Technique

A posterior viewing portal is placed through a puncture incision approximately 2 cm inferior and 1 cm medial to the posterolateral corner of the acromion. The joint is bluntly entered with an obturator and cannula, and the arthroscopic camera is inserted into the joint. Inflow of the lavage fluid is usually through the camera cannula. Some surgeons choose to mix a small quantity epinephrine with the arthroscopic lavage fluid to aid in hemostasis (see also Chap. 7 for control of the surgical field). The arthroscopic fluid may be infused using a pump or gravity.

An anterior working portal can then be established lateral to the coracoid process in the rotator interval between the supraspinatus and subscapularis tendons. Insertion of a spinal needle into the joint before making a puncture incision usually localizes the position of this portal. The joint is then bluntly entered with an obturator. A cannula is often used for this portal to maintain joint distention and easy access. Arthroscopy of the glenohumeral joint allows visualization of the articular surfaces of the humeral head and glenoid, the shoulder capsule and ligaments, the long head of the biceps, the glenoid labrum, and the articular surface of the rotator cuff.

After complete visualization of the glenohumeral joint, the subacromial region can also be viewed if the surgeon suspects pathology in this area. In this case each cannula is withdrawn from the joint and redirected into the subacromial space without removing the cannula from the skin. Often an additional portal is made directly lateral and inferior to the acromion, again using needle localization. Structures in the subacromial space are often difficult to see without using a shaver to resect bursal tissue, which can be thick or inflamed. Arthroscopy of the subacromial space allows visualization of the bursal surface of the rotator cuff, the undersurface of the acromion, the distal clavicle, and the acromioclavicular joint. Portals are closed with sutures.

Anesthetic Considerations
(See Also Chap. 7)

The surgery is frequently done with a nerve block as the sole anesthetic. For this purpose single-injection, interscalene block (ISB), or cervical paravertebral block (CPVB) is used (see Chap. 23). Keep in mind that the onset of CPVB can be substantially longer than that of interscalene block (30 to 45 min).

If general anesthesia is used, we typically place a single-injection nerve block before induction of anesthesia if indicated. Anesthesia is induced and maintained with propofol. If a nerve block is not used for intraoperative analgesia, we use remifentanil infusion intraoperatively and an opiate, such as morphine directly postoperatively.

Postoperative Analgesia

Please also refer to Chap. 7. Diagnostic shoulder arthroscopy is not typically painful and nothing but oral analgesics is required. If there is pain, it would be because of fluid extravasation and swelling and it is short-lived. A single-injection interscalene or cervical paravertebral block (see Chap. 23) is usually all that is required. Continuous nerve block is not indicated for diagnostic shoulder arthroscopy.

Associated Medications

One dose of preoperative antibiotics is given intravenously (see Chap. 3).

Postoperative Care

Diagnostic arthroscopy of the shoulder is usually performed as an outpatient procedure. The patient's arm is placed in a sling, and activity depends on the pathology identified and treated during the procedure. Patients are usually referred to physical therapy for rehabilitation postoperatively.

Arthroscopic Bankart
for Instability Repair

Indications and anatomic considerations

Arthroscopic instability repair is indicated for patients with persistent symptoms of pain, instability, or both, which are related to excessive shoulder laxity. These patients have usually undergone physical therapy and other nonoperative treatments. Surgery is performed to repair a detached capsulolabral structure, to tighten capsular laxity, or both (Fig. 17-1). Preoperatively, anatomic considerations include the direction of shoulder instability. Also, patients can develop bony abnormalities that affect the surgery, such as acute fracture or erosion of the

glenoid rim from dislocation and subluxation. Also, a Hill-Sachs lesion of varying size can be present (Fig. 17-2). This is an impaction fracture on the posterior aspect of the humeral head due to dislocations.

Patient Profile

Patients with shoulder instability are typically in their second to fourth decade and usually healthy and active in recreational activities and sports. These patients have often suffered a traumatic injury to the shoulder, such as a dislocation requiring reduction.

Special Biomechanics

Care is taken in positioning the shoulder during this procedure to avoid over- or undertightening. The patient may be placed in the beach chair position or in the lateral decubitus position.

Surgical Technique

Before preparing the shoulder for surgery, both shoulders should be examined under anesthesia to evaluate the degree of laxity. Routine shoulder arthroscopy is performed to evaluate for detachment of the labrum from the glenoid. A capsulolabral detachment at the anteroinferior aspect of the glenoid is often referred to as a Bankart lesion. If a Bankart lesion is identified, any fibrous tissue or damaged labrum that will not contribute to the repair is debrided using a shaver. The glenoid rim is abraded with the shaver or a burr so that blood reaches the repair site to promote healing.

Suture anchors are placed into the glenoid rim to secure the labrum. An accessory anterior or anterolateral portal must often be created to allow placement of these anchors. Once the anchors are placed, the sutures are passed through the labral tissue using arthroscopic penetrating and suture-passing devices. The sutures are then tied using arthroscopic knot-tying techniques.

If excessive laxity of the capsule is present, sutures can be placed into the capsule arthroscopically and then tied in order to fold over or imbricate the capsule and eliminate the laxity. This is referred to as capsular plication. Portals are closed with sutures.

Anesthetic Considerations
(Also Refer to Chap. 7)

Surgery for stabilization can be done with a nerve block as sole anesthetic, using an ISB or CPVB (see Chap. 23). If CPVB is used, the onset time for surgical anesthesia may be between 30 and 45 min.

We typically place a continuous ISB or CPVB before general anesthesia is induced and maintained with propofol. If a peripheral nerve block is not used for the management of intraoperative pain, we use a continuous infusion of remifentanil in combination with propofol. A

Arthroscopic Rotator Cuff Repair

Indications and Anatomic Considerations

Arthroscopic rotator cuff repair (ARCR) is indicated for patients with full-thickness rotator cuff tears or partial rotator cuff tears involving more than 50 percent of the thickness of the rotator cuff (Fig. 17-4). These patients experience pain, weakness, or both and usually have not benefited from treatments such as physical therapy, anti-inflammatory medications, and subacromial injection.

Patient Profile

Patients are typically in their fifth decade or beyond. There is an association between rotator cuff tear and cigarette smoking, with obvious anesthetic implications.

Positioning on the Operating Table

Patients are positioned for arthroscopy in the beach chair or lateral decubitus position.

Surgical Technique

Routine shoulder arthroscopy is performed. The glenohumeral joint and the articular surface of the rotator cuff are evaluated, and any damaged cuff tissue that will not contribute to the repair is debrided. The arthroscope is then placed into the subacromial space to inspect the bursal side of the rotator cuff. Subacromial decompression is performed with an acromioplasty if needed.

One or more accessory lateral portals are placed to facilitate mobilization and repair of the cuff. The cuff is often retracted after a tear and must be mobilized to allow repair of its anatomic insertion site on the greater tuberosity of the humerus. Releasing fibrotic tissue superiorly and inferiorly to the cuff with an arthroscopic shaver, elevator, or radiofrequency wand mobilizes the rotator cuff.

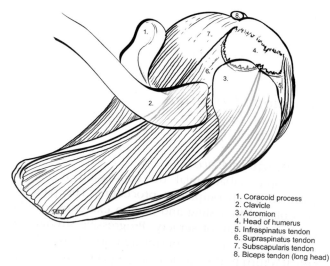

1. Coracoid process
2. Clavicle
3. Acromion
4. Head of humerus
5. Infraspinatus tendon
6. Supraspinatus tendon
7. Subscapularis tendon
8. Biceps tendon (long head)

Figure 17-4. Rotator cuff tear, viewed from above.

The insertion site is then debrided of fibrotic tissue to expose bleeding bone, which will promote healing of the repair.

When the cuff can be advanced to its insertion site, suture anchors are placed in the bone so that the cuff tissue can be secured. The sutures are then passed and the knots tied using arthroscopic techniques. A longitudinal split in the rotator cuff tendon can be closed using a technique called "margin convergence," in which one side of the tendon is sutured to the other. Once all the knots have been tied, the shoulder is moved through a full range of motion to ensure that the repair is secure.

Portals are left to close by secondary intention or are closed with sutures.

Anesthetic Considerations

Anesthetic considerations, control of bleeding in the surgical field, and postoperative pain control are the same as for arthroscopic Bankart repair, discussed above (see also Chap. 7). Rotator cuff repair is typically very painful and continuous peripheral nerve block is indicated for well into the postoperative period. We therefore place a CCPVB preoperatively (see Chap. 23), but a CISB is as effective and is widely used (see Chap. 23). The same applies here as is described for the open Bankart repair.

Associated Medications

One dose of preoperative antibiotics is given intravenously (see Chap. 3).

Postoperative Care

The arm is placed in a sling. Pendulum passive motion exercises are gradually instituted immediately after surgery. The patient then progresses to active-assisted and active range-of-motion exercises after 4 to 6 weeks. Progressive rotator cuff strengthening is started 6 to 8 weeks postoperatively. Patients may expect improved shoulder function and reduced pain after 4 to 12 months.

Mini-Open Rotator Cuff Repair

Indications and Anatomic Considerations

Open or mini-open rotator cuff repair is indicated for patients with full-thickness rotator cuff tears or partial tears that involve more than 50 percent of the thickness of the rotator cuff. The choice between an ARCR and a mini-open repair depends on the surgeon's preference, previous experience, and skills with arthroscopic surgery as well as the patient's previous surgical history. Mini-open treatment refers to repair of a rotator cuff tear through a 4- to 6-cm incision after an arthroscopy has been used to identify the tear and perform subacromial decompression if needed. Open rotator cuff repair is performed through a larger incision, usually without an initial arthroscopy.

Positioning on the Operating Table

The patient is positioned as for arthroscopy in the beach chair or lateral decubitus position. The arthroscopic and open parts of the operation can be performed in the beach chair position, but the open part of the procedure cannot be performed in the lateral decubitus position; the patient must therefore be repositioned after the arthroscopy. This repositioning may require reprepping and redraping of the patient.

Surgical Technique

A routine shoulder arthroscopy is performed. The glenohumeral joint and the articular surface of the rotator cuff are evaluated, and any damaged cuff tissue that will not contribute to the repair is debrided. The arthroscope is then placed into the subacromial space to inspect the bursal side of the rotator cuff. Subacromial decompression is performed if needed.

The location of the rotator cuff tear is determined, and a skin incision of approximately 5 cm is made in line with the deltoid muscle fibers beginning at the lateral edge of the acromion and extending distally. The deltoid fascia is exposed and incised, and the deltoid muscle is split in line with its fibers. Care must be taken to avoid splitting the deltoid more than 5 cm lateral to the acromion to prevent injury to the axillary nerve. The rotator cuff is exposed deep to the deltoid muscle. A part of the subdeltoid bursa must often be resected to expose the rotator cuff tendon.

A blunt instrument is used to dissect fibrous tissue superficially and deep to the rotator cuff to mobilize the tendon. The insertion site on the greater tuberosity is debrided of fibrous tissue to leave a bleeding bed of bone so as to promote healing. Once the tendon can be advanced to its insertion site, suture anchors or drill holes are placed in the bone so that the cuff tissue can be secured. The sutures are then placed into the rotator cuff tendon and tied. When all the knots have been tied, the shoulder is moved through a full range of motion to ensure that the repair is secure.

The subcutaneous tissues are closed with absorbable sutures and the skin is closed with an absorbable running subcuticular suture, interrupted skin sutures, or staples. Arthroscopic portals are left to close by secondary intention, or they are closed with sutures.

Anesthetic Considerations

Anesthetic considerations and postoperative pain control are the same as for arthroscopic Bankart repair, discussed above (see also Chap. 7). This is typically very painful surgery and a continuous peripheral nerve block is indicated for well into the postoperative period. We typically place a

CCPVB preoperatively (see Chap. 23), but a CISB is as effective and is widely used (see Chap. 23). What is described above for the open Bankart repair applies here.

Associated Medications

One dose of preoperative antibiotics is given intravenously.

Postoperative Care

The arm is placed in a sling, and these patients are usually kept in hospital for overnight observation and pain management. Pendulum and passive motion exercises are performed for the first 6 weeks. Progressive active-assisted and active motion and rotator cuff–strengthening exercises are started 6 to 8 weeks postoperatively. Patients may expect a return to full activity after 6 to 12 months.

▶ SPORT INJURIES TO THE KNEE JOINT

General Considerations

One of the most common complications of knee surgery is injury to the neural structures around the joint. Incisions are generally made to avoid nerve injury, but they are often near the nerves and retracting them is necessary to protect them from injury. With incisions for medial meniscal repair or medial collateral ligament (MCL) surgery, the prepatellar branch of the saphenous nerve and the saphenous nerve itself are in danger. With anterior incisions [patellar tendon (PT) graft for anterior cruciate ligament (ACL) reconstruction], the prepatellar branch of the saphenous nerve is almost always cut, leading to lateral numbness of the knee. Compression around the knee with postoperative bracing is a problem because of little padding around the fibular head and the peroneal nerve. It is therefore important to protect this area.

Knee Arthroscopy

Indications and Anatomic Considerations

Diagnostic knee arthroscopy is indicated for the evaluation of intraarticular pathology in patients in whom a diagnosis is based on clinical examination and history and the usual diagnostic tests are uncertain.

Patient Profile

Patients who undergo knee arthroscopy can fall within any age group, but they are often very active recreationally.

Positioning on the Operating Table

The patient is positioned supine and, depending on the surgeon's preference, the foot of the bed may be dropped and one or both legs may be placed in a leg holder, or the bed may remain flat. Some surgeons use a tourniquet and some do not.

Surgical Technique

A puncture is made in the skin overlying the anterolateral joint line at the lateral aspect of the patellar tendon and a blunt trocar and cannula are inserted into the joint. An arthroscopic camera is inserted into the joint through this cannula and the condition of the joint is evaluated. An inferomedial portal is then made at the joint line just medial to the patellar tendon. This portal is used as a working opening for the insertion of arthroscopic instruments. Often a third portal is made in the suprapatellar pouch, either superomedially or superolaterally, for fluid inflow or outflow.

The arthroscope and a probe are used to assess the articular cartilage, the menisci, and the cruciate ligaments. Arthroscopic portals are either left open to close by secondary intention or they are closed with sutures.

Anesthetic Considerations

Anesthetic techniques that have been used successfully for knee arthroscopy vary from subarachnoid block to combined femoral and sciatic nerve block to femoral nerve block combined with general anesthesia to general anesthesia or intraarticular injection of local anesthetic agents and local injection at the portholes. All these techniques have their supporters, but ultimately the choice depends on the patient, the surgeon, the institution, and the anesthesiologist. Patients will be satisfied with almost any technique as long as they are not hurt by it, but some patients prefer to be fully conscious and see what the surgeon finds during arthroscopy, while others prefer to be unconscious.

We use a "default" technique, which we adjust to the situation and the patient's requirements and wishes. This technique includes preoperative femoral nerve block followed by general anesthesia induced and maintained with propofol and mechanical ventilation of the lungs with air enriched with oxygen via an LMA. If there seem to be any problems with or contraindications to the LMA, we insert an endotracheal tube, using neuromuscular blocking agents or alfentanil to do so.

Analgesia

Postoperative analgesic requirements are typically low, but oral or parenteral analgesics may be necessary for a few hours after the surgery, especially if a single-injection nerve block has been done preoperatively. If a medial meniscectomy was done during arthroscopy, the femoral nerve block should be sufficient to treat the pain; but if a lateral meniscectomy was done, a sciatic nerve block would most probably be required, since this nerve sup-

plies the lateral part of the proximal tibia. The proximal medial aspect of the tibia receives most of its nerve supply from the femoral nerve.

Associated Medications

One dose of preoperative antibiotics is given intravenously.

Postoperative Care

No activity restrictions are placed on a patient following diagnostic arthroscopy. Patients may prefer to use crutches for a short period after surgery in order to bear weight comfortably. Patients usually resume normal activities within 4 to 6 weeks after surgery.

Treatment of Meniscal Pathology

Indications and Anatomic Considerations

Operative treatment of a meniscus tear is indicated for patients with a persistently locked knee or with intermittent catching or locking of the knee that does not resolve with treatment such as physical therapy. Meniscus repair is indicated for acute, unstable tears that involve the well-vascularized peripheral part of the meniscus and which do not demonstrate degeneration of the meniscal tissue. Partial meniscectomy is indicated for unstable tears that are not repairable.

Patient Profile

Patients undergoing knee arthroscopy and treatment of meniscal injury can fall within any age range, but they are usually very active.

Positioning on the Operating Table

The patient is positioned supine. Depending on the surgeon's preference, the foot of the operating table may be dropped and one or both legs may be placed in a leg holder, or the table may remain flat. Some surgeons use a tourniquet and some do not.

Surgical Procedure

A diagnostic arthroscopy of the knee is performed (see above) and a decision is made about the stability of the meniscus tear and whether it will require resection or repair. If partial meniscectomy is chosen, arthroscopic cutting instruments and shavers are used to resect the unstable part of the meniscus and smooth its contour. If meniscal repair is chosen, one of several different surgical techniques may be used, including "inside out," "outside in," and "all inside." All three techniques begin with debridement of the peripheral edge of the tear until bleeding tissue is exposed.

The inside-out technique begins with intraarticular preparation of the meniscus for repair. This is followed by an open surgical approach to the knee capsule on the posteromedial or posterolateral side of the joint, depending on the location of the meniscal tear. Care is taken to place retractors that protect the neurovascular structures from injury. Sutures on long needles are passed through the meniscus under arthroscopic visualization and retrieved by an assistant through the open incision. Sutures are then tied on the outside of the capsule to secure the repair. This technique allows repair of meniscal tears in the middle and posterior thirds of the meniscus and provides the strongest repair. However, it has the disadvantage of requiring an assistant and an additional incision.

The outside-in technique begins with intraarticular preparation of the meniscus and is followed by an open surgical approach to the knee capsule on the side of the joint with the meniscal tear through a 1- to 2-cm incision. Retractors are placed to avoid injury to neurovascular structures. Cannulated needles are passed from the capsule into the joint to reduce the meniscus, sutures are passed through the needles into the joint, and the needles are removed. The sutures are then tied inside the joint and over the capsule to secure the repair. This technique allows repair of the anterior and middle thirds of the meniscus.

The all-inside technique begins with intraarticular preparation of the meniscus. A 70-degree arthroscope is then used to visualize the posterior compartment and an accessory posterior portal is placed on the side of the knee with the meniscal tear. This portal is then used to pass sutures, using a specialized cannulated instrument, and knots are tied using arthroscopic techniques. As an alternative, multiple new fixation devices are available that allow all-inside repairs without the need for passing sutures and accessory portals. All-inside techniques are best suited for peripheral tears of the posterior third of the meniscus. They have the advantage of minimizing the risk of neurovascular injury and preventing unwanted capsular plication, which might restrict the range of knee motion.

Surgical incisions are closed with sutures, and arthroscopic portals are either closed with sutures or allowed to close by secondary intention.

Anesthetic Considerations
Anesthetic considerations and analgesic management are similar to those for diagnostic arthroscopy.

Associated Medications
One dose of preoperative antibiotics is given intravenously.

Postoperative Care
Patients are usually discharged on the day of surgery. After partial meniscectomy, patients are allowed to increase their activities gradually as tolerated, with minimal restrictions. Physical therapy is often prescribed to help in strengthening the knee and its motions. Patients

are advanced to full activities as tolerated. After meniscal repair, for 4 to 6 weeks, the patient's leg is placed in a brace that is locked in extension for bearing weight and is limited to 90 degrees of knee flexion to protect the repair. Progressive increases in bearing weight and range of motion are begun after 6 weeks, with most patients returning to full activity after 4 to 6 months.

Osteochondral Autograft Transfer and Microfracture

Indications and Anatomic Considerations
Microfracture and osteochondral autograft transfer (OAT) is indicated for the treatment of symptomatic osteochondral defects in the load-bearing portions of the knee joint, most commonly on the femoral condyles, the trochlea, or the patella. Microfracture and OAT can be used to treat defects up to 2 cm in area (also of the ankle joint). Microfracture is usually reserved for smaller chondral defects.

Patient Profile
Patients undergoing knee arthroscopy and treatment of osteochondral injury can fall within any age range, but they are often young and very active recreationally.

Positioning on the Operating Table
The positioning of the patient is as described for meniscal pathology.

Surgical Technique
A diagnostic knee arthroscopy is performed to evaluate the cartilage lesion, measure its size, and assess its position in relation to weight-bearing surfaces. If microfracture is chosen, the lesion is prepared by removing any loose or fragmenting cartilage. The defect is debrided of the calcified cartilage layer to the level of the subchondral bone, using curettes or a shaver. Stable peripheral margins of the lesion are created circumferentially. Microfracture picks are then used to puncture 2- to 3-mm holes in the subchondral bone, where intramedullary elements can egress into the defect and are transformed into fibrocartilage, which fills the defect.

The OAT procedure harvests osteochondral plugs from a part of the joint that does not bear weight and moves them to the symptomatic load-bearing portion of the joint (Fig. 17-5). The cartilage in the lesion is debrided until a stable border remains. The lesion is then measured to determine the size of autograft bone plugs that will be needed. A coring reamer is used to create recipient sites of chosen size in the defect. A similar reamer is then used to harvest appropriately sized bone plugs from the anterolateral aspect of the lateral femoral condyle anterior to the sulcus terminalis or from the border of the intercondylar notch. The bone plugs are then

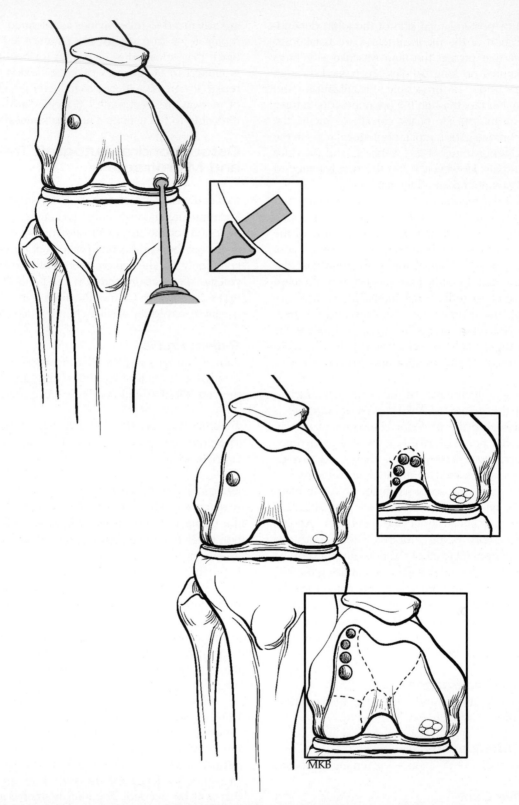

Figure 17-5. Osteochondral autograft transfer and microfracture (OAT).

tamped into the holes created in the defect to create a "mosaicplasty" of transplanted cartilage. This procedure can usually be performed through arthroscopic portals, but an open surgical approach may be necessary to improve exposure.

Surgical incisions are closed with sutures and arthroscopic portals are either closed with sutures or allowed to heal by secondary intention.

Anesthetic Considerations

Anesthetic considerations and analgesic management are similar to those for diagnostic arthroscopy, above. If an open incision is needed, a continuous femoral block is placed preoperatively. The catheter can be removed the day after surgery if the pain is manageable with oral analgesics, or, failing this, the patient can be discharged from the hospital with the femoral catheter and continuous femoral block in place (see Chaps. 20 and 21).

Associated Medications

One dose of preoperative antibiotics is given intravenously.

Postoperative Care

If the whole procedure is done arthroscopically, the patient is discharged home. If an open incision is needed for the procedure, the patient is generally admitted for overnight recovery and pain management. Range-of-motion exercises are begun immediately. Weight bearing is restricted and often a continuous passive motion machine is used until approximately 6 weeks postoperatively. The incorporation of autografts can be monitored on radiographs, CT scan, or MRI. Patients can expect a return to full activity after approximately 6 to 12 months, depending on the size of the treated area.

Autologous Chondrocyte Implantation

Indications and Anatomic Considerations

Autologous chondrocyte implantation (ACI) is indicated for treatment of symptomatic osteochondral defects in the load-bearing portions of the knee joint. This technique can be applied to lesions that are too large for treatment with OATS or microfracture.

Patient Profile

Patients undergoing knee arthroscopy and treatment of osteochondral injury can fall within any age range, but they are often young and very active recreationally.

Positioning on the Operating Table

The positioning of the patient is as described in the discussion of meniscal pathology above.

Surgical Technique

Autologous chondrocyte implantation is a staged procedure. In the first stage, a biopsy specimen of normal articular cartilage is obtained and sent to a laboratory, where the chondrocytes are grown in culture. When the cultured chondrocytes are ready, the second stage is performed, in which the chondrocytes are implanted under a periosteal patch that covers the defect.

The first stage also includes diagnostic arthroscopy to evaluate the lesion. The lesion may be debrided during the first stage, but an additional debridement must be done in the second stage so that the bony bed of the lesion is bleeding to promote healing.

The production of cultured chondrocytes takes approximately 6 weeks to complete, but the specimens can be stored for months to years prior to reactivation and growth of cells. When the cells are ready, the second procedure is performed (Fig. 17-6).

An arthrotomy is performed to expose the cartilage defect, and the defect is debrided until the edges are stable and bleeding bone is present in the bed. A piece of periosteum is harvested from the anteromedial surface of the

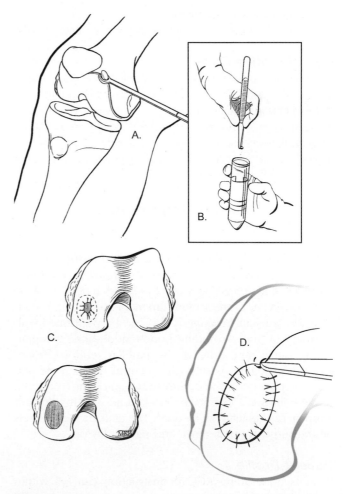

Figure 17-6. Autologous chondrocyte implantation (ACI).

proximal tibia and sutured over the defect. Before the last stitch is placed, the cultured chondrocytes are injected into the defect under the bony patch and the final suture is then placed. The incisions are closed with sutures.

Anesthetic Considerations

A variety of anesthetic techniques are used with good results. Our "default" technique includes preoperative continuous femoral nerve block. This is followed by general anesthesia induced and maintained with propofol and mechanical ventilation of the lungs with air enriched with oxygen via an LMA. If there seem to be any problems with the LMA or contraindications to its use, we insert an endotracheal tube (ETT). We use short-acting neuromuscular blocking agents or alfentanil to place the ETT.

Analgesia

Postoperative pain may be severe and is typically treated by keeping the continuous femoral block in place for a few days or as long as the patient requires it. Patients are typically discharged from the hospital with the catheters and continuous femoral blocks in situ (see Chaps. 20 and 21).

Associated Medications

One dose of preoperative antibiotics is given intravenously.

Postoperative Care

The patient is usually kept in the hospital overnight. A specific rehabilitation protocol involving restricted weight bearing, continuous passive motion, and progressive strengthening and range-of-motion exercises is begun on the day of surgery. Patients usually do not bear weight for the first 4 to 6 weeks and can expect a return to normal activity after approximately 6 to 18 months.

Anterior Cruciate Ligament Reconstruction

Indications and Anatomic Considerations

The indication for ACL reconstruction is recurrent episodes of knee instability in a knee with a deficient ACL. Tears of the ACL are seldom amenable to repair; reconstruction is usually required. This can be performed with a variety of grafts including bone-tendon-bone autograft (using the central third of the patellar tendon), bone-tendon autograft (using the central portion of the quadriceps tendon), and hamstrings autograft (using the semitendinosus and gracilis muscle tendons). In addition, a variety of allografts can be used. The graft choice depends on the surgeon's preference and patient factors.

Patient Profile

Patients undergoing ACL reconstruction can fall within any age range, but they usually are between their second and sixth decades. These patients are often young and very active recreationally.

Positioning on the Operating Table

The patient's positioning is as described in the discussion of meniscal pathology, above.

Surgical Technique

An examination under anesthesia is performed to confirm ACL insufficiency. Most surgeons will then proceed to harvest a graft unless the diagnosis remains uncertain, in which case a diagnostic arthroscopy will be performed first.

Patellar tendon is harvested through an anterior longitudinal incision over the medial border of the patellar tendon. The tendon is exposed and measured, and the central third is harvested with attached patellar and tibial bone blocks. The graft is then taken to the back table and fashioned to fit through appropriately sized bone tunnels in the tibia and femur.

A hamstrings harvest is performed through an anteromedial longitudinal incision midway between the tibial tubercle and the pes anserinus insertion. The sartorius fascia is incised to expose the semitendinosus and gracilis tendons, and the tendons are freed from their fascial attachments. A tendon stripper is passed over the tendon and up into the posterior thigh to harvest the tendon from the muscle belly. A scalpel is used to elevate the distal insertion of the tendon from the bone with a flap of periosteum. The graft is then taken to the back table and prepared to allow passage through tunnels in the tibia and femur.

While an assistant is preparing the graft, knee arthroscopy is performed. If additional injuries such as meniscal tears or chondral injuries are identified, they are treated at this time. Next, a femoral notchplasty is performed to debride the torn ACL and ensure that the femur will not impinge on the graft. The ACL grafts are placed in the knee using tunnels drilled through the proximal tibial and the lateral femoral condyle. The openings of these tunnels are in the knee joint at the anatomic attachment sites of the ACL. A guidewire is positioned in the tibia and overdrilled to create the tibial tunnel. Another guidewire is placed through the tibial tunnel into the femur and overdrilled to create the femoral tunnel. The femoral guidewire is advanced through the soft tissue of the anterolateral thigh and used to pull the graft into position through the tibial tunnel. Graft fixation is then performed using one of a variety of techniques (Fig. 17-7).

The graft harvest site is then closed with sutures and the arthroscopic portals are closed with sutures or allowed to heal by secondary intention.

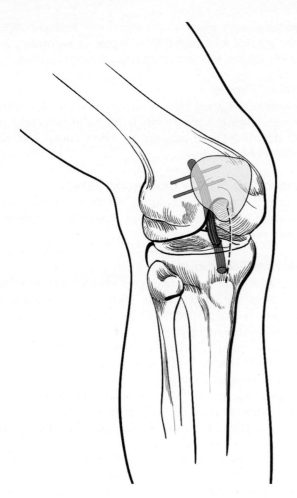

Figure 17-7. Anterior cruciate ligament (ACL) reconstruction.

Anesthetic Considerations
The anesthetic considerations are as described in the previous section (see "Autologous Chondrocyte Implantation").

Analgesia
Postoperative pain may be severe and is typically treated by keeping the continuous femoral block in place for a few days or as long as the patient requires it. These patients are typically discharged from the hospital with the catheters and continuous femoral blocks in situ (see Chaps. 20 and 21).

Associated Medications
One dose of preoperative antibiotics is given intravenously.

Postoperative Care
Patients may go home on the day of surgery or be kept in the hospital overnight, depending on the surgeon's preference. Range-of-motion and strengthening exercises are begun on the day of surgery, and patients are usually allowed to bear weight on the limb immediately unless other concomitant procedures preclude it. Rehabilitation is progressive over several months; a return to normal activities usually occurs 6 to 12 months after surgery.

Posterior Cruciate Ligament Reconstruction

Indications and Anatomic Considerations
Reconstruction of the posterior cruciate ligament (PCL) is indicated for treatment of symptomatic instability following PCL rupture that does not improve with physical therapy or for PCL rupture associated with injury to another knee ligament. Possible graft choices include the central third of the patellar tendon or quadriceps tendon autograft, hamstrings autograft, or allograft. Tibial fixation may be performed through a bone tunnel or by using the inlay technique.

Patient Profile
Patients undergoing PCL reconstruction can fall within any age range but usually are between their second and sixth decades. These patients are often young and very active recreationally.

Positioning on the Operating Table
For tibial bone tunnel fixation, the patient is positioned supine, as for a knee arthroscopy. For the inlay technique, the patient will need to be placed in a prone or semilateral decubitus position to allow access to the posteromedial aspect of the joint. A tourniquet is often used for this procedure.

Surgical Technique
If an autograft is used, the graft will be harvested as described for ACL reconstruction. While an assistant is preparing the graft, knee arthroscopy is performed. If additional injuries such as meniscal tears or chondral injuries are identified, these are treated at this time.

The femoral and tibial attachments of the PCL are debrided. An accessory posteromedial portal is usually used to aid in visualizing the tibial attachment of the PCL on the posterior aspect of the tibial eminence.

For the tibial tunnel technique, a guidewire is positioned in the tibia, using a drill guide, and overdrilled to the diameter of the graft. Fluoroscopic guidance is often used for this part of the procedure to confirm the location of the tunnel and to decrease the risk of injury to the posterior neurovascular structures.

For the inlay procedure, a posterormedial approach to the knee is used. A right-angle incision is made with the horizontal part in line with the posterior knee crease and the vertical part extending distally in line with the semimembranosus muscle tendon. The interval between the semimembranosus and the medial head of the gastrocnemius muscles is developed to expose the popliteus muscle. This muscle is then split to expose the tibial attachment site of the PCL on the posterior aspect of the proximal tibia. The graft is then positioned at the tibial attachment site and secured with screws.

Another guidewire is placed through the tibial tunnel into the femur and overdrilled to create the femoral tunnel. The femoral guidewire is advanced through the soft tissue of the anterolateral thigh and used to pull the graft into position through the tibial tunnel. The graft is then fixed by using one of a variety of techniques.

The graft harvest site is then closed with sutures and the arthroscopic portals are closed with sutures or allowed to heal by secondary intention.

Anesthetic Considerations

The anesthetic considerations are as described in previous sections (see "Autologous Chondrocyte Implantation," etc.).

Analgesia

Postoperative pain may be severe and is usually treated by keeping the continuous femoral block in place for a few days or as long as the patient requires it. These patients are usually discharged from the hospital with the catheters and continuous femoral blocks in situ (see Chaps. 20 and 21). The effects of the sciatic block normally lasts into the second postoperative day; continuous sciatic block is seldom required.

Associated Medications

One dose of preoperative antibiotics is given intravenously.

Postoperative Care

These patients may be kept in the hospital for overnight observation or discharged the same day. This surgery's proximity to the posterior neurovascular structures increases the risk of nerve injury, and monitoring overnight is therefore prudent. A postoperative brace is often employed and range-of-motion exercise initiated within the first 2 weeks after surgery. The patient's weight-bearing status is variable depending on the surgeon's preference and concomitant procedures performed. Return to normal activities is expected in 6 to 12 months after surgery.

Medial Collateral Ligament Reconstruction

Indications and Anatomic Considerations

Medial collateral ligament (MCL) repair or reconstruction is indicated for treatment of symptomatic instability that does not improve with physical therapy or for MCL injury associated with injury to another knee ligament. While acute injuries are amenable to repair or reconstruction, chronic injuries will generally require reconstruction.

Patient Profile

Patients undergoing MCL reconstruction can fall within any age range but are usually between their second and fifth decades. These patients are often young and very active recreationally.

Positioning on the Operating Table

Patients are positioned supine on the operating table. A tourniquet is sometimes used, depending on the surgeon's preference.

Surgical Technique

If reconstruction is planned, graft choices may include a hamstrings autograft or an allograft. If intraarticular pathology is suspected, the procedure may begin with diagnostic arthroscopy.

A longitudinal incision is made on the medial aspect of the knee centered over the joint line. The pes anserinus and semimembranosus tendons are isolated and the MCL is exposed. The MCL originates proximally on the medial femoral condyle and inserts distally on the tibia approximately 6 cm distal to the joint line deep to the pes anserinus tendons.

If the injury is acute, a midsubstance tear can be repaired with sutures and an avulsion can be repaired with suture anchors, staples, or screws. The repair may then be reinforced by suturing to the semimembranosus fascia or by augmentation with a local hamstrings tendon graft or an allograft. Chronic injuries usually require augmentation with a graft. The graft is secured with screws and washers, staples, or by using a bone tunnel technique. The incisions are closed with sutures.

Anesthetic Considerations

The anesthetic considerations are as previously described (see "Autologous Chondrocyte Implantation," above).

Analgesia

Postoperative pain may be severe and is usually treated by keeping the continuous femoral block in place for a few days or as long as the patient requires it. These patients are usually discharged from the hospital with the catheters and continuous femoral blocks in situ (see Chaps. 20 and 21).

Associated Medications

One dose of preoperative antibiotics is given intravenously.

Postoperative Care

These patients may be kept in hospital for overnight observation or discharged home on the same day. The patient is placed in a hinged knee brace in the operating room and range-of-motion exercises are begun within 2 weeks of surgery. The patient may bear weight with crutches while wearing the brace, and progressive strengthening is performed. Return to normal activities is expected in 6 to 12 months.

Lateral Collateral Ligament/Posterolateral Corner Repair or Reconstruction

Indications and Anatomic Considerations

Lateral collateral ligament (LCL) or posterolateral corner (PLC) repair or reconstruction is indicated for the treatment of symptomatic instability after physical therapy has been tried or when this instability is associated with another knee ligamentous injury requiring surgical treatment. Repair is reserved for acute injuries, although many surgeons now advocate reconstruction of all injuries, whether acute or chronic.

Patient Profile

Patients undergoing LCL reconstruction can fall within any age range but are usually between their second and fifth decades. These patients are often young and very active recreationally.

Positioning on the Operating Table

The patient is positioned supine on the operating table with a bump under the affected side to allow better access to the lateral side of the knee. A tourniquet is sometimes used, depending on the surgeon's preference.

Surgical Technique

Direct repair of the LCL and PLC is often possible. If reconstruction is chosen, an allograft is generally used. If associated intraarticular pathology is suspected, diagnostic arthroscopy is performed at the beginning of the procedure. Injury of the LCL and PLC is usually associated with injuries of other ligaments, such as the ACL or PCL tears, which are treated at the same time.

A curved, longitudinal incision is made on the lateral aspect of the knee with the knee flexed. The incision is centered over the joint line and placed just anterior to the biceps femoris tendon. The peroneal nerve is isolated deep to the biceps femoris tendon in the proximal aspect of the wound. The nerve is exposed as it courses distally around the fibular head and is protected.

The fascia lata is incised longitudinally and mobilized to allow access anteriorly and posteriorly to the lateral femoral condyle and joint line. The origins of the lateral collateral and popliteofibular ligaments are exposed on the femur, and the fibular head is exposed.

The femoral and tibial attachment sites of the lateral collateral and popliteofibular ligaments are exposed and identified. If the ligament tissue is healthy and the injury is acute, repair can be performed at this time by using a combination of sutures, suture anchors, and possibly screws or staples. If reconstruction is going to be performed, drill holes are placed in the femur and fibula at attachment sites of the ligaments and fixation is performed using interference screws, staples, or screws and washers.

The wound is closed with sutures and the leg is placed in a hinged knee brace.

Anesthetic Considerations

The anesthetic considerations are as previously described (see "Autologous Chondrocyte Implantation," above).

Analgesia

Postoperative pain may be severe and is typically treated by keeping the continuous femoral block in place for a few days or as long as the patient requires it. These patients are typically discharged from the hospital with the catheters and continuous femoral blocks in situ (see Chaps. 20 and 21). The effects of the sciatic block typically last into the second postoperative day; continuous sciatic block is seldom required.

Associated Medications

One dose of preoperative antibiotics is given intravenously.

Postoperative Care

These patients may be kept in hospital for overnight observation or discharged on the same day. Patients do not bear weight for 4 to 6 weeks postoperatively and begin range-of-motion exercises on the day of surgery. Return to normal activities is anticipated in 6 to 12 months.

High Tibial Osteotomy

Indications and Anatomic Considerations

High tibial osteotomy (HTO) is indicated for the treatment of symptomatic medial compartment osteoarthritis that does not respond to nonoperative measures. In addition, HTO can be used to unload the medial compartment in patients with varus knees who undergo cartilage resurfacing procedures or to correct varus malalignment in patients with ACL insufficiency in order to decrease the chance of rerupture.

Patient Profile

Patients undergoing HTO can fall within any age range but usually are between their third and sixth decades. These patients are often very active recreationally.

Positioning on the Operating Table

Patients are positioned supine on the operating table. A tourniquet is generally used during the procedure. This procedure requires bone graft, which can be iliac crest autograft, allograft, or bone graft substitute.

Surgical Technique

Preoperative templating is performed using full-length radiographs of the lower extremities while bearing weight in order to determine the degree of correction needed.

HTO may be performed in two ways, opening wedge and closing wedge. For opening-wedge HTO, a longitudinal incision is made on the anteromedial aspect of the proximal tibia just distal to the knee joint and midway between the tibial tubercle and the insertion of the pes anserinus. The dissection is continued down to the bone, and the periosteum is incised longitudinally just medial to the tubercle. The periosteum is elevated to expose the entire tibia from anterior to posterior in the incision.

A guidewire is advanced across the tibia in the direction of the osteotomy and its position checked with fluoroscopy. A saw and osteotomes are then used to perform the osteotomy, with care taken not to damage the posterior or posterolateral neurovascular structures. The osteotomy is not completed on the lateral side of the tibia so as to allow the bone to hinge open and to obviate the need for lateral fixation.

In performing an opening-wedge osteotomy, a metallic wedge opener is malleted into the osteotomy site to match the predetermined degree of correction. The limb alignment is checked by visual inspection and may be confirmed with fluoroscopy. A plate and screws are then used to fix the osteotomy site. A wedge of bone graft is placed into the osteotomy site and the wound is closed with sutures (Fig. 17-8).

For a closing-wedge HTO, the incision is made on the anterolateral aspect of the proximal tibia. The anterolateral tibia is exposed. The proximal fibula is also exposed and can be simply cut or a small section can be removed. The proximal tibiofibular joint is incised. Two osteotomy cuts that meet at the medial edge of the tibia are then made across the tibia. These cuts remove a wedge of bone, the size of which is determined by preoperative measurements. The bone edges proximal and distal to the removed wedge are then brought together and fixed with a plate and screws.

The lateral closing wedge is close to the fibular head and violates the anterior compartment; therefore, there is increased risk of peroneal nerve neuropraxia and anterior compartment syndrome.

Anesthetic Considerations

The anesthetic considerations are as described previously. A continuous femoral nerve block and a continuous

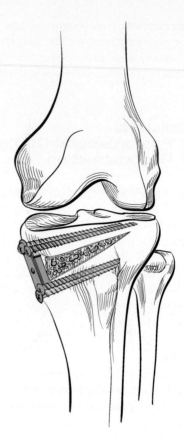

Figure 17-8. High tibial osteotomy (HTO).

sciatic nerve block are required for this surgery (see Chaps. 26 and 27).

Analgesia

Postoperative pain may be severe and is usually treated by keeping the continuous blocks in place for a few days or as long as the patient requires it. Patients are usually discharged from the hospital with the catheters and continuous blocks in place (see Chaps. 20 and 21). The effects of sciatic block normally last into the second postoperative day; continuous sciatic block is often required. There should be no hesitation in placing a continuous proximal sciatic block preoperatively if it is suspected that it may be required, since it is easier to remove a catheter if not required than to place one postoperatively. Also, the chances of needing it are greater than the chances of not needing it.

Associated Medications

One dose of preoperative antibiotics is given intravenously.

Postoperative Care

Patients usually stay in the hospital overnight after surgery. They do not bear weight for 6 weeks following the procedure in order to allow the osteotomy site to heal. Range-of-motion exercises are started on the day of surgery.

Tibial Tubercle Transfer

Indications and Anatomic Considerations
Tibial tubercle transfer (TTT) is indicated for treatment of patellofemoral maltracking or recurrent patellar dislocations.

Patient Profile
Patients undergoing tibial tubercle transfer can fall within any age range but usually are between their second and sixth decades. These patients are often very active recreationally.

Positioning on the Operating Table
The patient is positioned supine on the operating table. A tourniquet is usually used for this procedure.

Surgical Technique
A longitudinal incision is made just lateral to the tibial tubercle on the anterolateral aspect of the knee, extending from the distal pole of the patella to the distal aspect of the tibial tubercle. The medial and lateral borders of the patellar tendon and tibial tubercle are exposed. The tibialis anterior muscle is elevated from the anterolateral aspect of the tibia to expose the bone.

Two drill bits are placed from anteromedial to posterolateral in the tibia at the proximal and distal extent of the tubercle and are left in place to guide the osteotomy. An oscillating saw and osteotomes are used to perform the osteotomy. The distal part of the osteotomy is not completed so that the bone can hinge at this point. Fixation is then performed using two cortical screws (Fig. 17-9). The screw positions may be checked with fluoroscopy. The incisions are closed with sutures.

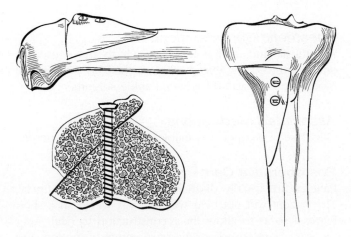

Figure 17-9. Tibial tubercle transfer (TTT).

Anesthetic Considerations
Anesthesia and analgesia for this procedure are similar to those for HTO and PCL surgeries.

Associated Medications
One dose of preoperative antibiotics is given intravenously.

Postoperative Care
Most patients stay in the hospital overnight following surgery. Patients do not bear weight for 4 to 6 weeks following the procedure in order to allow the osteotomy site to heal. Range-of-motion exercises are begun on the day of surgery.

▶ SPORTS INJURIES TO THE ANKLE JOINT

General Considerations

One of the most important considerations following foot and ankle surgery is the fact that casts or braces may compress the area of the fibular head and peroneal nerve. In addition, the circumferential dressing becomes a potential problem if it does not allow for postoperative swelling. Therefore close monitoring and attention to these will prevent complications, particularly in the face of an anesthetized foot and ankle.

Ankle Arthroscopy

Indications and Anatomic Considerations
Ankle arthroscopy is indicated for the treatment of intraarticular ankle pathology including loose bodies, osteochondral lesions, and anterior impingement. In addition, it can be used as an adjunct to other procedures such as ankle arthrodesis.

Patient Profile
Patients undergoing ankle arthroscopy can be of any age, but many are athletic individuals in their second to fourth decades.

Positioning on the Operating Table
Patients are most often placed supine on the operating table. Because traction is applied during the procedure to distract the ankle joint, it is helpful to place the patient in a slight Trendelenburg position for counter-traction. Occasionally, patients may be placed in the prone position to allow better access to the posterior aspect of the joint. A tourniquet is sometimes used during this procedure.

Surgical Technique

No portals are placed directly anterior to the joint so as to avoid injury to the neurovascular structures. An anteromedial portal is placed at the joint line just medial to the tibialis anterior tendon. An anterolateral portal is made just lateral to the extensor digitorum longus and peroneus tertius tendons. Care is taken to palpate the superficial peroneal nerve under the skin to avoid injuring it during portal placement.

Both the anteromedial and anterolateral portals must be used in turn as viewing portals to visualize the entire joint adequately. Instruments can be inserted through a portal when it is not used for viewing. Intraarticular pathology is identified and treated, and arthroscopic instruments are removed from the joint. The portals are closed with sutures or left to heal by secondary intention.

Anesthetic Considerations

Single-injection popliteal sciatic block (see Chap. 27) with saphenous (or femoral) nerve block (see Chap. 26) is ideal as the sole anesthetic for this surgery. Sedation can be adjusted to suit the individual patient. It is sometimes necessary to combine the block(s) with general anesthesia, which can be induced before or after placement of the block, depending on the preference of the anesthesiologist and the patient and the institutional protocol (see also Chap. 12). It should be pointed out here again that the saphenous nerve is not only a cutaneous nerve but also supplies the medial aspects of the ankle joint (see Chaps. 12 and 28).

General anesthesia is typically induced and maintained with propofol and mechanical ventilation of the lungs with air enriched with oxygen via an LMA. If a block is not used, we use a continuous intravenous infusion of remifentanil for intraoperative analgesia. If there seems to be any problems with or contraindications to the LMA, we place an ETT. We use short-acting neuromuscular blocking agents or alfentanil to place the ETT.

Analgesia

Postoperative analgesia requirements are low; the single-injection block is usually sufficient. This is followed by oral analgesics, usually opiate-combination drugs that should be started before the effects of the blocks wear off. Continuous nerve blocks are not required unless more extensive surgery is to be done.

Associated Medications

One dose of preoperative antibiotics is given intravenously.

Postoperative Care

Most patients are discharged on the day of surgery. The type of intraarticular pathology and the operation per-formed determines the patient's weight-bearing status. Range-of-motion exercises are usually begun on the day of surgery.

Lateral Ankle Reconstruction

Indications and Anatomic Considerations

Lateral ankle reconstruction is indicated for the treatment of painful lateral ankle instability that is refractory to conservative treatment and of recurrent lateral ankle sprains.

Patient Profile

Patients are usually active individuals in their second to fourth decades.

Positioning on the Operating Table

The patient is placed in a lazy lateral position with the operative side up to allow access to the posterolateral aspect of the ankle joint. A tourniquet is often used for this procedure.

Surgical Technique

A curvilinear incision is made over the distal aspect of the fibula at the level of the ankle joint. The lateral ankle capsule is exposed and elevated from its fibular attachment, and the anterior talofibular and calcaneofibular ligaments are identified and mobilized. The lateral aspect of the extensor retinaculum is also identified and mobilized to allow augmentation of the repair.

A high-speed burr or rongeur is used to roughen the surface of the bone where the ligaments will be secured. Suture anchors are then placed in the distal fibula at the site of attachment of the anterior talofibular ligament and calcaneal fibular ligament and, with the ankle in an everted position, the ligaments are sutured tightly to the bone. The extensor retinaculum is sutured to the repair for additional strength. The tissues are closed with sutures and the leg is placed in a short leg cast.

Anesthetic Considerations

Anesthesia and analgesia are similar to those used in ankle arthroscopy except that saphenous or femoral block is not indicated for lateral ankle surgery.

Associated Medications

One dose of preoperative antibiotics is given intravenously.

Postoperative Care

Patients are usually discharged on the day of surgery. The patient will not bear weight for 4 weeks in a short leg cast so as to allow the reconstruction to heal. After the cast is removed, progressive range-of-motion and strengthening exercises are begun.

Peroneal Tendon Exploration

Indications and Anatomic Considerations

Peroneal tendon exploration is indicated for symptomatic peroneal tendon tears or tendon instability that does not respond to nonoperative treatment such as immobilization or orthotic use.

Patient Profile

Patients with peroneal tendon pathology can be of any age. The majority are in their second to sixth decades.

Positioning on the Operating Table

Patients are placed in the semilateral position to allow access to the posterolateral aspect of the ankle joint. A tourniquet is often used during this procedure.

Surgical Technique

A curvilinear incision is made along the posterolateral border of the fibula following the course of the peroneal tendons. The posterolateral border of the fibula is exposed and inspected for damage to the superior peroneal retinaculum, the tissue that covers the fibular groove and contributes to the stability of the tendons. In addition, the depth of the fibular groove is evaluated, because a shallow groove promotes tendon instability. The tendons are then exposed and examined for the presence of anomalies, tears, or degeneration. Abnormal tissue is debrided and torn tissue repaired. A groove-deepening osteotomy may be performed if necessary.

If tendon repair, retinaculum repair, or groove deepening is performed, the wound is closed with sutures and the leg is placed in a short leg cast.

Anesthetic Considerations

Anesthesia and analgesia are similar to those used in ankle arthroscopy except that saphenous or femoral block is not indicated for lateral ankle surgery.

Associated Medications

One dose of preoperative antibiotics is given intravenously.

Postoperative Care

Most patients are discharged on the day of surgery. After debridement only, patients may begin bearing weight as tolerated in a supportive boot. After tendon or retinaculum repair or groove deepening, patients will have a short leg cast fitted and will not bear weight for 4 to 6 weeks.

Achilles' Tendon Repair

Indications and Anatomic Considerations

Achilles' tendon repair is indicated for the treatment of acute Achilles' tendon rupture. Although acute ruptures may be treated nonoperatively with cast immobilization, the rate of recurring rupture is lower with surgical treatment.

Patient Profile

The patient who presents with an Achilles' tendon rupture is typically in his or her late thirties or early forties, is slightly overweight, and participates in a strenuous sport that is not a regular activity. This condition can, however, occur at any age.

Positioning on the Operating Table

The patient is positioned prone on the operating table. A tourniquet is placed on the thigh.

Surgical Technique

A longitudinal incision is made slightly medial to the tendon, over the area of the rupture. The paratenon is incised and retracted to expose the tendon. Damaged tissue that will not contribute to the repair is excised. Running, locking sutures are placed in the proximal and distal ends of the tendon and tied. The repair is reinforced with additional sutures as needed. The wound is closed with sutures.

Anesthetic Considerations

Anesthesia and analgesia are similar to those used in ankle arthroscopy except that saphenous or femoral block is not indicated for lateral ankle surgery, although femoral or saphenous nerve block would make the tourniquet tolerable. If general anesthesia is also used, endotracheal intubation is required for airway management.

Associated Medications

One dose of preoperative antibiotics is given intravenously.

Postoperative Care

Most patients are discharged on the day of surgery. The ankle is splinted in plantarflexion for the first 2 weeks and the patient is kept from bearing weight. The ankle is gradually moved to a plantigrade position over the next 4 weeks until weight bearing is permitted. Progressive strengthening and range-of-motion exercises are continued, with most patients returning to full activity after 6 to 12 months.

Also refer to Chap. 12 for other major ankle surgery.

SUGGESTED FURTHER READING

Coughlin MJ, Mann, RA. *Surgery of the Foot and Ankle,* 7th ed. St. Louis: Mosby, 1999.

Craig EV. The shoulder, in *Master Techniques in Orthopaedic Surgery,* 2d ed. Philadelphia: Lippincott Williams & Wilkins, 2004.

DeLee J, Drez D, Miller MD. *DeLee & Drez's Orthopaedic Sports Medicine: Principles and Practice*, 2d ed. Philadelphia: Saunders, 2003.

LaPrade RF, Johansen S, Wentorf FA, et al. An analysis of an anatomical posterolateral knee reconstruction: An in vitro biomechanical study and development of a surgical technique. *Am J Sports Med* 32:1405–1144, 2004.

Lo IK, Burkhart SS. Current concepts in arthroscopic rotator cuff repair. *Am J Sports Med* 31:308–324, 2003.

McGinty JB, Burkhart SS. *Operative Arthroscopy*, 3d ed. Philadelphia: Lippincott Williams & Wilkins, 2003.

Morrison DS, Schaefer RK, Friedman RL. The relationship between subacromial space pressure, blood pressure, and visual clarity during arthroscopic subacromial decompression. *Arthroscopy* 11(5):557–560, 1995.

Nunley JA, Pfeffer GB, Sanders RW, Trepman E. *Advanced Reconstruction Foot & Ankle*. Rosemont, IL: American Academy of Orthopaedic Surgeons, 2004.

Rockwood CA, Matsen FA III. *The Shoulder*, 2d ed. Philadelphia: Saunders, 1998.

PART III

Regional Anesthesia for Orthopaedic Surgery

CHAPTER 18

Commonly Used Drugs and Equipment for Continuous Regional Anesthesia

PETER VAN DE PUTTE/MARTIAL VAN DER VORST

▶ INTRODUCTION

This chapter is not intended to represent an exhaustive overview of the pharmacologic text on all the drugs used for regional anesthesia but rather to offer a practical review of the minimal information required, especially for continuous peripheral nerve blocks. Readers are referred to pharmacology texts or the extensive list of references at the end of this chapter for complete detailed overviews. For continuous postoperative pain management, long-acting local anesthetic agents are mostly used. New local anesthetics, such as ropivacaine and levobupivacaine, have a reduced toxic potential compared to bupivacaine. This is important, because using continuous infusions may increase the risk of drug accumulation.

▶ REVIEW OF THE PHARMACOLOGY OF SOME LOCAL ANESTHETIC AGENTS

Ropivacaine is less toxic than bupivacaine at equipotent doses.[1] Several in vitro studies have shown that ropivacaine produces less block in heavily myelinated (motor) fibers and has a faster onset of block in lightly myelinated (sensory) fibers than bupivacaine. This provides a better differential blocking effect than that of bupivacaine.[2–4] Levobupivacaine is a new local anesthetic agent that may have a lower cardiotoxicity profile than the racemic mixture

bupivacaine.[5] In healthy volunteers, levobupivacaine produced significantly less depression of cardiac output than bupivacaine.[6] Lidocaine, in contrast, has a shorter duration of action and is less toxic than long-acting agents. This makes it a possible alternative for bupivacaine, levobupivacaine, and ropivacaine.[7–9] However, the denser motor block, the rapid development of tachyphylaxis[10] with lidocaine, and the good safety profile of newer drugs make lidocaine not the first choice for continuous infusions.[11] An advantage of ropivacaine is that its action stops sooner than that of bupivacaine after discontinuation of an infusion. This information may be useful during continuous blocks in trauma situations, because a blocked limb may mask the pain associated with a compartment syndrome, which should not be masked, since it is an early warning symptom.[12]

Potency

Experimental and clinical evidence suggest that ropivacaine is equipotent to bupivacaine when used in peripheral nerve blockade.[13–15] Studies have demonstrated that 30 to 40 mL of ropivacaine 0.5% produces a pattern of brachial plexus anesthesia broadly equivalent to that provided by 30 to 40 mL of bupivacaine 0.5%, whether administered via the subclavian perivascular,[16] the axillary,[17,18] or the interscalene[19] route. In patients undergoing lower arm surgery, McGlade et al.[20] concluded that 30 mL of ropivacaine (0.5%) or bupivacaine (0.5%) is equally effective for axillary brachial plexus block in terms of the onset time, motor blockade, and overall success rate. However, the duration of residual blockade was significantly longer with bupivacaine (6.8 versus 16 h). Using the same volume of local anesthetic for interscalene block, Klein et al.[21] compared 0.5% and 0.75% ropivacaine and 0.5% bupivacaine in patients undergoing shoulder surgery. They were not able to show any differences in success rate, onset of sensory or motor blocks, or the duration of analgesia among the three groups.

Metabolism and Systemic Toxicity of Local Anesthetic Drugs during Continuous Infusion

With the infusion of local anesthetic agents over a longer period, the accumulation of drugs and their metabolites may be important. In plasma, ropivacaine is mainly bound to alfa-1-acid glycoprotein (AAG), an acute-phase protein that increases gradually postoperatively[22] and may not reach a maximum until the sixth to twelfth postoperative day.[23-25] This postoperative increase in plasma AAG concentrations enhances the protein binding of ropivacaine and its metabolite, pipecoloxylidine, causing an increasing difference between total and unbound plasma concentrations.[26] In 1989, Tuominen et al.[27] suggested that the rise in AAG probably increases binding of bupivacaine to plasma proteins, which diminishes the risk of systemic toxicity in spite of a high total drug concentration.[28] During continuous interscalene block, the total plasma concentration of ropivacaine increased slightly but the unbound fraction decreased with time, reflecting an increase in the degree of plasma protein binding.[29]

The use of a large initial interscalene dose of bupivacaine (150 to 200 mg or 30 to 40 mL of 0.5%) followed by a continuous interscalene infusion of bupivacaine of 12.5 to 22.5 mg/h for 24 and 48 h (500 to 800 mg/24 h) is not likely to cause toxic plasma levels.[30-33] The main reason for this is the unchanged or decreasing plasma levels of free bupivacaine as the result of the increased AAG concentration.[34,35] After a 48-h interscalene infusion of ropivacaine at 18 mg/h (9 mL/h of 0.2%), the mean unbound plasma concentrations of ropivacaine and 3-OH-2',6'-pipecoloxylidine (PPX) were lower (0.026 and 0.12 mg/L)[36] than after a 72-h postoperative epidural ropivacaine infusion of 20 mg/h (0.06 and 0.4 mg/L)[37] and remained below believed theoretical threshold levels for systemic toxicity.[38]

Because toxic drug concentrations in the central nervous system (CNS) and heart are believed to be closely related to unbound plasma concentrations, the concentration of the unbound fraction may be a better indicator of potential toxicity than total plasma concentrations. The CNS toxicity threshold for unbound bupivacaine is believed to be 0.3 mg/mL and for unbound ropivacaine 0.6 mg/L.[39] The toxic threshold for levobupivacaine is unknown.

An increase in protein binding of ropivacaine and bupivacaine can result in a decrease in the total plasma clearance. This should have little or no effect on the clearance of the unbound plasma fraction, which mainly depends on the hepatic enzyme capacity. This may explain why unbound plasma concentrations remain relatively stable after 12 to 24 h,[40] in contrast to increasing total concentrations during continuous postoperative epidural infusion of ropivacaine.[41]

Ropivacaine undergoes extensive hepatic metabolism after intravenous administration, with only 1 percent of the drug appearing unchanged in the urine.[42] As ropivacaine is eliminated with an intermediate to low hepatic extraction ratio, its rate of elimination should depend on the unbound plasma concentration.[43] The major metabolite identified in the urine is 3-OH-ropivacaine, probably conjugated with glucuronic acid.[44] Agents, which inhibit the isoenzyme CYP1A2, affect the pharmacokinetic profile of ropivacaine.[45,46] Another metabolite of ropivacaine is PPX, which is a minor metabolite after a single dose[47] but a major metabolite during epidural infusion. Epidural infusion of ropivacaine over 72 h caused PPX plasma concentrations approaching that of ropivacaine, while unbound PPX concentrations were approximately eight to nine times higher than unbound ropivacaine concentrations.[48] After a 48-h continuous interscalene infusion of ropivacaine (0.2%) at 9 mL/h, unbound ropivacaine and PPX concentrations were lower than after a 72-h epidural infusion and remained below the theoretical threshold levels for systemic toxicity.[49]

In uremic patients, the enhanced absorption of ropivacaine into the circulation after axillary brachial plexus block, the increased binding to AAG, and the reduced urinary excretion of the metabolites led to larger total plasma concentrations of ropivacaine and its main metabolites.[50] Renal function is not important in the elimination of ropivacaine, since its excretion in the urine is minimal. However, renal function is important in the elimination of PPX and 3-OH-ropivacaine. Renal insufficiency may therefore be responsible for accumulation of these compounds. Caution should be exercised when large doses of ropivacaine are administered to patients with impaired renal function during continuous infusion.[51]

Only a small fraction (6%) of intravenously administered bupivacaine is excreted unchanged in the urine of humans.[52] The metabolites of bupivacaine are 4-hydroxybupivacaine (4-OHB) and desbutylbupivacaine (DBB) and are less toxic than bupivacaine.[53] During infusion of 0.25% bupivacaine for continuous interscalene brachial plexus block, there was a slow but significant increase in the plasma concentrations of bupivacaine and of DBB over 12 and 24 h of infusion.[54,55]

Neurotoxicity and Myotoxicity

Ropivacaine seems to be relatively free of neurotoxicity. Detailed histologic studies in guinea pigs and dogs also indicate that ropivacaine does not cause inflammation in peripheral nerves or the spinal cord.[56] It has been suggested that ropivacaine is significantly less painful on injection than bupivacaine.[57-59]

There is convincing experimental evidence that skeletal muscle is damaged by exposure to local anesthetic agents.[60-62] Although this occurs very rarely in the clinical use of these agents, it can be serious when it does occur. Myotoxicity should be suspected when localized muscle dysfunction and tenderness follow anesthetic injection.[63] Biopsy (using procaine for local anesthesia) aids in differential diagnosis, and magnetic resonance spectroscopy might be used to establish the diagnosis noninvasively.[64] Myotoxicity can be clinically relevant after a single injection and more so after repeated administration.[65-69] This suggests a potential risk of destroying muscle and nerve tissue in patients treated with frequent injections of 0.5% bupivacaine.[70] In animal studies local anesthetic agent myotoxicity is worse after repeated administration of large volumes. Therefore doses that may be safe for single-injection in patients may not be safe for repeat administration.[71]

In pigs, continuous peripheral nerve blockades with the long-acting local anesthetics bupivacaine and ropivacaine, in equipotent concentrations, cause fiber necrosis in skeletal muscle.[72] In comparison with ropivacaine, bupivacaine causes significantly more muscle damage and apoptosis in skeletal muscle cells (see Chap. 32). High concentrations of bupivacaine[73,74] and the use of epinephrine[75] are associated with increased myotoxicity and should be avoided if injections are to be made into or adjacent to muscle.[76]

Central Nervous System Toxicity

Case reports suggest that plasma concentrations of levobupivacaine or ropivacaine that are toxic to the CNS do not produce cardiotoxic effects.[77-79] It is therefore important to be aware of CNS toxicity symptoms after injection. These symptoms include numbness of the tongue, metallic taste, light-headedness, visual disturbances, and muscular twitching. More serious signs include convulsions, coma, respiratory arrest, and finally cardiovascular depression.[80,81]

A wide variety of animal experiments and several double-blind, randomized, controlled volunteer studies have shown that levobupivacaine and ropivacaine are significantly less toxic than bupivacaine. The central neurotoxicity of levobupivacaine is intermediate between that of ropivacaine and bupivacaine when administered at the same dosage and rate, and ropivacaine-induced cardiac arrest appears to be more responsive to treatment than that caused by bupivacaine or levobupivacaine.[82-86]

Scott et al.[87] demonstrated that ropivacaine caused fewer CNS symptoms and was at least 25% less toxic than bupivacaine in regard to the dose tolerated. The maximum tolerated unbound arterial plasma concentration was twice as high after ropivacaine than after bupivacaine. Muscular twitching occurred more frequently after bupivacaine. The time for all symptoms to disappear was shorter after ropivacaine. Levobupivacaine is also significantly less toxic to the CNS than bupivacaine. Convulsions with levobupivacaine occurred at a higher concentration and were of briefer duration.[88]

Cardiac Toxicity

Ropivacaine appears to be less cardiotoxic than equal concentrations of racemic bupivacaine, probably because of its faster dissociation from cardiac sodium channels,[89] but it seems to be more cardiotoxic than lidocaine.[90] Bupivacaine is more cardiodepressing and arrhythmogenic than either ropivacaine or lidocaine.[91]

Cardiac signs of toxicity such as dysrhythmia, bradycardia, and hypotension occurred at significantly higher doses of ropivacaine than bupivacaine.[92] Bupivacaine increased QRS width in the presence of sinus rhythm compared with placebo and ropivacaine. Bupivacaine reduced both left ventricular systolic and diastolic function compared with placebo, while ropivacaine reduced only systolic function. At doses producing CNS symptoms, cardiovascular changes, such as depression of conduction and diastolic function, were less pronounced with ropivacaine than with bupivacaine.[93]

Reports of cardiovascular toxicity after accidental intravascular administration of ropivacaine are extremely rare. A case report[94] described severe cardiac dysrhythmia, which developed in a patient with an unbound venous plasma ropivacaine concentration of 1.5 mg/L.

Huang et al.[95] compared the cardiovascular effects of intravenous bupivacaine and levobupivacaine, in sheep. Both drugs depressed the myocardium similarly, but myocardial depression was overshadowed by CNS excitation; levobupivacaine was less likely to cause fatal arrhythmias than bupivacaine. Bardsley et al.[96] confirmed the lower cardiotoxicity of levobupivacaine in humans. In particular the negative inotropic effect for levobupivacaine was less than that for bupivacaine.

Stewart et al.[97] compared the cardiotoxicity of ropivacaine and levobupivacaine and found that both produced similar cardiovascular effects when infused intravenously at equal dosages and infusion rates.

Summary

Ropivacaine and bupivacaine are equipotent over a wide range of concentrations when used in peripheral nerve blockade.

Ropivacaine is less cardiotoxic and causes less CNS toxicity than the same concentrations of bupivacaine.

The threshold for CNS toxicity is higher for ropivacaine than for bupivacaine.

Ropivacaine has advantages over bupivacaine in that the former causes CNS toxicity symptoms before cardiotoxic signs and that it has a higher survival rate than the latter after a massive overdose.

The more rapid clearance of ropivacaine, its more predictable duration of blockade, faster block onset, and less pain on injection are advantages that make ropivacaine the preferred long-acting local anesthetic.

Local Anesthetic Adjuvants

Epinephrine

Epinephrine shortens the onset time of nerve block, causes the block to be denser, increases its duration, and decreases local anesthetic blood concentrations by causing vasoconstriction and relative ischemia to the nerve.[98,99] Because of this ischemia, epinephrine is a possible risk factor for the development of peripheral nerve injury,[100] and we do not recommend its routine use. It may be handy as a marker of intravascular injection and it may reduce the toxic potential and increase the duration of action of short-acting and fast-absorbed drugs such as mepivacaine and lidocaine. Good nerve block techniques (see later) will shorten block onset time, higher concentrations of relatively safe drugs will improve the "density" of a block if that is required, and continuous peripheral block will increase the duration of the block in a controllable manner.

Clonidine

Extrapolating the concept of "balanced analgesia" introduced by Kehlet,[101] some authors advocate adding clonidine[102] and/or opioids[103] to the continuous peripheral nerve block solution. Clonidine prolongs duration of action of local anesthetic agents after single injection brachial plexus block.[104] This may also be true for continuous peripheral nerve block, although the logic of extending the duration of action of the drugs used during a continuous nerve blocks escapes the present authors.

Three mechanisms of action of clonidine can be proposed. Although it is disputed, clonidine may cause local vasoconstriction, thus prolonging local anesthetic action by decreasing the systemic absorption.[105,106] Second, clonidine may have local anesthetic activity.[107] Finally, clonidine could have a potentiating effect on local anesthetics. However, the most common adverse effect of clonidine (orthostatic hypotension) places the patient at risk of falling and injury. Furthermore, the possibility of low oxyhemoglobin levels that may occur in patients who receive clonidine may limit its use in outpatients.[108] A recent study failed to demonstrate better postoperative analgesia when 1 µg/mL of clonidine was added to ropivacaine (0.2%) for continuous femoral nerve block[109] or in continuous infraclavicular perineural infusion.[110] The addition of even 2 µg/mL of clonidine to an interscalene perineural ropivacaine infusion does not provide a clinically relevant improvement in breakthrough pain intensity, local anesthetic consumption, opioid requirements, sleep quality, or satisfaction score.[111]

Opioids

In a systematic review[112] and a metanalysis by Picard et al.,[113] it was concluded that there is no evidence for a clinically significant beneficial effect of added opioids during peripheral nerve blocks. The use of opioids does not seem to be warranted. In all trials, however, large doses of high-concentration local anesthetic agents were used. This may have masked the augmentative effect of the opioids.[114] Regional anesthesia with local anesthetic agents produces excellent analgesia with very few side effects compared to intravenous or subcutaneous opioids. Adding opioids to the local anesthetic agents may largely cause a loss of this advantage.

▶ INFUSION PUMPS

A pump that can provide a basal infusion as well as patient-controlled boluses is ideal for patient controlled regional anesthesia (PCRA). In this way, anesthesia can be tailored to provide a minimal basal rate to lengthen the duration of infusion maximally,[115] while breakthrough pain can be treated or prevented with boluses before physical therapy. Moreover, PCRA offers adequate analgesia with a lower consumption of local anesthetic agent as was proven in numerous trials.

For ambulant PCRA, battery-powered electronic and nonelectronic disposable pumps are available. The ideal infusion pump should be disposable, electronic, refillable, completely and easily programmable with both basal and bolus capabilities, and reprogrammable. The pump should be lightweight, allow monitoring of medication delivery through a digital readout screen, and come with a carrying case for ambulant patients. The pump that seems to answer these requirements is the PainPump2 BlockAid (Stryker Instruments, Kalamazoo, MI).

Nonelectronic Disposable Pumps

These pumps are classified into elastomeric-, spring-, or vacuum-powered. An elastomeric pump is a device with a distensible bulb inside a protective bulb, a filling port, delivery tubing, and a filter. It does not require special care or reprogramming; it is also simple to use, disposable, and potentially cheaper. Recent studies showed that there are fewer technical problems and greater patient and nurse satisfaction with these pumps.[116,117] Because of this and because they provide freedom of movement, they have also been used in children.[118] However, these pumps have limitations. There is no way to detect whether and how much local anesthetic is delivered or how much is left in the reservoir. Since there is no high-pressure alarm, detecting and correcting an occlusion in the catheter is difficult. When a pump with a low working pressure is used, the catheter can become occluded (25 percent in Iskandar's study).[119] Furthermore, the rate of drug delivery cannot be adjusted to the patient's needs. Ilfeld et al. investigated the accuracy of pump delivery in six PCRA-pumps (spring-, elastomeric-, and electronically powered) and found that both elastomeric- and spring-powered pumps infused at higher than expected rates initially, with infusion volume decreasing over the duration of the infusion period.[120] Increased ambient temperature increased the infusion rates by 5 to 10 percent in certain pumps. Low air pressure led to a decreased infusion rate in some pumps.[121] Therefore atmospheric pressure changes—as, for example, in airplanes—has some effect on fluid delivery.[122]

Electrical Pumps

There are a few nonelectrical disposable pumps available that provide continuous infusion and patient-controlled boluses, but only electronic pumps provide the desired profile. In principle, patients, who are often very weak, cannot provide the energy that is needed to inject the patient-controlled bolus. This situation prevents nonelectrical pumps from being ideal. However, most electronic pumps are complex and have to be reprogrammed in case of a too dense or insufficient block. Moreover, these pumps are usually nondisposable and expensive. They can get lost, particularly in an ambulatory setting, with financial hardship for the patient. This problem has been addressed by providing the patient with a self-addressed prepaid envelope to mail the pump back.[123] Ilfeld et al.[124] described the use of small, lightweight, reprogrammable pumps for which the programming instructions can be telephonically explained to the patient. This system allows a progressive decrease in the patient's basal infusion rate as the pain gets less, which not only decreases the risk of local anesthetic toxicity but also allows a longer period of infusion without the need to refill the pump.

Refer to the recent review article by Ilfeld et al. regarding continuous peripheral nerve blocks at home for more details concerning drugs and infusion pumps.[125]

For needles and catheter systems, see Chap. 20.

REFERENCES

1. Dony P, Dewinde V, Vanderick B, et al. The comparative toxicity of ropivacaine and bupivacaine at equipotent doses in rats. *Anesth Analg* 91:1489–1492, 2000.
2. Bader AM, Datta S, Flanagan H, et al. Comparison of bupivacaine and ropivacaine-induced conduction blockade in the isolated rabbit vagus nerve. *Anesth Analg* 68:724–727, 1989.
3. Rosenberg PH, Heinonen E. Differential sensitivity of A and C nerve fibres to long-acting amide local anesthetics. *Br J Ansth* 55:63–67, 1983.
4. Wildsmith JA, Brown DT, Paul D, et al. Structure-activity relationships in differential nerve block at high and low frequency stimulation (abstr). *Br J Anaesth* 63:444–452, 1989.
5. Foster RH, Markham A. Levobupivacaine: A review of its pharmacology and use as a local anesthetic. *Drugs* 59:551–579, 2000.
6. Bardsley H, Gristwood R, Baker H, et al. A comparison of the cardiovascular effects of levobupivacaine and rac-bupivacaine following intravenous administration to healthy volunteers. *Br J Clin Pharmacol* 46:245–249, 1998.
7. Casati A. Pharmacology of local anesthetics, in Chelly JE, Casati A, Fanelli G, (eds.): *Continuous Peripheral Nerve Block Techniques. An illustrated Guide.* New York: Mosby, 2001:29–36.
8. Brown DL, Ransom DM, Hall JA, et al. Regional anesthesia and local anesthetic-induced systemic toxicity: Seizure frequency and accompanying cardiovascular changes. *Anesth Analg* 81:321–328, 1995.
9. Dony P, Dewinde V, Vanderick B, et al. The comparative toxicity of ropivacaine and bupivacaine at equipotent doses in rats. *Anesth Analg* 91:1489–1492, 2000.
10. Choi RH, Birknes JK, Popitz-Bergez FA, et al. Pharmacokinetic nature of tachyphylaxis to lidocaine: Peripheral nerve blocks and infiltration anesthesia in rats. *Life Sci* 61:177–184, 1997.
11. Bardsley H, Gristwood R, Baker H, et al. A comparison of the cardiovascular effects of levobupivacaine and rac-bupivacaine following intravenous administration to healthy volunteers. *Br J Clin Pharmacol* 46:245–240, 1998.
12. Ilfeld BM, Morey TE, Enneking FK. Continuous infraclavicular brachial plexus block for postoperative pain control at home: A randomized, double-blinded placebo-controlled study. *Anesthesiology* 96:1297–1304, 2002.
13. Whiteside J. Regional anesthesia with ropivacaine (letter). *Reg Anesth Pain Med* 25:659, 2000.
14. Bertini L, Benedetto PD. Equipotency of ropivacaine and bupivacaine in peripheral nerve block (letter). *Reg Anesth Pain Med* 25:659–660, 2000.
15. Bertini L, Tagariello V, Mancini S, et al. 0.75% and 0.5% ropivacaine for axillary brachial plexus block: A clinical comparison with 0.5% bupivacaine. *Reg Anesth Pain Med* 24:514–518, 1999.
16. Hickey R, Hoffmann J, Ramamurthy S. A comparison of ropivacaine 0.5% and bupivacaine 0.5% for brachial plexus block. *Anesthesiology* 74:639–642, 1991.

17. Bertini L, Tagariello V, Mancini S, et al. 0.75% and 0.5% ropivacaine for axillary brachial plexus block: A clinical comparison with 0.5% bupivacaine. *Reg Anesth Pain Med* 24:514–518, 1999.

18. McGlade DP, Kalpokas MV, Mooney PH, et al. A comparison of 0.5% ropivacaine and 0.5% bupivacaine for axillary brachial plexus anesthesia. *Anaesth Intens Care* 126:515–520, 1998.

19. Klein SM, Greengrass RA, Steele SM, et al. A comparison of 0.5% bupivacaine, 0.5% ropivacaine, and 0.75% ropivacaine for interscalene brachial plexus block. *Anesth Analg* 87:1316–1319, 1998.

20. McGlade DP, Kalpokas MV, Mooney PH, et al. A comparison of 0.5% ropivacaine and 0.5% bupivacaine for axillary brachial plexus anesthesia. *Anaesth Intens Care* 126:515–520, 1998.

21. Klein SM, Greengrass RA, Steele SM, et al. A comparison of 0.5% bupivacaine, 0.5% ropivacaine, and 0.75% ropivacaine for interscalene brachial plexus block. *Anesth Analg* 87:1316–1319, 1998.

22. Rosenberg PH, Pere P, Hekali R, et al. Plasma concentrations of bupivacaine and two of its metabolites during continuous interscalene brachial plexus. *Br J Anaesth* 66:25–30, 1991.

23. Erichsen CJ, Sjövall J, Kehlet H, et al. Pharmacokinetics and analgesic effect of ropivacaine during continuous epidural infusion for postoperative pain relief. *Anesthesiology* 84:834–842, 1996.

24. Aronsen KF, Ekelund G, Kindmark CO, et al. Sequential changes of plasma proteins after surgical trauma. *Scan J Clin Lab Invest* 29:127–136, 1972.

25. Wulf H, Winckler K, Maier C, et al. Pharmocokinetics and protein binding of bupivacaine in postoperative epidural analgesia. *Acta Anesthesiol Scand* 32:530–534, 1988.

26. Burm AG, Stienstra R, Brouwer RP, et al. Epidural infusion of ropivacaine for postoperative analgesia after major orthopedic surgery: Pharmacokinetic evaluation. *Anesthesiology* 93:395–403, 2000.

27. Tuominen M, Haasio J, Hekali R, et al. Continuous interscalene brachial plexus block: Clinical efficacy, technical problems and bupivacaine plasma concentrations. *Acta Anesthesiol Scand* 33:84–88, 1989.

28. Tucker GT. Pharmacokinetics of local anaesthetics. *Br J Anaesth* 58:717–731, 1986.

29. Ekatodramis G, Borgeat A, Huledal G, et al. Continuous interscalene analgesia with ropivacaine 2 mg/mL after major shoulder surgery. *Anesthesiology* 98:143–150, 2003.

30. Tuominen M, Pitkanen M, Rosenberg PH. Postoperative pain relief and bupivacaine plasma levels during continuous interscalene brachial plexus block. *Acta Anesthesiol Scand* 31:276–278, 1987.

31. Tuominen M, Haasio J, Hekali R, et al. Continuous interscalene brachial plexus block: Clinical efficacy, technical problems and bupivacaine plasma concentrations. *Acta Anesthesiol Scand* 33:84–88, 1989.

32. Rosenberg PH, Pere P, Hekali R, et al. Plasma concentrations of bupivacaine and two of its metabolites during continuous interscalene brachial plexus. *Br J Anaesth* 66:25–30, 1991.

33. Pere P, Tuominen M, Rosenberg PH. Cumulation of bupivacaine, desbutylbupivacaine and 4-hydroxybupivacaine during and after continuous interscalene brachial plexus block. *Acta Anesth Scand* 35:647–650, 1991.

34. Tucker GT. Pharmacokinetics of local anaesthetics. *Br J Anaesth* 58:717–731, 1986.

35. Rosenberg PH, Pere P, Hekali R, et al. Plasma concentrations of bupivacaine and two of its metabolites during continuous interscalene brachial plexus. *Br J Anaesth* 66:25–30, 1991.

36. Ekatodramis G, Borgeat A, Huledal G, et al. Continuous interscalene analgesia with ropivacaine 2 mg/mL after major shoulder surgery. *Anesthesiology* 98:143–150, 2003.

37. Burm AG, Stienstra R, Brouwer RP, et al. Epidural infusion of ropivacaine for postoperative analgesia after major orthopedic surgery: Pharmacokinetic evaluation. *Anesthesiology* 93:395–403, 2000.

38. Ekatodramis G, Borgeat A, Huledal G, et al. Continuous interscalene analgesia with ropivacaine 2 mg/mL after major shoulder surgery. *Anesthesiology* 98:143–150, 2003.

39. Knudsen K, Beckman Suurküla M, Blomberg J, et al. Central nervous and cardiovascular effects of i.v. infusions of ropivacaine, bupivacaine and placebo in volunteers. *Br J Anaesth* 78:507–514, 1977.

40. Burm AG, Stienstra R, Brouwer RP, et al. Epidural infusion of ropivacaine for postoperative analgesia after major orthopedic surgery: Pharmacokinetic evaluation. *Anesthesiology* 93:395–403, 2000.

41. Erichsen CJ, Sjövall J, Kehlet H, et al. Pharmacokinetics and analgesic effect of ropivacaine during continuous epidural infusion for postoperative pain relief. *Anesthesiology* 84:834–842, 1996.

42. Halldin MM, Bredberg E, Angelin B. et al. Metabolism and excretion of ropivacaine in humans. *Drug Metab Dispos* 24:962–968, 1996.

43. Erichsen CJ, Sjövall J, Kehlet H, et al. Pharmacokinetics and analgesic effect of ropivacaine during continuous epidural infusion for postoperative pain relief. *Anesthesiology* 84:834–842, 1996.

44. Halldin MM, Bredberg E, Angelin B. et al. Metabolism and excretion of ropivacaine in humans. *Drug Metab Dispos* 24:962–968, 1996.

45. Ekström G, Gunnarsson UB. Ropivacaine, a new amide-type local anesthetic agent, is metabolized by cytochrome P450 1A and 3A in human liver microsomes. *Drug Metab Dispos* 24:955–956, 1996.

46. Arlander E, Ekström G, Alm C, et al. Metabolism of ropivacaine in humans is mediated by CYP1A2 and to a minor extent by CYP3A4: An interaction study with fluvoxamine and ketoconazole as in vivo inhibitors. *Clin Pharmacol Ther* 64:484–491, 1998.

47. Halldin MM, Bredberg E, Angelin B. et al. Metabolism and excretion of ropivacaine in humans. *Drug Metab Dispos* 24:962–968, 1996.

48. Burm AG, Stienstra R, Brouwer RP, et al. Epidural infusion of ropivacaine for postoperative analgesia after major orthopedic surgery: Pharmacokinetic evaluation. *Anesthesiology* 93:395–403, 2000.

49. Ekatodramis G, Borgeat A, Huledal G, et al. Continuous interscalene analgesia with ropivacaine 2 mg/mL after major shoulder surgery. *Anesthesiology* 98:143–150, 2003.

50. Pere P, Salonen M, Jokinen M, et al. Pharmacokinetics of ropivacaine in uremic and nonuremic patients after axillary brachial plexus block. *Anesth Analg* 96:563–569, 2003.

51. Pere P, Salonen M, Jokinen M, et al. Pharmacokinetics of ropivacaine in uremic and nonuremic patients after axillary brachial plexus block. *Anesth Analg* 96:563–569, 2003.

52. Reynolds F. Metabolism and excretion of bupivacaine in man: A comparison with mepivacaine. *Br J Anaesth* 43:33–37, 1971.

53. Rosenberg PH, Heavner J. Acute toxicity of bupivacaine and desbutylbupivacaine in the rat (ASA abstract). *Anesthesiology* 73:3A:A817, 1990.

54. Rosenberg PH, Pere P, Hekali R, Tuominen M. Plasma concentrations of bupivacaine and two of its metabolites during continuous interscalene brachial plexus. *Br J Anaesth* 66:25–30, 1991.

55. Pere P, Tuominen M, Rosenberg PH. Cumulation of bupivacaine, desbutylbupivacaine and 4-hydroxybupivacaine during and after continuous interscalene brachial plexus block. *Acta Anesth Scand* 35:647–650, 1991.

56. Lew E, Vloka JD, Hadzic A. Ropivacaine for peripheral nerve blocks: Are there advantages? *Tech Reg Anesth Pain Mgt* 5:56–59, 2001.

57. Akerman B, Hellberg IB, Trossvik C. Primary evaluation of the local anesthetic proporties of the amino-acid agent ropivacaine (LEA 103). *Acta Anesthesiol Scand* 32:571–578, 1988.

58. Luchetti M, Magni G, Marraro G. A prospective randomized double-blinded controlled study of ropivacaine 0.75% versus bupivacaine 0.5%-mepivacaine 2% for peribulbar anesthesia. *Reg anesth Pain Med* 25:195–200, 2000.

59. Krishnan SK, Benzon HT, Siddiqui T, et al. Pain of intramuscular injection of bupivacaine, ropivacaine, with and without dexamethasone. *Reg Anesth Pain Med* 25:615–619, 2000.

60. Benoit PW, Belt WD. Some effects of local anesthetic agents on skeletal muscle. *Exp Neurol* 34:264–278, 1972.

61. Benoit PW. Reversible skeletal muscle damage after administration of local anesthetics with and without epinephrine. *J Oral Surg* 36:198–201, 1978.

62. Foster AH, Carlson BM. Myotoxicity of local anesthetics and regeneration of the damaged muscle fibers. *Anesth Analg* 59:727–736, 1980.

63. Hogan Q, Dotson R, Erickson S, et al. Local anesthetic myotoxicity: A case and review. *Anesthesiology* 80:942–947, 1994.

64. Newman RJ, Radda GK. The myotoxicity of bupivacaine, a 31P n.m.r. investigation. *Br J Pharmacol* 79:395–399, 1983.

65. Benoit PW. Microscarring in skeletal muscle after repeated exposures to lidocaine with epinephrine. *J Oral Surg* 36:530–533, 1978.

66. Parris WC, Dettbarn WD. Muscle atrophy following nerve block therapy. *Anaesthesiology* 69:289, 1988.

67. Salama H, Farr AK, Guyton DL. Anesthetic myotoxicity as a cause of restrictive strabismus after scleral buckling surgery. *Retina* 20:478–482, 2000.

68. Hogan Q, Dotson R, Erickson S, et al. Local anesthetic myotoxicity: A case and review. *Anesthesiology* 80:942–947, 1994.

69. Sadeh M, Czyzewski K, Stern L. Chronic myopathy induced by repeated bupivacaine injections. *J Neurol Sci* 67:229–238, 1993.

70. Kytta J, Heinonen E, Rosenberg PH, et al. Effects of repeated bupivacaine administration on sciatic nerve and surrounding muscle tissue in rats. *Acta Anesthesiol Scand* 30:625–629, 1986.

71. Hogan Q, Dotson R, Erickson S, et al. Local anesthetic myotoxicity: A case and review. *Anesthesiology* 80:942–947, 1994.

72. Zink W, Seif C, Bohl JRE, et al. The acute myotoxic effects of bupivacaine and ropivacaine after continuous peripheral nerve blockades. *Anesth Analg* 97:1173–1179, 2003.

73. Kytta J, Heinonen E, Rosenberg PH, et al. Effects of repeated bupivacaine administration on sciatic nerve and surrounding muscle tissue in rats. *Acta Anesthesiol Scand* 30:625–629, 1986.

74. Benoit PW, Belt WD. Some effects of local anesthetic agents on skeletal muscle. *Exp Neurol* 34:264–278, 1972.

75. Benoit PW. Reversible skeletal muscle damage after administration of local anesthetics with and without epinephrine. *J Oral Surg* 36:198–201, 1978.

76. Hogan Q, Dotson R, Erickson S, et al. Local anesthetic myotoxicity: A case and review. *Anesthesiology* 80:942–947, 1994.

77. Scott DB, Lee A, Fagan D, et al. Acute toxicity of ropivacaine compared with that of bupivacaine. *Anesth Analg* 69:563–569, 1989.

78. Reiz S, Nath S. Cardiotoxicity of local anaesthetic agents on cardiac conduction and contractility. *Reg Anesth* 6:55–61, 1681.

79. Ala-Kokko TI, Löppönen A, Alahuhta S. Two instances of central nervous system toxicity in the same patient following repeated ropivacaine-induced brachial plexus block. *Acta Anesthesiol Scand* 44:623–626, 2000.

80. Breslin DS, Martin G, Macleod DB, et al. Central nervous system toxicity following the administration of levobupivacaine for lumbar plexus block: A report of two cases. *Reg Anesth Pain Med* 28:144–147, 2003.

81. Crews J, Rohman TE. Seizure after levobupivacaine for interscalene brachial plexus block. *Anesth Analg* 96:1188–1190, 2003.

82. Morrison SG, Dominguez JJ, Frascarlo P, et al. A comparison of the electrocardiographic cardiotoxic effects of racemic bupivacaine, levobupivacaine, and ropivacaine in anesthetized swine. *Anesth Analg* 90:1308–1314, 2000.

83. Ohmura S, Kawada M, Ohta T, et al. Systemic toxicity and resuscitation in bupivacaine, levobupivacaine, or ropivacaine-infused rats. *Anesth Analg* 93:743–748, 2001.

84. Scott DB, Lee A, Fagan D, et al. Acute toxicity of ropivacaine compared with that of bupivacaine. *Anesth Analg* 69:563–569, 1989.

85. Knudsen K, Beckman Suurküla M, Blomberg J, et al. Central nervous and cardiovascular effects of i.v. infusions of ropivacaine, bupivacaine and placebo in volunteers. *Br J Anaesth* 78:507–514, 1977.

86. Bardsley H, Gristwood R, Baker H, et al. A comparison of the cardiovascular effects of levobupivacaine and rac-bupivacaine following intravenous administration to healthy volunteers. *Br J Clin Pharmacol* 46:245–240, 1998.

87. Scott DB, Lee A, Fagan D, et al. Acute toxicity of ropivacaine compared with that of bupivacaine. *Anesth Analg* 69:563–569, 1989.

88. Huang YF, Pryor ME, Mather LE, et al. Cardiovascular and central nervous system effects of intravenous levabupivacaine and bupivacaine in sheep. *Anesth Analg* 86:797–804, 1998.

89. Clarkson CW, Hondeghem LM. Mechanism for bupivacaine depression of cardiac conduction: Fast block of sodium channels during the action potential with a slow recovery from block during diastole. *Anesthesiology* 62:396–405, 1985.

90. McClellan KJ, Faulds D. Ropivacaine: An update of its use in regional anesthesia. *Drugs* 60:1065–1093, 2000.

91. Pitkanen M, Feldman HS, Arthur GR, et al. Chronotropic and inotropic effects of ropivacaine, bupivacaine, and lido-caine in the spontaneously beating and electrically paced isolated, perfused rabbit heart. *Reg Anesth* 17:183–192, 1992.

92. Cuignet O, Dony P, Gautier P, et al. Comparative toxicity of ropivacaine and bupivacaine at equipotent dose in rats (abstr. A 370). *Eur J Anaesthesiol* 19:113, 2000.

93. Knudsen K, Beckman Suurküla M, Blomberg J, et al. Central nervous and cardiovascular effects of i.v. infusions of ropivacaine, bupivacaine and placebo in volunteers. *Br J Anaesth* 78:507–514, 1997.

94. Ruetsch YA, Fattinger KE, Borgeat A. Ropivacaine-induced convulsions and severe cardiac dysrhythmia after sciatic block. *Anesthesiology* 90:1784–1786, 1999.

95. Huang, YF, Pryor ME, Mather LE, et al. Cardiovascular and central nervous system effects of intravenous lev-abupivacaine and bupivacaine in sheep. *Anesth Analag* 86:797–804, 1998.

96. Bardsley H, Gristwood R, Baker H, et al. A comparison of the cardiovascular effects of levobupivacaine and rac-bupivacaine following intravenous administration to healthy volunteers. *Br J Clin Pharmacol* 46:245–249, 1998.

97. Stewart J, Kellett N, Castro D. The central nervous system and cardiovascular effects of levobupivacaine and ropiva-caine in healthy volunteers. *Anesth Analg* 97:412–416, 2003.

98. Bernards CM, Kopacz DJ. Effects of epinephrine on lido-caine clearance in vivo: A microdialysis study in humans. *Anesthesiology* 91:962–968, 1999.

99. Weber A, Fournier R, Van Gessel E, et al. Epinephrine does not prolong the analgesia of 20 mL ropivacaine 0.5% or 0.2% in a femoral three-in-one block. *Anesth Analg* 93:1327–1331, 2001.

100. Selander D, Brattsand R, Lundborg G, et al. Local anes-thetics: Importance of mode of application, concentration and adrenaline for the appearance of nerve lesions. An experimental study of axonal degeneration and barrier damage after intrafascicular injection or topical applica-tion of bupivacaine (Marcain). *Acta Anesthesiol Scand* 23:127–136, 1979.

101. Khelet H. Surgical stress: The role of pain and analgesia. *Br J Anaesth* 63:189–195, 1989.

102. Iskandar H, Bernard A, Ruel-Raymond J, et al. The anal-gesic effect of interscalene block using clonidine as an analgesic for shoulder arthroscopy. *Anesth Analg* 96:260–262, 2003.

103. Singelyn FJ, Seguy S, Gouverneur JM. Interscalene brachial plexus analgesia after open shoulder surgery: Continuous versus patient-controlled infusion. *Anesth Analg* 89:1216–1220, 1999.

104. Singelyn FJ, Gouverneur JM, Robrt A. A minimum dose of clonidine added to mepivacaine prolongs the duration of anesthesia and analgesia after axillary brachial plexus block. *Anesth Analg* 83:1046–1050, 1996.

105. Langer S, Duval N, Massingham R. Pharmacologic and therapeutic significance of alpha-adrenorecetor subtypes. *J Cardiovasc Pharmacol* 7:1–8, 1985.

106. Eledjam JJ, Deschodt J, Viel E, et al. Brachial plexus block with bupivacaine: Effects of added alpha-adrenergic ago-nists: Comparison between clonidine and epinephrine. *Can J Anaesth* 38:870–875, 1991.

107. Starke K, Wagner J, Schürmann HJ. Adrenergic neuron blockade by clonidine: Comparison with guanethidine and local anesthetics. *Anesth Analg* 74:719–725, 1992.

108. Bernard JM, Macaire P. Dose-range effects of clonidine added to lidocaine for brachial plexus block. *Anesthesiology* 87:277–284, 1997.

109. Manzoni P, Spreafico E, Mamo D, et al. 0.2% ropivacaine for continuous femoral nerve block after major knee surgery: A pilot study. *Minerva Anesthesiol* 70:531, 2004.

110. Ilfeld BM, Morey TE, Enneking FK. Continuous infraclav-icular perineural infusion with clonidine and ropivacaine compared with ropivacaine alone: A randomized double-blind, controlled study. *Anesth Analg* 97:706–712, 2003.

111. Ilfeld BM, Morey TE, Thannikary LJ, et al. Clonidine added to a continuous interscalene ropivacaine perineural infusion to improve postoperative analgesia: A randomized, double-blind, controlled study. *Anesth Analg* 100:1172–1178, 2005.

112. Murphy DB, McCartney CJ, Chan VW. Novel analgesic adjuncts for brachial plexus block: A systematic review. *Anesth Analg* 90:1122–1128, 2000.

113. Picard P, Tramèr M, McQuay H, et al. Analgesic efficacy of peripheral opioids: A qualitative systematic review of ran-domized controlled trials. *Pain* 72:309–318, 1997.

114. Liu SS, Salinas FV. Continuous plexus and peripheral nerve blocks for postoperative analgesia. *Anesth Analg* 96:263–272, 2003.

115. Ilfeld BM, Morey TE, Wright TW, et al. Continuous inter-scalene brachial plexus block for postoperative pain con-trol at home: A randomized, double-blinded, placebo controlled study. *Anesth Analg* 96:1089–1095, 2003.

116. Capdevila X, Macaire P, Aknin P, et al. Patient-controlled perineural analgesia after ambulatory orthopedic surgery: A comparison of electronic versus elastomeric pumps. *Anesth Analg* 96:414–417, 2003.

117. Sawaki Y, Parker RK, White PF. Patient and nurse evalua-tion of PCA delivery systems for postoperative pain man-agement. *J Pain Sympt Mgt* 7:443–453, 1992.

118. Dadure C, Pirat P, Raux O, et al. Peripoperative continuous peripheral nerve blocks with disposable infusion pumps in

children: A prospective descriptive study. *Anesth Analg* 97:687–690, 2003.

119. Iskandar H, Rakotondriamihary S, Dixmerias F, et al. Analgesia using continuous axillary block after surgery of severe hand injuries: Self-administration versus continuous injections. *Ann Fr Anesth Reanim* 17:1099–1103, 1998.

120. Ilfeld BM, Morey TE, Enneking FK. Portable infusion pumps used for continuous regional analgesia: Delivery rate accuracy and consistency. *Reg Anesth Pain Med* 28:424–432, 2003.

121. Mizuuchi M, Yamakage M, Iwasaki S, et al. The infusion rate of most disposable, non-electric infusion pumps decreases under hypobaric conditions. *Can J Anesth* 50:657–662, 2003.

122. Ilfeld BM, Morey TE, Enneking FK. New portable infusion pumps: Read advantages or just more of the same in a different package? *Reg Anesth Pain Med* 29:371–376, 2004.

123. Ilfeld BM, Morey TE, Wright TW, et al. Interscalene perineural ropivacaine infusion: A comparison of two dosing regimens for postoperative analgesia. *Reg Anesth Pain Med* 39:9–16, 2004.

124. Ilfeld BM, Enneking FK.: A portable mechanical pump providing over four days of patient-controlled analgesia by perineural infusion at home. *Reg Anesth Pain Med* 27:100–104, 2002.

125. Ilfeld BM, Enneking FK. Continuous peripheral nerve blocks at home: A review. *Anesth Analg* 100:1822–1833, 2005.

CHAPTER 19

Electrical Nerve Stimulation for Regional Anesthesia

BAN CHI-HO TSUI/DOMINIQUE HOPKINS

► INTRODUCTION

Electrical stimulation is the most commonly used method to localize nerves before the injection of a local anesthetic in performing regional anesthesia. The electrical nerve stimulator (ENS) produces an electrical current that depolarizes the nerve membrane and causes contraction of the effector muscles or sensory stimulation of the relevant area. This confirms the proximity of a needle to the nerve. To use the ENS effectively, a basic understanding of the electrophysiologic principles involved is necessary.

► HISTORICAL BACKGROUND

Although electrical stimulation gained wide acceptance in regional anesthesia only over the last two decades, this technique was first described by von Perthes in 1912.[1] Beginning in 1955, a number of researchers further improved it. Pearson described the localization of nerves with motor responses by electrical stimulation with an insulated needle,[2] Greenblatt and Denson described the use of a portable transistorized nerve stimulator with pulsed variable output,[3] and Montgomery et al. demonstrated that ordinary uninsulated needles could be used, albeit with a higher current.[4] Finally, in the 1980s, Ford, Pither, and Raj emphasized the important characteristics of the ENS and described the performances of insulated and uninsulated needles.[5,6]

► ELECTROPHYSIOLOGY OF NERVE STIMULATION

The ENS excites nerves by producing an electrical current that induces a flow of ions through the nerve membrane and initiates an action potential (Fig. 19-1). The characteristics of the electrical impulse affect its ability to stimulate nerve fibers. In addition, the distance from the nerve, polarity, and type of the electrode used also greatly influence the quality of stimulation.

Effects of the Characteristics of Impulse

Intensity

When a square pulse of current is applied to a nerve, a charge (Q) is delivered that is equal to the product of the intensity (I) of the applied current and the duration (t) of the current pulse:

$$Q = I \times t$$

When intensity is plotted against duration, a typical stimulation or excitability curve is obtained, with the relationship $I = \mathrm{Ir}\,(1 + C/t)$, with two important parameters:

1. The rheobase (Ir), which is the minimum current intensity, required to stimulate the nerve
2. The chronaxy (C), which is the minimum duration of the pulse required to stimulate the nerve when the intensity of the current is twice the rheobase

Cathode

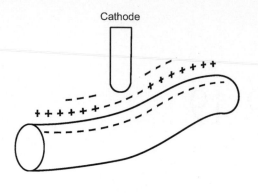

Anode

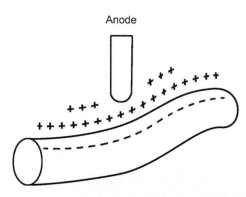

Figure 19-1. Preferential cathodal stimulation. A stimulating current applied via the cathode creates an area of depolarization of the nerve membrane around the electrode, whereas when applied via the anode, it creates an area of hyperpolarization and decreased excitability.

Duration

The rheobase and chronaxy demonstrate that it is not possible to stimulate a nerve by applying a current below a threshold intensity, regardless of the pulse duration, nor by applying a current below a threshold duration, regardless of its intensity.[7]

It has been observed that the larger the fiber, the easier it is to stimulate it and the shorter its chronaxy.[8,9] Different types of nerve fibers can be stimulated by varying the electrical pulse widths. Large A-alpha motor fibers with chronaxies of 50 to 100 μs can be stimulated without stimulating the smaller A-delta and C fibers (responsible for pain transmission), with chronaxies of about 150 and 400 μs, respectively.[9,10] By using a minimal current and a short pulse, a twitch of the muscles supplied by the motor fibers can be produced without causing pain, since the sensory fibers need a longer pulse for stimulation. However, more recent data suggest that the duration of the pulse is not important in causing pain or discomfort during electrostimulation.[11,12] The main causes of discomfort seem to be related to the withdrawal and repositioning of the stimulating needle,[13] the

strength of the elicited muscle contraction, and high intensities of the stimulating current.[11]

A short pulse can be used as a sensitive indicator of the distance between needle and nerve.[5] When the needle tip is touching the nerve, the duration of the stimulating current has only a moderate effect on the minimal intensity required. However, when the needle tip is remote from the nerve, the pulse duration becomes very important. When the tip of the needle is 1 cm away from the nerve, instead of touching it, a tenfold increase in the current is required with a 40-μs pulse to cause stimulation. If the pulse is lengthened to 1 ms, the necessary increase in current is only twofold.

Rate of Change

Finally, it may not be possible to stimulate a nerve fiber no matter how strong the stimulus if it is applied too slowly. A prolonged subthreshold stimulus or a slowly rising current may reduce nerve excitability by inactivating sodium conductance before the depolarization reaches the threshold.[14] This is known as "accommodation" of nerve fibers. To avoid accommodation, square waves of current are used to keep the rising time very short.

Relationship between Current Intensity and Distance from the Nerve

The closer the stimulating electrode is to a nerve, the lower the current intensity necessary for its excitation, as stated in Coulomb's law:

$$I = k(i/r^2)$$

where I is the current required, k is a constant, i is the minimal current, and r is the distance from the nerve. Since the relationship is the inverse of the square of the distance, a very high current is needed when the electrode is far from the nerve, and much less is needed as the electrode comes closer to the nerve. It is calculated that the current intensity necessary to stimulate a nerve is 0.1 mA when the electrode is right on the nerve, 2.5 mA when the electrode is 0.5 cm away from the nerve, and 40 mA when the electrode is 2 cm away.[10] In the clinical context, these higher currents may be sufficient to cause microshock if they are applied directly to the heart and become painful by directly stimulating nerve endings in the surrounding tissues.

Preferential Cathodal Stimulation

If two electrodes are placed on a nerve and a direct electrical current is made to flow through them, the nerve fiber is stimulated at the *cathode* (negative electrode) and becomes more resistant to excitation at the *anode* (positive electrode) (Fig. 19-1).[15] The negative current from the cathode reduces the voltage immediately outside the membrane. Consequently, the voltage difference across the membrane is decreased, causing an area of depolarization and an action potential. Conversely, at the anode, the injection of positive charges outside the nerve membrane increases the voltage difference across the membrane, causing hyperpolarization and a decrease in excitability (Fig. 19-1). Cessation of an anodal current may, however, overshoot the membrane potential in the depolarizing direction. This rebound may be large enough to initiate an action potential. If the anode instead of the cathode is used as the stimulating electrode to elicit a motor response, three to four times more current is required.[5,11,16]

Types of Electrodes/Needles

The needle is an extension of the stimulating electrode. Two types of stimulating needles can be used for this purpose: (1) electrically insulated or (2) uninsulated. Their properties and the geometries of the electrical fields they produce are quite different (Fig. 19-2).[6,17,18]

Insulated Needles

The shafts of insulated needles are covered with a layer of nonconducting material (e.g., Teflon), leaving the tip

bare. On stimulation, the pattern of the current density is a sphere around the tip of the needle (Fig. 19-2). Because of the small conducting area, there is a high current density at this point, and a low threshold current is sufficient to localize the nerve. Insulated needles with a cutting bevel are normally used. This type of needle requires a threshold current of about 0.5 to 0.7 mA and a pulse width of 100 μs to stimulate a nerve when it is approximately 2 to 5 mm away. More sophisticated needles have a pinpoint electrode tip, where both the shaft and the bevel are insulated and only the very tip of the needle can conduct the current.[19] The pinpoint electrode concentrates the entire stimulus current in this very small area, allowing for even more precise localization of the nerve with very low threshold currents, such as only 0.2 mA with a 100-μs pulse.

Uninsulated Needles

Uninsulated needles transmit the current throughout their entire length (Fig. 19-2). These needles require higher minimal currents than insulated ones, generally in excess of 1 mA, to excite a nerve.[6] The maximum current density is at the needle tip with a zone extending up the needle shaft.[17] With these needles, it is more difficult to localize the nerve accurately with low current intensities. As the needle tip moves further past the nerve, the required current remains constant because of continuous stimulation by the shaft.[6] Thus, "false localization" may occur due to stimulation of the nerve by the shaft instead of the tip of the needle.

▶ THE MODERN ELECTRICAL NERVE STIMULATOR

The electrical characteristics of the ENS that contribute to the successful localization of a peripheral nerve include the following.[5,20]

Constant and Linear Current Output

With the newer type of ENS, the current output may be set in milliamperes (intensity) or in nanocoulombs (charge). The relationship nC = mA × μs is obtained from $Q = I \times t$. (For example, a 2-mA current applied for 50 μs provides a 100-nC charge; the same current applied for 300 μs provides a 600-nC charge.)

Ideally, the current output of the ENS (intensity or charge) should remain unaffected by changes in the resistance of the entire circuit, such as those arising from tissue, needles, connectors, etc., and should also remain constant throughout a wide range of resistances. In the past, most commercially produced nerve stimulators utilized a constant voltage system. However, since it is the current and not the voltage that stimulates the nerve,

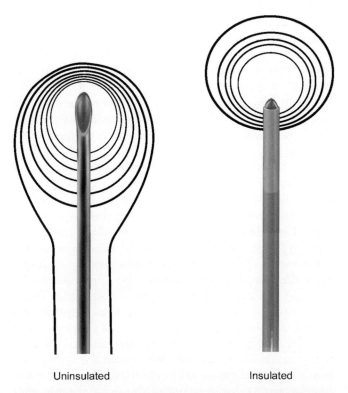

Uninsulated   Insulated

Figure 19-2. Current contour lines around uninsulated and insulated needles. Computer simulation of the electrical field around the tips of insulated and uninsulated needles. (*Adapted from Bashein et al.,*[17] *with permission.*)

new models now deliver a constant current in spite of changes in resistance. A linear current output, especially in the lower range, is also an important feature of the ENS. With a nonlinear output, a small movement of the dial in setting the current strength may result in a large change in intensity. A nerve stimulator with low- and high-output ranges will often have a linear output in the low range (0 to 5 mA) and a logarithmic output in the high range of intensities (as when it is used to monitor neuromuscular blockade). Current delivery, especially in the low-intensity range, was variable with older ENS models,[5,21,22] but newer models with constant and linear output circuitry deliver current with greater accuracy.

Variable Pulse Width

The duration of the delivered electrical pulse is an important element in neurostimulation because, apart from determining the amount of charge delivered, pulse width plays a role in the selectivity and precision of stimulation, as described earlier. Most nerve stimulators deliver an electrical pulse width of 100 or 200 μs for stimulating motor nerves as their default settings. However, more sophisticated devices can provide variable pulse widths from 50 to 1 ms.

Clearly Marked Polarity of the Electrodes

With the newer types of ENS, the cathode has a specialized male connector designed to fit into the female conducting portion of the stimulating needle. This serves two purposes: it avoids confusion between the electrodes and provides greater safety by eliminating any exposed "live" connection. The cathode should preferably be the stimulating electrode, as it is three to four times more effective than the anode in producing depolarization of the nerve membrane.[5,11,16]

Variable Pulse Frequency

With newer ENS models, the frequency of the delivered electrical pulse can be changed. The optimal is between 0.5 and 4 Hz, and most users select a frequency of 1 or 2 Hz.

▶ PRACTICAL CONSIDERATIONS OF PERIPHERAL NERVE BLOCKS

Previously, it was thought that, to prevent direct stimulation of muscles via local flow of the current, the returning electrode (which should be the anode or positive electrode) had to be positioned on the patient's skin at least 20 cm away from the site of stimulation.[23] However, new data suggest that the site is not critical. With a constant-current-output ENS, changing the position

of the returning electrode from a remote location to 5 cm away from the stimulation site did not result in any change in the grade of the motor response or in the current required to maintain it.[11]

The stimulating needle is connected to the cathode and the area where the needle is to be inserted is disinfected. The needle is advanced through the skin and the stimulator is turned on at the relatively high intensity of 2 to 3 mA, with a pulse of 100 to 200 μs. Under these conditions, an electrical charge large enough to excite the nerve is delivered while the needle is still at some distance from it without causing discomfort to the patient. Once contractions of the appropriate muscle group are elicited, the needle tip is likely to be 1 to 2 cm away from the nerve.[10] The needle is advanced further and, if the strength of the twitches increases, the current intensity is decreased. The current is gradually reduced until the smallest response is observed. The needle is moved until a muscle twitch is visible with a minimal current, usually around 0.5 mA. Until recently, there were no available data regarding the optimal current necessary to localize nerves. It has been postulated that stimulation at currents higher than 0.5 mA may result in block failure because the needle tip is too far from the nerve,[24] while stimulation at currents lower than 0.2 mA may possibly increase the risk of intraneural injection. In a recent study, Hadzic et al. showed that the minimal current necessary to produce a clearly visible twitch, without movement of the extremity, was about 0.3 mA with a 100-μs duration.[11] They suggested that it was unnecessary to search for a nerve response at currents lower than 0.2 mA (100 μs) since, under these conditions, all their blocks (femoral and interscalene) were successful with a small volume of local anesthetic. These values may not apply to the placement of perineural catheters.[25]

In diabetic and elderly patients, some nerves may have a higher threshold, and it may be necessary to start with a higher current.[10] After aspirating to check that the needle tip is not in a blood vessel, a test dose of 1 to 2 mL of local anesthetic is injected. If the needle is positioned correctly, the muscle twitch should disappear almost immediately.[3,19,23,26] This phenomenon, commonly known as the "Raj test," can also be demonstrated by injecting similarly small volumes of saline or air.[26] Previously, the disappearance of the muscle twitch was attributed to the physical displacement of the nerve from the stimulating needle tip by the injected fluid.[5] However, Tsui et al. recently demonstrated that this phenomenon is best explained in electrical terms and is not entirely due to displacement of the nerve.[27] Only after successful aspiration and injection tests is the full dose of local anesthetic slowly administered.

In stimulating purely sensory nerves, the position of the needle tip near the nerve is confirmed when the patient reports a radiating paresthesia with every pulse in the distribution of the nerve. The sensation should be felt at low current as for a motor block but preferably using a longer, 300-μs to 1-ms pulse width.[10,28]

▶ NEW ASPECTS OF ELECTRICAL STIMULATION

Peripheral Nerve Block

New Understanding of Nerve Stimulation

As described above, a small volume of local anesthetic or normal saline abolishes the muscle twitch induced by a low current (0.5 mA) during nerve stimulation. Despite years of clinical use of nerve stimulation in regional anesthesia, the electrophysiologic effect of such injections on nerve conduction has remained unexplained until recently. In a porcine model, Tsui et al. demonstrated that the injection of 0.9% NaCl abolished the motor response, while a subsequent injection of 5% dextrose in water (D$_5$W) reestablished effective stimulation.[27] An accompanying in vitro experiment showed that injections of solutions such as 0.9% NaCl or 5% D$_5$W cause a change in the electrical field at the needle-tissue interface (Fig. 19-3). It was concluded that the injection of electrically conducting solutions (saline or local anesthetic) increases the conductive area surrounding the stimulating needle tip. This causes a decrease in the current density surrounding a target nerve, which is therefore no longer stimulated. This suggests that effective nerve stimulation is sensitive to changes that occur at the needle-tissue interface, such as a change in the angle of

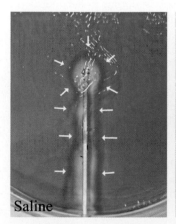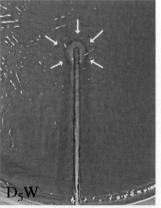

Figure 19-3. Gel electrophoresis: changes in the electrical field with injection of ionic (saline) and nonionic (D$_5$W) solutions. (*From Tsui et al.,*[27] *with permission.*) Arrows show the margin of the clear zone/electrical field. Left: An insulated needle after normal saline injection. Right: An uninsulated needle after D$_5$W injection.

the needle or injection of local anesthetic. The net effect appears to be a change in the current density at the tip of the needle or the path of the electric current, which affects the motor response.[20]

In view of these studies, further work will be needed to establish a new, acceptable current range for motor responses after dilating the perineural spaces with conducting solutions as commonly performed for the placement of perineural catheters. It is not certain, however, whether this "dilating of the perineural spaces" in fact does actually take place. On the other hand, one may use a nonconducting solution, such as D$_5$W, instead of saline, for dilating perineural spaces.[27] Future studies are also warranted to determine the merit of using nonconducting injections in peripheral nerve blocks.

Percutaneous Electrode Guidance (PEG) and "Nerve Mapping"

In recent years, percutaneous location of nerves via transcutaneous stimulation has been used to identify the optimal point on the skin for insertion of the block needle. Several types of cutaneous stimulating electrodes have been tried. These include a modified (0.5-cm diameter) electrocardiograph electrode,[25] the negative electrode of the nerve stimulator,[28,29] and a stub needle.[30–32] A cylindrical electrode with a 0.5-mm metallic tip has also been used successfully to guide the block needle via a central 22-gauge hole.[32] Recently, the tip of the actual stimulating needle has been used directly.[33] The smaller the electrode, the greater the current density applied to the skin and the greater the effect on the tissue.

Capdevila et al. described PEG using the same needle for both prelocation and nerve blockade.[33] The tip of the needle is gently pressed on the patient's skin surface and moved around until a motor response is obtained by using an initial transcutaneous current of 5 mA with a 200-μs pulse width. The stimulating current is then reduced to the minimum intensity required to produce a visible motor response. When the optimal location of the nerve is identified, the needle is inserted at 90 degrees through the skin and a 2-mA current of 100-μs duration is applied. As the required motor response is elicited, the needle depth is adjusted and the current intensity decreased until the muscle twitches are still visible at 0.5 mA. The median value of the minimal transcutaneous current needed to stimulate the nerves of the axillary brachial plexus is 2 to 3 mA. This method of percutaneous electrode guidance is said to be simple, reliable, noninvasive, and painless.

▶ CENTRAL NEURAXIAL BLOCKS

Electrostimulation is now well accepted for identifying peripheral nerves in performing regional anesthesia.[26] In recent years, the same technique has been applied to central neuraxial blocks and has been shown to be a safe, reliable, and easy-to-use method to monitor and confirm correct placement of epidural catheters.[34] Although both aspiration of the epidural catheter and standard test doses (e.g., 3 mL of 1.5% lidocaine with 1:200,000 epinephrine) can detect misplaced subarachnoid or intravascular catheters, many examples of false-positive and false-negative results are associated with these tests.[35] In addition, verification of proper epidural catheter placement is not possible with either of these techniques. Previously, it was thought that radiologic imaging was the only way to confirm that a catheter was located in the epidural space prior to local anesthetic injection.[36] However, recent advances in epidural anesthesia have demonstrated that electrical stimulation (the Tsui test) may be a reliable technique for this purpose.[37-48]

▶ ADVANTAGES OF NEUROSTIMULATION: DOES IT MAKE A DIFFERENCE?

Intuitively, a greater success rate and enhanced safety of the blocks should be expected with ENS. Compared with other methods of nerve localization, such as paresthesia, there is no need to rely on the patient's reports in localizing motor or mixed nerves, and the more accurate placement of the needle should decrease the risk of intraneural injections. In spite of these considerations, earlier clinical studies have claimed that the success rate of blocks performed with neurostimulation was not increased.[3,49] However, the ENS was found to be superior to a radiographic technique in blocking the obturator nerve.[24] Sciatic nerve blocks performed with the ENS were also shown to have a greater success rate than with the paresthesia technique.[49,50] For axillary blockade of the brachial plexus, when only a single nerve is stimulated, the success rate appears to be similar to that of the more traditional transarterial or paresthesia techniques.[51,52] This is not the case, however, when multiple nerves are stimulated. Greater chances of successful block and shorter onset times are reported with multistimulation.[13,53-55] The expected improved safety of the ENS technique has not been convincingly demonstrated either, in spite of the fact that it makes the search for paresthesia and arterial puncture obsolete.[29,56-59]

The novel approach of electrical stimulation for central neuraxial block is promising. It appears to have the potential, not only to detect all possible locations of epidural placement but also to guide the catheter/needle to a specific target epidural location.[37,45] In conjunction with a good loss of resistance technique, careful aspiration, and the use of a test dose, the ENS should improve the safety and success rate of epidural anesthesia.

REFERENCES

1. von Perthes G. Uber Leitungsanasthesis unter Zuhilfenahme Elektrischer Reizung. *Munch Med Wochenschr* 47:2545–2548, 1912.
2. Pearson RB. Nerve block in rehabilitation: A technic of needle localization. *Arch Phys Med Rehabil* 36:631–633, 1955.
3. Greenblatt GM, Denson JS. Needle nerve stimulator locator: Nerve blocks with a new instrument for locating nerves. *Anesth Analg* 41:599–602, 1962.
4. Montgomery SJ, Raj PP, Nettles D, et al. The use of the nerve stimulator with standard unsheathed needles in nerve blockade. *Anesth Analg* 52:827–831, 1973.
5. Ford DJ, Pither CE, Raj PP. Electrical characteristics of peripheral nerve stimulators: Implication for nerve localization. *Reg Anesth* 9:73–77, 1984.
6. Ford DJ, Pither C, Raj PP. Comparison of insulated and uninsulated needles for locating peripheral nerves with a peripheral nerve stimulator. *Anesth Analg* 63:925–928, 1984.
7. Lapicque L. *L'excitabilite en fonction du temps: La chronaxie, sa signification et sa mesure.* Paris: Presses Universitaires de France, 1926.
8. Ganong WF. Excitable tissues: Nerve, in *Review of Medical Physiology.* Los Altos, CA: Lange, 1999:47–59.
9. Guyton AC, Hall JE. Membrane potentials and action potentials. *Textbook of Medical Physiology.* Philadelphia: Saunders, 1996:57–71.
10. Pither CE, Raj PP, Ford DJ. The use of peripheral nerve stimulators for regional anesthesia: A review of experimental characteristics, technique, and clinical applications. *Reg Anesth* 10:49–58, 1985.
11. Hadzic A, Vloka JD, Claudio RE, et al. Electrical nerve localization: Effects of cutaneous electrode placement and duration of the stimulus on motor response. *Anesthesiology* 100:1526–1530, 2004.
12. Koscielniak-Nielsen ZJ, Rassmussen H, Jepsen K. Effect of impulse duration on patients' perception of electrical stimulation and block effectiveness during axillary block in unsedated ambulatory patients. *Reg Anesth Pain Med* 26:428–433, 2001.
13. Sia S, Bartoli M, Lepri A, et al. Multiple-injection axillary brachial plexus block: A comparison of two methods of nerve localization–nerve stimulation versus paresthesia. *Anesth Analg* 91:647–651, 2000.
14. Kimura J. Facts, fallacies, and fancies of nerve stimulation techniques, in Kimura J (ed): *Electrodiagnosis in Diseases of Nerve and Muscle: Principles and Practice.* Philadelphia: Davis, 1989:139–166.
15. Hodgkin AL. The subthreshold potentials in a crustacean nerve fibre. *Proc R Soc Lond* 126:87, 1938.
16. Tulchinsky A, Weller RS, Rosenblum M, et al. Nerve stimulator polarity and brachial plexus block. *Anesth Analg* 77:100–103, 1993.
17. Bashein G, Haschke RH, Ready LB. Electrical nerve location: Numerical and electrophoretic comparison of insulated vs uninsulated needles. *Anesth Analg* 63:919–924, 1984.
18. Pither CE, Ford DJ, Raj PP. Peripheral nerve stimulation with insulated and uninsulated needles: Efficacy of characteristics. *Reg Anesth* 9:42–43, 1984.

19. Galindo A. A special needle for nerve blocks. *Reg Anesth* 5:12–13, 1980.
20. Kaiser H, Niesel HC, Hans V. Fundamentals and requirements of peripheral electric nerve stimulation. A contribution to the improvement of safety standards in Regional Anesthesia]. *Reg Anesth* 13:143–147, 1990.
21. Barthram CN. Nerve stimulators for nerve location: Are they all the same? A study of stimulator performance. *Anaesthesia* 52:761–764, 1997.
22. Hadzic A, Vloka J, Hadzic N, et al. Nerve stimulators used for peripheral nerve blocks vary in their electrical characteristics. *Anesthesiology* 98:969–974, 2003.
23. Raj PP, Banister R. Peripheral nerve stimulators for nerve blocks, in Raj PP, De Andres J, Grossi P, Banister R, Sala-Blanch X (eds): *Textbook of Regional Anesthesia*. New York: Churchill Livingstone, 2002:251–268.
24. Magora F, Rozin R, Ben-Menachem Y, et al. Obturator nerve block: An evaluation of technique. *Br J Anaesth* 41:695–698, 1969.
25. Wehling MJ, Koorn R, Leddell C, et al. Electrical nerve stimulation using a stimulating catheter: What is the lower limit? *Reg Anesth Pain Med* 29:230–233, 2004.
26. Raj PP, Rosenblatt R, Montgomery SJ: Use of the nerve stimulator for peripheral blocks. *Reg Anesth* 5:14–21, 1980.
27. Tsui BC, Wagner A, Finucane B. Electrophysiologic effect of injectates on peripheral nerve stimulation. *Reg Anesth Pain Med* 29:189–193, 2004.
28. Shannon J, Lang SA, Yip RW, et al. Lateral femoral cutaneous nerve block revisited. A nerve stimulator technique. *Reg Anesth* 20:100–104, 1995.
29. Hadzic A. Peripheral nerve stimulators: Cracking the code—one at a time. *Reg Anesth Pain Med* 29:185–188, 2004.
30. Ganta R, Cajee RA, Henthorn RW. Use of transcutaneous nerve stimulation to assist interscalene block. *Anesth Analg* 76:914–915, 1993.
31. Bosenberg AT, Raw R, Boezaart AP. Surface mapping of peripheral nerves in children with a nerve stimulator. *Pediatr Anaesth* 12:398–403, 2002.
32. Urmey WF, Grossi P. Percutaneous electrode guidance: A noninvasive technique for prelocation of peripheral nerves to facilitate peripheral plexus or nerve block. *Reg Anesth Pain Med* 27:261–267, 2002.
33. Capdevila X, Lopez S, Bernard N, et al. Percutaneous electrode guidance using the insulated needle for prelocation of peripheral nerves during axillary plexus blocks. *Reg Anesth Pain Med* 29:206–211, 2004
34. Tsui BCH, Finucane B. Epidural stimulator catheter. *Reg Anesth Pain Med* 6:150–154, 2002.
35. Mulroy MF, Norris MC, Liu SS. Safety steps for epidural injection of local anesthetics: Review of the literature and recommendations. *Anesth Analg* 85:1346–1356, 1997.
36. Stevens RM. Neuraxial blocks, in Brown DL (ed): *Regional Anesthesia and Analgesia*. Philadelphia: Saunders, 1996: 319–356.
37. Tsui BC, Gupta S, Finucane B. Confirmation of epidural catheter placement using nerve stimulation. *Can J Anaesth* 45:640–644, 1998.
38. Tsui BC, Gupta S, Finucane B. Detection of subarachnoid and intravascular epidural catheter placement. *Can J Anaesth* 46:675–678, 1999.
39. Tsui BC, Gupta S, Finucane B. Determination of epidural catheter placement using nerve stimulation in obstetric patients. *Reg Anesth Pain Med* 24:17–23, 1999.
40. Tsui BC, Guenther C, Emery D, et al. Determining epidural catheter location using nerve stimulation with radiological confirmation. *Reg Anesth Pain Med* 25:306–309, 2000.
41. Tsui BC, Gupta S, Emery D, et al. Detection of subdural placement of epidural catheter using nerve stimulation. *Can J Anaesth* 47:471–473, 2000.
42. Tsui BC, Seal R, Koller J, et al. Thoracic epidural analgesia via the caudal approach in pediatric patients undergoing fundoplication using nerve stimulation guidance. *Anesth Analg* 93:1152–1155, 2001.
43. Tamai H, Sawamura S, Kanamori Y, et al. Thoracic epidural catheter insertion using the caudal approach assisted with an electrical nerve stimulator in young children. *Reg Anesth Pain Med* 29:92–95, 2004.
44. Tsui BCH, Wagner A, Finucane B. The threshold current in the intrathecal space to elicit motor response is lower and does not overlap that in the epidural space: A porcine model. *Can J Anaesth* 51:690–695, 2004.
45. Tsui BCH, Wagner A, Cave D, et al. Threshold current for an insulated epidural needle in pediatric patients. *Anesth Analg* 99:694–696, 2004.
46. Tsui BCH, Wagner A, Cunningham K, et al. Threshold current of an insulated needle in the intrathecal space in pediatric patients. *Anesth Analg* 100:662–665, 2005.
47. Tsui BCH, Seal R, Entwistle L. Thoracic epidural analgesia via the caudal approach using nerve stimulation in an infant with CATCH22. *Can J Anaesth* 46:1138–1142, 1999.
48. Tsui BCH, Bateman K, Bouliane M, et al. Cervical epidural analgesia via a thoracic approach using nerve stimulation guidance in an adult patient undergoing elbow surgery region. *Reg Anesth Pain Med* 29:355–360, 2004.
49. Smith BL. Efficacy of a nerve stimulator in regional analgesia: Experience in a resident training programme. *Anaesthesia* 31:778–782, 1976.
50. Smith BE, Allison A. Use of a low-power nerve stimulator during sciatic nerve block. *Anaesthesia* 42:296–298, 1987.
51. Forte TE, Lee KI, Galindo A, et al. Use of a nerve stimulator for peripheral nerve blocks. *Anesthesiology* 68:315–317, 1988.
52. Goldberg ME, Gregg C, Larijani GE, et al. A comparison of three methods of axillary approach to brachial plexus blockade for upper extremity surgery. *Anesthesiology* 66:814–816, 1987.
53. Baranoswski AP, Pither CE. A comparison of three methods of axillary brachial plexus anesthesia. *Anaesthesia* 45:362–365, 1990.
54. Bouaziz H, Narchi P, Mercier FJ, et al. Comparison between conventional axillary block and a new approach at the midhumeral level. *Anesth Analg* 84:1058–1062, 1997.
55. Lavoie J, Martin R, Tetrault JP. Axillary plexus block using a peripheral nerve stimulator: Single or multiple injections. *Can J Anaesth* 37:S39, 1990.
56. Auroy Y, Narchi P, Messiah A, et al. Serious complications related to regional anesthesia: Results of a prospective survey in France. *Anesthesiology* 87:479–486, 1997.

57. Eisenach JC. Regional anesthesia: Vintage Bordeaux (and Napa Valley). *Anesthesiology* 87:467–469, 1997.

58. Fanelli G, Casati A, Garancini P, et al. Nerve stimulator and multiple injection technique for upper and lower limb blockade: Failure rate, patient acceptance, and neurologic complications. Study Group on Regional Anesthesia. *Anesth Analg* 88:847–852, 1999.

59. Auroy Y, Benhamou D, Bargues L, et al. Major complications of regional anesthesia in France: The SOS Regional Anesthesia Hotline Service. *Anesthesiology* 97:1274–1280, 2002.

CHAPTER 20

Continuous Peripheral Nerve Blocks

ANDRÉ P. BOEZAART

► INTRODUCTION

It is generally accepted that peripheral nerve blocks and neuraxial block are superior to all other modalities for the treatment of acute pain, especially postoperative pain. The problem, however, is that acute postoperative pain usually outlasts single-injection peripheral nerve blocks. This fact stimulated the development of continuous peripheral nerve blocks (CPNBs).

Long-acting local anesthetic agents have also received attention, but the problem with this concept is that side effects will also last as long as the anesthetic effects. Furthermore, one will not be able to alter the effects once established. Continuous nerve block via a perineural catheter, on the other hand, can be discontinued or the infusion changed if unwanted effects or side effects occur. The main emphasis in developing this method during the past decade has been to place catheters accurately to ensure effectiveness and to reduce secondary block failure. These aims have now been achieved and the new focus is on the appropriate use of CPNBs and infusion strategies, especially for ambulatory care.

Two techniques are currently used to place perineural catheters: the nonstimulating catheter technique as described by Steele et al.[1] and the stimulating catheter technique as described by Boezaart et al.[2] With the nonstimulating catheter technique, an insulated needle (usually a Tuohy needle) is inserted near a nerve with the aid of a nerve stimulator. Saline or a local anesthetic agent is then injected to "expand" the perineural space and a standard epidural catheter (usually a multiorifice catheter) is advanced through the needle. This technique is relatively easy to perform and usually provides a good primary block (local anesthetic agent injected through the needle), but the success rate of the secondary block (infusion through the catheter) has been disappointing for some blocks.

With the stimulating catheter technique, an insulated needle (typically a Tuohy needle) is inserted close to a nerve, making using of a nerve stimulator. A catheter with an electrically conductive connection to the tip of the catheter (a spring wire[2] or a steel stylet[3]) is then inserted through the needle, while stimulating the nerve via the catheter to ensure accurate positioning. The main local anesthetic dose and continuous infusion is injected through the catheter. This technique is more difficult to perform and the primary success rate equals that of the nonstimulating technique, but it is thought to have better secondary block success owing to more accurate catheter placement.[4]

► THE BASIC TECHNIQUES

Historical Overview and Future Trends

F. Paul Ansbro[5] has often been credited with the first use of a continuous nerve block in 1946, although he did not use a perineural catheter. He inserted a blunt needle lateral to the subclavian artery in contact with the first rib after eliciting paresthesia in the patient's arm. He then secured the needle by inserting it through a cork and strapping the cork to the skin with adhesive tape. The needle was connected with a rubber tube to a 10-mL

Luer-lock syringe for repeated injections of local anesthetic agent. The objective of the continuous nerve block was to increase the duration of action of the 1% procaine used. Ansbro presented 27 patients in whom the average duration of the anesthesia was 2 h, ranging from 90 min to 4 h and 20 min. This was a significant improvement over the usual 15-min duration obtained with a single injection of 1% procaine.

Interestingly, two of the earliest recorded uses of electrical nerve stimulation for peripheral nerve block[3] and neuraxial block,[6] in 1949 and 1951, respectively, were intended to assist in the accurate placement of catheters for continuous block and not for needle placement. Stanley and Lili-Charlotte Sarnoff, a husband-and-wife team, pioneered the use of nerve stimulation for continuous peripheral perineural and subarachnoid block for the accurate placement of catheters.

In the middle of the polio epidemic of the late 1940s and early 1950s, the Sarnoffs worked on the development of the "Electrophrenic Respirator" at the Harvard School of Public Health.[7] This device was capable of eliciting breathing by stimulating the phrenic nerve transcutaneously in cases of bulbar polio in which respiration could not be established by the iron lung. At the time, the couple's daughter, Daniela, was stricken by bulbar polio and saved by this method. This event made worldwide news under the headline "The Device [that] Cheats Death."

Armed with this knowledge and his previous experience of the precise placement of intrathecal catheters with nerve stimulation,[6] Dr. Sarnoff was confronted by a patient suffering from intractable hiccups.[3] He placed a "prolonged peripheral nerve block" catheter to continuously and accurately block the phrenic nerve by stimulating the phrenic nerve via the catheter. In his description of the technique, he stated that

> The accurate placement of the tip of the needle and catheter is important to the success of the procedure....we adapted a previously described method of electrical localization of catheters to the purpose...by applying an electrical potential to the tip of the catheter by way of its stylet in the subarachnoid space. The same principle was used in localizing the tip of the needle in relation to the phrenic nerve in this study.

This early use of nerve stimulation in nerve block was thus for the accurate placement of a catheter for continuous block of a motor nerve—the phrenic nerve. Although the nonstimulating catheter technique is often referred to as the "classic technique," this is indeed incorrect, since the stimulating technique is in actual fact the "classic" technique.

Years later, in 1995, after the use of nerve stimulators for single-injection blocks of peripheral nerves and for placing neuraxial blocks (although the latter has never been popularized), the technique of placing catheters for CPNBs by stimulating the nerve via both the needle and the catheter has been "reinvented."[2,8]

In the 30 years after the first descriptions by the Sarnoffs, the main focus in the development of CPNBs was on the upper extremity, and mainly to improve blood flow by sympathetic block for reimplantations of traumatically amputated parts of the upper limb. Most of the authors used variations of the axillary perivascular technique in the 1970s and 1980s.[9–12] For example, during the Angola Civil War in 1975, the present author, as anesthesiologist for the "Number 1 Forward Surgical Unit," used a cut-down technique onto the axillary artery and, under direct vision, placed a central line catheter in the perivascular space to manage the pain due to severe war injuries of the hand and arm (see Chap. 34). The justification for all these techniques in the 1970s and 1980s was mainly to achieve sympathetic block and improved blood flow. At the time, the analgesia was almost viewed as an additional "bonus," but it was not the primary focus until the early 1990s.

During the next decade, the 1990s, the emphasis shifted toward the use of continuous nerve blocks to manage acute postoperative pain. This was, among other factors, driven by the quest for cost-effective ambulatory surgery following the exponential explosion of medical inflation in the mid- to late-1980s. Because of the efficiency and relative safety of neuraxial nerve blocks, the lower extremity received little attention during the early development, and the main focus was on continuous interscalene blocks.[13–16] All these authors used the nonstimulating catheter technique.

Later on, during the 1990s, the question was being asked whether CPNBs made any difference to the outcome of surgery. Francois Singelyn and coworkers[17] addressed this question in Belgium by demonstrating that continuous femoral nerve block for total knee replacement is superior to patient-controlled intravenous morphine and epidural analgesia in managing postoperative pain. They also demonstrated fewer complications and earlier and better rehabilitation. This work was repeated and its results confirmed by Capdevila[18] in France and Chelly[19] in the United States.

A frustrating problem with perineural catheters was inaccurate catheter placement and, therefore, secondary block failure. This was highlighted by the work of Ganapathy[20] and Klein,[21] and it became clear that patients could not be sent home with catheters in place unless anesthesiologists learned how to place catheters for continuous nerve blocks accurately. It was shown[21] that discharging patients from the hospital with continuous nerve blocks that failed after the primary block had worn off doubled costs instead of saving them because patients had to be readmitted to treat their acute pain. A description of the "stimulating catheter" or the "reinvention" of the Sarnoff technique followed in 1995[2] and 1999.[8]

It is now well understood how to place perineural catheters so that they will function well with very little or no secondary failure, and the emphasis from the start of the twenty-first century has been on management strategies for infusions through these catheters. Borgeat et al.[22] pioneered the use of patient-controlled regional anesthesia, and Ilfeld and colleagues published numerous papers on continuous infusion strategies for ambulatory patients.[23-26] The great success reported by Ilfeld et al. may be attributed to their use of stimulating catheters. The main early drive toward ambulatory management of postoperative pain came from Grant and colleagues at Duke University.[27] The use of ultrasound for CPNB placement is not yet well established and is currently undergoing preliminary evaluation.

The aim now should be the design of the appropriate infusion strategies and use of continuous nerve blocks most appropriate for the specific surgery being performed. Outcome studies should be the main research focus. Although little research has been published in this regard, it should become clearer which blocks are best suited to different surgical procedures and the difference they ultimately make, if any. For example, it is most likely not appropriate to do a continuous infraclavicular block for painful wrist and elbow surgery. Although the primary block may work well and block all three brachial plexus cords necessary for complete analgesia of the wrist and elbow, the catheter settles on one cord only—for example, the posterior cord. The result is that in the subsequent days, when low infusion volumes and concentrations are used, the patient will suffer severe pain in the areas supplied by the two cords that are not blocked. Another example is the use of continuous sciatic nerve block for major ankle surgery without a continuous femoral nerve block to provide analgesia in the distribution of the important saphenous branch to the ankle joint and medial side of the lower leg and foot. Some anesthesiologists are using continuous psoas compartment block for war injuries to the lower limb distal to the knee (see Chap. 34). It is probably an "overkill" approach in civilian practice to block the saphenous nerve, but it can certainly be justified in operational war conditions, where facilities may be in short supply and manpower issues prevail. Furthermore, it is probably inappropriate to use CPNBs for relatively painless surgery such as carpal tunnel decompression, finger amputation, and digital nerve repair.[28] It is expected that clinical research will clarify all these issues over the next 10 years. We need objective evidence to establish the most appropriate infusion strategies and the most suitable continuous blocks for each specific surgical situation (see Chap. 21).

The Nonstimulating Catheter Technique

An insulated Tuohy needle (e.g., Contiplex B Braun, Bethlehem, PA; Vygon, Less Ullis, France; and Alphaplex, Sterimed, Saarbrucen, Germany) is connected to a nerve stimulator. The needle is inserted at the required site and advanced until an appropriate motor response is elicited with a current output of 0.3 to 0.5 mA, 2 Hz, and 100 to 300 μs. The needle is attached via tubing to a syringe to aspirate for blood or cerebrospinal fluid in order to avoid intravascular or intrathecal injection. The needle is maintained in the required position and saline or local anesthetic agent with or without epinephrine is injected in divided doses. A 19- or 20-gauge standard epidural catheter is then advanced 5 to 10 cm past the distal end of the needle, the needle is removed, and the catheter is secured with medical adhesive spray, Steri-Strips (3M Health Care, St. Paul, MN), or transparent occlusive dressing. Different authors have described various local anesthetic agent regimens, but generally a relatively large bolus dose is injected through the needle followed by an infusion of a more dilute concentration and smaller volume of local anesthetic agents through the catheter and various patient-controlled bolus dosages.

The Stimulating Catheter Technique

A nerve stimulator set to 1 to 1.5 mA is attached to an insulated Tuohy needle (e.g., StimuCath, Arrow International, Reading PA; or Stimulong Plus, Pajunk, Geisingen, Germany) and the nerve or plexus appropriate for the surgery is approached. When the correct motor response is elicited, the needle is advanced until a brisk motor response is elicited with a current output of 0.3 to 0.5 mA and a pulse width between 100 to 300 μs at a frequency of 1 to 2 Hz. The needle is then held steady in this position and, without injecting any drug or saline through the needle, the nerve stimulator is clipped to the proximal end of the catheter and the catheter advanced through the needle. The elicited motor response should be similar to that elicited by stimulating via the needle. The catheter is advanced beyond the distal end of the needle and the motor response should still remain unchanged. If the motor response changes, the catheter is carefully withdrawn into the shaft of the needle and the needle's position is changed slightly by rotating clockwise or counterclockwise or moving it a few millimeters inward or outward. The catheter is then advanced again. This process is repeated by making small changes to the needle after careful catheter withdrawal until the desired motor response is elicited when the catheter is advanced. The catheter is then advanced 3 to 5 cm along the appropriate nerve.

Ultrasound-Guided Blocks

Ultrasound holds some promise for the placement of continuous nerve blocks. It is fairly well established for single-injection nerve blocks.[29] Although Sutherland has proposed the use of ultrasound for the accurate placement of continuous sciatic nerve blocks,[30] much work still needs to be done before this can be accepted as an alternative method for the placement of continuous nerve blocks. A problem with ultrasound is that, although it works well for superficial nerves, the depth of penetration of most affordable ultrasound probes is not sufficient to identify deeper nerves, especially in very obese patients. This problem will no doubt be addressed as more advanced technology becomes available. Ultrasound is ultimately likely to be a valuable addition to nerve stimulation but will probably not replace it, just as ultrasound did not replace x-rays.

Catheter Fixation

Catheter dislodgment causes problems, and various methods of fixating catheters have been described. Most authors now tunnel the catheter subcutaneously,[8,31,32] and this has virtually eliminated the problem of dislodgment. Various methods of tunneling a catheter have been described, but most of them are variations of the following.

There are basically two approaches to tunneling the catheter: (1) tunneling without a "skin bridge" and (2) tunneling with a "skin bridge." Leaving a skin bridge makes catheter removal easier and is normally done for a short-term (1- to 7-day) catheterization, while tunneling without a skin bridge is typically used for long-term infusions (>7-day) catheterization and has the potential advantage of preventing infection. The first method may be associated with more leakage at the skin-bridge area, while the latter may make catheter removal more difficult.

With one commonly used technique, the inner steel stylet of the Tuohy needle is used as a guide. If a skin bridge is wanted, it enters the skin 2 to 3 mm from the catheter exit site or through the catheter exit site (taking special care not to damage the catheter) if a skin bridge is not wanted. The stylet is then advanced subcutaneously for approximately 8 to 10 cm. The Tuohy needle is then "railroaded" back over the stylet, the stylet is removed, and the distal end of the catheter is advanced retrogradely through the needle. The needle is removed and the catheter tunneled. If a skin bridge is left, a small piece of plastic or silicone tubing can be inserted to protect the skin under the skin bridge.

Various authors have used different adhesive materials, such as medical adhesive spray, Steri-Strips, and transparent occlusive dressings successfully.[27]

General Considerations for Perineural Catheters

- Since an indwelling catheter is left in place for some time, strict sterile procedures are necessary for insertion. The catheter should be covered with a transparent dressing to enable daily inspection of the catheter exit site and skin-bridge area for early signs of infection (see Chap. 21).
- Catheters should not be removed before full sensation has returned to the limb. If the patient's pain is still intolerable after the infusion is stopped, a bolus of the local anesthetic agent should be injected and the infusion restarted for a further 24 h. If the pain is manageable with oral analgesic, the catheter can be removed (see Chap. 21).
- Radiating pain experienced during removal of a catheter should be approached with caution.
- Because the whole limb is likely to be insensitive for the duration of a continuous block, the ulnar nerve at the level of the elbow, the radial nerve at the midhumeral level, and the common peroneal nerves at the fibular head should be specifically protected from injury or pressure for the duration of the block (see Chap. 32).
- Patients with continuous blocks should always use a properly fitted arm sling to prevent traction injury to the brachial plexus or injury to the radial nerve.
- If a stimulating catheter is used, it should never be cut. The catheter has an inner wire that keeps it together; cutting this causes the catheter to fall apart and makes its removal very difficult.
- The needle should never be manipulated while the catheter still protrudes beyond its tip. This may cause shearing of the catheter.
- A leg brace should be worn if a continuous femoral nerve block is in place to prevent falling due to quadriceps muscle paralysis.

▶ COMPLICATIONS OF PERINEURAL CATHETERS

Complications of perineural catheters for continuous nerve blockade are rare and probably less than those for single-injection nerve blocks,[31] although large comparative studies have not yet been reported. The most common problems associated with continuous nerve blockade are technical ones, including failed blocks or incomplete analgesia, which does seem to become less as the use of stimulating catheters increases; catheter dislodgment, which seems to be largely solved with catheter tunneling; and leakage around the catheter entry site. This last problem is probably more frequent if a skin bridge is used during tunneling.

Nerve Injury

Complications due to nerve injury are usually secondary to insensitivity of the limb (see Chap. 32). The nerves most commonly injured by this are the ulnar, radial, and common peroneal nerves, owing to compression by ill-fitting slings and braces or compression of the ulnar nerve on the bed in the supine patient. Nerve injury due to traction, diathermy, and direct injury during surgery is often unfairly attributed to nerve blocks. Severe permanent nerve injury caused by continuous nerve blockade has not yet been reported, although surgical damage to nerves has recently been shown to be much more common than originally thought.[32] Transient neurologic damage has mainly been reported for continuous interscalene blocks[31] and 0.5 percent of continuous axillary blocks.[33] In a personal as yet unpublished series of 4700 continuous interscalene blocks, this author encountered 14 incidents of transient nerve damage, which presented with burning pain in the forearm. Of these 14 patients, 10 were scheduled for arthroscopic capsulotomy for primary adhesive capsulitis, or "frozen shoulder." Since the interscalene approach was abandoned and the continuous cervical paravertebral block used as routine first choice for shoulder surgery by this author, this complication has not been encountered in a personal series of well over 2000 cases.

Furthermore, it is my practice not to offer any preoperative nerve blocks to patients scheduled for shoulder surgery if patients suffer pain, paresthesia, or dysesthesia distal to the elbow. Bona fide shoulder pathology does not usually cause pain or dysesthesia distal to the elbow. This pain is most likely caused by existing brachial plexitis, and it may be prudent to err on the side of safety in such patients by offering them a postoperative nerve block after the shoulder pathology has become clear. This is especially relevant if the patient was scheduled for subacromial decompression, in which case a continuous cervical paravertebral block can be performed postoperatively if shoulder pathology was found and treated, if deemed necessary by the patient (see Chap. 23).

Infection

Capdevila and colleagues reported their experience with 1416 CPNBs[34] (Table 20-1), while Boezaart et al. reported on their early experience with 256 cervical paravertebral blocks[35] (Table 20-2). These reports represent what can typically be expected from CPNBs.

Colonization of catheters by bacteria can be expected to occur in roughly 28 percent of cases if prophylactic antibiotics are not used.[34] Infection, defined as redness, swelling, or pus around the catheter entry site, can be expected to be present in 3[34] to 5 percent[35] of cases. Bacterial species found include *Staphylococcus epidermidis* (61 percent, mostly found in interscalene catheters), gram-negative bacilli (22 percent, mainly associated with femoral nerve blocks), and *Staphylococcus aureus* (17 percent).[34] The incidence is not known if prophylactic antibiotics are used, as is often the case with orthopaedic surgery, but it is expected to be lower. Risk factors for local inflammation are patients in intensive care units, males, catheter duration longer than 48 h, absence of prophylactic antibiotics, diabetes, and femoral nerve blockade.[34] Catheters should be removed and appropriate antibiotics prescribed when signs of infection are present.

Associated Unwanted Nerve Blockade

A comparison was made between the Winnie paresthesia interscalene blocks (group I), stimulating needle

▶ **TABLE 20-1.** MEAN DURATION OF CATHETER USE 66.2 ± 36.3 H

Complication	*n*	%
Total catheters	1461	100%
Diaphragmatic paralysis	2	5% (of 256 CISB)
Recurrent laryngeal nerve paralysis	2	5% (of 256 CISB)
Epidural migration of catheter	3	8% (of 256 CISB)
Retroperitoneal catheter placements	1	0.2% (of 20 CLPVB)
Neuropathy	3	0.2% (of total catheters)
Intravenous catheter migration	1	0.07% (of total catheters)
Transient paresthesia and dysesthesia	21	1.4% (of total catheters)
Persistent motor block	31	2.2% (of total catheters)
Complete sensory block during infusion	42	1.9% (of total catheters)
Technical problems	253	17% (of total catheters)
Pain relief failure	47	3.2% (of total catheters)

CISB = continuous interscalene block; CLPVB = continuous lumbar paravertebral block.
SOURCE: *Capdevila et al.,[34] with permission.*

▶ **TABLE 20-2.** MEAN DURATION OF CATHETER USE 41.7 ± 14.7 H

Complication	*n*	%
Total CCPVB	256	100%
Horner's syndrome	103	40%
Dyspnea requiring no treatment	20	8%
Dyspnea requiring treatment	0	0%
Catheter-site infection	13	5%
Posterior neck pain at catheter entry site	56	22%
Posterior neck pain requiring catheter removal	16	6%
Supraclavicular hematoma	3	1%
Contralateral spread after bolus	11	4%
Contralateral spread after 6 h	0	0%
Bothersome "dead feeling" of arm	21	8%
Residual block after 2 weeks	10	4%
Residual block after 3 weeks	0	0%

CCPVB = continuous cervical paravertebral block.
SOURCE: *Boezaart et al.,[35] with permission.*

single-injection interscalene blocks (group II), and continuous interscalene blocks using a stimulating catheter (group III).[8] The authors reported 85 percent complete phrenic nerve blocks in the first group compared to 35 percent in the second group and 20 percent in the group receiving continuous interscalene blocks. Other common nerves that are incidentally blocked are the recurrent laryngeal nerve and the superficial cervical plexus, but these pose no problems.

Total spinal anesthesia has been associated with continuous lumbar paravertebral blockade.[36] Recurrent brachial plexus neuropathy in a diabetic patient after shoulder surgery and a continuous interscalene block has been reported.[37]

Complications Due to Drug Effects

Toxic drug effects during continuous infusion have not yet been described, but this can be expected. Acute myotoxic effects of local anesthetic agents have been described after continuous peripheral nerve blockade with bupivacaine and ropivacaine in a porcine model.[38] Compared with bupivacaine, which caused both muscle fiber necrosis and apoptosis, the tissue damage caused by ropivacaine was significantly less severe than that with bupivacaine in experimental animals.

Pain during Catheter Placement

All catheters (and all nerve blocks, for that matter) are placed under some form of anesthesia: some under general anesthesia, some under regional anesthesia, and other under local anesthesia. In dentistry and ophthalmology, nerve blocks are even placed under topical anesthesia. In this respect, the practitioner should not be rigid but instead choose the technique appropriate for each individual patient. The placement of catheters

for CPNBs should never be painful or uncomfortable. I believe that the most common cause for pain with CPNB placement is anxiety, which can be adequately dealt with by administering adequate dosages of anxiolytic agents, such as midazolam 0.015 to 0.15 mg/kg. Propofol is commonly used, but practitioners should be cautioned, since this drug may cause the patient to be "unruly" at low doses and, at higher doses, to lose consciousness, causing airway embarrassment.[39]

Furthermore, when appropriate (for example, in the case of children, in cases of very painful conditions or very anxious patients), the catheter can be placed under general anesthesia. There is no guidance from the literature as to whether this may increase the incidence of complications or side effects of CPNBs, but I contend that placing blocks under general anesthesia in certain circumstances may even be less hazardous, since the patient will not move during needle and catheter placement.

The area where the CPNB is to be placed should be anesthetized thoroughly before the catheter is inserted. For example, a regional block of the superficial cervical plexus, slowly injected with a fine needle, can be performed before a continuous interscalene block is attempted.[8] Similarly, a field block down to the pars intervertebralis (or articular column) of the sixth cervical vertebra should be done before a continuous cervical paravertebral block is performed.[35] It should go without saying that the area of intended catheter tunneling should be appropriately anesthetized before tunneling is undertaken.

Other rare and minor complications of perineural catheters have been reported, although none seem to be due to long-term continuous exposure of the nerves to local anesthetic agents or the presence of the catheter on or near the nerves.

► CONCLUSION

Perineural catheters for CPNBs have developed from pure motor blockade for intractable hiccups, through upper limb sympathetic blocks to enhance blood flow following reimplantation surgery, to sensory blocks for the ambulatory management of acute pain. Over the years the techniques and equipment have improved, and it is now possible to place catheters for CPNBs accurately and thus virtually eliminate secondary block failure. Although not yet sufficiently investigated, it seems that complications of CPNBs are rare and, if present, are mild and occur following the initial, relatively large dose of local anesthetic agent, while the patient is usually still under the care of the anesthesiologist. It is never necessary to hurt patients during catheter placement, and infusion strategies can and should be tailored to the individual requirements of each patient.

It is important that the patient's well-being and pain relief improve continuously each day after surgery. It is therefore inappropriate to remove catheters prematurely before pain is manageable with oral or parenteral analgesics.

REFERENCES

1. Steele SM, Klein SM, D'Frcole FJ, et al. A new continuous catheter delivery system (letter). *Anesth Analg* 87:28, 1988.
2. Boezaart AP, de Beer JF. Accurate placement of a catheter for selective continuous interscalene brachial plexus nerve block (abstr V14). *World Congress of Anesthesiologists*, Sydney Australia, 1996.
3. Sarnoff ST, Sarnoff LC. Prolonged peripheral nerve block by means of indwelling plastic catheter. Treatment of hiccup. *Anesthesiology* 12:270–277, 1951.
4. Salinas FV, Neal JM, Sueda LA, et al. Prospective comparison of continuous femoral nerve block with nonstimulating catheter placement versus stimulating catheter-guided perineural placement in volunteers. *Reg Anesth Pain Med* 29:212–220, 2004.
5. Ansbro FP. A method of continuous brachial plexus block. *Am J Surg* 71:716–722, 1946.
6. Sarnoff SJ. Functional localization of intraspinal catheters. *Anesthesiology* 11:360–366, 1950.
7. Sarnoff, SJ, Hardenbergh E, Whittenberger JL. Electrophrenic respiration. *Science* 108:482, 1948.
8. Boezaart AP, de Beer JF, Du Toit C, et al. A new technique of continuous interscalene nerve block. *Can J Anaesth* 46:275–281, 1999.
9. Selander D. Catheter technique in axillary plexus block. *Acta Anaesthesiol Scand* 21:324–329, 1977.
10. Manriquez RG, Pallares V. Continuous brachial plexus block for prolonged sympathectomy and control of pain. *Anesth Analg* 57:28–130, 1978.
11. Sada T, Kobayashi T, Murakami S. Continuous axillary brachial plexus block. *Can Anaesth Soc J* 30:201–205, 1983.
12. Ang ET, Lassale B, Goldfarb G. Continuous axillary brachial plexus block: A clinical and anatomical study. *Anesth Analg* 63:680–684, 1984.
13. Haasio J, Tuominen M, Rosenberg PH. Continuous interscalene brachial plexus block during and after shoulder surgery. *Ann Chirurg Gynaecol* 79:103–107, 1990.
14. Rosenberg PH, Pere P, Hekali R, et al. Plasma concentrations of bupivacaine and two of its metabolites during continuous interscalene brachial plexus block. *Br J Anaesth* 66:25–30, 1991.
15. Pere P, Tuominen M, Rosenberg PH. Cumulation of bupivacaine, desbutylbupivacaine and 4-hydroxybupivacaine during and after continuous interscalene brachial plexus block. *Acta Anaesthesiol Scand* 35:647–650, 1991.
16. Koh DLH, Lim BH. Postoperative continuous interscalene brachial plexus blockade for hand surgery. *Ann Acad Med Singapore* 24(Suppl):3S–7S, 1995.
17. Singelyn FJ, Deyaert M, Joris D, et al. Effects of intravenous patient-controlled analgesia with morphine, continuous epidural analgesia, and continuous three-in-one on postoperative pain and knee rehabilitation after unilateral total knee arthroplasty. *Anesth Analg* 87:88–92, 1998.
18. Capdevila X, Barthelet Y, Biboulet P, et al. Effects of perioperative analgesic technique on the surgical outcome and duration of rehabilitation after major knee surgery. *Anesthesiology* 19:8–15, 1999.
19. Chelly JE, Greger J, Gebhard R, et al. Continuous femoral blocks improve recovery and outcome of patients undergoing total knee arthroplasty. *J Arthroplasty* 16:436–445, 2001.
20. Ganapathy S, Wasserman RA, Watson JT, et al. Modified continuous femoral three-in-one block for postoperative pain after total knee arthroplasty. *Anesth Analg* 89:1197–1202, 1999.
21. Klein SM, Steele SM, Nielsen KC, et al. The difficulties of ambulatory interscalene and intra-articular infusions for rotator cuff surgery: A preliminary report. *Can J Anesth* 50:265–259, 2003.
22. Borgeat A, Schäppi B, Biasca N, et al. Patient-controlled analgesia after major shoulder surgery. *Anesthesiology* 87:1343–1347, 1997.
23. Ilfeld BM, Morey TE, Wright TW, et al. Interscalene perineural ropivacaine infusion: A comparison of two dosing regimens for postoperative analgesia. *Reg Anesth Pain Med* 29:1–3, 2004.
24. Ilfeld BM, Morey TE, Enneking FK. Infraclavicular perineural local anesthetic infusion: A comparison of three dosing regimens for postoperative analgesia. *Anesthesiology* 100:395–402, 2004.
25. Ilfeld BM, Thannikary LJ, Morey TE, et al. Popliteal sciatic perineural local anesthetic infusion: A comparison of three dosing regimens for postoperative analgesia. *Anesthesiology* 101:970–977, 2004.
26. Ilfeld BM, Enneking FK. Continuous peripheral nerve blocks at home: A review. *Anesth Analg* 100:1822–1833, 2005.
27. Grant SA, Nielsen KC, Greengrass RA, et al. Continuous peripheral nerve block for ambulatory surgery. *Reg Anesth Pain Med* 26:209–214, 2001.

28. Rawal N, Allvin R, Axelsson K, et al. Patient-controlled regional analgesia (PCRA) at home. *Anesthesiology* 96:1290–1296, 2002.

29. Sutherland ID. Continuous sciatic nerve infusion: Expanded case report describing a new approach. *Reg Anesth Pain Med* 23:496–501, 1998.

30. Sandhu NS, Capan LM. Ultrasound-guided infraclavicular brachial plexus block. *Br J Anaesth* 89:254–259, 2002.

31. Borgeat A, Ekatodramis G, Kalberer F, Benz C. Acute and non-acute complications associated with interscalene block and shoulder surgery: A prospective study. *Anesthesiology* 95:875–880, 2001.

32. Boardman ND III, Cofield RH. Neurologic complications of shoulder surgery. *Clin Orthop* 368:44–53, 1999.

33. Bergman B, Hebl J, Kent J, et al. Neurologic complications of 405 consecutive continuous axillary catheters. *Anesth Analg* 96:247–252, 2003.

34. Capdevila X, Pirat P, Bringuier S, et al. Continuous peripheral nerve blocks on hospital wards after orthopedic surgery: A multicenter prospective analysis of their efficacy and incidences and characteristics of adverse events in 1,416 patients. *Anesthesiology* 103:1035–1045, 2005.

35. Boezaart AP, De Beer JF, Nell ML. Early experience with continuous cervical paravertebral block using a stimulating catheter. *Reg Anesth Pain Med* 28(5):406–413, 2003.

36. Lekhak B, Barley C, Conacher ID, et al. Total spinal anaesthesia in association with insertion of a paravertebral catheter. *Br J Anaesth* 86:280–282, 2001.

37. Horlocker TT, O'Driscoll SW, Dinapoli RP. Recurring brachial plexus neuropathy in a diabetic patient after shoulder surgery and continuous interscalene block. *Anesth Analg* 91:688–690, 2000.

38. Zink W, Seif C, Bohl JRE, et al. The acute myotoxic effects of bupivacaine and ropivacaine after continuous peripheral nerve blockades. *Anesth Analg* 97:1173–1179, 2003.

39. Boezaart AP, Berry RA, Nell ML, van Dyk AL. A comparison of propofol and remifentanil for sedation and limitation of movement during periretrobulbar block. *J Clin Anesth* 6:422–426, 2001.

CHAPTER 21

Continuous Peripheral Nerve Block Infusion Strategies and Catheter Care

PETER VAN DE PUTTE/MARTIAL VAN DER VORST

► INTRODUCTION

Continuous peripheral nerve block (CPNB) provides superior postoperative analgesia compared to single-injection nerve block and intravenous opioids.[1,2] It has been shown to be particularly effective in treating pain after shoulder surgery.[3]

This chapter reviews the general principles of postoperative infusions and the dose regimens and infusion strategies that have been used for the different peripheral nerve blocks.

Although CPNB is relatively new and research in this field is continuing, its importance in outpatient analgesia has already been established by the growing number of publications on this issue. Advantages include decreased length of hospital stay, better rehabilitation and patient satisfaction, and higher cost-effectiveness.[4]

► PATIENT SELECTION

A good understanding of the surgical approach and the expected intensity of pain is essential in choosing an analgesic strategy. Surgical considerations, such as active or passive mobilization for rehabilitation, are also important. For example, diagnostic arthroscopy of the shoulder, hip, knee, or ankle (with or without debridement of soft tissue) or limited hand or foot surgery causes only mild to moderate and short-lived postoperative pain that is easily treated with single-injection nerve blocks or oral analgesics.

Ligament reconstructions; mobilization of a frozen knee or shoulder; extensive foot, ankle, or hand surgery; arthroplasty; and other procedures on the other hand are good indications for CPNB (Table 21-1). The different blocks and proposed infusion strategies are summarized in Table 21-1.

► CATHETER CARE

Visit the patient daily.

Inspect catheter entry site daily.

Inspect surgical dressing and surgical wound if appropriate.

Protect ulnar, radial, and common peroneal nerves from pressure.

Ensure that arm sling or leg brace is properly fitted.

Measure, evaluate, and record visual analogue scale (VAS) for pain, motor function, proprioception, and blood flow of the anesthetized limb.

Attend to the patient's general well-being.

This list summarizes the daily care of the patient with an indwelling catheter.

► CATHETER REMOVAL (FIG. 21-1)

General Principles

Catheter removal is a sterile procedure.

Catheters should be removed only after full sensation has returned to the limb. This may eliminate

► **TABLE 21-1.** PROPOSED CONTINUOUS BLOCKS AND INFUSION STRATEGIES FOR COMMON SURGICAL PROCEDURES*†

Surgical Procedure	Suggested Continuous Block	Suggested Infusion Strategy* (Note: adjust individually to suit patient requirements)
Total shoulder arthroplasty (Hemi-shoulder arthroplasty) Rotator cuff repair Anterior Bankart repair SLAP repair Shoulder arthrodesis Latarjet stabilization procedure Subscapularis repair	CCPVB* CISB	POB, 0.5% bupivacaine or 0.5–0.75% ropivacaine, 20–40 mL CI, 0.2% ropivacaine at 5 mL/h PCRA, 0.2% ropivacaine 10 mL with 60-min lockout time
Scapular fractures and surgery Humeral fractures and surgery Radial fractures and surgery Ulnar fractures and surgery	CCPVB* CISB	
Total elbow arthroplasty Total wrist arthroplasty	CCPVB* CICB CAxB	
Elbow arthrodesis Wrist arthrodesis	CCPVB* CICB CAxB	
Upper limb reimplantation surgery	CCPVB* CICB CAxB	
Major upper limb trauma (significant risk of compartment syndrome; beware fractures around elbow)	CCPVB* CICB CAxB	
Arthroscopic capsulotomy for frozen shoulder	CCPVB	POB, 0.5% bupivacaine or 0.5–0.75% ropivacaine, 20 mL CI, 0.1% ropivacaine at 0–5 mL/h (preserve motor function) PCRA, 0.1% ropivacaine 10 mL with 60-min lockout time (bolus higher concentration before physical therapy if necessary)
Latissimus dorsi transfer	CCPVB	POB, 0.5% bupivacaine or 0.5–0.75% ropivacaine, 20–40 mL CI, 0.2% ropivacaine at 5 mL/h PCRA, 0.2% ropivacaine 10 mL with 60-min lockout time
Unilateral thoracotomy	CTPVB (thoracic epidural)	
Major unilateral breast surgery	CTPVB (add lateral pectoral nerve block)	
Revision total hip arthroplasty (continuous peripheral nerve block probably not indicated for primary hip arthroplasty. Consider CSE)	CLPVB (CSE)* (epidural)	
Pelvic osteotomy		

Hip fracture	CFNB (combine with unilateral spinal for surgery)	
Femoral fracture (Significant risk of compartment syndrome. Beware fractures around knee.)	CFNB (combine with unilateral spinal for surgery)	
Tibial fracture (Significant risk of compartment syndrome. Beware fractures around knee)	CSSNB (CFNB additionally required for saphenous nerve)	
Fibular fracture	CSSNB (CFNB not additionally required)	
Anterior cruciate ligament reconstruction	CFNB (if hamstring muscle is harvested for graft, SI sciatic nerve block required)	
Posterior cruciate ligament reconstruction	CSSNB (CFNB additionally required)	POB, 0.5% bupivacaine or 0.5–0.75% ropivacaine, 20–40 mL CI, 0.2% ropivacaine at 5 mL/h PCRA, 0.2% ropivacaine 10 mL with 60-min lockout time (Split POB between blocks and use 5 mL/h for each block)
Total knee arthroplasty	CFNB (area behind knee sometimes requires SI sciatic nerve block)	POB, 0.5% bupivacaine or 0.5–0.75% ropivacaine, 20–40 mL CI, 0.1% ropivacaine at 5 mL/h (preserve motor function) PCRA, 0.1% ropivacaine 10 mL with 60-min lockout time
Ankle fusion (arthrodesis)	CSSNB* CPSB (CFNB additionally required for saphenous nerve)	POB, 0.5% bupivacaine or 0.5–0.75% ropivacaine, 20–40 mL CI, 0.2% ropivacaine at 5 mL/h PCRA, 0.2% ropivacaine 10 mL with 60-min lockout time (Split POB between blocks and use 5 mL/h for each block)
Subtalar fusion (arthrodesis)	CSSNB* CPSB (CFNB not additionally required)	POB, 0.5% bupivacaine or 0.5–0.75% ropivacaine, 20–40 mL CI, 0.2% ropivacaine at 5 mL/h PCRA, 0.2% ropivacaine 10 mL with 60-min lockout time
Total ankle arthroplasty	CSSNB* (CFNB additionally required for saphenous nerve)	POB, 0.5% bupivacaine or 0.5–0.75% ropivacaine, 20–40 mL CI, 0.2% ropivacaine at 5 mL/h PCRA, 0.2% ropivacaine 10 mL with 60-min lockout time (Split POB between blocks and use 5 mL/h for each block)

CAxB = continuous axillary block; CCPVB = continuous cervical paravertebral block; CFNB = continuous femoral nerve block; CI = continuous infusion; CICB = continuous infraclavicular block; CISB = continuous interscalene block; CLPVB = continuous lumbar paravertebral block; CPSB = continuous popliteal sciatic nerve block; CSE = combined spinal/epidural; CSSNB = continuous subgluteal sciatic nerve block; CTPVB = continuous thoracic paravertebral block; PCRA = Patient-controlled regional anesthesia; POB = preoperative bolus; SI = single injection; SLAP = superior labrum anterior and posterior.

*Preference of these authors.

†Instructional movies of all the above blocks can be viewed on *http://www.RAEducation.com* or *http://uianesthesia.com/rasci*.

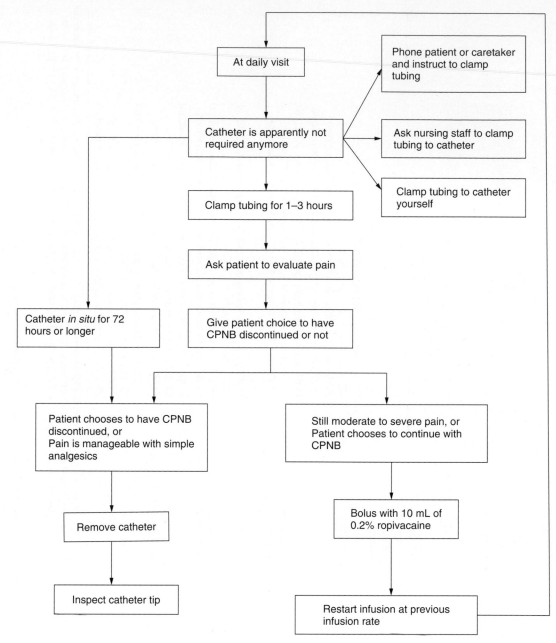

Figure 21-1. Timing of catheter removal.

ABBREVIATIONS: CPNB = continuous peripheral nerve block.

the theoretical possibility of nerve damage if a catheter has curled around a nerve.

"Stimulating" catheters should never be cut, especially not nerve-stimulating catheters, since cutting causes it to "fall apart" and the pieces can subsequently be left behind in the patient.

The timing of the catheter removal is presented in Fig. 21-1.

Examples of Typical Periods of Usage

Rotator cuff repair	2 to 4 days
Frozen shoulder	3 to 7 days
Total shoulder arthroplasty	3 to 5 days
Hemi–shoulder arthroplasty	2 to 4 days
Bankart repair	1 to 3 days
Elbow arthroplasty	3 to 5 days
Wrist arthroplasty	3 to 5 days
Hip arthroplasty	1 to 2 days
Knee arthroplasty	2 to 5 days
Ankle arthroplasty	2 to 5 days
Anterior cruciate ligament	1 to 3 days

Catheter removal technique is as follows:

This is a sterile procedure.
Remove transparent dressings.
Clean skin with suitable antiseptic.

Remove catheter end by gently pulling on the catheter while pulling the skin in the opposite direction.

If skin bridge is present, first remove the distal end of the catheter from the skin bridge while anchoring proximal end.

Keep the distal end from touching surrounding areas.

Remove the rest of catheter.

Inspect the catheter tip for completeness.

There is a theoretical possibility that a catheter can coil around a nerve. This should cause radiating pain during attempts to remove the catheter. For this reason, catheters should be removed only after full sensation has returned to the limb and preferably by trained personnel. Ilfeld et al.[5] reported a case in which the caretaker was not able to remove an infraclavicular catheter. The patient reported acute radiating pain when slight traction was exerted on the catheter. Fluoroscopy did not reveal a knot in the catheter, and it was removed surgically. Inspection at the time of surgery revealed a misshapen catheter tip, but the patient did not suffer any consequences. We believe the reported management of this extremely rare complication to be correct in such a situation.

▶ INFUSION STRATEGIES

General Principles

There are three basic regimens to provide continuous peripheral nerve block analgesia: fixed basal rate, fixed basal rate plus bolus doses, and boluses only. The last two regimens can be defined as patient-controlled regional analgesia (PCRA) systems. This is a drug delivery system aimed at controlling acute pain by using negative feedback technology in a closed-loop system in which the patient plays an active role. It overcomes the inadequacies of traditional analgesic protocols, which are due to the marked differences in pharmacokinetics of analgesics from one patient to another. Patients can control the analgesic dose in such a way as to balance pain relief with the side effects they are willing to tolerate. Patients usually choose less than the available total dose of analgesic.[6]

The optimal method of administration is yet to be determined, but preliminary evidence indicates that a basal background infusion with boluses provides equivalent or superior analgesia, improved patient satisfaction, and less consumption of local anesthetic as compared with a continuous infusion[7] or bolus dosing alone.[8,9] The use of bolus doses allows the patient to reinforce the block rapidly shortly before physiotherapy. If only boluses are used, patients experience more difficulty in sleeping[10] but might use less local anesthetic.[11]

Rawal offered a convincing argument for the use of bolus doses only.[12] Because the analgesic needs of individuals differ greatly and the duration of a single-dose local anesthetic varies considerably, PCRA by bolus doses on demand may be preferable to continuous infusion because it satisfies individual needs. Patient-controlled boluses permit patients to maintain adequate analgesia regardless of changes in pain intensity. A possible disadvantage of the bolus only technique may be either too dense a motor block after the bolus or too weak a sensory block before the next bolus. Another important factor that must be considered is the sleep disturbances that may occur when a basal infusion is not given.

After administration of the initial preoperative bolus dose of the local anesthetic agent, 10 to 15 mL/h of the local anesthetic, divided between the continuous infusion and the PCRA, can be given. If large bolus doses are used (e.g., 10 mL), the lockout time can be kept at 60 min. With smaller boluses (2 to 5 mL), a lockout time of 20 to 30 min can be used.

After 1 or 2 days of continuous infusion, as the postoperative pain decreases, the local anesthetics can be decreased as well. The progressive decrease of the basal infusion rate and concentration of local anesthetic agent not only decreases the risk of local anesthetic toxicity but also lowers the need to refill the infusion reservoir. Another strategy would be to refill the half empty reservoir with saline after every 24 h. This will halve the concentration of local anesthetics every day, as the need for analgesia decreases and the need for motor function increases.

The different limb infusion strategies as used by various authors are summarized in Tables 21-2*A* and 21-2*B*.

Infusion Strategies in the Upper Limb

Interscalene Block

There are a large number of postoperative infusion strategies, the use of which depend very much on the desired effect. For example, a rotator cuff repair, where early motor function is undesirable, would require a large volume and high concentration of local anesthetic followed by a high infusion rate of relatively highly concentrated drug and none or few patient-controlled bolus doses. Adhesive capsulitis or frozen shoulder, on the other hand, would require a smaller volume and lower concentration of initial bolus drug, since motor function and participation by the patient in physical therapy is desirable. This is followed by a low infusion volume at low concentration, but a greater volume and concentration PCRA for physical therapy sessions.[13]

Most authors give an initial bolus of 20 to 40 mL ropivacaine (0.5 to 0.75%) or bupivacaine (0.5%). Epinephrine (1:400,000) is sometimes added to indicate inadvertent intravascular injection. Continuous infusions of bupivacaine 0.25% at a rate of 0.25 mg/kg/h can be used. The mean plasma concentration of bupivacaine after 48 h of infusion is statistically significantly higher than after 24 h but remains below 2 μg/mL,[14] which is

▶ **TABLE 21-2A.** UPPER LIMB INFUSION STRATEGIES USED BY VARIOUS AUTHORS

Author	Aim of Study	Number of Patients per Group	Surgery	Duration	Initial Bolus	Postoperative Strategy	Results/Comments
Borgeat[1] 1997	PCA IV vs PCA ISB	40 (20 IV, 20 ISB)[p,r]	Shoulder arthroplasty, rotator cuff repair	48 h	30 mL bupi 0.4%	I: bupi 0.15% C: 5 mL/h B: 3–4 mL LO: 20 min	Higher satisfaction in ISB group (p <0.05); Less pain in ISB group at 12 and 18 h (p < 0.05); Less side effects (vomiting, pruritus) in ISB group
Borgeat[2] 1998	PCA IV vs PCA ISB	60 (30 IV, 30 ISB)[p,r]	Shoulder arthroplasty, rotator cuff repair	48 h	30 mL ropi 0.75%	I: ropi 0.2% C: 5 mL/h B: 3–4 mL LO 20 min	Higher satisfaction in ISB group (p <0.05); Less pain in ISB group at all times except 42 h (p < 0.05); Less side effects (nausea, pruritus) in ISB group (p < 0.05)
Lierz[3] 1998	CISB left and C axillary cath right	1[cr]	Phantom pain	6 d	20 mL ropi 0.2% on each side	I: ropi 0.2% 4 mL/h for 2 days, 6 mL/h next 4 days	Good pain relief; No toxic reaction; No motor block
Singelyn[4] 1999	Search for dose sparing infusion technique in ISB C vs C+B vs B	60 (20 C, 20 C+B, 20 B)[p,r,db]	Rotator cuff repair, total shoulder arthroplasty	48 h	20 mL bupi 0.25% + epi	I: bupi 0.125% + suf + CI 1. C: 10 mL 2. C: 5 mL + B: 2.5 mL; LO: 30 min 3. B 5 mL; LO 30 min	36% reduction in LA in group 2; Sensory block in 1 and 2 better than in 3 (p < 0.001); Less analgesics in 1 and 2 (p < 0.01); Side effects comparable in the 3 groups
Klein[5] 2000	CISB ropi 0.2% vs saline 0.9% Outpatients	40 (22 ropi, 18 placebo)[r,db,pc]	Open cuff, biceps tendonesis	24 h	30 mL ropi 0.5% + epi + CI	I: ropi 0.2% C: 10 mL/h	Decreased pain in ropi group (p = 0.001); 50% reduction M+ consumption (p = 0.001); MTSC ropi 1.04 +/– 0.5 µg/mL after 24 h
Borgeat[6] 2000	PCA IV vs PCA ISB with ropi 0.2%	33 (15 IV, 18 ISB)[p,r]	Shoulder arthroplasty, rotator cuff repair	48 h	30 mL ropi 0.75%	I: ropi 0.2% C: 5 mL B: 3–4 mL LO: 20 min	Less pain in ISB at 12 and 24 h (p < 0.05); More nausea/vomiting in IV group (p < 0.05); Similar effects on respiratory function
Borgeat[7] 2001	PCA CISB: ropi 0.2% vs bupi 0.15%: effects on hand motor function	60[p,r,db]	Major open shoulder surgery	48 h	40 mL ropi 0.6% or bupi 0.5%	I: ropi 0.2% or bupi 0.15% C: 5 mL/h B: 4 mL LO: 20 min	Similar pain control; Better preservation of strength in the hand and less paresthesia in the fingers in ropi group

Reference	Study	N patients	LA bolus	Duration	Infusion	Results
Ilfeld[8] 2002	Interscalene catheter Outpatients	1 (77 years old)cr	38 mL mepi 0.5% + epi + Cl	98 h	I: ropi 0.2% C: 6 mL/h B: 2mL LO: 20 min	No postoperatively opioid requirements No side effects VAS at rest 0; during physiotherapy 2–3/10
Ilfeld[9] 2003	ISB Ropi 0.2% vs saline 0.9% Outpatients	20 (10 ropi, 10 placebo)r,db,pc	40 mL mepi 1.5% + epi + Cl	48 h	I: ropi 0.2% C: 8 mL/h B: 2 mL LO: 15 min	Decreased pain in ropi group ($p < 0.001$) Decreased opioid requirements ($p < 0.001$)
Nielsen[10] 2003	Interscalene catheter Outpatients	4cr	30–40 mL ropi 0.5% + epi	72 h	I: ropi 0.2% C: 10 mL/h	2 pts VAS 0, no opioid requirements 2 pts with 1 episode of breakthrough pain which led to increase rate to 12 mL/h No adverse effects (nausea in 2 pts not related to ropi)
Casati[11] 2003	CISB 0.5% levobupivacaine vs 0.5% ropivacaine	50 (25 levo, 25 ropi)p,rdb	30 mL ropi or levo 0.5%	24 h	I: levo 0.125% or ropi 0.2% C: 6 mL/h B: 2 mL LO: 15 min; max 3/h	Similar postoperative analgesia Similar recovery of motor block Reduced LA volume consumed in levo group
Casati[12] 2003	CISB Lido vs ropi	40 (20 lido, 20 ropi)p,rdb	30 mL lido 1.5% or ropi 0.5%	24 h	I: Lido 1% or ropi 0.2% C: 6 mL/h B: 2 mL LO: 15 min; max 3/h	Better postoperative pain relief, lower needs for rescue analgesia and faster recovery of postoperative motor function in ropi group
Klein[13] 2003	CISB vs continuous intra-articular block Outpatients	17 (9 CISB, 8 CIA)p,r	40 mL ropi 0.5%	48 h	I: ropi 0.2% C: 10 mL	No satisfactory analgesia probably due to inaccurate catheter placement, poor information of the patient, use of slow onset opioids as escape medication
Boezaart[14] 2003	Evaluation continuous cervical paravertebral block	256p,o	30 mL ropi 0.5%		I: ropi 0.2% C: 0.1 mL/kg/h B: 10 mL on demand	Use of a stimulating catheter VAS 0.27 +/- 1.04 to 0.78 +/- 1.56 for the first 48h; 3.8 +/- 2.1 at 60 h; 3.5 +/- 2.4 at 14 days High patient satisfaction (91%)
Borgeat[15] 2003	Evaluation CISB, lateral modified approach	700p,o	30–50 mL ropi 0.5%	1.5–5 d (3.2 d)	I: ropi 0.2% C: 5 mL/h B: 4 mL LO: 20 min	High patient satisfaction Low rates of infection and neurologic complications
Ekatodramis[16] 2003	CISB with 6 vs 9 mL/h ropi 0.2%	24p,o	30 mL ropi 0.75%	48 h	I: ropi 0.2% C: 6 or 9 mL/h	Similar pain scores at rest Excellent pain relief 43% (6 mL) vs 63% (9 mL)

(Continued)

Author	Aim of Study	Number of Patients per Group	Surgery	Duration	Initial Bolus	Postoperative Strategy	Results/Comments
Ilfeld[17] 2004	CISB, high C and low B vs Low C and high B Outpatients	24[p,rdb] (12 C8, 12 C4)	Moderately painful shoulder surgery	3 d	40 mL mepi 1.5% + epi + CI	I: ropi 0.2% C: 8 mL/h; B: 2 mL; LO: 1 h C: 4 mL/h; B: 6 mL; LO: 1 h	Increased breakthrough pain incidence and intensity, sleep disturbances and decrease analgesia satisfaction in C4 group.
Gauman[18] 1988	CAB	20°	Elbow, wrist surgery; revascularization, reimplantation	3.7 d (longest 11.5 d)	45 mL bupi 0.5% + epi	I: bupi 0.125% C: 4–8 mL/h	Excellent pain relief No LA toxicity
Mezzatesta[19] 1997	AB: C vs B	20 (10C, 8 B)[p,r]	Major upper limb surgery	38–98 h	7 mg/kg Lido 1.5% + epi	I; bupi 0.25% + epi C-group: 0.25 mg/kg/h B-group: 0.25 mg/kg every h	Plasma bupi levels lower in B group. No difference in postoperative analgesia or motor block degree.
Iskandar[20] 1998	AB C vs B	42[p,r] (C 21, PCA 21)	Hand trauma		15–20 mL bupi 0.25%	I: bupi 0.25% C-group: 0.1 mL/kg/h B-group: 0.1 mL/kg; LO:1 h	Reduced amount LA, higher satisfaction and less opioid consumption in B-group.
Mak[21] 2000	AB	1[cr]	Pain, fibrosis after hand crush injury	6 d	20 mL ropi 0.2%	I: ropi 0.2% C: 3 mL/h B:1 mL LO: 10 min; max 10 mg/h	Marked reduction in pain. No major complications. Total cumulative dose was 904 mg (6.79 mg/h)
Vranken[22] 2000	CAB Outpatients	6°	Neuropathic pain (Pancoast tumor)		40 mL bupi 0.25%	I: bupi 0.25% C: 4 mL/h	Significant reduction in pain, increase in performance skills and quality of life. No side effects
Rawal[23] 2002	AB bupi 0.125% vs ropi 0.125% Outpatients	60[p,r, db] (29 ropi, 31 bupi)	Hand and wrist surgery	3 d	20 mL mepi 1.5%	I: bupi or ropi 0.125% B: 10 mL LO: 1 h	Satisfaction ropi group 81% vs 52% in bupi group on D0, 79% vs 83% on POD1 Numbness in fingers 6.9% in ropi group vs 29% in bupi group
Turkoglus[24] 2003	AB C vs B	29[p,r]	Hand surgery		40 mL ropi 0.75%	I: ropi 0.2% C-group: 0.25 mg/kg/h B-group: 0.25 mg/kg; LO: 1 h	Higher pain scores (p < 0.001), higher analgesic consumption (p < 0.001) and higher incidence of numbness of the fingers in C-group

Study	Block/drug	N	Surgery	Duration	Local anesthetic	Infusion	Results
Ilfeld[25] 2002	ClcB ropi 0.2% vs saline 0.9%	30[p,r, db] (15 ropi 15 saline)	Moderately painful upper extremity surgery	3 d	50mL 1.5% mepi + NaHCO$_3$ 5 mEq + epi + Cl	I: ropi 0.2% or saline 0.9% C: 8 mL/h B: 2 mL LO: 20 min	Less pain ($p < 0.001$), reduced opioid consumption ($p < 0.001$), less sleep disturbances ($p < 0.001$) and higher satisfaction ($p < 0.002$) in ropi group.
Ilfeld[26] 2004	ClcB: comparison of 3 regimens Outpatients	30[p,r,db] (10,10,10)	Moderately painful upper extremity surgery	3 d	50 mL 1.5% mepi + epi + Cl	I: ropi 0.2% 1: C: 12 mL/h + B: 0.05 mL 2: C: 8 mL/h + B: 4 mL 3: C: 0.3 mL/h + B: 9.9 mL	C + B (Group 2) optimizes analgesia while minimizing oral analgesic used compared to groups 1 and 3

AB = axillary block; B = bolus; CI = Clonidine; C = continuous; d = day; Epi = epinephrine; h = hour; I = infusion; IcB = Infraclavicular block; IV = intravenous; ISB = Interscalene block; LO = lock out; Mepi = mepivacaine; Min = minutes; MTSC = mean total serum concentration; PCA = patient-controlled analgesia; Ropi = ropivacaine; cr = case report; db = double blinded; o = observational; pc = placebo controlled; p = prospective; r = randomized.

1. Borgeat A, Schäppi B, Biasca N, Gerber C. Patient-controlled analgesia after major shoulder surgery: patient-controlled interscalene analgesia versus patient-controlled analgesia. Anesthesiology 87:1343–1347, 1997.
2. Borgeat A, Tewes E, Biasca N, Gerber C. Patient-controlled interscalene analgesia with ropivacaine after major shoulder surgery: PCIA versus PCA. Br J Anesth 81:603–605, 1998.
3. Lierz P, Schroegendorfer K, Choi S, et al. Continuous blockade of both brachial plexus with ropivacaine in phantom pain: A case report. Pain 78(2):135–137, 1998.
4. Singelyn FJ, Seguy S, and Gouverneur JM. Interscalene brachial plexus analgesia after open shoulder surgery: Continuous versus patient-controlled infusion. Anesth Analg 89:1216–1220, 1999.
5. Klein SM, Grant SA, Greengrass RA, et al. Interscalene brachial plexus block with a continuous catheter insertion system and a disposable infusion pump. Anesth Analg 91:1473–1478, 2000.
6. Borgeat A, Perschak H, Bird P, et al. Patient-controlled interscalene analgesia with ropivacaine 0.2% versus patient-controlled intravenous analgesia after major shoulder surgery. Anesthesiol 92:102–108, 2000.
7. Borgeat A, Kalberer F, Jacob H, et al. Patient-controlled interscalene analgesia with ropivacaine 0.2% versus bupivacaine 0.15% after major open shoulder surgery: The effect on hand motor function. Anesth Analg 92(1):218–223, 2001.
8. Ilfeld BM, Enneking FK. A portable mechanical pump providing over four days of patient-controlled analgesia by perineural infusion at home. Reg Anesth Pain Med 27:100–104, 2002.
9. Ilfeld BM, Morey TE, Wright TW, et al. Continuous interscalene brachial plexus block for postoperative pain control at home: A randomized, double-blinded, placebo-controlled study. Anesth Analg 96:1089–1095, 2003.
10. Nielsen KC, Greengrass RA, Pietrobon R, et al. Continuous interscalene brachial plexus blockade provides good analgesia at home after major shoulder surgery—Report of four cases. Can J Anesth 50:57–61, 2003.
11. Casati A, Borghi B, Fanelli G, et al. Interscalene brachial plexus anesthesia and analgesia for open shoulder surgery: A randomized, double-blinded comparison between levobupivacaine and ropivacaine. Anesth Analg 96:253–259, 2003.
12. Casati A, Vinciguerra F, Scarioni M, et al. Lidocaine versus ropivacaine for continuous interscalene brachial plexus block after open shoulder surgery. Acta Anaesthesiol Scand 47:355–360, 2003.
13. Klein SM, Steele SM, Nielsen KC, et al. The difficulties of ambulatory interscalene and intra-articular infusions for rotator cuff surgery: A preliminary report; Can J Anesth 50:265–269, 2003.
14. Boezaart AP, De Beer, JF, Nell ML. Early experience with continuous cervical paravertebral block using a stimulating catheter. Reg Anest Pain Med 28:406–413, 2003.
15. Borgeat A, Dullenkopf A, Ekatodermis G, Nagy L. Evaluation of the lateral modified approach for continuous interscalene block after shoulder surgery. Anesthesiology 99:436–442, 2003.
16. Ekatodramis G, Borgeat A, Huledal G, et al. Continuous interscalene analgesia with ropivacaine 2 mg/mL after major shoulder surgery. Anesthesiology 98:143–150, 2003.
17. Ilfeld BM, Morey TE, Wright TW, et al. Interscalene perineural ropivacaine infusion: A comparison of two dosing regimens for postoperative analgesia. Reg Anesth Pain Med 29:9–16, 2004.
18. Gaumann DM, Lennon RL, Wedel DJ. Continuous axillary block for postoperative pain management. Reg Anesth 13:77–82, 1988.
19. Mezzatesta JP, Scott DA, Schweitzer SA, Selander, DE. Continuous axillary brachial plexus block for postoperative pain relief. Intermittent bolus versus continuous infusion. Reg Anesth 22:357–362, 1997.
20. Iskandar H, Rakotondriamihary S, Dixmerias F, et al. Analgesia using continuous axillary block after surgery of severe hand injuries: Self-administration versus continuous injections. Ann Fr Anesth Reanim 17:1099–1103, 1998.
21. Mak PH, Tsui SL, Ip WY, Irwin MG. Brachial plexus infusion of ropivacaine with patient-controlled supplementation. Can J Anaesth 47:903–906, 2000.
22. Vranken JH, Zuurmond WW, de Lange JJ. Continuous brachial plexus block as a treatment for the Pancoast syndrome. Clin J Pain 16:327–333, 2000.
23. Rawal N, Allvin R, Axelsson K, et al. Patient-controlled regional analgesia at home: Controlled comparison between bupivacaine and ropivacaine brachial plexus analgesia. Anesthesiology 96:1290–1296, 2002.
24. Turkoglu K. Comparison of patient-controlled analgesia and continuous infusion with 0.2% ropivacaine in brachial plexus analgesia after hand surgery. Reg Anesth Pain Med 28 (suppl) nr 62:52, 2003.
25. Ilfeld BM, Morey, TE, Enneking FK. Continuous infraclavicular brachial plexus block for postoperative pain control at home: A randomized, double-blinded placebo-controlled study. Anesthesiology 96:1297–1304, 2002.
26. Ilfeld BM, Morey TE, Enneking FK. Infraclavicular perineural local anesthetic infusion: A comparison of three dosing regimens for postoperative analgesia. Anesthesiology 100:395–402, 2004.

▶ **TABLE 21-2B.** LOWER LIMB INFUSION STRATEGIES USED BY VARIOUS AUTHORS

Author	Aim of Study	Number of Patients per Group	Surgery	Initial Bolus	Postoperative Strategy	Results/Comments
Singelyn,[1] 1997	PCA IV vs. cont popliteal sciatic	60 & 45 p nr	Foot surgery	30 mL mepi 1% + epi 1:200,000	I: bupi 0.125% + suf 0.1 µg/mL + cl 1 µg/mL C: 7 mL/h	Superior analgesia and decreased incidence of side effects vs. IV PCA ($p < 0.005$) 25% kinked or broken catheter
Singelyn,[2] 1998	CFA vs. IV PCA or CEA	15, 15, & 15 p r	TKA	37 mL bupi 0.25% + epi 1:200,000	I: bupi 0.125% + suf 0.1 µg/mL + cl 1 µg/mL C: 10 mL/h	CFA vs. IV PCA: Improved analgesia ($p = 0.04$) 20% decrease in hospital stay ($p < 0.05$)
Capdevila,[3] 1999	CFA vs. IV PCA or CEA	20, 17, & 19	TKA	25 mL lido 2% + epi 1:200,000 + morphine 2 mg	I: lido 1% + morphine 30 µg/mL, cl 2 µg/mL C: 0.1 mL/kg/h	CFA vs. CEA: comparable analgesia CFA vs. IV PCA: improved analgesia ($p < 0.01$) Fewer side effects
Singelyn,[4] 1999	CFA vs. CEA or IV PCA	1142, 64, & 132 p nr	THA		I: bupi 0.125% + suf 0.1 µg/mL + cl 1 µg/mL C: 10 mL/h	Comparable analgesia between three regimens CFA with lower side effects vs. IV PCA and CEA
Ganapathy,[5] 1999	Fascia iliaca compartment analgesia	saline 20 bupi 0.1:20 bupi 0.2:22 p r	TKA	20 mL bupi 0.2% via needle and 10 mL via catheter	I: saline, bupi 0.1% or bupi 0.2% C: 10 mL/h	Bupi 0.2% gave decreased morphine consumption vs. saline ($p < 0.05$). Only 40% of catheters correctly placed
Chudinov,[6] 1999	Continuous psoas compartment vs. IV PCA	20 & 20 p r	Hip fracture		I: bupi 0.25% + epi 1:200,000 at 1–2 mg/kg/8 h when VAS > 3/10	Improved analgesia and patient satisfaction in psoas group vs. IV PCA ($p < 0.05$)
Chelly,[7] 2001	CFA vs. CEA or IV PCA	29, 30, & 33 p nr	TKA		I: ropi 0.2% C: 12 mL/h	CFA vs. CEA: comparable analgesia CFA vs. IV PCA: improved analgesia, fewer side effects, decreased hospital stay ($p < 0.05$)
Grant,[8] 2001	Continuous lumbar, femoral and sciatic	5, 35, & 35	All kinds of orthopaedic procedures	Lumbar and femoral: 30 mL ropi 0.5% Sciatic: 20 mL ropi 0.5%	I: ropi 0.2% C: 10 mL/h	Patients were discharged after 20-mL bolus of ropi 0.5% + epi 1:400,000
Capdevila,[9] 2002	Cont psoas compartment vs. saline	18	THA	0.4 mL/kg ropi 0.2%	I: ropi 0.2% C: 0.15 mL/kg/h	Optimal analgesia, few side effects
Ilfeld,[10] 2002	Cont popliteal sciatic	15 & 15 r db pc	Surgery distal to the knee	50 mL mepi 1.5% + epi 125 µg + cl 100 µg + sodium bicarbonate 5 meq	I: ropi 0.2% C: 8 mL/h B: 2 mL LO: 20 min	Excellent analgesia, significant decrease in sleep problems, opioid use and side effects ($p < 0.05$)

Author, Year	Study	Surgery	N, design	LA	Infusion	Outcome
Di Benedetto,[11] 2002	Cont subgluteus sciatic vs. popliteal	Foot surgery	30 & 30 p r	20 mL ropi 0.75%	I: ropi 0.2% C: 5 mL/h B: 10 mL LO: 60 min	Effective analgesia in both approaches
Di Benedetto,[12] 2002	Cont subgluteus sciatic PCA vs. cont infusion	Foot and ankle	25 & 25 p r	20 mL ropi 0.75%	I: ropi 0.2% C: 10 mL/h Or C: 5 mL/h B: 5 mL LO: 60 min	Good analgesia in both groups Lower consumption of local anesthetic agent in PCA group ($p < 0.0005$)
Pham-Dang,[13] 2003	Continuous blocks ISB, axillary, femoral, midfemoral (130 in total)		47 fem & 19 midfem	10 mL ropi 0.75%	I: ropi 0.2% C: 2–5 mL/h B: 5–10 mL LO: 30 min	Using in situ stimulable catheter increases success rate in catheter placement

B = bolus; bupi = bupivacaine; C = continuous; CEA = continuous epidural anesthesia/analgesia; CFA = continuous femoral anesthesia/analgesia; Cl = clonidine; cont = continuous; cr = case report; db = double-blind; Epi = epinephrine; I = infusion; l = infusion; ISB = interscalene block; IV = intravenous; LO = lockout; mepi = mepivacaine; nr = nonrandomized; o = observational study; p = prospective; pc = placebo-controlled; PCA = patient-controlled analgesia; r = randomized; ropi = ropivacaine; THA = total hip arthroplasty; TKA = total knee arthroplasty.

[1]Singelyn F, Aye F, Gouverneur JM. Continuous popliteal sciatic block: An original technique to provide postoperative analgesia after foot surgery. *Anesth Analg* 84:383–386, 1997.

[2]Singelyn FJ, Deyaert M, Joris D, et al. Effect of intravenous patient-controlled analgesia with morphine, continuous epidural analgesia and continuous three-in-one block on postoperative pain and knee rehabilitation after unilateral knee arthroplasty. *Anesth Analg* 87:88–92, 1998.

[3]Capdevila X, Barthelet Y, Biboulet P, et al. Effects of perioperative analgesic technique on the surgical outcome and duration of rehabilitation after major knee surgery. *Anesthesiology* 91:8–15, 1999.

[4]Singelyn FJ, Gouverneur JM. Postoperative analgesia after total hip arthroplasty : IV PCA with morphine, patient-controlled epidural analgesia or continuous 3-in-1 block—A prospective evaluation by our acute pain service in more than 1300 patients. *J Clin Anesth* 11:550–554, 1999.

[5]Ganapathy S, Wasserman R, Watson JT, et al. Modified continuous femoral three-in-one block for postoperative pain after total knee arthroplasty. *Anesth Analg* 89:1197–1202, 1999.

[6]Chudinov A, Berkenstadt H, Salai M, et al. Continuous psoas compartment block for anesthesia and perioperative analgesia in patients with hip fractures. *Reg Anesth Pain Med* 24:563–568, 1999.

[7]Chelly JE, Greger J, Gebhard R, et al. Continuous femoral nerve blocks improve recovery and outcome of patients undergoing total knee arthroplasty. *J Arthrop* 16:436–445, 2001.

[8]Grant SA, Nielsen KC, Greengrass RA, et al. Continuous peripheral nerve block for ambulatory surgery. *Reg Anesth Pain Med* 26:209–214, 2001.

[9]Capdevila X, Macaire P, Dadure C, et al. Continuous psoas compartment block for anesthesia and perioperative analgesia after hip arthroplasty: New landmarks, technical guidelines, and clinical evaluation. *Anesth Analg* 94:1606–1613, 2002.

[10]Ilfeld B, Morey T, Wang RD, et al. Continuous popliteal sciatic nerve block for postoperative pain control at home: A randomized, double-blinded, placebo controlled study. *Anesthesiology* 97:959–965, 2002.

[11]Di Benedetto P, Casati A, Bertini L, et al. Postoperative analgesia with continuous sciatic nerve block after foot surgery: A prospective randomized comparison between the popliteal and subgluteus approaches. *Anesth Analg* 94:996–1000, 2002.

[12]Di Benedetto P, Casati A, Bertini L. Continuous subgluteus sciatic nerve block after orthopedic foot and ankle surgery: Comparison of two infusion techniques. *Reg Anesth Pain Med* 27:168–172, 2002.

[13]Pham-Dang C, Kick O, Collet T, et al. Continuous peripheral nerve blocks with stimulating catheters. *Reg Anesth Pain Med* 28:83–88, 2003.

generally accepted as the toxic blood level. One must be aware that if a postoperative infusion is given after a preoperative bolus of 150 to 210 mg bupivacaine, it will cause toxic bupivacaine plasma levels.[15]

Borgeat et al.[16] demonstrated that PCRA with ropivacaine (0.2%) or bupivacaine (0.15%) provided similar pain relief after major shoulder surgery. They also showed that smaller concentrations than these do not produce adequate postoperative pain control in this situation. Furthermore, ropivacaine (0.2%) through an interscalene catheter caused less motor impairment than bupivacaine 0.15% but equivalent analgesia. Infusions of 0.2% ropivacaine into a brachial plexus sheath at a rate of 10 mL/h for 24 h[17] or 6.8 mg/h for 1 week (total cumulative dose 904 mg)[18] were not associated with any signs or symptoms of toxicity.

Casati et al.[19] compared levobupivacaine (0.125%) to ropivacaine (0.2%) for continuous interscalene nerve block after open shoulder surgery. Patients receiving levobupivacaine required a smaller volume of drug during the 24 h of PCRA. There was no difference between the two drugs in postoperative analgesia or in the recovery of motor function.

Potent analgesic effects have been demonstrated for ropivacaine (0.2%) in ambulatory patients receiving a basal infusion of 8 mL/h and 2-mL patient-controlled bolus doses available every 20 min.[20] This was also demonstrated with 4 mL/h and a 6-mL bolus every hour.[21] However, patients experienced an increase in the frequency and intensity of breakthrough pain and sleep disturbances, and they were less satisfied with the latter regimen.

Axillary Block

Selander et al.[22] first described the technique and reported a relatively high percentage of inadequate blocks (27 percent) for surgery. In a review article, Liu and Salinas concluded that in contrast with the documented benefits of continuous interscalene analgesia, definitive benefits have not been established for continuous axillary brachial plexus block.[4]

A study by Salonen et al. also leads to the conclusion that continuous axillary block may not be effective for postoperative analgesia.[23] They compared the analgesic efficacy of three infusion regimens through an axillary catheter for surgery of the hand or forearm. Patients received a continuous infusion of ropivacaine 0.1%, ropivacaine 0.2%, or saline. The initial block with 5 mg/kg ropivacaine (injected volume ranged from 42 to 60 mL) provided postoperative analgesia for approximately 10 h. However, none of the infusions relieved the patients' pain adequately. A possible reason for the failure may be inaccurate placement of the catheter tip.

Infraclavicular Block

For moderately painful surgery of the upper limb, continuous infraclavicular nerve blocks have significantly reduced pain and opioid consumption as well as improved sleep, with increased patient satisfaction.[21] The combination of a continuous infusion and boluses provided optimal analgesia while minimizing oral analgesics as compared with basal- or bolus-only regimens.[10]

A continuous infusion of 5 to 8 mL/h of 0.2% ropivacaine with 2 to 4 mL PCRA boluses every 20 min results in a high level of patient satisfaction.[24]

Cervical Paravertebral Block

In a prospective study, Boezaart et al.[13] performed continuous cervical paravertebral block on 256 patients for pain relief after 14 different shoulder operations. Immediately after an initial bolus of 30 mL 0.5% ropivacaine (maximum 0.5 mL/kg), a continuous ropivacaine (0.2%) infusion at 0.1 mL/kg/h was started. The infusion rates were adjusted over the first 24 h to obtain optimal analgesia and minimal motor block. In the case of "breakthrough" pain, an additional bolus of 10 mL ropivacaine 0.2% was injected through the catheter. This was permitted every 30 min, up to a maximum of three bolus injections per 6-h period. This regimen provided excellent results, with early return of motor function; however, it is anticipated that self-administration of analgesics should yield even better results for breakthrough pain than when analgesia is administered by nurses.

Infusion Strategies of the Lower Limb

Femoral Nerve Block

A femoral nerve block with a single injection of 20 mL of bupivacaine (0.5%) may provide effective analgesia for 18 to 24 h.[25] Some authors have even reported effective analgesia up to 48 h after total knee arthroplasty (TKA) with a 30-mL bolus of ropivacaine (0.25%).[26]

A consistent problem with femoral nerve block has been inaccurate catheter placement. The older "blind" placement techniques, such as the "3-in-1" technique or the "sub-iliaca fascia" technique have all yielded disappointing results but can now largely be replaced with the "stimulating" catheter technique. The current authors use 20 to 40 mL of ropivacaine (0.5 to 0.75%) or bupivacaine (0.5%) as an initial bolus, followed by an infusion of ropivacaine (0.2%) at 5 mL/h and PCRA boluses of 10 mL every 60 min. This seems to be successful, but comparative studies are needed to verify it.

Psoas Compartment Block
(Lumbar Plexus Block)

Capdevila et al.[27] studied the efficacy of continuous psoas compartment analgesia after total hip arthroplasty (THA). An initial loading dose of ropivacaine (0.2%, 0.4 mL/kg) was injected. Chelly et al.[28] successfully used a 30-mL bolus injection of a mixture of mepivacaine (1.5%) and ropivacaine (0.75%) in 13 patients with acetabular fractures, while Kaloul et al.[29] used a 30-mL bolus dose of ropivacaine (0.5%) with epinephrine 1:200,000.

Sciatic Nerve Block

Most authors use a 30-mL bolus injection to achieve analgesia. White[30] used bupivacaine (0.25%), while Zaric[31] used ropivacaine (0.5%) and Ilfeld[32] used a 50-mL bolus of the shorter-acting mepivacaine (1.5%). Most authors use ropivacaine (0.2%) for continuous postoperative infusion rates ranging from 5 to 10 mL/h[33] and 5- to 10-mL PCRA doses. Ilfeld infused 8 mL/h with a 2-mL PCRA bolus every 20 min.

Pediatric Infusion Strategies

In recent years, the growing use of continuous regional anesthetic techniques in adults has led to the increasing use of these techniques in children (see Chap. 31).[34] Due to the anatomy of the nerves (small diameters, short distances between the Ranvier nodes), large volumes and low concentrations are the key in pediatric nerve block.[35] One must, however, remember that there is a higher risk of toxicity in infants due to their immature metabolic systems and the lower albumin and alpha$_1$-glycoprotein levels. The different infusion strategies in children are summarized in Table 21-3.

▶ **TABLE 21-3.** INFUSION STRATEGIES IN CHILDREN

Author	Technique	Number of Patients	Bolus Dose	Continuous Infusion	Comment
Johnson[36]	Continuous femoral nerve	3		Bupi 0.125%: 0.375 mg/kg/h	Safe bupi plasma levels
Paut et al.[37]	Continuous fascia iliaca	20	Bupi 0.25% with epi: 0.62 mL/kg	Bupi 0.1%: 0.135 mL/kg/h	No severe side effects, safe bupi plasma levels
Sciard et al.[38]	Continuous lumbar plexus	2	Ropi 0.2% and mepi 1.5%, equal mixture	Ropi 0.2% at 0.17 and 0.2 mL/kg/h respectively	Good analgesia, no side effects
Dadure et al.[39]	Continuous infraclavicular	2	Ropi 0.5% and lido 1% with 1:200,000 epinephrine, equal mixture: 0.5 mL/kg	Ropi 0.2% - 0.1 mL/kg/h	Optimal analgesia without adverse effects
Dadure et al.[40]	Continuous psoas compartment	15	Ropi 0.5% and lido 1% with 1:200,000 epinephrine, equal mixture: 0.5 mL/kg	Ropi 0.2% 0.1 mL/kg/h	Effective analgesia with few adverse effects
Dadure et al.[41]	Axillary, femoral, popliteal catheters	25	Bupi 0.25% and lido 1% with 1:200,000 epinephrine, equal mixture: 0.5 mL/kg	Ropi 0.2% 0.1 mL/kg/h	Study with disposable pumps, satisfactory pain scores without major adverse events
Dadure et al.[42]	Continuous axillary and popliteal sciatic	1 (13 kg)	Bupi 0.25% and ido 1% with epinephrine 1:200,000:6 mL in each catheter	Bupi 0.125% at 2 mL/h in each catheter	Two catheters in one patient, no problems
Ivani et al.[43]	Continuous lateral sciatic	1		Ropi 0.2% 0.4 mg/kg/h with clonidine 0.12 µg/kg/h	Perfusion during 21 days, complete pain relief

bupi = bupivacaine; mepi = mepivacaine; ropi = ropivacaine.

▶ PROBLEMS WITH CONTINUOUS NERVE BLOCKS

Pain during Continuous Peripheral Nerve Block (Fig. 21-2)

If the CPNB and PCRA do not control the operative pain satisfactorily, the infusion should be stopped for 2 to 6 h. The pain can then be reevaluated and the patient given the choice as to whether the perfusion should be continued or not. If the patient chooses to continue, a bolus injection of 10 mL of ropivacaine (0.2%) can be given and the infusion continued at the previous rate. If the patient wants the infusion to be stopped, the catheter must be removed and alternative analgesia provided.

If there is severe pain during physical therapy, the patient should receive a full bolus dose 1 h before the next session. If there is pain at the catheter entry site, cold compression must be applied to the site and a nonsteroidal anti-inflammatory drug (NSAID) can be administered. The pain must be reevaluated 2 h later; if pain is still experienced, the patient should be given the choice of whether to continue the perfusion or not. If not, the catheter will have to be removed and alternative analgesia provided. This applies to all situations when complications may make it necessary to replace a catheter or stop infusion by catheter altogether.

Pain at the Catheter Insertion Site

Tenderness or pain at the puncture site can result from irritation, due to movement of the catheter or from inflammation and infection. In exceptional cases, pain can result from local anesthetic–induced toxicity.[44] In

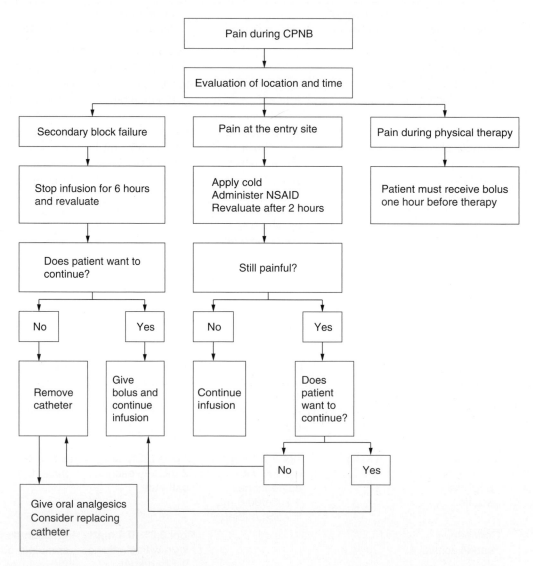

Figure 21-2. Proposed approach of pain during continuous peripheral nerve block.
ABBREVIATIONS: CPNB = continuous peripheral nerve block; NSAID = nonsteroidal anti-inflammatory drug.

using a continuous paravertebral block, one should take care to avoid penetration of the paraspinal extensor muscles of the neck and insert the catheter between the levator scapulae and trapezius muscle.[45]

If the patient experiences pain at the puncture site, inspect it. If there is irritation, give a NSAID or similar agent and apply cold compression to the site. Do a follow-up if the site is still painful:

> Stop the infusion for 6 h and give the patient the choice of having the catheter removed.
>
> Provide the patient with alternative analgesics if the catheter is removed; otherwise give a bolus of 10 mL of 0.2% ropivacaine or 0.25% bupivacaine and continue the infusion at the previous rate.
>
> If the entry site is infected, remove the catheter, use oral analgesia, and consider antibiotic treatment.

Catheter Dislodgment

The frequency of catheter dislodgement reported in the literature varies between 0 and 20 percent.[46] Paradoxically, good analgesia may even increase the chance of dislodgement because the patient moves and turns more freely.

Tunnelling the catheter subcutaneously can prevent dislodgment. A dislodged catheter must be removed and replaced or alternative analgesic agents must be given. This implies a return to the hospital if the patient is cared for at home. Migration of a catheter after correct placement has not been reported.[47] Give the patient the choice of having the catheter replaced (keep in mind that stimulating muscles in an operated region can cause severe pain) or treatment with an alternative analgesic regimen.

Bacterial Colonization, Inflammation, or Infection

Previous reports have failed to demonstrate a relationship between the duration of catheter use and bacterial culture of the catheter tip.[48,49] Cuvillon et al.[50] found femoral catheter colonization in 57 percent and bacteremia in 1.5 percent of the cases after 48 h. In a multicenter study involving 1416 perineural catheters at different anatomic locations, Bernard et al.[51] documented a colonization rate of 28 percent; 3 percent had signs of local inflammation, and infection was found in 0.7 percent, which was similar to the findings of Borgeat et al.[20] In these patients, local pain, redness, and indurations were noted after 3 to 4 days. Despite this high number of positive cultures of catheter tips, the risk of local or systemic infection seems to be very small in postoperative patients.[52] This may be due to the routine prophylactic use of antibiotics in patients undergoing orthopaedic surgery. At present, there are no definitive recommendations regarding continuous use of catheters and routine antibiotic prophylaxis. If strict aseptic surgical conditions are maintained, preliminary results indicate that the incidence of infection of perineural catheters is low.[50] If infection is suspected or likely, remove the catheter and take a pus swab of the entry site for culture. Prescribe antibiotics in consultation with the surgeon if appropriate and treat the patient with an alternative analgesic regimen.

Free Blood Aspirated from Catheter

Klein et al.[47] reported one case where a catheter had blood-tinged fluid on aspiration after 24 h. It is not clear whether this was from intramuscular placement, blood in the brachial plexus sheath, or inadvertent vascular cannulation. Before discharge from the recovery room, the correct placement of the catheter tip must be confirmed, especially when early discharge from the hospital is planned. The position of catheters can be confirmed by testing the extent of the block after infusing analgesic through the catheter or by injecting epinephrine through the catheter as a marker for intravascular cannulation. An alternative is to visualize the location of the catheter tip radiographically. However, determining the location of the catheter tip may be difficult with this technique. The use of stimulating catheters can probably reduce the misplacement of the catheter tip. However, the absence of blood in aspirates, no effect on heart rate after a test dose of epinephrine, and the injection of the primary (initial bolus) and secondary block (continuous infusion) form the mainstays of protection against intravascular catheter tips. If such a misplacement does occur, discontinue the infusion, remove the catheter, and treat the patient with alternative analgesics. Consider replacing the catheter.

Kinking, Knotting, and Shearing

Manipulation of catheters through needles can lead to catheter damage, weakening, and eventually shearing. This can happen while advancing the catheter through the needle[53] or while removing the guidewire from the catheter with the needle still in situ.[54] A catheter fragment can therefore remain in the body. This may necessitate surgical removal, although in some situations it may be wise to leave the fragment. The use of stimulating catheters may increase the degree to which they are manipulated in order to optimize catheter position. This may possibly increase the potential for shearing. Catheters, especially long ones, may kink.[55] Knotting of the catheter is extremely rare but it can happen during insertion, making its surgical removal necessary.[56,57] Knotting is more common when the catheter is threaded more then 10 cm past the needle tip. This can theoretically also cause the catheter to curl around the nerve, making its removal a problem.

REFERENCES

1. Tuominen M, Haasio J, Hekali R, Rosenberg PH. Continuous interscalene brachial plexus block: Clinical efficacy, technical problems and bupivacaine plasma concentrations. *Acta Anesthesiol Scand* 33:84–88, 1989.

2. Lehtipalo S, Koskinen LO, Johansson G, et al. Continuous interscalene brachial plexus block for postoperative analgesia following shoulder surgery. *Acta Anaesthesiol Scand* 43:258–264, 1999.

3. Borgeat A, Tewes E, Biasca N, et al. Patient-controlled interscalene analgesia with ropivacaine after major shoulder surgery: PCIA versus PCA. *Br J Anesth* 81:603–605, 1998.

4. Liu SS, Salinas FV. Continuous plexus and peripheral nerve blocks for postoperative analgesia. *Anesth Analg* 96:263–272, 2003.

5. Ilfeld BM, Morey TE, Enneking FK. Infraclavicular perineural local anesthetic infusion: A comparison of three dosing regimens for postoperative analgesia. *Anesthesiology* 100:395–402, 2004.

6. Scherpereel P. Patient controlled analgesia. *Ann Fr Anesth Reanim* 10:269–283, 1991.

7. Iskandar H, Rakotondriamihary S, Dixmerias F, et al. Analgesia using continuous axillary block after surgery of severe hand injuries: Self-administration versus continuous injections. *Ann Fr Anesth Reanim* 17:1099–1103, 1998.

8. Singelyn FJ, Seguy S, Gouverneur JM. Interscalene brachial plexus analgesia after open shoulder surgery: Continuous versus patient-controlled infusion. *Anesth Analg* 89:1216–1220, 1999.

9. Mezzatesta JP, Scott DA, Schweitzer SA, et al. Continuous axillary brachial plexus block for postoperative pain relief. Intermittent bolus versus continuous infusion. *Reg Anesth* 22(4):357–362, 1997.

10. Ilfeld BM, Morey TE, Enneking FK. Infraclavicular perineural local anesthetic infusion: A comparison of three dosing regimens for postoperative analgesia. *Anesthesiology* 100:395–402, 2004.

11. Turkoglu K. Comparison of patient controlled analgesia and continuous infusion with 0.2% ropivacaine in brachial plexus analgesia after hand surgery. *Reg Anesth Pain Med* 28(suppl 62):52, 2003.

12. Rawal N, Allvin R, Axelsson K, et al. Patient-controlled regional analgesia at home: Controlled comparison between bupivacaine and ropivacaine brachial plexus analgesia. *Anesthesiology* 96:1290–1296, 2002.

13. Boezaart AP, De Beer JF, Nel ML. Early experience with continuous cervical paravertebral block using a stimulating catheter. *Reg Anesth Pain Med* 28:406–413, 2003.

14. Pere P, Tuominen M, Rosenberg PH. Cumulation of bupivacaine, desbutylbupivacaine and 4-hydroxibupivacaine during and after continuous interscalene brachial plexus block. *Acta Anesth Scand* 35(7):647–650, 1991.

15. Haasio J, Tuominen M, Rosenberg PH. Continuous interscalene brachial plexus block during and after shoulder surgery. *Ann Chir Gynaecol* 79(2):103–107, 1990.

16. Borgeat A, Kalberer F, Jacob H, et al. Patient-controlled interscalene analgesia with ropivacaine 0.2% versus bupivacaine 0.15% after major open shoulder surgery: The effect on hand motor function. *Anesth Analg* 92(1):218–223, 2001.

17. Klein SM, Greengrass RA, Gleason DH, et al. Major ambulatory surgery with continuous regional anesthesia and a disposable infusion pump. *Anesthesiology* 91:563–565, 1991.

18. Mak PH, Tsui SL, Ip WY, Irwin MG. Brachial plexus infusion of ropivacaine with patient-controlled supplementation. *Can J Anaesth* 47(9):903–906, 2000.

19. Casati A, Borghi B, Fanelli G, et al. Interscalene brachial plexus anesthesia and analgesia for open shoulder surgery: A randomized, double-blinded comparison between levobupivacaine and ropivacaine. *Anesth Analg* 96:253–259, 2000.

20. Borgeat A, Dullenkopf A, Ekatodermis G, Nagy L. Evaluation of the lateral modified approach for continuous interscalene block after shoulder surgery. *Anesthesiology* 99(2):436–442, 2003.

21. Ilfeld BM, Morey TE, Wright TW, et al. Interscalene perineural ropivacaine infusion: A comparison of two dosing regimens for postoperative analgesia. *Reg Anesth Pain Med* 29:9–16, 2004.

22. Selander D. Catheter techniques in axillary plexus block. *Acta Anaesthesiol Scand* 21:324–329, 1977.

23. Salonen MHA, Haasio J, Bachmann et al. Evaluation of efficacy and plasma concentrations of ropivacaine in continuous axillary brachial plexus block: High dose for surgical anesthesia and low dose for postoperative analgesia. *Reg Anesth Pain Med* 25:47–51, 2000.

24. Ilfeld BM, Morey TE, Enneking FK. Continuous infraclavicular brachial plexus block for postoperative pain control at home: A randomized, double-blinded placebo-controlled study. *Anesthesiology* 96:1297–1304, 2002.

25. Hirst GC, Lang SA, Dust WN, et al. Femoral nerve block: Single injection versus continuous infusion for total knee arthroplasty. *Reg Anesth* 21:292–297, 1996.

26. Ng HP, Cheong KF, Lim A, et al. Intraoperative single-shot 3-in-1 femoral nerve block with ropivacaine 0.25%, ropivacaine 0.5% or bupivacaine 0.25% provides comparable 48-hr analgesia after unilateral total knee replacement. *Can J Anesth* 48:1102–1108, 2001.

27. Capdevila X, Macaire P, Dadure C, et al. Continuous compartment block for postoperative analgesia after total hip arthroplasty: New landmarks, technical guidelines and clinical evaluation. *Anesth Analg* 94;1606–1613, 2002.

28. Chelly JE, Casati A, Al-Samsam T, et al. Continuous lumbar plexus block for acute postoperative pain management after open reduction and internal fixation of acetabular fractures. *J Orthop Trauma* 17:362–367, 2003.

29. Kaloul I, Guay J, Côté C, et al. The posterior lumbar plexus (psoas compartment) block and the three-in-one femoral nerve block provide similar postoperative analgesia after total knee replacement. *Can J Anesth* 51:45–51, 2004.

30. White PF, Issioui T, Skrivanek GD, et al. The use of a continuous popliteal sciatic nerve block after surgery involving the foot and the ankle: Does it improve the quality of recovery? *Anesth Analg* 97:1303–1309, 2003.

31. Zaric D, Boysen K Christiansen J, et al. Continuous popliteal sciatic nerve block for outpatient foot surgery: A randomized controlled trial. *Acta Anaesthesiol Scand* 48:337–341, 2004.

32. Ilfeld BM, Morey TE, Wang RD, et al. Continuous popliteal sciatic nerve block for postoperative pain control at home. *Anesthesiology* 97:959–965, 2002.

33. Pernot M, Graff D, Pierron A, et al. Continuous popliteal sciatic nerve block for foot surgery in 531 patients: Efficacy and adverse effects. *Eur J Anaesthesiol* 21(Suppl): A-450, 2004.

34. Ivani G, Tonetti F. Postoperative analgesia in infants and children: New developments. *Minerva Anestesiol* 70:399–403, 2004.

35. Bosenberg A, Ivani G. Regional anaesthesia: Children are different (editorial). *Paediatr Anaesth* 8:447–450, 1998.

36. Johnson C. Continuous femoral nerve blockade for analgesia in children with femoral fractures. *Anaesth Intens Care* 22:281–283, 1992.

37. Paut O, Sallaberry M, Schreiber E, et al. Continuous fascia iliaca compartment block in children: A prospective evaluation of plasma bupivacaine concentrations, pain scores and side effects. *Anesth Analg* 92:1159–1163, 2001.

38. Sciard D, Matuszczak M, Gebhard R, et al. Continuous posterior lumbar plexus block for acute postoperative pain control in young children. *Anesthesiology* 95:1521–1523, 2001.

39. Dadure C, Raux O, Troncin R, et al. Continuous infraclavicular brachial plexus block for acute pain management in children. *Anesth Analg* 97:691–693, 2003.

40. Dadure C, Raux O, Gaudard P, et al. Continuous psoas compartment blocks after major orthopedic surgery in children: A prospective computed tomographic scan and clinical studies. *Anesth Analg* 98:623–628, 2004.

41. Dadure C, Pirat P, Raux O, et al. Peripoperative continuous peripheral nerve blocks with disposable infusion pumps in children: A prospective descriptive study. *Anesth Analg* 97:687–690, 2003.

42. Dadure C, Acosta C, Capdevila X. Perioperative pain management of a complex orthopedic surgical procedure with double continuous nerve blocks in a burned child. *Anesth Analg* 98:1653–1655, 2004.

43. Ivani G, Codipietro L, Gagliardi F, et al. A long-term continuous infusion via a sciatic catheter in a 3-year-old boy. *Paediatr Anaesth* 13:718–721, 2003.

44. Hogan Q, Dotson R, Erickson S, et al. Local anesthetic myotoxicity: A case and review. *Anesthesiology* 80:942–947, 1994.

45. Boezaart AP, Koorn R, Rosenquist RW. Paravertebral approach to the brachial plexus: An anatomic improvement in technique. *Reg Anesth Pain Med* 28:241–244, 2003.

46. Cuvillon P, Ripart J, Lalourcey L, et al. The continuous femoral nerve block catheter for postoperative analgesia: Bacterial colonization, infectious rate and adverse effects. *Anesth Analg* 93:1045–1049, 2001.

47. Klein SM, Grant SA, Greengrass RA, et al. Interscalene brachial plexus block with a continuous catheter insertion system and a disposable infusion pump. *Anesth Analg* 91:1473–1478, 2000.

48. Tuominen M, Rosenberg PH, Kalso E. Blood levels of bupivacaine after single dose, supplementary dose and during continuous infusion in axillary plexus block. *Acta Anaesthesiol Scand* 27(4):303–306, 1983.

49. Manriquez RG, Pallares V. Continuous brachial plexus block for prolonged sympathectomy and control of pain. *Anesth Analg* 57:128–130, 1978.

50. Cuvillon P, Ripart J, Lalourcey L, et al. The continuous femoral nerve block catheter for postoperative analgesia: Bacterial colonization, infectious rate and adverse effects. *Anesth Analg* 93:1045–1049, 2001.

51. Bernard N, Pirat P, Branchereau S, et al. Continuous peripheral nerve blocks in 1416 patients: A prospective multicenter study measuring incidences and characteristics of infectious adverse events (abstr). *Anesthesiology* 93:1045–1049, 2002.

52. Gaumann DM, Lennon RL, Wedel DJ. Continuous axillary block for postoperative pain management. *Reg Anesth* 13:77–82, 1998.

53. Coventry DM, Timperley J. Perineural catheter placement: Another potential complication (letter). *Reg Anesth Pain Med* 29:174–175, 2003.

54. Lee B, Goucke CR. Shearing of a peripheral nerve catheter. *Anaesth Analg* 95:760–761, 2002.

55. Singelyn FJ. Continous popliteal sciatic nerve block: An original technique to provide postoperative analgesia after foot surgery. *Anesth Analg* 84:383, 1997.

56. MacLeod D. Knotted peripheral nerve catheter (letter). *Reg Anesth Pain Med* 28:487–488, 2003.

57. Rudd K, Hall PJ. Knotted femoral nerve catheter. *Anaesth Intens Care* 32:282–283, 2004.

CHAPTER 22

The Use of Ultrasound for Peripheral Nerve Blocks

VINCENT W. S. CHAN

▶ INTRODUCTION

Peripheral nerve blocks for orthopaedic surgery are usually performed without visual guidance, relying mainly on surface anatomic landmarks and electrical stimulation to localize nerves. It is therefore not surprising that regional anesthesia may fail. Incorrect placement of needles and local anesthetic account for most failures, especially in patients without clear anatomic landmarks. Moreover, multiple trial-and-error attempts to place a needle can frustrate the operator, cause unwarranted pain to the patient, and waste time in the operating room.

Diagnostic and therapeutic imaging has become commonplace in medicine. Image-guided navigation systems allow delicate procedures (e.g., brain surgery) to be performed with precision and safety. The use of ultrasound to localize nerves for regional anesthesia is a new concept.[1,2] Ultrasound is a more attractive option than magnetic resonance imaging (MRI) or computed tomography (CT) because it is readily available in the operating room, poses no radiation hazard, and is more economical than these other modalities. Potential disadvantages of ultrasound include user-dependency, inaccurate imaging due to operator inexperience, and prolonged technical training for some operators.

▶ PRINCIPLES OF ULTRASOUND

Ultrasound waves have a frequency greater than 20,000 cycles per second (20 kHz), and those used in clinical medicine are in the higher megahertz (MHz) range.[3]

When an electrical current is applied to an array of piezoelectric (quartz) crystals on the ultrasound transducer, electrical energy is converted into mechanical energy. The mechanically deformed crystals send ultrasound waves through body tissues that each possess different acoustic impedances. The waves are attenuated (loss of amplitude with depth), reflected, and/or scattered. When "backscatter" echo waves are returned to the transducer, the sound waves are transformed into electrical currents, which generate after signal processing an ultrasound image.

Ultrasound waves travel at a speed of 1540 m/s in the body; they pass easily through fluids but poorly through bone and air. Information obtained from reflected ultrasound waves is translated into a two-dimensional image of white echoes of varying intensity, representing different degrees of echogenicity on a black background. Hypoechoic structures with high water content (e.g., vessels and cysts) appear dark and black on the screen due to weak reflection of ultrasound waves. Hyperechoic structures (e.g., fat, bone, pleura) appear bright and white due to strong reflection of sound waves back to the transducer. Knowing the speed of sound in tissue and the time of echo return, the distance between the probe and the target structure can be calculated.

▶ NERVE IMAGING

Scanning probes come in different sizes, shapes, and frequencies. Curved probes provide a wider field of view than linear probes of the same size. High-frequency probes in the range of 10 to 15 MHz provide high axial resolution of 250 to 500 μm and are more suitable for imaging superficial neural structures (within 3 to 4 cm from the skin) than lower-frequency probes (2 to 5 MHz), but tissue penetration is limited. Image quality is also influenced by ultrasound machine functionality. Some cart-based units (e.g., Philips HDI 5000) provide real-time compound imaging. This is an advanced feature that scans and captures different views of a structure before software reconstruction into a full image of high resolution. Compact handheld ultrasound units (e.g., SonoSite TITAN), although they have no compound imaging capability, are attractive alternatives because they offer many of the sophisticated features, such as, color Doppler, tissue harmonic imaging, and memory storage, but cost significantly less. Images of the interscalene region obtained with both types of ultrasound machines are shown in Fig. 22-1.

Nerve fibers coalesce to form a fascicle and fascicles group together to form a nerve. The nerve sonogram shows echotexture, with fascicles being hypoechoic (or hypoechogenic) and the surrounding connective tissues being hyperechoic (or hyperechogenic), representing the interfascicular and superficial epineurium.[4] The perineurium that surrounds a single nerve is generally beyond the sonographic resolution.

Many factors can influence nerve echogenicity. The first is nerve composition; i.e., the proportion of hypoechoic

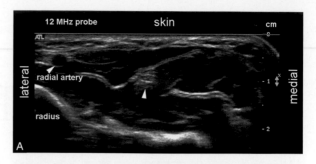

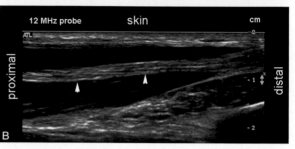

Figure 22-2. Images of the median nerve in the forearm. Arrowheads indicate nerve. *A.* With the probe and ultrasound beam positioned perpendicular to the nerve, a transverse (short-axis, cross-sectional) view of the nerve, which appears round or oval, is obtained. *B.* A beam parallel to the course of the nerve showing a longitudinal view.

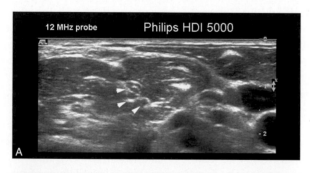

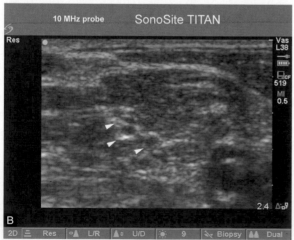

Figure 22-1. Images of the interscalene region. Arrowheads indicate nerves. *A.* Image captured by a machine with a compound imaging feature. *B.* Image captured by a machine without compound imaging.

nerve fascicle to hyperechoic connective tissue. Second is the angle of the transducer beam that reaches the nerve or the concept of anisotropy. For example, when a significant proportion of the reflected echoes do not return to the transducer because of an angulated beam, a nerve structure may appear hypoechoic while the same structure would appear hyperechoic when the beam is perpendicular. Third, echogenicity varies with the anatomic region that is scanned. Nerves appear predominantly hypoechoic in the interscalene and supraclavicular regions but hyperechoic in the infraclavicular and popliteal regions.

Nerve images can be captured by ultrasound in two views, transverse and longitudinal. With the probe and ultrasound beam positioned perpendicular to the nerve, a transverse (short-axis, cross-sectional) view of the nerve, which appears round or oval, will be obtained (Fig. 22-2*A*). A beam parallel to the course of the nerve will generate a longitudinal view, which shows a characteristic fascicular pattern, especially in peripheral nerves (Fig. 22-2*B*).

▶ ULTRASOUND IMAGING OF THE BRACHIAL PLEXUS

Linear high-frequency probes in the range of 10 to 15 MHz are best for scanning in the upper limb to locate the brachial plexus and its branches. It is technically easiest to scan perpendicular to the nerve to capture a transverse view of the nerve. Hypoechoic fascicles can be seen interspersed with hyperechoic epineurium (connective) tissue.[5,6] The probe orientation most useful for brachial plexus imaging is shown in Fig. 22-3.

In the interscalene region, it is best to scan with a linear 10- to 15-MHz probe in the axial oblique plane at approximately the cricoid cartilage level and over the sternocleidomastoid muscle while the subject's head is slightly turned to the contralateral side. Moving the probe slowly in the cephalad-caudad direction will show the best possible transverse view of the cervical nerve roots or proximal trunks of the brachial plexus. The transverse sonogram (Fig. 22-4) shows the sternocleidomastoid muscle as a triangular structure, just underneath the skin surface. Deep to the sternocleidomastoid muscle are the anterior and middle scalene muscles, with the brachial plexus sandwiched between them. The nerves, usually one to three in number, are oval to round, and seen as predominantly hypoechoic (dark) with a rim and sometimes with internal punctate hyperechoic echoes (Fig. 22-4). Medial to the brachial plexus are the carotid artery, internal jugular vein, and thyroid gland. When scanned more cephalad, the cervical roots can be seen exiting the neural foramina and the transverse processes of the cervical vertebrae. When scanned more caudad, nerves are seen traveling peripherally toward the skin surface in the interscalene groove (i.e., toward the top of the screen if your probe is properly extended).

At the supraclavicular region, it is also best to scan with a linear 10- to 15-MHz probe in the coronal oblique plane. Because the supraclavicular fossa is limited in size, a smaller probe is ideal. The probe is moved incrementally

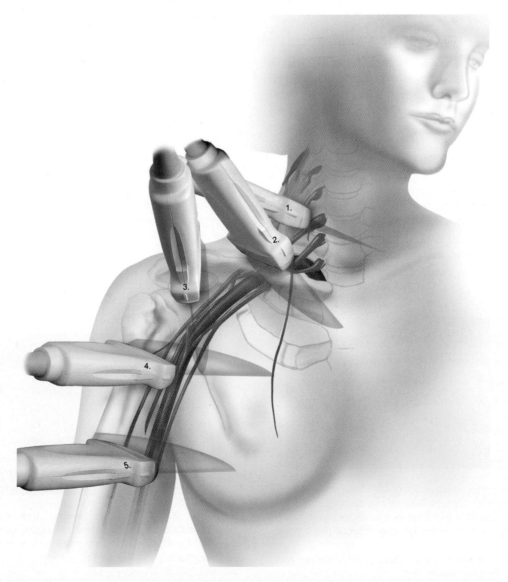

Figure 22-3. The probe orientations most useful for brachial plexus imaging are shown here.

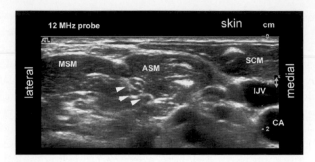

Figure 22-4. Transverse sonogram. The sternocleidomastoid muscle is shown as a triangular structure just underneath the skin surface, with the apex pointing laterally.

ABBREVIATIONS: ASM = anterior scalene muscle; CA = carotid artery; IJV = internal jugular vein; MSM = middle scalene muscle; SCM = sternocleidomastoid muscle.

in the medial and lateral direction and then tilted in the dorsal and ventral direction to search for the best possible transverse view of the brachial plexus trunks or divisions. The supraclavicular image most commonly shows nerves as a cluster of hypoechoic nodules (resembling a bunch of grapes) lateral, posterior, and often cephalad to the round, pulsating, hypoechoic subclavian artery lying on top of the hyperechoic first rib (Fig. 22-5). When moved medially, the probe shows the anterior scalene muscle and subclavian vein. When angled dorsally and medially, the probe shows the hyperechoic pleural lining, which fluctuates with respiration.

At the infraclavicular region immediately medial and inferior to the coracoid process, one can capture the transverse view of the brachial plexus at the cord level using a linear or curved 4- to 7-MHz probe positioned in the parasagittal plane. A lower-frequency probe is usually required because of the thickness of the pectoralis major and minor muscles immediately underneath the

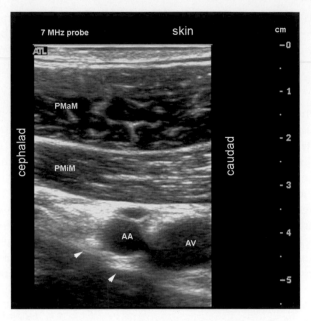

Figure 22-6. The cords of the brachial plexus (*arrowheads*) are deep to the muscles in the infraclavicular region, immediately medial and inferior to the coracoid process.

ABBREVIATIONS: AA = axillary artery; AV = axillary vein; PMaM = pectoralis major muscle; PMiM = pectoralis minor muscle.

skin. Deep to the muscles are the cords of the brachial plexus (arrowheads), which appear hyperechoic, surrounding the round pulsatile axillary artery, which is cephalad to the axillary vein (Fig. 22-6). The lateral and posterior cords are most commonly found cephalad and posterior, respectively, to the axillary artery. The medial cord may be found in between the axillary artery and vein, but it is not always visible on ultrasound.

At the axillary region, it is best to scan with a linear 10- to 15-MHz probe perpendicular to the axillary fold

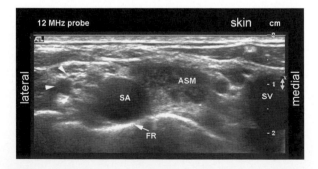

Figure 22-5. The supraclavicular image showing nerves (*arrowheads*) as a cluster of hypoechoic nodules lateral, posterior, and cephalad to the round, pulsating, hypoechoic subclavian artery lying on top of the hyperechoic first rib.

ABBREVIATIONS: ASM = anterior scalene muscle; FR = first rib; SA = subclavian artery; SV = subclavian vein.

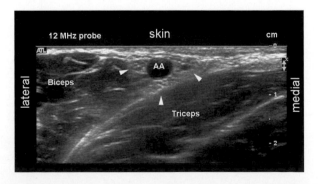

Figure 22-7. In the axilla, the three terminal branches representing the median, ulnar, and radial nerves (*arrowheads*) are only 1 cm or less from the skin surface.

ABBREVIATIONS: AA = axillary artery.

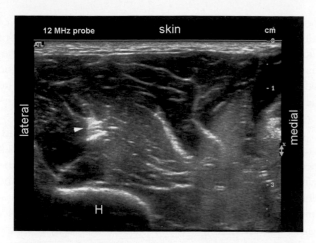

Figure 22-8. The radial nerve at the elbow (*arrowhead*).

ABBREVIATIONS: H = humerus.

while the subject's arm is abducted to a 90-degree angle. Terminal branches of the brachial plexus are found surrounding the pulsatile axillary artery. The axillary veins (one or two in number) are easily collapsible and are often found more superficial and medial to the artery. Nerves in the axilla are round to oval and hypo-echoic, with internal hyperechoic echoes presumably representing the epineurium. Most commonly identified are two to three terminal branches representing the median, ulnar, and radial nerves (arrowheads) only 1 cm or less from the skin surface (Fig. 22-7). The biceps and coracobrachialis muscles are lateral to the axillary artery in an outstretched arm and the triceps muscle is deep to the artery. Terminal branches of brachial plexus in the axilla are highly variable in location.[7]

Peripheral nerves appear hyperechoic and can be tracked on ultrasound from the arm to the hand.[8] Commonly seen are the musculocutaneous nerve in the biceps muscle, the radial nerve at the elbow (arrowhead in Fig. 22-8), the median nerve from the elbow all the way to the wrist and the ulnar nerve at the olecranon fossa and the wrist.

▶ ULTRASOUND IMAGING OF THE LUMBOSACRAL PLEXUS

Imaging in the lower limb may require high-frequency probes in the 10- to 15-MHz range or lower-frequency probes in the 5- to 7-MHz range (curved or linear), depending on superficial or deep nerve location, respectively. The principle of imaging is the same; i.e., it is technically easiest to scan perpendicular to the nerve to capture a transverse view of the nerve, which invariably appears hyperechoic in the lower limb.

At the femoral region immediately below the inguinal crease, a transverse view of the femoral nerve shows a hyperechoic superficial triangular structure when a 10- to 15-MHz probe is used.[9] It is situated laterally to the femoral artery and vein at approximately the same depth (Fig. 22-9). It is difficult to scan the course of the femoral nerve above the inguinal crease because the neurovascular bundle is buried under the anterior abdominal wall muscles. Branches of the femoral nerve may be seen when scanned distally.

Ultrasound scanning of the sciatic nerve below the buttock is a rather simple procedure, but scanning above the buttock is more difficult because the nerve is deep in the pelvis. The sciatic nerves, located in the subgluteal and popliteal regions, are relatively superficial and available for scanning.

The subgluteal approach to the sciatic nerve was first described by Raj et al.[10] and later modified by Sutherland[11] and Sukhani et al.[12] At this location, it is best to use a 10- to 15-MHz probe for a preliminary scan and change to a lower frequency probe (7 MHz) if the nerve is more than 4 cm from the skin surface. The nerve is commonly seen as a hyperechoic elliptical structure deep to muscle layers, the gluteus maximus muscle superficially, the biceps femoris muscle medially, and the iliotibial tract laterally (Fig. 22-10).

Further down in the popliteal region around the midthigh, it is best to scan with a 7-MHz probe because the sciatic nerve is more than 4 cm deep at this location. A transverse view of the sciatic nerve (arrowhead in Fig. 22-11) shows a predominantly hyperechoic structure with internal hypoechoic shadows, that are likely the fascicles. This structure is consistently superficial to the femur, lateral to the popliteal artery, deep to the semitendinosus and semimembranosus muscles medially and the biceps femoris muscle laterally. When scanning distally toward the popliteal crease, it is common to observe branching of the sciatic nerve into the tibial and peroneal components.

Distal peripheral nerves in the lower extremity can be easily visualized using a 10- to 15-MHz probe, since they

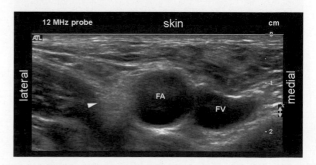

Figure 22-9. The femoral nerve (*arrowhead*) is lateral to the femoral artery (FA) and vein (FV) at approximately the same depth.

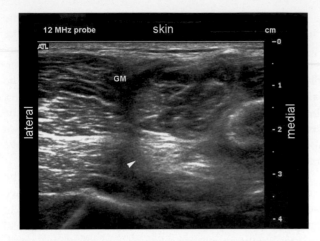

Figure 22-10. The sciatic nerve in the subgluteal region is commonly seen as a hyperechoic elliptical structure deep to muscle layers, the gluteus maximus muscle (GM) superficially, the biceps femoris muscle medially, and the iliotibial tract laterally.

are located superficially.[13] Again, they appear predominantly hyperechoic with internal hypoechoic shadows.

► ULTRASOUND-GUIDED NERVE BLOCK TECHNIQUE

A number of studies have been published on ultrasound-guided nerve block for interscalene,[14,15] supraclavicular,[16–18] infraclavicular,[19–21] axillary,[7,22] femoral,[23,24]

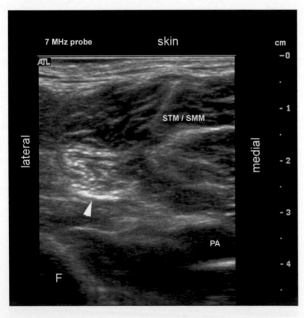

Figure 22-11. Transverse view of the sciatic nerve (*arrowhead*) in the popliteal region.

ABBREVIATIONS: F = femur; PA = popliteal artery; STM/SMM = semitendinosus/semimembranosus muscles.

popliteal,[25,26] and peripheral[27,28] locations. The ease of ultrasound-guided nerve block depends on a number of factors, including the operator's ability to locate the nerve, handle the probe in one hand and the needle in the other, utilize coordinated hand movement to align the needle with the probe, and use the ultrasound machine properly (e.g., focus, contrast, and gain adjustment).

There are two common techniques for ultrasound-guided nerve blocks. The first aligns and moves the block needle along the long axis of the ultrasound probe in line with the ultrasound beam (Fig. 22-12*A*). In this way, the needle can be visualized as a hyperechoic line in real time when it is advanced (Fig. 22-12*B*). Incorrect needle-probe alignment will show the needle shaft only partially, and this can be misinterpreted as the needle tip.

The second technique aligns the needle perpendicular to the probe (Fig. 22-13*A*). In this position, the ultrasound beam captures only a transverse view of the needle as a hyperechoic dot on the screen (Fig. 22-13*B*). The actual location of the needle tip is difficult to visualize

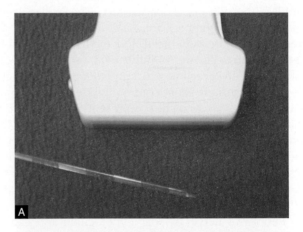

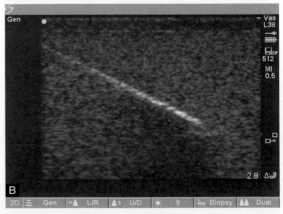

Figure 22-12. There are two common techniques for ultrasound-guided nerve blocks. The first (*A*) aligns and moves the block needle along the long axis of the ultrasound probe in line with the ultrasound beam. In this way, the needle can be visualized (*B*) as a hyperechoic line in real time when it is advanced.

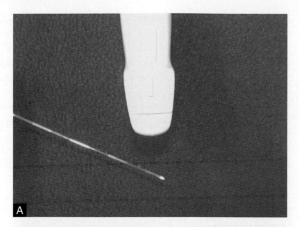

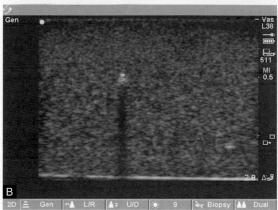

Figure 22-13. There are two common techniques for ultrasound-guided nerve blocks. The second technique (A) aligns the needle perpendicular to the probe. In this position, the ultrasound beam captures only a transverse view of the needle as a hyperechoic dot on the screen (B).

moment by moment, despite scanning the needle perpendicularly along its shaft. Most often, observed tissue and nerve movement during needle advancement give some indication of the needle tip location. The author recommends the technique of longitudinal needle-probe alignment for single injection (Fig. 22-12) and perpendicular needle-probe alignment for catheter insertion (Fig. 22-13).

Probe preparation before nerve block is important. To maintain sterile conditions, the ultrasound probe is placed inside a sterile plastic sheath. To ensure a firm skin contact and avoid air artifacts, the probe covering is smoothed to remove any wrinkles and conductivity gel is generously layered between the probe and skin. Before inserting the needle, a preliminary ultrasound examination is recommended to check (1) nerve location and anatomic variation; (2) vital structures (e.g., vessels and pleura) adjacent to the target nerves so as to avoid puncturing them; and (3) the optimal needle path to the target nerve in order to minimize attempts to insert the needle correctly.

After ultrasound-guided localization of the nerve and needle advancement to the target, it is important to determine the identity of the nerve by using a nerve stimulator. Although it is easy to visualize nerves with ultrasound, it can be difficult to identify a specific root, trunk, or branch of the plexus accurately with ultrasound alone because of anatomic variation. This is especially true in the supraclavicular and axillary regions when a cluster of nerves is seen. With electrical stimulation and appropriate motor responses, one can positively identify and anesthetize the required nerve.

Finally, ultrasound visualization while local anesthetic is injected is invaluable because it provides continuous visual guidance, unlike nerve stimulation, where signs of needle-nerve contact disappear quickly after several milliliters of local anesthetic have been injected. Generally speaking, circumferential spread of the local anesthetic seen with ultrasound indicates a complete block as opposed to a partial block when anesthetic spread is asymmetrical. To ensure a circumferential spread, it is possible to move the needle halfway during injection to that part of the nerve deficient in local anesthetic.

Ultrasound can also assist catheter placement by identifying the nerve location and visualizing local anesthetic spread during injection.[26] Unfortunately, ultrasound cannot help to guide the catheter into the sheath compartment. Because catheters generally curl up as they are advanced, multiple cross-sectional views of a catheter are captured on ultrasound; thus the position of the catheter tip cannot be determined accurately.

At present there are few randomized controlled trials to demonstrate the usefulness of ultrasound in nerve block. Williams et al. have suggested that ultrasound guidance improves the quality of supraclavicular block when combined with neurostimulation when compared to neurostimulation alone.[18] Sandhu and coworkers have suggested that ultrasound-guided nerve blocks cost less than the conventional nerve stimulator technique.[21] So far no study has examined the risk of nerve injury.

▶ SUMMARY

Preliminary results showing that ultrasound imaging can be a valuable tool for peripheral nerve blocks are encouraging. Future outcome data to define the safety and success associated with ultrasound-guided nerve blocks are pending.

REFERENCES

1. De Andres J, Sala-Blanch X. Ultrasound in the practice of brachial plexus anesthesia. *Reg Anesth Pain Med* 27:77–89, 2002.
2. Peterson MK, Millar FA, Sheppard DG. Ultrasound-guided nerve blocks. *Br J Anaesth* 88:621–624, 2002.

3. Kossoff G. Basic physics and imaging characteristics of ultrasound. *World J Surg* 24:134–142, 2000.

4. Silvestri E, Martinoli C, Derchi LE, et al. Echotexture of peripheral nerves: Correlation between US and histologic findings and criteria to differentiate tendons. *Radiology* 197:291–296, 1995.

5. Demondion X, Herbinet P, Boutry N, et al. Sonographic mapping of the normal brachial plexus. *AJNR* 24:1303–1309, 2003.

6. Sheppard DG, Iyer RB, Fenstermacher MJ. Brachial plexus: Demonstration at US. *Radiology* 208:402–406, 1998.

7. Retzl G, Kapral S, Greher M, et al. Ultrasonographic findings of the axillary part of the brachial plexus. *Anesth Analg* 92:1271–1275, 2001.

8. Beekman R, Visser LH. High-resolution sonography of the peripheral nervous system: A review of the literature. *Eur J Neurol* 11:305–314, 2004.

9. Gruber H, Peer S, Kovacs P, et al. The ultrasonographic appearance of the femoral nerve and cases of iatrogenic impairment. *J Ultrasound Med* 22:163–172, 2003.

10. Raj PP, Parks RI, Watson TD, et al. A new single-position supine approach to sciatic-femoral nerve block. *Anesth Analg* 54:489–493, 1975.

11. Sutherland ID. Continuous sciatic nerve infusion: Expanded case report describing a new approach. *Reg Anesth Pain Med* 23:496–501, 1998.

12. Sukhani R, Candido KD, Doty R Jr, et al. Infragluteal-parabiceps sciatic nerve block: An evaluation of a novel approach using a single-injection technique. *Anesth Analg* 96:868–873, 2003.

13. Peer S, Kovacs P, Harpf C, et al. High-resolution sonography of lower extremity peripheral nerves: Anatomic correlation and spectrum of disease. *J Ultrasound Med* 21:315–322, 2002.

14. Perlas A, Chan VW, Simons M. Brachial plexus examination and localization using ultrasound and electrical stimulation: A volunteer study. *Anesthesiology* 99:429–435, 2003.

15. Martinoli C, Bianchi S, Santacroce E, et al. Brachial plexus sonography: A technique for assessing the root level. *AJR* 179:699–702, 2002.

16. Kapral S, Krafft P, Eibenberger K, et al. Ultrasound-guided supraclavicular approach for regional anesthesia of the brachial plexus. *Anesth Analg* 78:507–513, 1994.

17. Chan VW, Perlas A, Rawson R, et al. Ultrasound-guided supraclavicular brachial plexus block. *Anesth Analg* 97:1514–1517, 2003.

18. Williams SR, Chouinard P, Arcand G, et al. Ultrasound guidance speeds execution and improves the quality of supraclavicular block. *Anesth Analg* 97:1518–1523, 2003.

19. Ootaki C, Hayashi H, Amano M. Ultrasound-guided infraclavicular brachial plexus block: An alternative technique to anatomical landmark–guided approaches. *Reg Anesth Pain Med* 25:600–604, 2000.

20. Sandhu NS, Capan LM. Ultrasound-guided infraclavicular brachial plexus block. *Br J Anaesth* 89:254–259, 2002.

21. Sandhu NS, Sidhu DS, Capan LM. The cost comparison of infraclavicular brachial plexus block by nerve stimulator and ultrasound guidance. *Anesth Analg* 98:267–268, 2004.

22. Reed J, Leighton S. Ultrasound facilitation of brachial plexus block. *Anaesth Intens Care* 22:499, 1994.

23. Marhofer P, Schrogendorfer K, Koinig H, et al. Ultrasonographic guidance improves sensory block and onset time of three-in-one blocks. *Anesth Analg* 85:854–857, 1997.

24. Marhofer P, Schrogendorfer K, Wallner T, et al. Ultrasonographic guidance reduces the amount of local anesthetic for 3-in-1 blocks. *Reg Anesth Pain Med* 23:584–588, 1998.

25. Sites BD, Gallagher J, Sparks M. Ultrasound-guided popliteal block demonstrates an atypical motor response to nerve stimulation in 2 patients with diabetes mellitus. *Reg Anesth Pain Med* 28:479–482, 2003.

26. Sinha A, Chan VW. Ultrasound imaging for popliteal sciatic nerve block. *Reg Anesth Pain Med* 29:130–134, 2004.

27. Gray AT, Schafhalter-Zoppoth I. Ultrasound guidance for ulnar nerve block in the forearm. *Reg Anesth Pain Med* 28:335–339, 2003.

28. Gray AT, Collins AB. Ultrasound-guided saphenous nerve block. *Reg Anesth Pain Med* 28:148, 2003.

CHAPTER 23

Blocks above the Clavicle

ANDRÉ P. BOEZAART/CARLO D. FRANCO

▶ INTRODUCTION

This chapter deals with the interscalene, cervical paravertebral, and supraclavicular blocks. There are many different versions of these blocks, but this discussion is limited to the blocks that the authors regularly do and which they feel have the best chance of success and the lowest rate of complications.

▶ APPLIED ANATOMY

Gross Anatomy

The brachial plexus is formed by five roots that originate in the ventral divisions of C5 through T1 (Fig. 23-1).[1] These roots converge over the first rib to form three trunks—upper, middle, and lower—which are stacked one on top of the other as they traverse the interscalene triangle. The triangle is formed between the anterior and middle scalene muscles and commonly known as the interscalene groove but in fact forms more of a triangle than a groove.

The anterior scalene muscle originates at the anterior tubercles of the transverse processes of C3–C6 and is inserted on the scalene tubercle on the upper surface of the first rib. The middle scalene muscle originates at the posterior tubercles of the transverse processes of C2–C7 and is inserted on the upper surface of the first rib behind the subclavian groove. The upper surface of the first rib therefore forms the base of the wide interscalene triangle. The subclavian artery is located within this triangle just anterior to the lower trunk of the brachial plexus.

While the roots of the plexus are long, the trunks are almost as short as they are wide, soon giving off anterior and posterior divisions as they approach the clavicle. Thus, there is a narrow window where the trunks can be accessed before they divide into six divisions and lose their compact arrangement. The divisions then form the three cords as they enter the axilla below the clavicle. The three cords are named according to their relationship with the axillary artery: posterior, lateral, and medial (Fig. 23-1). Finally, the terminal branches are formed from the cords, lateral to the pectoralis minor muscle.

Successful brachial plexus blockade requires the identification and block of the appropriate roots, trunks, cords, and peripheral nerves for the proposed surgery.[2] Accurate identification of the correct nerve bundles and avoiding injection on incorrect nerves may provide higher success rates if the single-stimulation technique of the infraclavicular block, for example, is followed.[3,4] It may also provide shorter latency periods if the multiple-stimulation technique[5] is chosen. In the case of blocks at the trunk level, it is also important to recognize false motor responses and to avoid injecting on these responses.[6]

Brachial Plexus Root Stimulation

Fifth, Sixth, and Seventh Cervical Roots (C5, C6, and C7)

Figure 23-1 shows that the fifth cervical root (C5) and the superior parts of the sixth and seventh cervical roots (C6 and C7) form most of the superior and middle trunk and all of the lateral cord of the brachial plexus. Fibers from the C5, C6, and C7 roots then end as the dorsal scapular nerve, suprascapular nerve, lateral pectoral nerve, musculocutaneous nerve, and part of the median nerve (Table 23-1). Electrical stimulation of only the C5 root, will therefore cause a motor response in any or

1. Phrenic nerve
2. Nerve to levator scapulae
3. Spinal accessory nerve
4. Dorsal scapular nerve
5. Suprascapular nerve
6. Superior trunk
7. Middle trunk
8. Inferior trunk
9. Long thoracic nerve
10. Nerves to longus colli and scalene muscles
11. Nerve to subclavius muscle
12. Lateral cord
13. Posterior cord
14. Medial cord
15. Lateral pectoral nerve
16. Medial pectoral nerve
17. Upper subscapular nerve
18. Lower subscapular nerve
19. Medial cutaneous nerve of arm
20. Medial cutaneous nerve of upper arm
21. Axillary nerve
22. Musculocutaneous nerve
23. Radial nerve
24. Median nerve
25. Ulnar nerve

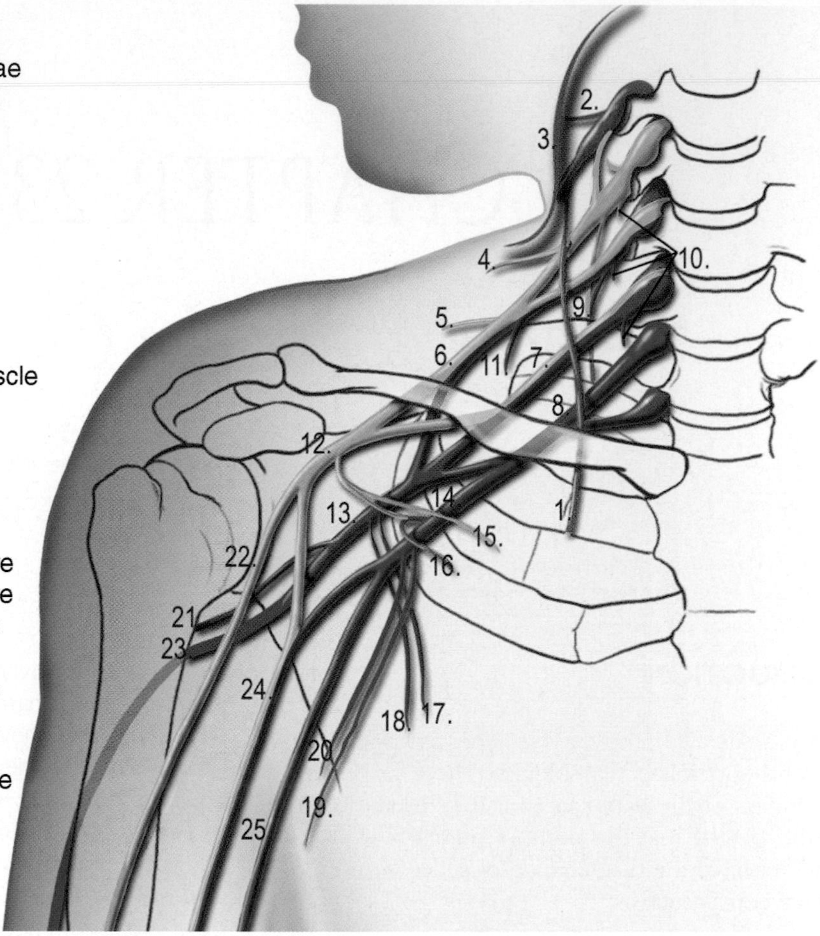

Figure 23-1. Schematic representation of the brachial plexus.

▶ **TABLE 23-1.** MOTOR RESPONSE DUE TO STIMULATION OF NERVES ORIGINATING FROM THE C5 ROOT

Roots	Trunks	Cords	Peripheral Nerves	Muscle	Motor Response
C5	Superior	Lateral	Nerve to scalene muscles	Anterior and middle scalene mm.	Bending of cervical spine forward and ipsilaterally, with slight rotation to the other side
			Long thoracic n.	Serratus anterior m.	Protraction (forward drawing) of the scapula
			Suprascapular n.	Infraspinatus m.	Glenohumeral extension
				Supraspinatus m.	Glenohumeral vertical abduction
			Lateral pectoral n.	Pectoralis major m.	Glenohumeral adduction
			Musculocutaneous n.	Biceps brachii m.	Elbow flexion
				Brachialis m.	Elbow flexion
			Median n.	Pronator teres m.	Pronation of the forearm
				Palmaris longus m.	Wrist flexion
				Flexor carpi radialis m.	Wrist flexion
				Flexor carpi radialis m.	Wrist abduction
				Flexor digitorum superficialis m.	Flexion fingers (MP and PIP joints)
				Lumbrical mm. I and II	Extension PIP and DIP joints
				Abductor pollicis brevis m.	Abduction and rotation thumb
				Opponens pollicis m.	Opposition thumb
			Anterior interosseous n.	Flexor pollicis longus m.	Flexion IP joint of thumb

DIP = distal interphalangeal; IP = interphalangeal; MP = metacarpophalangeal; PIP = proximal interphalangeal.

all of the muscles supplied by the above nerves. These muscles are the rhomboid, rotator cuff, pectoralis major, and biceps brachii muscles. Also included are the pronators of the forearm, superficial flexors of the forearm, first and second lumbricals of the hand, and abductor of the thumb. Electrical stimulation of the C6 and C7 roots will cause motor responses in the muscles supplied by nerves branching off the posterior cord. These muscles are the deltoid muscle (axillary nerve), extensors of the arm (radial nerve) (Table 23-2), and also any combination of the above muscles supplied by the nerves branching from the lateral cord (Table 23-1).

Eighth Cervical and First Thoracic Roots (C8 and T1)

The roots of C8 and T1 continue to form the inferior trunk (Fig. 23-1). Fibers coming from C8 join the posterior and medial cords, while fibers of the T1 root form the medial cord. Electrical stimulation of the inferior trunk will cause contractions of all or some of the muscles supplied by nerves branching off the posterior cord (Table 23-2) but will mainly affect the muscles supplied by the nerves from the medial cord (Table 23-3). These are the pectoralis minor muscle (medial pectoral nerve) and muscles supplied by the ulnar nerve (flexor carpi ulnaris, ulnar side of flexor digitorum profundus, adductor pollicis, flexor pollicis, the interossei muscles of the hand, the third and fourth lumbricals and flexors, and flexor and opponens digiti minimi) (Table 23-3).

Summary

Electrical stimulation of the superior three roots of the brachial plexus (C5, C6 and C7)—as is seen with cervical paravertebral block for shoulder surgery—will result mainly in motor responses of the posterior and anterior shoulder girdle muscles and flexor and extensor muscles of the proximal arm.

Electrical stimulation of the inferior two roots of the brachial plexus (C8 and T1), as is seen with cervical paravertebral block for wrist surgery, will result mainly in motor responses in the deep flexor muscles of the hand.

▶ **TABLE 23-2.** MOTOR RESPONSE DUE TO STIMULATION OF NERVES ORIGINATING FROM THE C6 AND C7 ROOTS

Roots	Trunks	Cords	Peripheral Nerves	Muscle	Motor Response
C6	Superior	Lateral	See Table 23-1	See Table 23-1	See Table 23-1
C7	Middle	Posterior	N to longus colli	Longus colli m.	Forward flexion of the neck
			N to scalene muscles	Anterior and middle scalene mm.	Bending of cervical spine forward and ipsilaterally, with slight rotation to the other side
			Axillary n.	Anterior deltoid m.	Glenohumeral flexion, horizontal abduction and medial rotation of humerus
				Posterior deltoid m.	Glenohumeral extension, horizontal abduction, and lateral rotation of humerus
				Teres minor m.	Glenohumeral extension
				Middle deltoid m.	Glenohumeral vertical abduction
			Radial n.	Brachioradialis m.	Elbow flexion
				Triceps brachii m.	Elbow extension
				Extensor carpi radialis longus m.	Wrist extension and abduction
			(Posterior interosseous n.)	Extensor digitorum m.	Extension MP, PIP, and DIP joints of fingers
			(Posterior interosseous n.)	Extensor indices m.	Extension MP, PIP and DIP joints of fingers
			(Posterior interosseous n.)	Extensor digiti minimi m.	Extension MP, PIP and DIP of fifth finger
			(Posterior interosseous n.)	Extensor pollicis brevis m.	Extension MP joint thumb
			(Posterior interosseous n.)	Extensor pollicis longus m.	Extension IP joint of thumb
			(Posterior interosseous n.)	Abductor pollicis longus m.	Abduction of thumb

DIP = distal interphalangeal;   IP = interphalangeal;   MP = metacarpophalangeal;   PIP = proximal interphalangeal.

▶ **TABLE 23-3.** MOTOR RESPONSE DUE TO STIMULATION OF NERVES ORIGINATING FROM THE C8 AND T1 ROOTS

Roots	Trunks	Cords	Peripheral Nerves	Muscle	Motor Response
C8	Inferior	Posterior	See Table 23-2	See Table 23-2	See Table 23-2
T1		Medial	N to scalene muscles	Anterior and middle scalene mm.	Bending of cervical spine forward and ipsilaterally, with slight rotation to the other side
			Medial pectoral n.	Pectoralis minor m.	Glenohumeral horizontal abduction
			Median n.	See Table 23-1	See Table 23-1
			Ulnar n.	Flexor carpi ulnaris m.	Wrist flexion and abduction
				Flexor digitorum profundus m. (medial)	Flexion DIP joints of fingers
				Dorsal interossei mm.	Flexion DIP joints of fingers
				Palmar interossei mm.	Flexion DIP joints and abduction of fingers
				Flexor digiti minimi brevis m.	Flexion MP joints of fifth finger
				Lumbrical mm. III and IV	Extension PIP and DIP joints
				Dorsal interossei mm.	Abduction fingers
				Abductor digiti minimi m.	Abduction fifth finger
				Opponens digiti minimi m.	Opposition fifth finger
				Adductor pollicis m.	Adduction and rotation of thumb
				Palmar interosseous I	Adduction and flexion of MP joint of thumb
				Opponens pollicis	Opposition thumb

DIP = distal interphalangeal; MP = metacarpophalangeal; PIP = proximal interphalangeal.

The limits of the nerve stimulator current output for blocks at the level of the roots have not yet been established. For example, Wehling and colleagues reported a case of successful cervical paravertebral block without any untoward sequelae after stimulating through a catheter at a current of 0.05 mA and 300 μs.[7]

Continuous blocks at the level of the roots of the brachial plexus seem to be ideal for major surgery to all three large joints of the upper arm, since they receive sensory innervation from the entire brachial plexus.

Stimulation of the Brachial Plexus Trunks

Nerve conduction studies have demonstrated that electrical stimulation of the proximal aspects of all three brachial plexus trunks results in a motor response mainly of the muscles supplied by the radial nerve (Table 23-2).[8] If the stimulating probe is moved to the distal part of the superior trunk of the brachial plexus, it will cause motor responses in the muscles supplied by the musculocutaneous nerve (flexion at the elbow by biceps contraction) and axillary nerve (abduction of the arm by deltoid contraction (Table 23-1). If the inferior part of the inferior trunk is stimulated, a flexor response will be observed in the hand owing to contraction of the muscles supplied by the median and ulnar nerves (Tables 23-1 and 23-3).

Nerve Stimulator Responses That Can Be Misleading in Performing Blocks above the Clavicle

In performing an interscalene block, it is also important to know those motor responses indicating that the wrong nerves are being stimulated. In the posterior triangle of the neck (behind the sternocleidomastoid muscle), there are five nerves that do not form part of the brachial plexus. If these nerves are stimulated, they cause misleading motor responses and are a frequent cause of failed blocks.

Stimulating the phrenic nerve will cause contraction of the diaphragm, which can clearly be seen as abdominal twitches. The trunks of the brachial plexus are approximately 1 cm posterior to the phrenic nerve, between the anterior and middle scalene muscles.

The dorsal scapular nerve, which originates from the C5 root, exits 1 cm further posteriorly between the middle and posterior scalene muscles (Fig. 23-1). This nerve supplies the rhomboid muscles, and its stimulation will cause medial and superior movements of the scapula. If the elbow is flexed and the patient's hand rests on his or her abdomen, the elbow may be fixed on the bed and medial movements of the scapula may be mistaken for abduction of the arm due to deltoid contractions. This could lead to failed block.

The suprascapular nerve originates from the superior trunk (Fig. 23-1). This nerve mainly supplies the muscles of the rotator cuff and causes internal rotation of the humerus when stimulated. As in the case of the dorsal scapular nerve, if the elbow is flexed and the patient's hand is on the abdomen, rotation of the humerus can create the false impression that the arm is abducting due to deltoid contractions. Electrical stimulation of the suprascapular nerve, therefore, also frequently leads to confusion, although if this nerve is stimulated, it is no longer a true interscalene (supraclavicular) block.

Further posterior is the nerve to the levator scapulae muscle, which originates from the cervical plexus (Fig. 23-1). Electrical stimulation of this nerve will cause a motor response in the levator scapulae muscle and subsequent elevation of the scapula. Stimulation of this nerve therefore, like stimulation of the dorsal scapular and suprascapular nerves, can cause confusion.

The accessory nerve is a cranial nerve and is further posterior, being superficial to the prevertebral layer of the deep cervical fascia, which forms the floor of the posterior triangle of the neck. It runs parallel and superficial to the levator scapulae muscle and perpendicular to the trapezius muscle, which it supplies (Fig. 23-1). Stimulation of this nerve causes contraction of the trapezius muscle, which elevates the scapula. Like the other three nerves mentioned above, electrical stimulation of this nerve can cause confusion and failed block.

Summary

Stimulation of the proximal portion of all three trunks causes a triceps motor response via the radial nerve.

Stimulation of the distal portion of the superior trunk causes a motor response in the biceps and deltoid muscles via the musculocutaneous and axillary nerves, respectively.

Stimulation of the inferior portion of the inferior trunk causes a flexor response in the hand.

Stimulation of the phrenic nerve means that the needle is located anterior to the anterior scalene and that it should be reoriented posteriorly in order to find the correct position.

There are four nerves posterior to the brachial plexus in the posterior triangle of the neck that may cause confusion and failed blocks. These are, from front to back, the dorsal scapular nerve, which supplies the rhomboid muscles; the suprascapular nerve, which innervates the rotator cuff muscles; the nerve to the levator scapulae muscle, which lifts the scapula; and the accessory nerve, which is a cranial nerve and innervates the trapezius muscle.

Blocks at the level of the trunks produce reliable anesthesia of the entire upper extremity distal to the shoulder, the only exception being the small area innervated by the intercostobrachial nerve.

▶ THE INTERSCALENE BLOCK

Introduction

The modern technique of interscalene block was introduced by Winnie in 1970 and soon became the standard technique for anesthesia and analgesia of the shoulder. It is usually not indicated for surgery of the upper extremity distal to the shoulder joint. Winnie realized that directing the needle medially could align it with the intervertebral foramen, resulting in severe injury. Thus he advised directing the needle somewhat caudad and posterior. Different authors have modified this technique even further. The method described in this chapter is the longitudinal approach, also called the lateral approach.[9,10] The continuous interscalene block is indicated for intra- and postoperative pain management in major shoulder surgery; for example, shoulder arthroplasty and rotator cuff repair.

Applied Anatomy (Fig. 23-2)

Surface Anatomy

The posterior border of the sternocleidomastoid muscle, the external jugular vein, and the clavicle are palpated and marked (Fig. 23-3). Before the needle is inserted, all the nerves in the posterior triangle of the neck can be mapped transcutaneously with a special probe or with the tip of the needle. For this purpose, the nerve stimulator output is typically set on 5 to 10 mA.

The phrenic nerve can be located immediately behind the sternocleidomastoid muscle at the level of the cricoid cartilage.

Moving the probe approximately 1 cm posteriorly will put it in contact with the C5 or C6 roots of the brachial plexus and elicit a biceps or triceps motor response.

Moving the probe a further 1 cm posteriorly will stimulate the dorsal scapular nerve, which innervates the rhomboid muscle.

Block Technique

Patient Positioning

The patient is positioned in the supine position with the head of the table slightly raised (to discourage venous congestion) and the patient's head turned slightly to the side not being blocked. The operator stands at the head, facing the patient's feet.

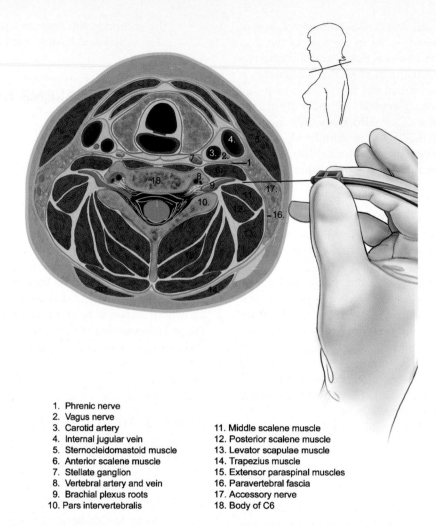

1. Phrenic nerve
2. Vagus nerve
3. Carotid artery
4. Internal jugular vein
5. Sternocleidomastoid muscle
6. Anterior scalene muscle
7. Stellate ganglion
8. Vertebral artery and vein
9. Brachial plexus roots
10. Pars intervertebralis
11. Middle scalene muscle
12. Posterior scalene muscle
13. Levator scapulae muscle
14. Trapezius muscle
15. Extensor paraspinal muscles
16. Paravertebral fascia
17. Accessory nerve
18. Body of C6

Figure 23-2. Oblique cross-section through the neck from the spinous process of C6 to the suprasternal notch, showing the anatomy of the neck for interscalene block.

Single-Injection Interscalene Block

Needle Insertion and Technique

The interscalene groove is palpated with the index and middle fingers at the intersection of posterior border of sternocleidomastoid and cricoid cartilage, 1 cm behind the muscle. These two fingers are now split, leaving the middle finger in the interscalene groove (Fig. 23-3). This causes congestion of the external jugular vein, which makes it easy to identify and, with the index finger, traction is applied to tighten the skin.

The nerve stimulator is typically set to 1 to 2 mA, 2 Hz, and a 100- to 300-μs pulse width. The needle is inserted behind the sternocleidomastoid muscle approximately midway between the clavicle and the mastoid process. It is aimed toward the brachial plexus, which is beneath the middle finger of the operator's left hand. The needle enters longitudinally to the neck and is typically aimed approximately at the midpoint of the clavicle on the ipsilateral side (Fig. 23-4). If the needle is too far anterior, the phrenic nerve will be stimulated and an unmistakable diaphragmatic motor response will be noticed. Moving the tip of the needle slightly posterior will cause either a triceps or biceps motor response.

If the needle is too far posterior, the dorsal scapular nerve will be encountered. This will be indicated by contractions of the rhomboid muscles (which can easily be mistaken for deltoid muscle contractions) and the needle must be redirected approximately 1 cm anterior.

The nerve stimulator's output is now decreased to approximately 0.3 to 0.5 mA and, with the brisk motor response still visible in the biceps or triceps muscles, the injection is started.

The interscalene block typically blocks the neurotomes supplied by the axillary, radial median, and musculocutaneous nerves (Fig. 23-5).

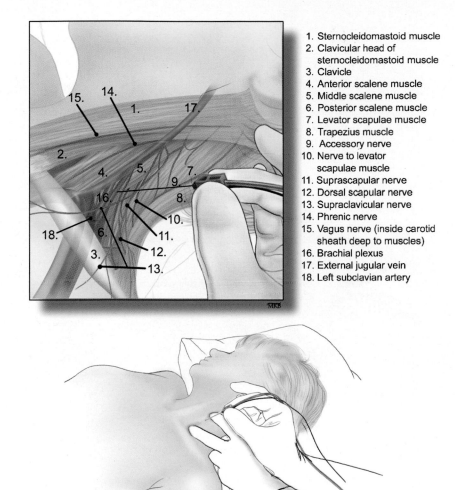

1. Sternocleidomastoid muscle
2. Clavicular head of sternocleidomastoid muscle
3. Clavicle
4. Anterior scalene muscle
5. Middle scalene muscle
6. Posterior scalene muscle
7. Levator scapulae muscle
8. Trapezius muscle
9. Accessory nerve
10. Nerve to levator scapulae muscle
11. Suprascapular nerve
12. Dorsal scapular nerve
13. Supraclavicular nerve
14. Phrenic nerve
15. Vagus nerve (inside carotid sheath deep to muscles)
16. Brachial plexus
17. External jugular vein
18. Left subclavian artery

Figure 23-3. Surface anatomy and positioning for interscalene block.

Continuous Interscalene Block

Needle Insertion
The needle placement is similar to that described for the single-injection interscalene block, the only difference being that a 17- or 18-gauge Tuohy needle is used (e.g., StimuCath, Arrow International, Reading PA).[6]

Catheter Placement
When the brachial plexus is identified by the appropriate motor responses at a current of 0.3 to 0.5 mA, the stylet of the needle is removed, the nerve stimulator is attached to the proximal end of the catheter, and the distal end is placed inside the needle shaft for advancement (See Chap. 20).[6]

Catheter Fixation
See Chap. 20.

Selection of Local Anesthetic Agent

Infusion strategies used by various authors are outlined in Chap. 21. Common choices are 20 to 40 mL of ropivacaine (0.5 to 0.75%) or 20 to 40 mL of bupivacaine (0.5%) as an initial bolus, followed by a continuous infusion of 5 mL/h of 0.2% ropivacaine or 0.25% bupivacaine. Patient-controlled boluses of 5 to 10 mL

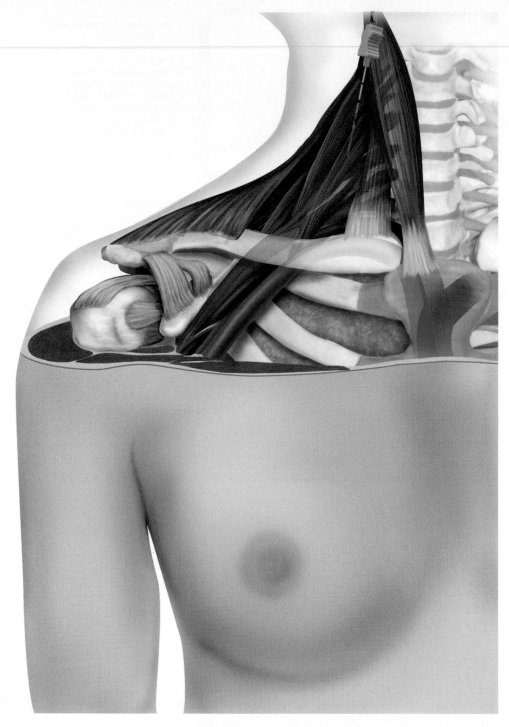

Figure 23-4. Three-dimensional anatomy of the interscalene block.

can be allowed with a lockout time of 60 to 240 min (see Chap. 21).

Potential Problems and Complications

Complications seem to be rare and in some cases result from injuries sustained after the limb has been rendered insensitive (see Chap. 32). For example, ulnar or radial nerve injuries due to compression by ill-fitting slings or splints and compression of the ulnar nerve at the elbow against a hard surface or for a prolonged time. Nerve traction, diathermy, and direct injury to nerves during surgery can also be unjustifiably blamed on the technique.

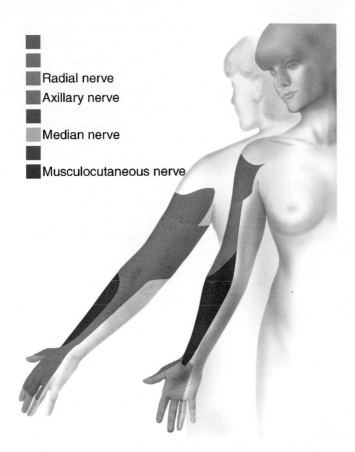

Radial nerve
Axillary nerve
Median nerve
Musculocutaneous nerve

Figure 23-5 (Plate 1). Peripheral nerve dermatomes blocked by the interscalene block.

Numerous rare complications due to perineural catheters have been reported, although none seems to be due to long-term continuous exposure of the nerves to local anesthetic agents or the presence of the catheter on or near the nerves. Capdevila and colleagues reported 13 (0.92 percent) major complications in their experience with 1416 continuous peripheral nerve blocks, which included two cases of diaphragmatic paralysis with acute respiratory failure and two cases of laryngeal and recurrent laryngeal nerve paralysis with swallowing difficulty. Boezaart et al.,[6] in a study comparing interscalene blocks performed either via a single injection with paresthesia or a single injection with nerve stimulator or continuous block with a stimulating catheter, reported 85 percent complete phrenic nerve blocks in the paresthesia group compared with 35 percent in the nerve stimulator group and 20 percent in the group with continuous interscalene block. Recurrent laryngeal nerve paralysis was reported in 20, 5, and 0 percent, respectively, with Horner's syndrome in 30, 0, and 0 percent, respectively. No nerve injuries were observed. Borgeat et al.,[9] in a prospective study, followed 521 patients for 9 months who had received an interscalene block. Of the 520 patients who completed the

study, 230 received an interscalene catheter. There was one case of pneumothorax (0.2 percent). The investigators actively questioned their patients for persistent paresthesia and dysesthesia and found that symptoms were present at 10 days in 74 patients (14 percent), at 1 month in 41 patients (7.9 percent), at 3 months in 20 patients (3.9 percent), and at 9 months in only 1 patient (0.2 percent), who had persistent dysesthesia. There were no reported cases of muscle weakness.

Minor complications—such as brachial plexus irritation caused by interscalene perineural catheters,[11] knotting,[12,13] and shearing[14] of peripheral perineural catheters—have been reported.

Special Considerations

It is important to realize that pain, paresthesia, and dysesthesia distal to the elbow are almost never symptoms of shoulder pathology. They frequently indicate existing brachial plexitis; thus care should be taken in patients presenting with shoulder pain and pain distal to the elbow, and perhaps it would be wise to avoid brachial plexus blocks in this type of patient.

Special care should also be taken with patients presenting with primary frozen shoulder or "adhesive capsulitis," since this condition is a fibromatosis such as that in Dupuytren's disease, which in itself should not be painful.[15–17] The pain of frozen shoulder may be due to traction on the brachial plexus due to rotation of the scapula, or it may even be an early manifestation of complex regional pain syndrome (CRPS).

The shoulder "freezes" with the shoulder in the functional position of forward flexion, abduction, and internal rotation. Carrying the arm at the side causes the scapula to rotate with "pseudowinging" of the scapula, a common sign of frozen shoulder. The patients will also frequently report pain relief if the arm is kept in the functional position. This rotation of the scapula may lengthen the distance from the vertebral column to the coracoid process and may cause traction to the brachial plexus. The area of maximal stress to the plexus is where it crosses the first rib. It is often postulated that it is this traction to the brachial plexus that causes the pain of adhesive capsulitis once the acute phase is over. It would therefore be wise to be cautious in offering these patients brachial plexus blocks in the area of the plexus–first rib crossing.

Special caution is also sometimes necessary when a patient is scheduled for subacromial decompression. The exact diagnosis of the shoulder pathology can often be unclear in the patient with brachial plexitis, who often presents with shoulder pain, and interscalene block may aggravate the pain. The key here may be pain distal to the elbow, which is not usually a symptom of bona fide shoulder pathology.

► THE CERVICAL PARAVERTEBRAL BLOCK

Introduction

The cervical paravertebral approach to the brachial plexus usually blocks all its roots and therefore the whole plexus. This block is a modification of the single-injection block that was originally described by Kappis in the 1920s[18] and modified by Pippa in 1990.[19] As originally described, this block never gained popularity, probably because penetration of the paraspinal extensor muscles of the neck made it painful.

We recently described a modified technique in which the needle is inserted in the "V" between the leva-tor scapulae and trapezius muscles at the level of the sixth cervical vertebra (Fig. 23-6).[20,21] This approach avoids penetration of the posterior paraspinal muscles and minimizes the pain associated with it. Since all the structures associated with complications of brachial plexus blockade (vertebral artery and vein, phrenic nerve, carotid and other major arteries, internal jugular vein, etc.) are anterior to the nerve roots in the neck, the original argument of Kappis that it is best to approach the roots posteriorly, where there are only muscles, remains valid (Fig. 23-6).

The onset of a cervical paravertebral block is relatively slow (30 to 45 min). If this block is used as sole anesthesia for shoulder surgery, it should be done well in advance of the operation.

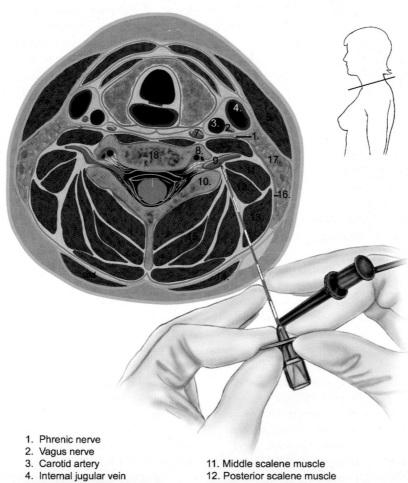

1. Phrenic nerve
2. Vagus nerve
3. Carotid artery
4. Internal jugular vein
5. Sternocleidomastoid muscle
6. Anterior scalene muscle
7. Stellate ganglion
8. Vertebral artery and vein
9. Brachial plexus roots
10. Pars intervertebralis
11. Middle scalene muscle
12. Posterior scalene muscle
13. Levator scapulae muscle
14. Trapezius muscle
15. Extensor paraspinal muscles
16. Paravertebral fascia
17. Accessory nerve
18. C6

Figure 23-6. Oblique cross section through the neck from the spinous process of C6 to the suprasternal notch, showing the anatomy of the neck for cervical paravertebral block.

Indications

Cervical paravertebral block is indicated for anesthesia and postoperative analgesia in all major operations on the upper extremities including all three of the major joints of the upper limb. It is especially suitable for patients in whom it is difficult to reach the brachial plexus trunks via the interscalene approach. Because the loss of resistance to air technique can also be used to ensure correct placement of this block, it is well suited to postoperative use or for people in whom muscle contraction due to nerve stimulation may be poorly tolerated; e.g., patients with fractures.

Applied Anatomy

Gross Anatomy

The vertebral artery and vein are situated in the transverse processes of the cervical vertebrae anterior to the brachial plexus roots. The approach described here avoids penetrating the extensor muscles of the neck by entering through the "window" at the level of apex of the "V" formed by the trapezius and levator scapulae muscles (Fig. 23-6).

Functional Neuroanatomy

Electrical stimulation of the upper roots of the brachial plexus will cause motor responses of the shoulder girdle and more lateral parts of the arm. Stimulation of the lower roots will cause motor responses in the hand and more distal and medial parts of the arm (Tables 23-1, 23-2, and 23-3).

Surface Anatomy

Needle entry is on a line connecting the dorsal spine of the sixth cervical vertebra to the suprasternal notch in the apex of the "V" formed by the anterior border of the trapezius muscle and the posterior border of the levator scapulae muscle (Fig. 23-7).

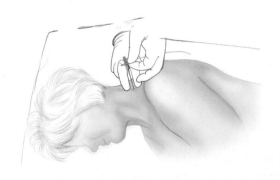

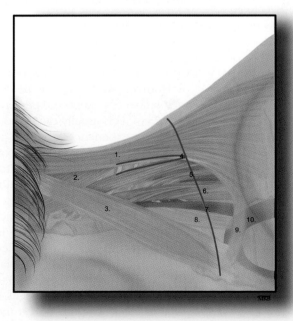

1. Trapezius muscle
2. Splenius muscle
3. Sternocleidomastoid muscle
4. Levator scapulae muscle
5. Posterior scalene muscle
6. Middle scalene muscle
7. Brachial plexus
8. Anterior scalene muscle
9. Clavicle
10. Subclavian artery

Figure 23-7. Surface anatomy and positioning for cervical paravertebral block.

Single-Injection and Continuous Block Technique

Patient Positioning

The patient is placed in the sitting or lateral decubitus position (the levator scapulae muscle is usually easier to identify if the patient is in the sitting position). The patient's neck is flexed slightly forward. The anesthesiologist stands behind the patient.

Needle Placement

Local anesthetic is injected in the skin and subcutaneous tissue all the way to the level of the pars intervertebralis (articular column) while the levator scapulae and trapezius muscles are pushed apart with the fingers of the nonoperative hand (Figs. 23-6 and 23-7). If use of a catheter is planned, the anticipated path of tunneling is also anesthetized at this stage. An insulated 17- or 18-gauge Tuohy needle is inserted and directed slightly mesiad, anterior and slightly caudad, aiming at the suprasternal notch while still keeping the trapezius and levator scapulae muscles apart (Figs. 23-6, 23-7, and 23-8).

The nerve stimulator is set to a current of 1 to 2 mA, a frequency of 2 Hz and a pulse width of 100 to 300 μs. The needle is advanced anteromedially and caudally until the transverse process of C6 or the pars intervertebralis (articular column) of the sixth cervical vertebra (C6) is encountered. The stylet of the needle is removed and a loss-of-resistance syringe is attached to the needle. While continuously testing for loss of resistance, the needle is walked off the bony structure laterally and gently advanced anteriorly. A distinct loss of resistance to air is usually felt simultaneously with the appearance of contraction of the shoulder muscles when the cervical paravertebral space is entered anterior to the middle scalene muscle, approximately 0.5 to 1 cm beyond the transverse process of the vertebra.

If a single-injection technique is used, the main dose of the local anesthetic is incrementally injected now. In most cases a volume of 20 to 40 mL is sufficient. The choice of local anesthetic will depend on the desired degree of motor blockade and the desired duration of action. In most cases, however, a catheter will be inserted to sustain the block into the postoperative period.

It is sometimes necessary to block the superficial cervical plexus to alleviate pain due to skin incisions made during shoulder surgery or arthroscopy, especially the posterior portal for arthroscopic surgery or the incision for a posterior Bankart repair.

Because the needle is inserted near to the ear, patients should be warned that they might hear a crunching sound as it enters the skin and advances through the subcutaneous tissues.

Catheter Placement

Proximity of the needle tip to the roots of the brachial plexus is indicated by a motor response, as described earlier, or by the patient's report of a sensory pulsation at a nerve stimulation output of approximately 0.5 mA. It can also be ascertained by loss of resistance to air. The needle is held steady while the loss of resistance syringe is removed. If a nonstimulating technique is used for catheter placement, a bolus injection is given through the needle and a standard epidural catheter pushed through it. If a stimulating catheter technique is used, the nerve stimulator lead is attached to the proximal end of the 19- or 20-gauge stimulating catheter and its distal end is inserted into the needle shaft (see Chap. 20).

The CCPVB, because it blocks all the roots of the brachial plexus, typically blocks all the neurotomes of the upper limb (Fig. 23-9). The area inside the upper arm (not indicated in Fig. 23-9) is usually also blocked due to caudad spread of local anesthetic agent in the paraspinal "gutter" toward T1.

Selection of Local Anesthetic Agent

An initial bolus of 20 to 40 mL of 0.5% bupivacaine, 0.5 to 0.75% ropivacaine, or 0.5% levobupivacaine may be used. When this approach is used for postoperative analgesia, this is usually followed by a continuous infusion of a lower concentration of the same drug; i.e., 0.25% bupivacaine, 0.2% ropivacaine, or 0.2% levobupivacaine at an infusion rate of 3 to 10 mL/h. In addition, boluses of patient-controlled regional anesthesia (PCRA) of 5 to 10 mL every 30 to 240 min may be used, depending on the clinical situation and keeping potential local anesthetic drug toxicity in mind (see Chap. 21).

Potential Problems and Complications

Experience with this block is limited. We published a report of our initial experience with 256 cases and we have continued to accumulate a growing experience over 4 years after that early report.[21]

Horner's syndrome can be expected in a relatively large number of patients (40 percent) (see stellate ganglion in Fig. 23-6). This usually causes no distress to the patients.

In our experience, about 8 percent of the patients complain of dyspnea in the recovery room. However, with oxygen supplementation, elevating the head of the bed, and reassurance, this should not pose any problems. The incidence of dyspnea can be expected to decrease to 2 percent after 6 h and zero after 12 h.

Infection at the catheter site is a potentially serious complication, especially if the block has been used for shoulder, elbow, or wrist arthroplasty. In the study mentioned above, 5 percent (in 13 of 256 cases) of the catheter entry sites showed signs of infection. This was limited to redness of the skin at the catheter entry site in 10 of 13 cases and involved a purulent discharge in 3 of 13 cases. *Staphylococcus aureus* and *Staph. epidermidis* were cultured in 7 of the 13 cases. These patients did not

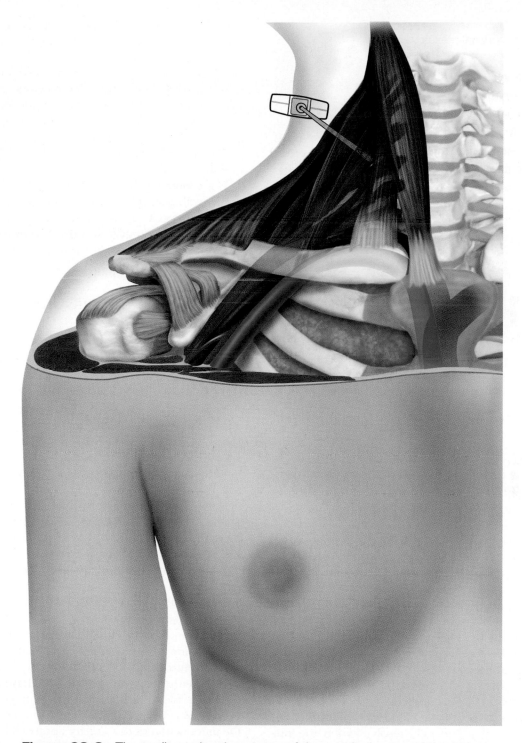

Figure 23-8. Three-dimensional anatomy of the cervical paravertebral block.

receive prophylactic antibiotics (see Chap. 3). If infection is suspected, the catheter should be removed and antibiotic therapy considered.

Posterior neck pain is a common complication with this block, but the incidence seems to decrease as the operator's experience increases. This complication was encountered in 56 of the 256 cases (22 percent), and all were in the first 100 cases in the early part of the study. All but 16 of the patients were successfully treated with nonsteroidal anti-inflammatory drugs, and in most cases there was no need to remove the catheters.

The subclavian artery, situated anterior to the brachial plexus, can be punctured by a posterior approach only if the plexus is penetrated. This is highly unlikely if the nerve stimulator is functional. This complication

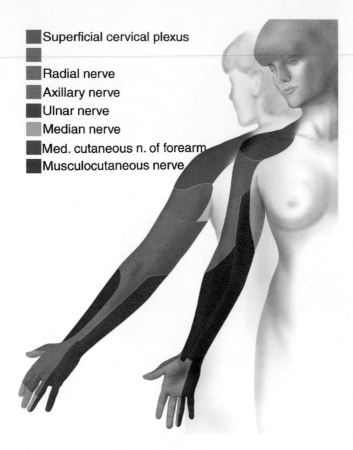

■ Superficial cervical plexus
■
■ Radial nerve
■ Axillary nerve
■ Ulnar nerve
■ Median nerve
■ Med. cutaneous n. of forearm
■ Musculocutaneous nerve

Figure 23-9 (Plate 2). Peripheral nerve dermatomes blocked by the cervical paravertebral and supraclavicular blocks. The part inside the upper arm is also likely to be blocked.

occurred in three patients in the above-mentioned series, and in every instance the nerve stimulator was defective. Defects of this kind are unlikely in modern nerve stimulators (see Chap. 19). Of the 256 patients in this series, 11 (4 percent) experienced numbness in the fingers of the contralateral hand. This was due to epidural spread of the local anesthetic agent (confirmed by MRI). It resolved in all the patients within 6 h without any respiratory or other sequelae.

It does seem that all side effects and complications can be expected to appear in the immediate postoperative period when the patient is still under the care of the anesthesiologist; they generally resolve when the primary block wears off and the low-volume continuous infusion takes effect. The complications thus far encountered with this block have been rare and generally mild. We have not documented any case of nerve injury and intrathecal injection.

Special Considerations

Catheter placement should be a sterile procedure because the catheter is a foreign object that will be left in situ for some time.

The catheter entry site should be covered with a transparent dressing to allow frequent and easy inspections.

This block is probably not indicated for surgery of the clavicle, since this bone receives its nerve supply from the cervical plexus. Acromioclavicular joint surgery probably falls into this category. If used for this type of procedure, an additional superficial cervical block should probably be done.

The cervical paravertebral block, and especially the continuous block, is relatively new and experience with it is still limited. It seems to be a promising alternative to continuous interscalene block for shoulder surgery and the continuous infraclavicular blocks for major elbow and wrist surgery.

▶ THE SUPRACLAVICULAR BLOCK

Introduction

The supraclavicular approach to the brachial plexus is a technique usually associated with rapid-onset, predictable, and dense anesthesia. This is because the block is performed at the level of the plexus trunks, where almost the entire sensory, motor, and sympathetic innervation of the upper arm is carried in just three nerve structures confined to a small space.

The supraclavicular block was introduced into clinical practice in Germany by Kulenkampff in 1911; a description of his technique appeared in the English literature in 1928.[22] Kulenkampff accurately described the plexus as being more compact in the neighborhood of the subclavian artery, where he believed a single injection could suffice to provide adequate anesthesia of the entire upper arm. Kulenkampff's technique was simple and in terms of landmarks and knowledge of the brachial plexus, it was sound. Unfortunately, his recommendation to introduce the needle toward the first rib in the direction of the spinous process of T2 or T3 carried an inherent risk of pneumothorax.

Nevertheless, with several modifications, the supraclavicular block remained a popular choice until the early 1960s. Eventually, the risk of pneumothorax and the introduction of the axillary approach by Accardo and Adriani in 1949[23] and especially by Burnham in 1958[24] marked the beginning of the decline of the supraclavicular block. The axillary approach introduced a good technique; however, it had its share of shortcomings (e.g., smaller area of anesthesia than supraclavicular, tendency to produce "patchy" blocks, and lower overall success rate), although it definitely posed no risk of pneumothorax. The axillary block received a big boost when, in 1961, De Jong published an article in *Anesthesiology* encouraging its use.[25] The study was based on cadaver dissections and included the now famous calculation of 42 mL as the volume needed to fill a cylinder 6 cm long, which according to De Jong "should be sufficient to completely bathe all branches of the brachial plexus." Coincidentally or not, the same journal contained a paper by Brand and Papper, out of New York, that compared axillary and supraclavicular techniques.[26] This is the source of the 6.1 percent rate of pneumothorax frequently quoted for supraclavicular block. In retrospect, these two articles were instrumental in turning the tide against the supraclavicular block.

In addition to the risk of pneumothorax, many authors cite the perceived complexity of supraclavicular block as the reason for not performing it more often. However, the advantages of a supraclavicular technique—namely its rapid onset, dense and predictable anesthesia, and high rate of success—are, according to Brown and colleagues, "unrivaled" by other techniques.[27] In our practice the supraclavicular approach is the cornerstone of upper extremity regional anesthesia.

Indications

The supraclavicular block can be used to provide anesthesia for any surgery on the upper extremity that does not involve the shoulder. It is a good choice for elbow, wrist, and hand surgery. The block is ideal for adult patients, but we also consider it in pediatric patients above 10 years of age on a case-by-case basis. This block is not performed bilaterally because of the potential risk of respiratory emergency due to pneumothorax or phrenic nerve block.

Applied Anatomy

Gross Anatomy
The gross anatomy is described in detail above.

Patient Positioning
The patient is placed in the semisitting position with the head turned slightly opposite to the side to be blocked. The ipsilateral shoulder is dropped, the elbow is flexed, and the forearm is made to rest in the patient's lap. If possible, the patient's wrist is supinated so that the fingers are free to move (Fig. 23-10).

Surface Anatomy
The point at which the lateral border of the sternocleidomastoid muscle meets the clavicle is marked as shown in Fig. 23-10. This point coincides with the anterior scalene muscle and is close to the pleural dome. This is the point of needle entrance to the "plumb-bob" technique. We prefer our point of needle entry to be away from this point by a distance we call the "margin of safety." This distance is about 2.5 cm lateral to the insertion of the sternocleidomastoid muscle to the clavicle or the width of the clavicu-lar head of the patient's sternocleidomastoid muscle. Because the trunks are short and have a steep direction, a larger safety margin will miss the trunks as well as the entire supraclavicular portion of the plexus. The point of needle insertion found this way should always fall close to the midpoint of the clavicle. Since the brachial plexus passes under the midpoint of the clavicle and because its direction is from medial to lateral as it descends in the neck, the plexus is slightly medial to its midpoint at 1 cm above the clavicle (Figs. 23-10 and 23-11).

The index finger of the palpating hand is placed right above the clavicle. The entrance point is immediately cephalad to the palpating finger and is marked by the arrow pointing toward the clavicle (Fig. 23-10). A second arrow is drawn on the skin over the clavicle caudad to the palpating finger and points cephalad toward it. Both arrows mark the direction in which the needle is advanced, as shown in Fig. 23-10.

Block Technique

Single-Injection Supraclavicular Block
A 5-cm, short-bevel, 22-gauge, insulated needle is used. A small skin wheal is raised and the stimulating needle is inserted first, perpendicular to the skin toward the plane of the plexus. After being advanced for a few millimeters, the needle is then turned caudad under the palpating finger in a direction parallel to the midline of the patient. The nerve stimulator is initially set at a current output of 0.8 mA,[28] a pulse width of 100 to 300 μs, and a frequency of 1–2 Hz.

Our clinical experience has shown that better results are obtained when flexion or extension motor responses in the fingers are obtained. These are often incorrectly called "median" and "radial" nerve responses, since these two nerves have not yet been formed at this level and their fibers are still present in all three trunks. When such a response in the fingers has been obtained, the injection is started without decreasing the output of the nerve stimulator. This is indeed the only block that we routinely inject at a higher current than 0.5 mA and at the same initial current. We have demonstrated in a randomized study that the block is equally successful at this current as it is at 0.5 mA.[28] The local anesthetic solution is then injected slowly.

If needle repositioning is necessary, the needle is redirected either anteriorly or posteriorly but exactly in the same original parasagittal plane (parallel to the patient's midline). The tip of the needle is always kept above the clavicle.

Intercostobrachial Nerve and Tourniquet
Most of the sensory innervation of the medial side of the arm is provided by the medial brachial cutaneous nerve, a branch of the medial cord of the brachial plexus. The

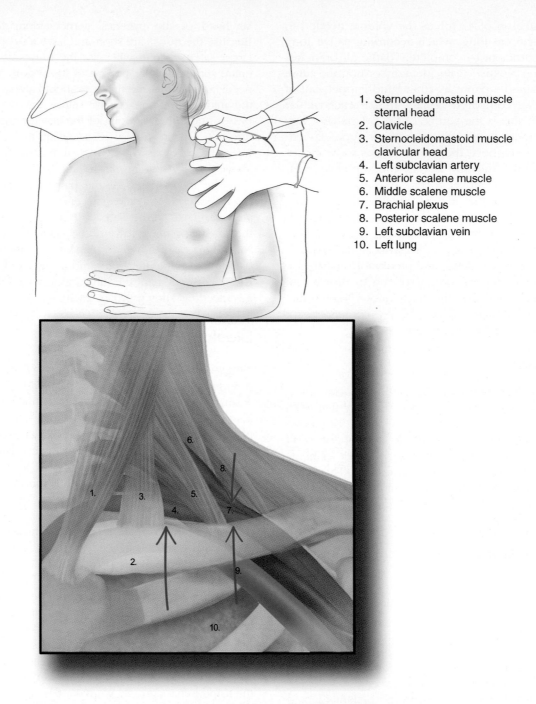

1. Sternocleidomastoid muscle sternal head
2. Clavicle
3. Sternocleidomastoid muscle clavicular head
4. Left subclavian artery
5. Anterior scalene muscle
6. Middle scalene muscle
7. Brachial plexus
8. Posterior scalene muscle
9. Left subclavian vein
10. Left lung

Figure 23-10. Surface anatomy and positioning for the supraclavicular block.

skin of the axilla and the uppermost portion of the medial side of the arm are supplied by the intercostobrachial nerve, which is the lateral branch of the second intercostal nerve (T2). This nerve can be blocked by a subcutaneous injection performed under the area of the axillary hair. However, because the supraclavicular block provides enough circumferential anesthesia of the arm, it is usually unnecessary to block this nerve only for the purpose of blocking tourniquet pain.

Continuous Supraclavicular Block

Traditionally the supraclavicular technique has not been considered suitable for placement of catheters. The great mobility of the neck at this location can easily cause accidental catheter dislodgement. Tunneling of the catheter to the infraclavicular level could help to make the catheter more stable, but there are not enough data available at this stage to recommend it.

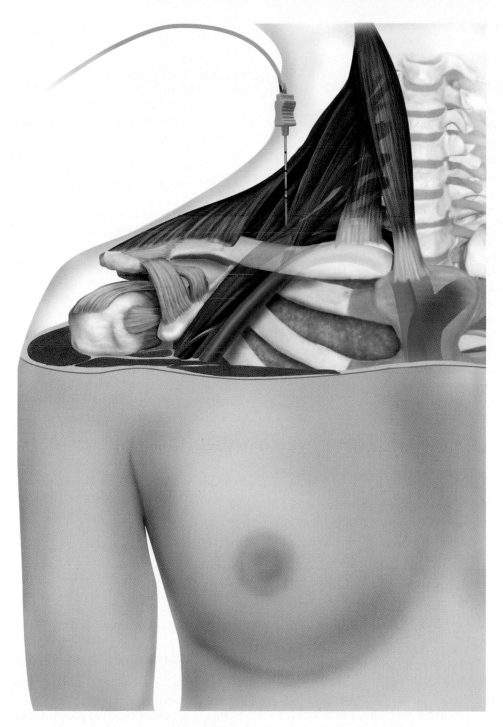

Figure 23-11. Three-dimensional anatomy of the supraclavicular block.

As it is the case with any continuous block, using aseptic technique, including a sterile field and sterile gloves, is important to avoid infection. A sterile clear dressing is used for easy inspection of the puncture site. The technique is the same as described for single-injection supraclavicular block. Because in this technique the needle approaches the plexus almost tangentially, it is easy to advance a catheter 3 to 5 cm beyond the needle tip while observing the unchanged brisk motor response if a stimulating catheter is being used.

The initial dose of local anesthetic is usually similar to that used for single-injection supraclavicular block, but it is injected through the catheter. A continuous infusion of 3 to 5 mL/h of a lower concentration of the same drug with or without patient-controlled boluses will yield good results (see Chap. 21).

The supraclavicular block provides a block of the neurotomes similar to that obtained by the cervical paravertebral block (Fig. 23-9).

Selection of Local Anesthetic Agent

We most commonly use 35 to 40 mL (1.5%) mepivacaine with 1:200,000 epinephrine, which provides about 3 to 4 h of surgical anesthesia. The same anesthetic solution without epinephrine provides about 2 to 3 h of surgical anesthesia. The authors have also used other local anesthetic agents—such as ropivacaine (0.5 to 0.75%), bupivacaine (0.5%), and levobupivacaine (0.625%)—when rapid onset was not important. These drugs provide good anesthesia lasting 5 to 8 h.

For continuous techniques, a bolus dose of about 10 to 15 mL of local anesthetic solution can be given followed by an infusion rate of 8 to 10 mL/h. A solution of 0.2% ropivacaine, 0.2% levobupivacaine, or 0.25% bupivacaine can be used for this purpose. Patient-controlled regional anesthesia can be added, allowing the patient to administer 3 to 5 mL every 30 min for breakthrough pain. If PCRA is added, the basal infusion is decreased to around 5 mL/h (see also Chap. 21).

Special Considerations

This approach brings back some of the simplicity of Kulenkampff's original technique but avoids directing the needle toward the pleura. The pleural dome is avoided by inserting the needle at some distance lateral to the insertion of the sternocleidomastoid muscle on the clavicle and by directing it parallel to the midline. On the other hand, the recognition that the trunks are supraclavicular when the shoulder is down makes bringing the needle below the clavicle unnecessary and eliminates the risk of penetrating the first intercostal space.

We do not recommend performing this particular block on heavily sedated or unconscious patients, since some authorities feel that the patient's reactions may provide important indications to prevent intraneural injection and other potentially catastrophic complications. Although there is no support for this notion in the literature, it is not necessary to have patients heavily sedated or unconscious to place this or most other blocks. Furthermore, low injection pressures and overall meticulous technique also probably minimizes the risk of intraneural injection. If undue pressure is felt at any point during injection, the needle should be withdrawn 1 to 2 mm and the situation reassessed.

Removal of a cast or splint before performing this block is not necessary as long as the fingers are visible.

Depending on the patient's weight, the palpating finger must exert different amounts of pressure on the deeper tissues. This maneuver helps bring the plexus closer to the skin and makes the trajectory of the needle shorter.

The needle should never be inserted deeper than 1 in. (2.5 cm) if a muscle twitch elicited from the brachial plexus is not present. A twitch elicited by stimulating one of the trunks, on the other hand, confirms the location of the needle close to the plexus, allowing for deeper penetration, if necessary, to obtain an appropriate muscle twitch.

Knowledge of anatomy is important for any peripheral block, but for the supraclavicular block it is one of the most crucial points. A supraclavicular block should not be attempted without a thorough knowledge of the brachial plexus and its important surrounding structures. Good anatomic knowledge, the use of simple landmarks, and meticulous technique can provide the operator with all the advantages of this block while significantly limiting the potential for complications.

Potential Problems and Complications

Pneumothorax

Most of the published cases of pneumothorax associated with supraclavicular block have been diagnosed within a few hours of the procedure and before patient's discharge from the hospital. Although a late presentation is rare, its occurrence has been commonly overemphasized in the literature. Based on the available literature, it can be said that pneumothorax associated with supraclavicular block is rare, often small, and occurs within a few hours following the procedure. In some rare instances its presentation can be delayed up to 12 h. In our experience, including over 3000 supraclavicular blocks over a period of 11 years, we have yet to demonstrate a single pneumothorax, suggesting that a sound anatomic technique minimizes this risk.

Other Complications

Blood vessel penetration and intravascular injections should be obvious and should have an incidence similar to that of all other brachial plexus blocks. Neural injury, as seems to be the case with most peripheral nerve blocks, is rare.

REFERENCES

1. Standring S (ed). *Gray's Anatomy: The Anatomical Basis of Clinical Practice*, 39th ed. New York: Elsevier, 2004: 801–942.
2. Borene SC, Edwards JN, Boezaart AP. At the cords, the pinkie towards: Interpreting infraclavicular motor response to neurostimulation. *Reg Anesth Pain Med* 29:125–129, 2004.

3. Kapral S, Jandrasits O, Schabernig C, et al. Lateral infraclavicular plexus block vs axillary block for hand and forearm surgery. *Acta Anaesthesiol Scand* 43:1047–1052, 1999.

4. Jandard C, Gentili ME, Girard F, et al. Infraclavicular block with lateral approach and nerve stimulation: Extent of anesthesia and adverse effects. *Reg Anesth Pain Med* 27:37–42, 2002.

5. Gaertner E, Estebe J-P, Zamfir A, et al. Infraclavicular plexus block: Multiple injections vs single injection. *Reg Anesth Pain Med* 27:590–594, 2002.

6. Boezaart AP, de Beer JF, du Toit C, et al. A new technique of continuous interscalene block. *Can J Anesth* 46:275–281, 1999.

7. Wehling MJ, Koorn R, Leddell C, et al. Electrical nerve stimulation using a stimulating catheter: What is the lower limit? *Reg Anesth Pain Med* 29:230–233, 2004.

8. Wilbourn AJ. Brachial plexus disorders, in Dyck PJ, Thomas PK (eds): *Peripheral Neuropathy*, 3d ed. Philadelphia: Saunders, 1993:921–922.

9. Borgeat A, Ekatodramis G. Anaesthesia for shoulder surgery. *Best Pract Res Clin Anesthesiol* 16:211–225, 2002.

10. Meier G, Büttner J. *Atlas der Peripheren Regionalenästesie.* Stuttgart: Georg Thieme Verlag, 2004.

11. Ribeiro FC, Georgousis H, Bertram RS, et al. Plexus irritation caused by interscalene brachial plexus catheter for shoulder surgery. *Anesth Analg* 82:870–872, 1996.

12. Hubner T, Gerber H. Knotting of a catheter in the plexus brachialis: A rare complication. *Anaesthetist* 52:606–607, 2003.

13. David M. Knotted peripheral nerve catheter. *Reg Anesth Pain Med* 28:487–488, 2003.

14. Lee BH, Goucke CR. Shearing of a peripheral nerve catheter. *Anesth Analg* 95:760–761, 2002.

15. Smith SP, Dvaraj VS, Bunker TD. The association between frozen shoulder and Dupuytren's disease. *J Shoulder Elbow Surg* 10:149–151, 2001.

16. Bunker TD, Anthony PP. The pathology of frozen shoulder: A Dupuytren-like disease. *J Bone Joint Surg [Br]* 77-B:677–683, 1995.

17. Müller LP, Müller LA, Happ J. Frozen shoulder: A sympathetic dystrophy? *Arch Orthop Trauma Surg* 120:84–87, 2000.

18. Kappis M. Weitere Erfahrungen mit der Sympathektomie. *Klin Wochnschr* 2:1441, 1923.

19. Pippa P, Cominelli E, Marinelli C, et al. Brachial plexus block using the posterior approach. *Eur J Anaesth* 7:411–420, 1990.

20. Boezaart AP. Continuous interscalene block for ambulatory shoulder surgery. *Best Pract Res Clin Anaesthesiol* 16:295–310, 2002.

21. Borene SC, Rosenquist RW, Koorn R, et al. An indication for continuous cervical paravertebral block (posterior approach to the interscalene space). *Anesth Analg* 97:898–900, 2003.

22. Kulenkampff D, Persky M. Brachial plexus anesthesia: Its indications, technique and dangers. *Ann Surg* 87:883–891, 1928.

23. Accardo N, Adriani J. Brachial plexus block: A simplified technique using the axillary route. *South Med J* 42:929–937, 1949.

24. Burnham P. Regional anesthesia of the great nerves of the upper arm. *Anesthesiology* 19:281–284, 1958.

25. De Jong R. Axillary block of the brachial plexus. *Anesthesiology* 22:215–225, 1961.

26. Brand L, Papper E. A comparison of supraclavicular and axillary techniques for brachial plexus blocks. *Anesthesiology* 22:226–229, 1961.

27. Brown DL, Cahill D, Bridenbaugh D. Supraclavicular nerve block: Anatomic analysis of a method to prevent pneumothorax. *Anesth Analg* 76:530–534, 1993.

28. Franco CD, Domashevich V, Voronov G, et al. The supraclavicular block with a nerve stimulator: To decrease or not to decrease, that is the question. *Anesth Analg* 98:1167–1171, 2004.

CHAPTER 24

Brachial Plexus Blocks below the Clavicle

ROBERT M. RAW

► INTRODUCTION

In 1973 Raj described the first infraclavicular block.[1] Since then, many infraclavicular approaches have been described. The distal four portions of the brachial plexus that are accessible to needles from an infraclavicular direction are (1) trunks lying over the first rib, (2) the divisions lying behind and immediately below the clavicle, (3) the cords lying medial to the tip of the coracoid process, and (4) the terminal branches of the brachial plexus lying toward the axilla.

Bazy's original 1921 description of an infraclavicular block was the inferolateral block of the trunks for the brachial plexus.[2] The continuous version of this block has been demonstrated in a video/DVD textbook[3] (see further on). The needle is inserted below the midpoint of the clavicle and directed retrograde, aiming superiorly, medially, and posteriorly toward Chassaignac's tubercle. The needle meets the brachial plexus at the trunks over the first rib.

Infraclavicular Blocks of the Brachial Plexus Divisions

Infraclavicular block is known as the vertical infraclavicular block (VIB) or vertical infraclavicular plexus (VIP) block. Described in 1995 by Kilka,[4] this block achieved popularity in Europe and is the most distal block still associated with potential phrenic nerve block.[5–7]

There are large anatomic variations in the position of the brachial plexus, which are due to differences in clavicular morphology or lung inflation. Greher[8] investigated this by ultrasound and demonstrated that the anatomic variations cause difficulty in performing the block and increase the risk of pneumothorax.[9,10]

Kilka recommended using the midpoint of the line between the surprasternal notch (jugular fossa) and the ventral process of the acromion,[11] with the needle insertion point 1 cm below the clavicle, and directed posteriorly. However, Greher found the ideal block point up to 8 mm more lateral than the one predicted by Kilka's landmarks. When the plexus is situated more medial to the midpoint of the clavicle (more likely in tall, slender patients), it is also shifted inferiorly, which likewise increases the risk of pneumothorax.

A major limitation of this approach is that the clavicle moves independently of the brachial plexus. It is best performed with the help of ultrasonography.

Infraclavicular Blocks of the Brachial Plexus Cords

Medial Block of the Cords of the Brachial Plexus

Raj originally named this the infraclavicular block, although it would be more correct to refer to it as the *medial block of the cords of the brachial plexus*.[1] In his early descriptions, Raj referred to blockade of the terminal branches of the brachial plexus, although the cords were actually blocked more often. This approach became popular for catheter insertion because it is easier to perform, more comfortable for the patient, and provides more reliable results.

One problem often experienced with this approach was isolated blockade of the musculocutaneous nerve, with failure to block the rest of the cord.[12]

Superomedial Block of the Cords of the Brachial Plexus

Borgeat proposed a modification of Raj's medial block of the cords by "shifting" the insertion point laterally.[13] He proposed an insertion point similar to that for the anterior block of the divisions but aimed the needle inferolaterally, along the brachial line, toward the axillary artery palpated in the axilla. The needle insertion point is at the midpoint of a line joining the suprasternal notch and the lateral edge of the acromion (approximately 1.5 cm medial to the needle insertion point used in the superior block of the brachial plexus cords, as discussed further on).

Klaastadt investigated this superomedial approach to the cords with MRI to define landmarks,[14] and recommended an angle of needle insertion of 65 degrees to the skin. These instructions based on the infraclavicular skin plane are not consistent, however, because skin planes vary considerably from one patient to another, depending on pectoral muscle mass, breast size, and obesity.

Anterior Block of the Cords of the Brachial Plexus

The permutations of technique are numerous. This approach is attributed to Whiffler, who used a non-nerve-stimulator technique and bony reference points and named the block the coracoid block.[15] Whiffler proposed a needle entry point 2 cm caudad and 1 cm medial to the inferior border of the coracoid with the needle directed posteriorly.

Wilson and Brown proposed a needle entry point 2 cm medial and 2 cm inferior to the edge of the coracoid process.[16] With magnetic resonant imaging (MRI), they demonstrated that most of the neuronal tissue lies behind the axillary artery. This remains the major limiting factor in all the anterior approaches, because the posterior cord, which is the best cord to block, is the least accessible cord by an anterior approach.

Infraclavicular blocks of the Brachial Plexus Terminal Branches

Medial Approach of the Terminal Branches of the Brachial Plexus

Jandard described the medial approach of the terminal branches technique and proposed the deltopectoral triangle as landmark for needle insertion. The precise point of needle entry was not described, but an accompanying illustration suggests a needle entry 4 cm medial to the tip of the coracoid and aimed toward the axillary artery in the axilla. This approach relies on soft tissue landmarks, which are not readily palpable in obese patients.

Superior Approach of the Terminal Branches of the Brachial Plexus

Sims described this approach in 1977 in an effort to improve on the medial approach to the brachial plexus cords.[17] He used the same needle entry point as for the superior block of the cords (see below) but aimed the needle laterally. This is essentially a block of the terminal branches of the brachial plexus, and the musculocutaneous nerve is the most likely nerve to be encountered first. Because it is outside the plexus sheath, this nerve may be blocked while other brachial plexus nerves are not blocked.

Transaxillary Block of the Cords of the Brachial Plexus

Krebs described the insertion of a catheter in the axilla and advanced approximately 13 cm proximally into the infraclavicular region.[18] This unusual approach never gained popularity and is used only rarely when alternate catheter approaches cannot be used.

Many other variations of the anterior approach to the brachial plexus cords have been proposed. The infraclavicular approaches proved popular and many practitioners have abandoned axillary blocks in their favor.

▶ THE SUPERIOR APPROACH TO THE BRACHIAL PLEXUS CORD BLOCK

Introduction

The pilot study of this approach was presented in 2003.[19] In 2004, Klaastadt et al. assessed this approach on the basis of MRI anatomic studies of 82 clinical cases.[20] They suggested that it would be optimal to block all three cords of the brachial plexus, particularly the posterior one (most important and largest of the three) and concluded that pneumothorax risk would be low. The present author has had personal experience with 1500 cases of the use of this block at his institution, with excellent results.

Klaastadt's MRI study revealed the mean distances from the skin to each cord.[14] As outlined in Table 24-1, this distance varies from 40 to 83 mm. For the particular parasagittal plane, he demonstrated that the pleura closest to the coracoclavicular trough was 75 mm from the skin and furthest at 161 mm. He also discovered that in 20 percent of his patients, the pleura was medial to the block plane (with no possibility of reaching lung). In 10 percent, the "window" to the lung was fully obstructed by the neurovascular structures or ribs. Considering this and the fact there is a muscle that defines needle depth, this block seems to pose very little risk of pneumothorax.

Klaastadt recommended that the needle be inserted at 15 degrees posterior to the coronal plane and not

▶ **TABLE 24-1.** CORRECTIVE ACTION IF FAULTY MOTOR RESPONSES ARE ENCOUNTERED DURING INFRACLAVICULAR BLOCK

Motor Response	Correction	To Find
Subscapularis and latissimus dorsi muscles	Move needle tip slightly anterior while maintaining the same depth	Posterior cord
Biceps muscle (musculocutaneous nerve)	Move needle tip slightly deeper	Posterior cord
Flexion and pronation of hand (medial and lateral cord responses)	Move needle tip 0.5 to 1.5 cm medial into a zone to where posterior cord is more accessible below and behind the lateral cord	Posterior cord
Extensor motor responses (posterior cord)	Move needle tip laterally toward B zone	Medial cord
Hand flexion (medial cord responses)	Move needle tip medial toward A zone	Lateral cord
Pectoral muscle response	Move needle tip posteriorly while maintaining the same depth	Any cord

deeper than 65 mm. However, our clinical experience suggests that in the majority of adults, the average angle of approach should be between 30 and 60 degrees. In infants and toddlers, the cords tend to be shallower and a needle entry at an angle parallel (at zero degrees) to the coronal plane seems to be common.

Patient Selection

Infraclavicular blocks can be used for all surgery of the arm and forearm distal to and including the elbow. It is, however, not suitable for surgery to the shoulder and upper arm.

▶ APPLIED ANATOMY

Gross Anatomy

The brachial plexus is formed by the anterior rami of nerves from the fifth cervical root (C5) through the first thoracic root (T1). These roots alternately fuse and bifurcate[21] (Fig. 23-1). The roots combine into three trunks at the lateral edge of the scalene muscles and pass over the first rib, where they lie posterior and superior to the subclavian artery. Each trunk then divides into anterior and posterior divisions behind the clavicle and lateral to the first rib. The three posterior divisions form the posterior cord, the anterior divisions of the upper and middle trunk form the lateral cord, and the anterior division of the lower trunk forms the medial cord. The cords then rearrange and embrace the axillary artery. Inferior to the coracoid process, the cords give off their final terminal branches (Fig. 23-1). The medial and lateral cords supply the muscles that cause flexion of the arm, while the posterior cord supplies the muscles that cause extension.

The cords are named medial, lateral, and posterior, according to their relation to the second part of the axillary artery, viewed as if the artery descended parallel to the long axis of the body (Fig. 24-1). The true position of the axillary artery is, however, at 45 degrees to the long axis of the body, and the lateral cord lies somewhat superior to the artery. The medial cord lies inferior to the artery, while the posterior cord is always posterior to the artery (Fig. 24-2).

The subclavian artery becomes the axillary artery lateral to the first rib; it is divided into three parts, the first part being medial to, the second part being behind, and the third part being lateral to the minor pectoral muscle near its attachment to the tip of the coracoid process. The anteromedial tip of the coracoid process is approximately 36 mm from the lateral cord of the brachial plexus and the axillary nerve lies approximately 7 mm closer.[22]

The medial cord is at first behind the first part of the axillary artery and winds inferiorly around the artery to reach its medial position at the second part of the axillary artery. The posterior cord at first lies adjacent to the lateral cord in a superoposterior position to the first part of the axillary artery before rotating around to the second part of the artery. The lateral cord is superoposterior and shifts toward its lateral position on the second part of the axillary artery.

There is often anatomic variation in the formation of the cords and their relationship to the second part of the axillary artery, but they mostly follow the trend of the described pattern. Thus, while the posterior cord is always posterior, the lateral and medial cords may rotate in their path toward the second part of the axillary artery.

The pectoral nerves are formed at the level of the trunks or divisions (Fig. 23-1) but keep close association with the medial and lateral brachial plexus cords, after which they are respectively named. The pectoral nerves turn anteriorly around and though the minor pectoral muscle and are connected by the Martin-Gruber communicating branch.[23]

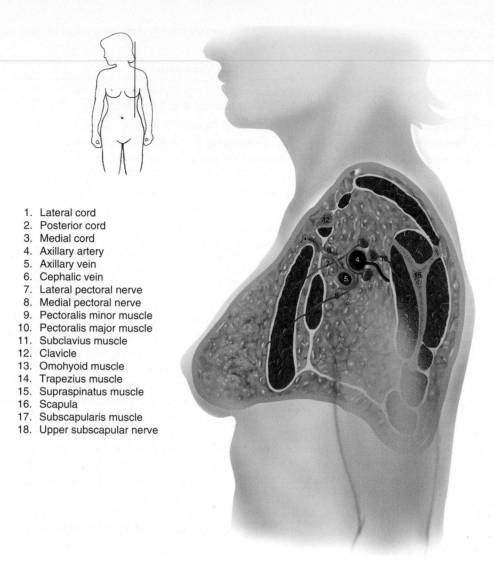

1. Lateral cord
2. Posterior cord
3. Medial cord
4. Axillary artery
5. Axillary vein
6. Cephalic vein
7. Lateral pectoral nerve
8. Medial pectoral nerve
9. Pectoralis minor muscle
10. Pectoralis major muscle
11. Subclavius muscle
12. Clavicle
13. Omohyoid muscle
14. Trapezius muscle
15. Supraspinatus muscle
16. Scapula
17. Subscapularis muscle
18. Upper subscapular nerve

Figure 24-1. Cross section through the coracoclavicular trough.

The important branches of the medial cord are the medial part of the median nerve, which crosses the front of the axillary artery, the terminal ulnar nerve, and the medial cutaneous nerves of the arm and the forearm (Fig. 23-1). The important branches of the lateral cord are the musculocutaneous nerve and the lateral part of the median nerve. The posterior cord gives off the axillary nerve posterior, the nerves to the subscapularis muscle and the latissimus dorsi muscle, and posterior to the axillary artery, the radial nerve. The latter is the largest nerve of the upper limb.

The musculocutaneous nerve branches off from the lateral cord inferior to the coracoid process (Fig. 23-1) and deviates superior from the plexus to enter the coracobrachialis muscle 3 to 7 cm inferolateral to the coracoid process.

The Brachial Plexus Sheath

The simple concept of a tubular brachial plexus sheath proposed by Winnie is no longer accepted. Thompson[24] convincingly demonstrated that the epineural septa form partitions that surround components of the brachial plexus. These septa of epineurium restrict the diffusion of injected fluids, and it is now accepted that not all the nerves of the plexus are within one surrounding sheath. However, in the case of infraclavicular blocks, the spread of a drug injected into one fascial compartment to another can be facilitated by injection of large volumes, which can spread proximally to where septa thin out. Large volumes can also create high hydrostatic pressures, which can force flow across septa or create large areas for gradual diffusion across septa. Alternately, the success of a block

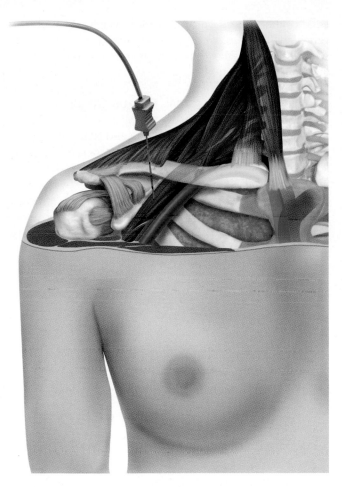

Figure 24-2. Three-dimensional view of the superior block of the brachial plexus cords.

and speed of onset can be improved by blocking multiple compartments by divided injection portions, following the multistimulation technique as popularized by Fanelli.[25]

Other Practical Anatomic Issues

THE MUSCULOCUTANEOUS NERVE

When infraclavicular injections of local anesthetic agents are given at the level of the terminal branches, confusion may arise. The musculocutaneous nerve may be missed while the other nerves are blocked, or it may be blocked while missing the other plexus nerves.[26] This also applies to blocks in the axilla (see Chap. 25) but potentially to all infraclavicular blocks where the needle is directed laterally. Because the musculocutaneous nerve separates from the lateral cord inferiorly to the coracoid process to enter the coracobrachialis muscle, which attaches to the tip of the coracoid process[27] it is preferable to block the musculocutaneous nerve proximally while it is still part of the lateral cord. In 4 percent of people, the median nerve and musculocutaneous nerves merge and follow the typical median nerve course[28]; in 8 percent of people, the musculocutaneous nerve does not penetrate the coracobrachialis muscle but passes anterior to it.

THE CONCEPT OF BOUNDARY-DEFINING MUSCLES

The pectoral nerves that innervate the minor and major pectoral muscles and the nerve to the subscapularis and latissimus dorsi muscles are useful aids in identifying the brachial plexus cords (Fig. 24-3). Unlike the erroneous classic description of the pectoral nerves, the superior, middle, and inferior pectoral nerves originate from the brachial plexus at the level of the divisions and the trunks.[24] They remain in the proximity of the plexus to the level of the cords and then turn anteriorly to pass around and through the minor pectoral muscle. Pectoral muscle contraction in isolation, therefore, indicates that the stimulating needle tip is anterior to the brachial plexus cords and needs to be moved posteriorly.

On the other side of the cords, three nerves directed posteriorly to the subscapular and the latissimus dorsi muscles originate from the posterior cord. A subscapular muscle contraction is seen as adduction of the arm and internal rotation of the humerus, or a latissimus dorsi muscle motor response is seen as a muscle twitch on the posterior aspect of the lateral chest wall. Seen in isolation, these indicate that the needle tip is posterior to the brachial plexus and needs to be directed more anteriorly. The anterior and posterior boundary-defining muscles also respond to cord stimulation, but then with movements of the arm.

Thus, when a stimulating needle has been inserted superiorly and toward the brachial plexus cords and a pectoral muscle twitch is observed alone without arm or hand movements, the depth of needle is correct, but the tip of the needle is too anterior in the coronal plane and should be directed more posteriorly. Similarly, if adduction or internal rotation of the humerus or a motor twitch of the posterior part of the lateral chest wall is seen without extension movements of the arm or hand, the needle is too far posterior and needs to be moved anteriorly at the same depth.

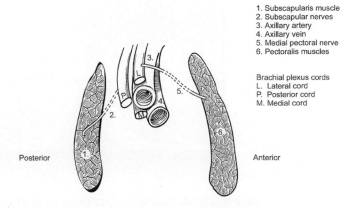

1. Subscapularis muscle
2. Subscapular nerves
3. Axillary artery
4. Axillary vein
5. Medial pectoral nerve
6. Pectoralis muscles

Brachial plexus cords
L. Lateral cord
P. Posterior cord
M. Medial cord

Figure 24-3. Boundary-defining muscles.

THE CORACOCLAVICULAR TROUGH

The coracoclavicular trough is bordered by bony structures on its superior and lateral sides. It can be identified by palpating the concave anterior edge of the lateral clavicle, abutting against the coracoid process on the lateral side. This bony trough has some correlation with the deltopectoral triangle, but it differs in that the deltopectoral triangle is a fascia-covered space between the pectoralis major and deltoid muscles just below the clavicle. Its apex points inferolaterally, and it is continuous with the sloping deltopectoral groove extending from the axilla. The deltopectoral triangle is seldom visible and is best seen after open dissection. The lateral edge of the deltopectoral triangle, when visible, generally coincides with the lateral edge of the upper coracoclavicular trough, although this varies with different degrees of muscle development, while the coracoclavicular trough remains consistent in the parasagittal plane (Fig. 24-4).

STABILITY OF THE BRACHIAL PLEXUS CORDS IN RELATION TO OTHER ANATOMY

The shoulder girdle is highly mobile and is firmly attached to the rest of the skeleton only at the sternoclavicular joint. It is able to swing through 360 degrees and most of the movements shift the clavicle and brachial plexus in opposite directions. However, the position of the brachial plexus relative to the pivotal point of the shoulder girdle remains constant. The lengths of the neck and clavicle

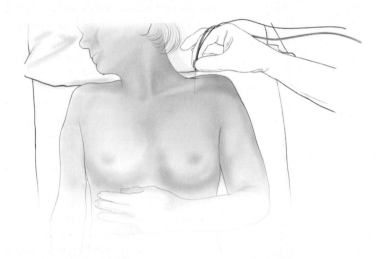

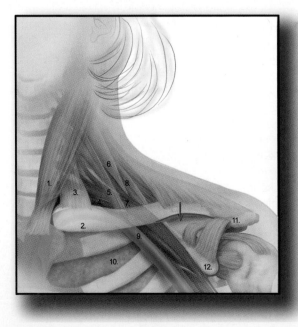

1. Sternocleidomastoid muscle sternal head
2. Clavicle
3. Sternocledomastoid muscle clavicular head
4. Left subclavian artery
5. Anterior scalene muscle
6. Middle scalene muscle
7. Brachial plexus
8. Posterior scalene muscle
9. Left subclavian vein
10. Left lung
11. Acromion
12. Coracoid process

Figure 24-4. Surface anatomy and positioning for the superior approach to the brachial plexus cord block.

vary considerably from one person to another, and people have varying degrees of chest inflation because of lung disease or obesity, which in turn elevates the sternum and the shoulder girdle to varying degrees. Nearly all infraclavicular block landmarks based on the midclavicular zone or soft tissue are therefore unreliable. Exceptions are those that relate to the second part of the brachial plexus cords around the second part of the axially artery and the coracoid process.

Functional Neuroanatomy

With blocks of the cords it is important to differentiate stimulation of a cord from stimulation of a terminal branch, when each may give similar muscle twitches. Differentiation can be achieved with a high stimulating current (e.g., 1.2 mA). If the needle is applied to a cord, all the motor fascicles in that cord will likely fire and many muscle groups will respond, but when it is applied to a terminal branch, it will cause a vigorous motor response in the group of muscles supplied by that nerve.

WATCH THE PINKIE (FIFTH DIGIT)

Borene et al. simplified the interpretation of upper limb motor responses to stimulation by pointing out that the pinkie (fifth digit) moves toward the cord being stimulated.[29] The anatomy of the brachial plexus is complex; it is difficult to remember which terminal nerves and muscles are supplied by each. Borene et al. proposed a simple way to identify the cord being stimulated. In applying a relatively high current (e.g., 1.0 to 1.5 mA) to evoke an action potential in the entire lateral cord, the pinkie will move laterally from the anatomic position (pronation). Posterior movement of the pinkie (extension) indicates posterior cord stimulation, while its medial movement (fifth finger flexion and ulnar deviation) indicates medial cord stimulation. This is best observed by using higher stimulating currents to ensure that all the motor fascicles of a cord are stimulated.

It is clear that finger flexion can differ according to which part of the cord forming the median nerve is stimulated. The lateral part of the median nerves controls the flexor muscles of the thumb and fingers two and three, while the medial portion of the median nerve controls the flexor muscles of fingers four and five (see Tables 23-1, 23-2, and 23-3).

BRACHIAL PLEXUS CORD SUBDIVISION

In order to understand the anatomy of the brachial plexus better, the cords may be regarded as having four zones extending from their formation below the clavicle to their terminal branches under the coracoid process. The zones may be named A, B, C, and T and are approximately 1.5 to 4 cm long and centered on the second part of the axillary artery. They represent patterns of nerve positions relative to each other and the axillary artery. An understanding of these zones may be helpful when it is difficult to locate a particular component.

In zone A, the cords are in a more posterior coronal plane of the axillary artery, typically in its first part. The medial cord still needs to swing inferiorly around to the "medial" position. The A zone is recognized by the medial cord seeming "invisible" to the stimulating needle because of the artery. The zone is also characterized by the fact that the posterior and lateral cords are very close to each other.

In zone B, the cords are in their classically named positions relative to the second part of the axillary artery, and typically this anatomy seems to apply to the majority of block attempts. The nerves that define the boundary to the muscles branch sharply away from this zone.

In zone C, the terminal branches start to form. The medial part of the median nerve originates here and tracks forward over the anterior aspect of the artery to meet its lateral part from the lateral cord. The ulnar nerve sometimes moves slightly posteriorly again and the musculocutaneous nerve is in the lateral position. The posterior cord seems "invisible" in zone C.

In the T (or terminal) zone, the cords of all the terminal branches have been formed. For the superior cord block, the musculocutaneous nerve (biceps motor response) seems prominent and far (over 4 mm) from all other structures. See Table 24-1 for corrective action.

Surface Anatomy (Landmarks)

Needle entry is in the superior part of the coracoclavicular trough described above. It remains strictly in the parasagittal plane and enters at an angle of 25 to 45 degrees to the patient's coronal plane (Fig. 24-4). Using a relatively high nerve stimulator output current (1.2 mA) a pectoral muscle twitch will indicate that the correct depth has been reached. Since this defines the caudal plane, the tip of the needle should now be redirected slightly posteriorly.

Block Technique

Patient Positioning

The patient is placed in the supine position with the head slightly turned to the contralateral side, the elbow flexed, and the hand placed on the abdomen. The anesthesiologist stands at the patient's head. The onset of this block is relatively fast; approximately 20 min should be allowed between completion of the block and surgery.

Single-Injection Superior Approach Infraclavicular Block

A 50- to 100-mm shallow-bevel insulated needle is used. It is connected to a nerve stimulator, set to an output of 1.2 mA, 100- to 300-ms pulse duration, and a frequency of 2 Hz. Needle entry is close to the clavicle in the coracoclavicular trough, aimed 15 degrees posteriorly to the coronal plane and advanced until arm muscle and anterior or posterior boundary muscle motor responses are observed.

It is important that the needle remain within the parasagittal plane, without medial or lateral deviation. Misdirection of the needle by 45 degrees medially represents the shortest route to lung and pleura, which at this level is 5 to 9 cm. Misdirecting the needle too far laterally may place it on the base of the coracoid bone, which is harmless, or in the terminal branches of the brachial plexus, causing incomplete nerve block. It is, however, permissible to vary the direction 5 degrees medially or laterally so as to seek a better cord subzone (see above).

After the correct cord is located with a brisk motor response at a current output of 0.3 to 0.5 mA, the local anesthetic agent can be injected.

Inject on One or Multiple Cords?

The present author recommends injecting all three cords individually for optimal block results. It is advisable to locate the posterior cord, as the largest cord, first and inject 20 mL of the drug; shortly after that, 10 mL is injected onto each of the other cords. If a third cord cannot be located, it is most likely the medial cord. This may be due to anatomic variations or the possibility that the cord is already blocked by the earlier drug injection. The remaining drug is then injected onto any other cord component that can be found.

CONTINUOUS SUPERIOR APPROACH TO THE INFRACLAVICULAR BLOCK

Like the single-injection infraclavicular block, the continuous block is used for surgery of the arm distal to the shoulder. Because major wrist and elbow surgery and pain management require all three of the cords to be blocked, the continuous infraclavicular block has proven disappointing. The reason is probably that while all three of the cords are blocked with the initial relatively large volume of anesthetic in the primary block, only the cord on which the catheter has been placed seems to be blocked by the smaller volume used in continuous infusion. To block the other two cords, then, requires relatively large-volume boluses of local anesthetic agent.

NEEDLE PLACEMENT FOR THE CONTINUOUS INFRACLAVICULAR BLOCK TECHNIQUE

The patient is placed in the supine position with the hand on the abdomen and the head turned slightly to the opposite side. After skin preparation, the area is covered with a sterile fenestrated transparent plastic drape.

The surface landmarks are similar to those used for the anterior single-injection infraclavicular block as described by Wilson and Brown,[30] 2 cm or one width of the patient's thumb medial and one width caudad of the coracoid process.

Catheter placement and fixation are as described in Chap. 20.

▶ SELECTION OF LOCAL ANESTHETIC AGENT

We use approximately 0.3 to 0.5 mL/kg (40 mL for a 100-kg patient) of 0.75% ropivacaine for single-injection infraclavicular blocks. For continuous infusions, we start with a similar bolus injection followed by an infusion of 0.2% ropivacaine at approximately 0.05 mL/kg/h (5 mL/h for a 100-kg patient) and patient-controlled boluses of 10 mL with a lockout time of 120 min (see Chap. 21).

Ilfeld et al. studied infraclavicular infusion protocols and found that they had the least breakthrough events at relatively high flow rates of 12 mL/h 0.2% ropivacaine compared to lower infusion rates and large boluses.[31] However, with 8 mL/h infusion and 4 mL of patient-controlled boluses, the infusion reservoir lasted longer and, despite some increased pain, patients felt more satisfied. They also found that the addition of clonidine to the local anesthetic infusions offered no benefit.[32] They also confirmed that patient-controlled infusions used at home greatly reduced opiate consumption and its associated side effects.[23]

Complications of Blocks of the Brachial Plexus Cords

Vascular Puncture and Intravascular Injection

Because of the arrangement of the nerves around the axillary artery and the proximity of the axillary vein lying inferiorly and slightly anterior, there is a danger of vascular penetration. All nerves have good blood supplies and no nerve block is exempt from the risk of intravascular injection. The cord blocks seem to have a remarkably low incidence of vascular complications. In one series of 100 cases of cord blocks, there were four cases of vascular puncture and one patient with symptoms of local anesthetic toxicity. Salazar.[33] encountered 0.6 percent vascular punctures in 360 cases. Jandard, using an anterior cord approach, found 5 percent of cases in which arterial puncture occurred before the nerves were reached.[34] In the study by Whiffler, the use of sharp needles was associated with an incidence of 50 percent vascular puncture.[35]

In our experience, when we use blunt needles and the superior approach to the block of the cords, vascular puncture is unusual. The artery's resistance to puncture by blunt needles may explain this, and the fact that the axillary vein lies further from the needle. All ultrasound studies demonstrate that blunt needles slip off arteries more easily than they penetrate them.

Phrenic and Other Nerve Block

In performing an anterior block of the divisions of the brachial plexus phrenic nerve block is possible because the approaches are similar.[6] However, the incidence of inadvertent phrenic nerve block is very low. A phrenic nerve block from a cord block approach seems impossible. One study showed no respiratory effect in 20 patients specifically assessed for diaphragm dysfunction after injecting 50 mL of local anesthetic agent via the superomedial approach to the brachial plexus cords.[26] After the injection of local anesthetic agent into six patients, using the anterior block of the cords of the brachial plexus, spread above the level of the clavicle never occurred, confirming that cord block approaches cannot block the phrenic nerve.[36] The development of hoarseness (recurrent laryngeal nerve block) and a Horner's syndrome (superior cervical–stellate ganglion) are similarly unlikely. In one series of 100 patients, using the anterior block of the divisions of the brachial plexus and a single 40-mL injection, the authors did, however, observe Horner's syndrome in four cases[37] but no clinical respiratory embarrassment. It is important to realize that the complications associated with blocks of the divisions are not necessarily also associated with blocks of the cords, Although both blocks being classified as infraclavicular blocks.

Pneumothorax

Pneumothorax has been associated with the anterior infraclavicular block of the divisions of the brachial plexus, the risk being approximately 0.2 to 0.7 percent.[38] An ultrasound study of the brachial plexus cords showed the shortest distance to the chest wall in a medial direction to be between 1.5 and 6 cm.[15] If a 100-mm needle is used and kept in the parasagittal plane and medial deviation is avoided, it is unlikely to reach the pleura, because anatomic studies show that the ribs and pleura are between 5 and 15 cm deeper than the nerve.

Other Complications

There is one case report of an obese patient who underwent a spontaneous shoulder dislocation while the anterior block of cords of brachial plexus for hand surgery was still in effect.[39] It was thought that there was probably unrecognized prior glenohumeral instability.

Intolerance to the Tourniquet following Infraclavicular Block

Upper arm tourniquets often cause discomfort of the medial aspect of the arm. Sensation in this part is mediated by the medial cutaneous nerve and the intercostobrachial nerve (T2 roots). These nerves are not included in the brachial plexus but they are easily blocked by subcutaneous injection of a local anesthetic agent across the medial aspect of the upper arm above the area where the tourniquet is to be applied.

▶ SPECIAL CONSIDERATIONS

Ultrasound and Infraclavicular Blocks (See Also Chap. 22)

It seems that the choice between ultrasonography and electrostimulation for infraclavicular blocks will depend on the decision to use a single injection outside the epineurium or multiple injections within the epineurium. These two approaches still lack formal comparison with respect to block quality; therefore no firm conclusions about their respective success rates, speed of onset, and outcomes can be drawn. However, the considered opinion of this author is that the best technique to locate the nerves may be a combination of nerve stimulation and ultrasound.

Single or Multiple Injections

Multiple-injection techniques offer faster onset in nerve blocks that are more complete and require smaller volumes of local anesthetic agent than single-injection infraclavicular blocks.[25] All studies of multiple injections indicate no increase in nerve or other tissue injuries. It seems that injuries to nonneural tissue all occur before the nerve is generally located. We recommend that all three cords be identified, if possible, and separately blocked. First, inject 20 mL of local anesthetic on the posterior cord, and then 10 mL on each of the other two cords. If one of the cords cannot be identified, then the remaining drug is injected on whichever cord is identified.

Infraclavicular Block in Children

This block should be encouraged for infants and children, in whom it is probably underutilized. De Jose et al. performed anterior infraclavicular blocks of the divisions of the brachial plexus (vertical infraclavicular block) on children.[40] They used a single-injection technique, accepted a motor response closest to the surgical field, and observed 4 percent Horner's syndromes but no other complications. All blocks were performed under general anesthesia, and in 25 percent of cases it took longer than 5 min to find the first motor nerve response. Two percent of cases showed evidence of block failure, but *all* cases had full analgesia on awakening after surgery.

We have performed the superior cord block on children and find it as easy as in adults, but with the difference that the cords are found more anteriorly than in adults.

REFERENCES

1. Raj PP. Infraclavicular brachial plexus block: A new approach. *Anesth Analg* 52:897–904, 1973.
2. Bazy L, Pauchet V, Labat GL (eds). *Anesthesie Regionale,* 3rd ed. France: Doin et Cie, 1921:222–225.
3. Boezaart AP. *Orthopaedic Regional Anesthesia.* DUD Iowa City, IA. 2004.
4. Kilka HG. Infraclavicular vertical brachial plexus blockade: A new method for anesthesia of the upper extremity: An anatomical and clinical study. *Anaesthetist* 44:339–344, 1995.
5. Heid FM. Transient respiratory compromise after infraclavicular vertical brachial plexus blockade. *Eur J Anaesth* 19:693–694, 2002.
6. Stadlmeyer W. Unilateral phrenic paralysis after vertical infraclavicular plexus blockade. *Anaesthetist* 49:1030–1033, 2000.
7. Gentili ME. Severe respiratory failure after infraclavicualr block with 0.75% ropivacaine: A case report. *J Clin Anesth* 14:459–461, 2002.
8. Greher M. Ultrasonographic assessment of topographic anatomy in volunteers suggest a modification of the infraclavicular vertical brachial plexus anatomy. *Br J Anesth* 88:632–636, 2002.
9. Stadlmeyer W. Unilateral phrenic paralysis after vertical infraclavicular plexus blockade. *Anaesthetist* 49:1030–1033, 2000.
10. Schupfer GK. Infraclavicular vertical plexus blockade: A safer alternative to the axillary approach? [letter] *Anesth Analg* 84:233, 1997.
11. Kilka HG. Infraclavicular vertical brachial plexus blockade. A new method for anesthesia of the upper extremity. An anatomical and clinical study. *Anaesthetist* 44:339–344, 1995.
12. Fitzgibbon DR. Selective musculocutaneous nerve block and infraclavicular brachial plexus blocks. *Reg Anesth* 20:239–241, 1995.
13. Borgeat A. An evaluation of the infraclavicular block via a modified approach of the infraclavicular brachial plexus block. *Reg Anesth Pain Med* 28:33–36, 2003.
14. Klaastadt O. A magnetic resonance imaging study of modifications to the infraclavicular brachial plexus block. *Anesth Analg* 91:929–933, 2000.
15. Whiffler K. Coracoid block: A safe and easy technique. *Br J Anesth* 53:845–848, 1981.
16. Wilson JL. Infraclavicular brachial plexus block: Parasagittal anatomy important to the coracoid technique. *Anesth Analg* 87:870–873, 1998.
17. Sims JK. A modification of landmarks for the infraclavicular approach to the brachial plexus block. *Anesth Analg* 56:554–555, 1998.
18. Krebs P. High continuous axillary–brachial plexus anesthesia: Comparison of new method with perivascular axillary–brachial plexus anesthesia. *Reg Anesth* 10:1–15, 1987.
19. Raw R. Workshop: Demonstration of 10 brachial plexus nerve block approaches. *Proceedings of the South African Society of Anaesthesia, National Annual Congress* February 2003.
20. Klaastadt O. A novel infraclavicular brachial plexus block: The lateral and sagittal technique developed by magnetic resonance imaging studies. *Anesth Analg* 98:252–256, 2004.
21. Sandring S (ed): *Gray's Anatomy,* 39th ed. New York: Elsevier.
22. Lo IK. Surgery about the coracoid: Neurovascular structures at risk. *Arthroscopy* 20:591–595, 2004.
23. Shu HS, Chantelot C, Oberlin C, et al. Martin-Gruber communicating branch: Anatomical and histological study. *Surg Radiol Anat* 21:115–118, 1992.
24. Thompson GE. Functional anatomy of the brachial plexus sheaths. *Anesthesiology* 59:117–122, 1983.
25. Fanelli G. Nerve stimulation and multiple injection techniques for upper and lower limb blockade: Failure rate, patient acceptance, and neurological complications. *Anesth Analg* 88:847–852, 1999.
26. Fitzgibbon DR. Selective musculocutaneous nerve block and infraclavicular brachial plexus blocks. *Reg Anesth* 20:239–241, 1995.
27. Eglseder WA. Anatomic variations of the musculocutaneous nerve of the arm. *Am J Orthop* 11:777–780, 1997.
28. Yang Z. The musculocutaneous nerve and its branches to the biceps and brachialis muscles. *J Hand Surg* 20A:671–675, 1995.
29. Borene S. At the chords, the pinkie towards interpreting infraclavicular motor response to neurostimulation. *Reg Anesth Pain Med* 29:125–129, 2004.
30. Wilson JL. Infraclavicular brachial plexus block: Parasagittal anatomy important to the coracoid technique. *Anesth Analg* 87:870–873, 1998.
31. Ilfeld BM. Infraclavicular perineural local anesthetic infusion: A comparison of three dosing regimens for postoperative analgesia. *Anesthesiology* 100:395–402, 2004.
32. Ilfeld BM. Continuous infraclavicular perineural infusion with clonidine and ropivacaine compared with ropivacaine alone: A randomised double blinded, controlled study. *Anesth Analg* 97:706–712, 2003.
33. Salazar CH. Infraclavicular brachial plexus block: Variation in approach and results of 360 cases. *Reg Anesth Pain Med* 24:411–416, 1999.
34. Jandard C. Infraclavicular block with lateral approach and nerve stimulation: Extent of anesthesia and adverse effects. *Reg Anesth Pain Med* 27:37–42, 2002.
35. Whiffler K. Coracoid block: A safe and easy technique. *Br J Anesth* 53:845–848, 1981.
36. Rodriguez J. Restricted infraclavicular distribution of the local anesthetic solution after infraclavicular brachial plexus block. *Reg Anesth Pain Med* 28:33–36, 2003.
37. Jandard C. Infraclavicular block with lateral approach and nerve stimulation: Extent of anesthesia and adverse effects. *Reg Anesth Pain Med* 27:37–42, 2002.
38. Neuberger M. Pneumothorax in vertical infraclavicular block of the brachial plexus: Review of a rare complication. *Anaesthetist* 49:901–904, 2000.
39. Rodriguez J. Shoulder dislocation after infraclavicular coracoid block. *Reg Anesth Pain Med* 28:351–353, 2003.
40. de Jose M. Vertical infraclavicular brachial plexus block in children: A preliminary study. *Paediatr Anaesth* 14:931–935, 2004.

CHAPTER 25

Nerve Blocks in the Axilla

ANDREW C. STEEL/WILLIAM HARROP-GRIFFITHS

▶ INTRODUCTION

"...this injection within the axilla is, to say the least, unsurgical, and is not to be recommended."

C. W. Allen, 1914

Brachial plexus nerve blockade was first described by Halsted in 1884. He exposed the roots of the brachial plexus in the neck surgically and, after freeing up the cords and peripheral nerves of the plexus, injected them under direct vision with a dilute solution of cocaine. This noticeably distended the roots and produced complete anesthesia of the upper extremity, allowing painless surgical intervention. Such a direct approach has met with an enthusiastic response from surgeons. In 1911, Hirschel described the first percutaneous technique for blocking the brachial plexus in the axilla. He made separate injections above and below the axillary artery with a four-inch needle directed into the apex of the axilla. He reported his success in three patients in the *Munich Medical Weekly* (this was well before the days of large, randomized, controlled studies). He advised that injection should be continued as the needle is advanced to ensure that "(blood) vessels are pushed aside to avoid entering them,"[1] a technique that many surgeons still seem to support today.

Hirschel's technique was based on an intimate knowledge of the anatomy of the axilla that he had gained from the performance of large numbers of mastectomies. Despite his report of a larger series of successful cases the following year, the technique was not widely accepted or favorably received by his peers. Allen wrote of the technique in 1914 that "it is far better, safer, and surer, as well as quite simple, to resort to the free exposure of the plexus above the clavicle and injection of each individual nerve by the intraneural method." Allen went

on to say "this injection within the axilla is, to say the least, unsurgical, and is not to be recommended."[2]

As so often happens, innovations that are rejected initially become widely embraced as new developments and experience win over skeptics. Over the next 50 years, many important contributions made the axillary brachial plexus block into the well-recognized technique of today.[3–9] We will mention but a few:

1921

Reding first reported that the nerves were "gathered into a bundle and surrounded by a common fascial sheath which contains and directs the course of the anesthetic solution."[3] He also demonstrated that the musculocutaneous nerve leaves the bundle at a higher level and therefore must be blocked separately.

1922

Labat suggested that to inject or even have a syringe of anesthetic attached to an advancing needle was dangerous and advocated aspiration tests before injecting.[4]

1949

Accardo and Adriani suggested that eliciting paresthesia in the distribution area of the four nerves to be blocked was essential before injecting in order to guarantee success.[5]

1961–1965

De Jong dissected many cadavers; from the average diameter of the sheath and assuming an even spread of anesthetic agent from injection site, he calculated that the average adult male would require 42 mL of anesthetic solution for a successful block.[6] De Jong later modified his technique by injecting a smaller volume (20 to 25 mL) into the sheath and 5 mL at the biceps tendon to block the musculocutaneous nerve separately.

1962

Eriksson[7] introduced the use of a tourniquet placed below the point of injection, believing that it would prevent distal spread of the local anesthetic solution from the desired site of action. This appears not to be the case anatomically, since Winnie showed that a tourniquet does not compress the sheath. Indeed, a finger pressing distally to the injection site is more efficient and better tolerated by the patient than a tourniquet.

1990s

Recent years have seen the axillary brachial plexus block develop beyond a single injection of local anesthetic high up in the axilla, with multiple injection techniques being advocated not only in the axilla but also lower down the humerus—the "midhumeral" technique. Notwithstanding claims of shorter onset times and higher success rates for these newer approaches, the single-injection technique remains much used.

The axillary brachial plexus block remains popular and is probably the most commonly used brachial plexus block in the world. This is not due to its rapid onset and high success rate, because they do not always compare favorably with those of other brachial plexus blocks, but because of its simplicity and safety. Its simplicity derives from the easily located landmark for injection: the arterial pulsation in the axilla. Its safety relates to the fact that of all the true brachial plexus blocks, it is the most remote from the pleura, the great vessels, and the neuraxis. The incidence of life-threatening complications should therefore be the lowest.

▶ APPLIED ANATOMY

"...in anatomy it is better to have learned and lost, than never to have learned at all."

W. Somerset Maugham

Although a detailed knowledge of the anatomy of the axilla is not absolutely essential for the safe and effective performance of the block, it is certainly no hindrance and should be gained. Those averse to detailed anatomic description may bypass it and go to the paragraph at the end of this section.

▶ GROSS ANATOMY

The brachial plexus enters the axilla as the lateral, medial, and posterior cords (Fig. 25-1). The axilla is a fat-filled pyramidal cavity between the upper thorax and the arm. It has an apex, a base, and four "walls"—lateral, medial, anterior and posterior. The apex of the axilla projects into the neck as the cervicoaxillary canal, through which the axillary blood vessels and brachial plexus cords pass. The first rib, the superior border of the scapula, the posterior border of the clavicle, and the medial aspect of the coracoid process form this canal. The base of the axilla is formed by the skin and axillary fascia between pectoralis major and latissimus dorsi muscles. It is convex, thus conforming to the shape of the armpit, and narrows from the lateral wall of the chest into the arm.

The anterior and posterior walls are easily palpable between forefinger and thumb. The anterior wall is formed by the pectoralis muscles, with a small contribution at the superior part by the covering of the clavipectoral fascia. The posterior wall is slightly lower than the anterior and is formed mainly by teres major muscle, with subscapularis above and latissimus dorsi below. The anterior and posterior walls converge laterally onto the palpable humeral intertubercular sulcus, the narrow lateral wall. The medial wall is formed by the first four ribs and their respective intercostal muscles and the upper part of the serratus anterior muscle.

The axilla contains the axillary vessels, the infraclavicular part of the brachial plexus and its branches, lateral branches of some intercostal nerves, many lymph nodes and vessels, loose adipose tissue, and often the "tail" of the breast. The axillary artery is a continuation of the subclavian artery and represents that part of the vessel between the outer border of the first rib and the inferior border of the teres major muscle, where its name changes from axillary artery to brachial artery. It is important to note that its direction changes with the position of the arm: it is almost straight when the arm is in abduction at 90 degrees and becomes more concave as the arm is raised or convex as the arm is lowered alongside the chest. The axillary vein, like the artery, is defined superiorly by the first rib and clavicle. Above the first rib, the subclavian vein does not lie within the neurovascular bundle as it is forming between the scalene muscles but rather is separated from the artery by the insertion of the anterior scalene muscle. However, as it passes over the first rib and under the clavicle, the subclavian vein in becoming the axillary vein does join the neurovascular bundle. Thus, parts of the plexus are sandwiched between artery and vein.

The passage of the subclavian artery under the clavicle, becoming the axillary artery, sees a significant change in the relationship between the artery and the brachial plexus. While the subclavian artery lies anterior and close to the trunks of the plexus and distal to the clavicle, the axillary artery lies more central to the three cords of the plexus. The first part of the artery is medial to the lateral and posterior cords and anterior to the medial cord. En route to the distal axilla, the cords rotate

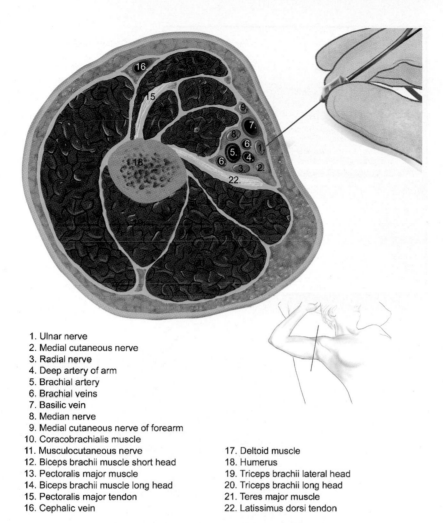

1. Ulnar nerve
2. Medial cutaneous nerve
3. Radial nerve
4. Deep artery of arm
5. Brachial artery
6. Brachial veins
7. Basilic vein
8. Median nerve
9. Medial cutaneous nerve of forearm
10. Coracobrachialis muscle
11. Musculocutaneous nerve
12. Biceps brachii muscle short head
13. Pectoralis major muscle
14. Biceps brachii muscle long head
15. Pectoralis major tendon
16. Cephalic vein

17. Deltoid muscle
18. Humerus
19. Triceps brachii lateral head
20. Triceps brachii long head
21. Teres major muscle
22. Latissimus dorsi tendon

Figure 25-1. Cross section through axilla.

around the artery, and as they pass behind the pectoralis minor muscle, their positions become truly medial, lateral, and posterior, as their names suggest.

Around the lateral edge of the pectoralis minor muscle the cords give rise to the terminal nerves of the plexus. It is only the median, radial, ulnar, and medial antebrachial cutaneous nerves that will continue with the artery and vein within the axillary sheath. The musculocutaneous and axillary nerves, two of the major terminal nerves, are not in the sheath at this level. They have left under cover of the pectoralis minor muscle at the level of the coracoid process. The musculocutaneous nerve enters the coracobrachialis muscle and continues down the arm within it (essentially parallel to the sheath). The axillary nerve leaves the sheath almost immediately after arising from the posterior cord.

Detailed anatomic description aside, the nub of it is that at the level at which the block is usually performed (approximately at the lateral border of pectoralis major), three nerves (median, ulnar, and radial) lie within the conceptual brachial plexus sheath along with the axillary

artery and the axillary vein (Fig. 25-1). The fourth "target nerve" of the axillary brachial plexus block, the musculocutaneous nerve, lies outside the sheath in the body of the coracobrachialis muscle.

▶ SURFACE ANATOMY

The landmarks for the axillary brachial plexus block are easily identified (Fig. 25-2). With the patient positioned supine, the upper arm externally rotated and abducted to 90 degrees, and the elbow flexed to 90 degrees, the following can be palpated to assist placement of the stimulating needle:

The groove between biceps brachialis and coracobrachialis muscles in front and the triceps muscle behind
The inferior border of the pectoralis major muscle
The pulsation of the axillary artery felt against the humerus

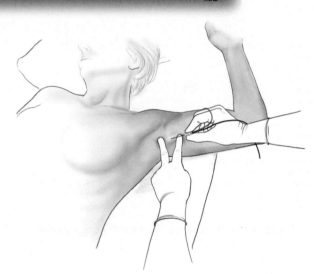

1. Deltoid muscle
2. Pectoralis major muscle
3. Pectoralis minor muscle
4. Latissimus dorsi muscle
5. Ulnar nerve
6. Brachial artery
7. Medial cutaneous nerve
8. Median nerve
9. Coracobrachialis muscle
10. Biceps muscle
11. Triceps muscle

Figure 25-2. Surface anatomy and positioning for axillary block.

The most difficult of these three is the palpation of the arterial pulse. Although anesthesiologists would like to think that they can palpate the pulse readily in almost all their patients, an inability to feel the pulse is quite common. In such cases, the use of the first two landmarks above, along with a little experience and luck, usually suffices to take the needle reasonably close to the nerves of the brachial plexus.

The patient position outlined above is thought to optimize the position of the axillary artery. Some texts recommend that the patient's hand be placed behind the head. Although this is a convenient position, the overabduction of the humerus that this involves may cause the head of the humerus to distort the axillary sheath and thereby impair proximal spread of the injected local anesthetic.

Anesthesiologists attempting the block should be aware that in a small number of patients the coracoid

head of the pectoralis major muscle might be congenitally absent. The groove normally formed with the coracobrachialis muscle will therefore also be absent, and the operator will have to rely on the palpation of the axillary pulse to position the nerve stimulator.

▶ FUNCTIONAL ANATOMY

A successful axillary brachial plexus block will provide excellent anesthesia and analgesia for the forearm and hand as well as anesthesia for the majority of operations on the elbow. However, it is of little use for operations on the upper arm and shoulder. Note that the skin underlying upper arm tourniquets will not be blocked with this approach; therefore other steps should be taken to ensure patient comfort if a tourniquet is used and the patient is to remain awake. Local anesthetic for the skin under the tourniquet is one option, as is the use of a forearm tourniquet for wrist and hand surgery; there is little argument against this apart from unfamiliarity with the technique.

In 1927, Labat proposed that the reason why brachial plexus blocks may often give patchy and delayed anesthesia in one or more nerves could be found in an appreciation of what he called the "minute anatomy."[4] Investigations using cadavers, ultrasound, computed tomography, and magnetic resonance imaging have furthered our understanding of the functional anatomy of the brachial plexus and axilla. We can now improve our techniques through a better understanding of where needles should be positioned and where the anesthetic agent is working.

The traditional view of the relationship between the three nerves and the axillary artery in the axillary sheath was simplicity itself: the median nerve lies anterior to the artery, the radial nerve posterior, and the ulnar nerve medial to the artery. Clinical practice suggests that these relationships are not always as constant as we would wish them to be. There is considerable variation in the anatomy. For example, at the usual level of an axillary block approach, the ulnar nerve has been found in the posteromedial position in 59 percent of volunteers scanned with ultrasound.[10] The radial nerve was found to be posterolateral in 38 percent and anterolateral in 20 percent, the median nerve to be anteromedial in 30 percent and posteromedial in 26 percent. It was also found that application of light pressure distally, a consistent maneuver in the technique, displaces nerves laterally, especially when they are positioned anterior to the axillary artery. There is also increasing evidence that the main nerves may be extensively subdivided in the axilla and that multiple axillary veins are not uncommon.

There is much discussion about the distribution of local anesthetic in the axillary sheath and, in particular, about whether it is free or limited when the blocks are performed. Thompson and Rorie found that fascial compartments exist for each nerve of the plexus and that these barriers limit circumferential (cross-sectional) spread of local anesthetic solutions.[11] Winnie et al. and Partridge et al. questioned the importance of these compartments and were proponents of the single-injection technique.[12,13] On the basis of studies with magnetic resonance imaging, Klaastad disagreed with Winnie and Partridge, concluding that distribution patterns correlated well with clinical effect and that there was not complete, uninhibited cross-sectional spread around the artery. Therefore a multiple-injection technique was necessary to ensure a successful block.[14] It is research of this sort, using increasingly detailed imaging techniques, that is driving the move toward multiple-injection techniques.

▶ PATIENT SELECTION

Indications

The block, as described above, is principally indicated for surgical procedures on the elbow, forearm, and hand. It is suitable for patients of all ages, having been used successfully in both neonates and the very elderly.[15] It can be used for elective, emergency, and trauma patients and is occasionally used to achieve analgesia in the field by first providers. Axillary approaches to the brachial plexus blockade have been well described and are well received in day surgery and ambulatory care patients.[16] The axillary approach is the lowest true brachial plexus block and has the lowest incidence of pneumothorax and phrenic nerve block. It is therefore popular for patients in whom these complications would be particularly undesirable or dangerous.

Contraindications

Axillary brachial plexus blockade shares common contraindications with most other peripheral nerve blocks, such as patient refusal and significant local sepsis. The technique is without doubt associated with a high incidence of arterial puncture and should perhaps be avoided in patients with coagulopathy. However, if a brachial plexus block is still deemed advantageous and if puncture occurs and a hematoma develops, the axillary artery can be directly compressed against a bone. Whether to perform an axillary brachial plexus block on a patient with coagulopathy should nevertheless be decided by an experienced clinician on an individual basis.

Patient Positioning

The best position for the ideal patient is described above and is illustrated in Fig. 25-2. Unfortunately, many patients do not conform to the ideal, but minor modifications in positioning can be made. Patients who find it hard to lie flat can be sat up to a moderate degree provided that the position of the arm can be maintained. Patients who find it hard to abduct their arms, as a result of arthritis or the pain of trauma, may not be suitable for an axillary brachial plexus block. Rather than struggle to perform a block in a patient whose arm is only slightly abducted, it may be wise to consider a brachial plexus block that is low in the plexus but does not require arm abduction, such as the coracoid approach to the brachial plexus.

▶ PROCEDURE

"Any technique which results in a good block without injury to the patient is a good technique."

D. Selander, 1987

After acquiring informed patient consent, gaining intravenous access, and after placing appropriate monitors, the block should be performed in a safe environment with the assistance of a trained assistant. The following equipment should be available:

25- or 50-mm block needle (insulated if a nerve stimulator is being used)

Local anesthetic for the skin, with syringe and 25-gauge needle

Two (or three) 20-mL syringes of local anesthetic mixture

Peripheral nerve stimulator or ultrasound device for nerve location

Sterile procedure pack, including gloves

The following description is of the performance of an axillary block using a peripheral nerve stimulator. Anesthesiologists using ultrasound nerve location will have to modify the technique. The anesthesiologist should sit or stand at the side of the patient. The authors favor the sitting position for performing peripheral nerve blocks in order to maintain as stable a base as possible in performing the injection. Palpate the landmarks and mark the position of the axillary artery if desired. Clean the skin with an antiseptic and place drapes as desired. Infiltrate local anesthetic over the axillary artery as high as reasonably possible in the axilla. Having given time for this to work, place the index and middle fingers of the nondominant hand over the artery just below the point of the insertion of the local anesthetic. Holding the block needle in the dominant hand, insert it just anterior or posterior to (above or below) the axillary artery.

There appear to be two schools of thought about the angle that the needle should make with the brachial plexus. Some anesthesiologists favor a near 90-degree angle (Fig. 25-1), while others try to align the needle with the long axis of the plexus (Fig. 25-2). Either is appropriate for a single-injection technique. However, we would argue that when the needle and plexus are aligned as much as is possible, plexus catheterization will be aided when continuous techniques are planned.

With an initial stimulating current of 1.0 mA and a stimulus duration of 0.1 ms, advance the needle. On a good day, you will be immediately rewarded with evoked contractions of muscles supplied by the target nerve. On a bad day, you may have to persist for some minutes before succeeding in identifying this endpoint. Table 25-1 provides an aide memoire for evoked contractions. The endpoint for nerve location is taken to be evoked contractions at a threshold current <0.5 mA. Thresholds <0.2 mA are thought to be associated with a high incidence of intrafascicular injection and should therefore be avoided.

Single-Injection Technique

Once an evoked contraction in one of the muscles supplied by one of the three nerves (ulnar, median, radial) within the axillary sheath is produced, the anesthesiologist should aspirate with the syringe to exclude intravascular needle placement. Pressure can then be exerted by the fingers of the nondominant hand on the sheath below the point of injection. It is important that aspiration precede pressure on the sheath, as the axillary vein may be collapsed by the pressure, so that no blood is aspirated in spite of intravenous placement. The first 1 mL of local anesthetic injection should be easy and painless and should lead to the disappearance of the evoked contractions. If these three criteria are not fulfilled, the injection should not proceed, the needle should be withdrawn, and the block should start all over again. If the criteria are fulfilled, the whole volume of local anesthetic should now be injected slowly and in incremental volumes while aspirating frequently and observing both the patient and the monitoring devices carefully.

Multiple-Injection Technique

The present authors favor the following approach. The needle is initially placed so as to go just above (anterior to) the artery in order to identify the median nerve. When contractions evoked by median nerve stimulation are produced at a current <0.5 mA, 10 mL of the local

▶ **TABLE 25-1.** AIDE MEMOIRE FOR NERVE STIMULATION

Nerve	Spinal Segments	Usual Sensory Distribution	Motor Distribution
Radial	C5–T1	Posterolateral surface of the arm, dorsum of hand and thumb	Extension of the arm (triceps), forearm (brachioradialis), wrist and digits, thumb abduction
Median	C6–T1	Anterolateral surface of the hand, dorsal tips of second, third, and half of fourth digits	Flexion of the forearm and digits; pronation
Ulnar	C8–T1	Medial surface of the hand, anterior and posterior	Contraction of flexor carpi ulnaris and thumb adduction
Musculocutaneous	C5–C7	Lateral surface of the forearm	Flexion of the arm at the elbow (biceps)

anesthetic solution is injected after negative aspiration. The needle is then withdrawn almost to the skin and is redirected so as to go just below (posterior to) the artery. Stimulation of the radial nerve is then sought and a further 10 mL of local anesthetic solution is injected. After this, the needle is manipulated so that it is placed behind (lateral to) the artery, and the ulnar nerve is located; a further 10 mL of local anesthetic injected. It is as easy as that—occasionally. In practice, the median nerve is usually easy to identify above the artery, but things often get more difficult when one is seeking the radial and ulnar nerves. As described above, their positions are very variable, and one nerve is often found when the other is being sought. It is common to experience difficulty in identifying one of these nerves when the other has already been found and blocked. It is reasonable to persist with attempts at identifying the target, but these attempts sometimes go unrewarded.

Other Techniques

Many clinicians still rely on more traditional techniques for axillary brachial plexus block. The use of paresthesia to identify correct needle placement is still acceptable practice in most countries and, in experienced hands, is associated with a high success rate and a low complication rate. Similarly, arterial transfixion or the "transarterial" technique has its proponents. In this technique, the artery is deliberately punctured with a needle and the needle is passed through the artery until no blood emerges from the needle. After negative aspiration, local anesthetic is injected; it is thereby deposited posterior to the artery but within the conceptual brachial plexus sheath. The needle is then withdrawn to a position just anterior to the artery and the remainder of the local anesthetic is injected. This deposition of local anesthetic "either side" of the artery can be associated with a high success rate. Deliberate arterial trauma does not appeal to many anesthesiologists, but the proponents of the transarterial technique point to the very low complication rate associated with axillary artery puncture.

Anesthesiologists who practice the multiple-injection technique should admit that they occasionally practice the "inadvertent transarterial technique"; the present authors certainly do. If having successfully identified, for instance, the median and the ulnar nerves and while searching for the radial nerve the artery is accidentally entered, it seems silly not to use the anatomic knowledge that the artery lies in close relation to the radial nerve. Local anesthetic injected behind the artery will usually block it, and it is often preferable to persist in attempts to find the nerve.

At the time of writing, the use of ultrasound imaging to perform axillary brachial plexus blocks is relatively new. However, there are already proficient performers of this technique who argue rationally that it offers effective visualization of the anatomy of the brachial plexus, the placement of the needle, and the distribution of the local anesthetic. Review articles are already emerging claiming that ultrasound techniques increase success rate, decrease onset time, decrease local anesthetic volumes, and increase safety.[17] Only time will tell whether these claims are valid.[18]

The Musculocutaneous Nerve

The musculocutaneous nerve lies outside the brachial plexus sheath in the axilla and, although it is possible to block this nerve by injecting large volumes (up to 60 mL) as a single injection of local anesthetic into the axillary sheath, separate block of the nerve is usually recommended. Blind injection of local anesthetic into the body of the coracobrachialis muscle anterior to the axillary artery may succeed, but it is easy to identify the nerve more accurately with a nerve stimulator, aiming to evoke contractions of the biceps muscle.

The Second Thoracic Dermatome

It is an inconvenience that the skin of the upper inner arm is not usually supplied by a nerve that forms part of the brachial plexus. This is particularly so because upper arm tourniquets can cause pain in this area when they have been in place for some time. Before leaping forward to block T2 (the second thoracic root), it is worth considering whether the surgery can be performed with a forearm tourniquet; many wrist and hand procedures are amenable to this, and it places the tourniquet in the distribution area of an axillary brachial plexus block. If this is not possible, local anesthetic injected subcutaneously over the axillary artery is said to be effective, although we favor a subcutaneous line of local anesthetic extending across the medial side of the arm high up in the axilla.

Choice of Technique

The clinician's own experience should guide him or her as to the choice of technique. However, when a nerve stimulator technique is used, there is sufficient evidence that twitch responses evoked by stimulation of the musculocutaneous and one of the median, radial, or ulnar nerves will provide the greatest chance of a successful block. In addition, this technique may cause the fewest adverse events and will not increase either the time required for the procedure or the onset of the block.[19–24] Clinicians will be guided by the success rates they achieve while trying out different approaches. Success may be defined objectively with scoring systems such as that suggested by Vester-Andersen.[25] However, simply put, complete success is the performance of a surgical procedure without anesthetic supplementation. Partial success requires supplementation, such as elbow nerve blocks or sedation, while complete failure usually necessitates conversion to general anesthesia.

► CATHETER PLACEMENT AND FIXATION

Continuous brachial plexus anesthesia was first described in 1946, but its popularity awaited the development of reliable plastic cannulas and catheters some 30 years later. The principal benefits to the patient from the placement of a catheter into the axillary sheath are the provision of excellent analgesia that can be prolonged for days or the possibility of administering repeated anesthetic doses without repeated needle insertions. The benefit to the anesthesiologist is that there are few complications and it is possible to align the inserting needle with the brachial plexus, thus facilitating catheter insertion (Fig. 25-2). Equipment designed for nerve catheter placement can be used, although catheters through which the nerves can be stimulated ("stimulating catheters") offer theoretical advantages in that the correct catheter position can be confirmed once the catheter is placed. The brachial plexus sheath at this level (axilla and perhaps at any level) is a concept more than a reality, and if a needle is "correctly" positioned as judged by nerve stimulation, it does not guarantee that the catheter passed several centimeters through it has been directed to the correct position. It is important to note that if a stimulating catheter is to be used, local anesthetic should not be injected down the introducing needle to initiate the nerve block, as this will impair the electrical function of the catheter.[26]

The placement of axillary brachial plexus catheters differs little in equipment or concept from the placement of other nerve plexus catheters. However, axillary brachial plexus catheters are prone to dislodgment, in large part because of the mobility of the skin in the axilla when the patient moves the arm. We have used a variety of sutures, adhesive tape, and biooclusive dressings to secure axillary catheters and prevent their dislodgment. We have decided that the best way of

avoiding accidental displacement of the catheter is by tunneling it subcutaneously to an area where the skin is not so mobile. This can be either distally down the arm on its medial or anterior aspect, provided that this does not interfere with a tourniquet, or anteriorly and superiorly to the skin over the anterior deltoid muscle.

► PHARMACOLOGIC CHOICE

Large volumes of local anesthetic are often used in performing axillary brachial plexus blocks, either as a single injection or particularly in performing multiple injections. It is often recommended that 40 mL, and up to 60 mL, of local anesthetic solution be injected. The anesthesiologist therefore must make sure that the total amount of local anesthetic drug does not exceed the accepted maximum dose for that particular patient, taking into account the patient's weight, age, and overall physical condition. The choice of local anesthetic will affect the onset and duration of the block, as will the addition of adjuncts such as epinephrine and sodium bicarbonate. Table 25-2 encapsulates the authors' experience.

► POTENTIAL PROBLEMS

"When there are problems with any regional technique, look for the cause first on the proximal end of the needle."

A.P. Winnie, 1983

Anesthesia-related nerve injury accounts for up to 16 percent of the total claims in the American Society of Anesthesiologists Closed Claims database. Of these, 19 percent involved the brachial plexus and only 9 percent of brachial plexus injuries were attributed to regional anesthetic techniques at the axilla.[26] Significant complications of the axillary approach are relatively rare, in large part because of the distance of the axilla from the pleura and the great vessels. Although the axillary approach shares several "generic" potential complications with all other nerve blocks, the following particular points are worthy of note.

TABLE 25-2. DRUGS AND DOSES FOR AXILLARY BRACHIAL PLEXUS BLOCK

Drug	Approximate Onset Time (min)	Approximate Block Duration (h)
Mepivacaine 1% (+epinephrine)	10–20	3–4
Lidocaine 1.5% (+epinephrine)	10–20	4–6
Ropivacaine 0.5%	20–25	6–8
Bupivacaine 0.375%	30–40	10–14
Levobupivacaine 0.375%	30–40	10–14

Infection

Although reports of significant infections resulting from axillary brachial plexus blocks are rare, the armpit is not a clean area and it behooves the anesthesiologist to attempt as aseptic a technique as possible. It is well worth resisting the temptation to shave the patient's armpit, as this may increase the risk of infection.

Vascular Complications

Arterial puncture is a sine qua non of the transarterial technique and is common with other single- and particularly multiple-injection techniques. The overall risk of the formation of a significant hematoma is small (up to 0.02 percent),[27] but most are inconsequential. However, hematomas may be implicated in the development of postoperative paresthesia and nerve injuries. The development of significant hematomas is much more likely in patients with coagulation abnormalities, so these disorders should be considered relative contraindications. Vascular injury is also rare but potentially dangerous. Transient vascular insufficiency occurs in up to 1 percent of patients,[28] resulting from vasospasm after arterial puncture or local anesthetic-induced vasoconstriction. Pseudoaneurysm formation and axillary artery dissection are other rare complications of brachial plexus blocks at the axilla.

Local Anesthetic Toxicity

Intravascular injection of local anesthetic was found to occur in 0.2 percent of patients undergoing transarterial axillary block in one study,[28] even with aspiration before injecting. As mentioned above, the vascular anatomy of the axillary sheath is variable and a number of blood vessels may exist within it. Large volumes of local anesthetic are often used; total drug doses may therefore approach the safe acceptable maximum. The frequency of seizures after the axillary approach to the brachial plexus is 1.2 to 1.3 per 1000 patients[29] (the numbers are 7.6 for interscalene and 7.9 for supraclavicular approaches). The risk of seizure after intravascular injection in brachial plexus anesthesia is exceeded only by that after caudal anesthesia.

Nerve Injury

The axillary approach to the brachial plexus does not seem to be associated with a significantly higher or lower incidence of short- or long-term nerve damage (see Chap. 32). Concerns that multiple injection techniques may be associated with a higher incidence of nerve damage have not yet been conclusively borne out by published data.[30] Hebl et al. evaluated the safety of regional versus general anesthesia in patients with preexisting ulnar neuropathy who had undergone ulnar nerve transposition. Their retrospective study included 360 patients, of whom 28 percent had surgery with an axillary block and the remainder general anesthesia alone. They found that although regional anesthesia techniques may theoretically place patients at an increased risk of neural damage, this did not seem to worsen neurologic outcome in ulnar transposition under axillary blockade. It is worth noting that only 10.1 percent of patients in the study received axillary blockade with a nerve stimulator technique. Hebl concluded that peripheral neuropathy should not be considered a contraindication to axillary block.[31]

▶ SPECIAL CONSIDERATIONS

The concentration focused on proximal brachial plexus blocks by the publication of an increasingly large number of new approaches may give the impression that the old and humble axillary brachial plexus block is an archaic technique. Nothing could be further from the truth. Its simplicity, safety, and enviable track record make it enduringly popular for novices and experts alike. If it suffers from anything, it is from familiarity and adverse publicity. Many claim that it has a slow onset and a high failure rate. Multiple-injection techniques and the use of ultrasound may increase onset time or, at the very least, may appear to increase onset time, as both may well take longer to perform than single-injection techniques. Success rates can be as high as 98.4 percent in experienced hands,[32] which compares favorably those any other brachial plexus blocks. In addition to all this, the axillary approach is an ideal technique whereby residents can learn the fundamentals of the safe practice of regional anesthesia. Although we have enjoyed many hours trying out new brachial plexus blocks, we always return to the axillary approach when safety, reliability, and a numb hand or forearm are sought.

REFERENCES

1. Hirschel G. Anesthesia of the brachial plexus for operations on the upper extremity [German]. *Münch Med Wochenschr* 58:1555–1556, 1911.
2. Allen CW. *Local and Regional Anaesthesia*. Philadelphia: Saunders, 1918:224–225.
3. Reding M. A new method of anesthesia for the upper extremity [French]. *Presse Med* 29:294–296, 1921.
4. Labat G. Brachial plexus block: Some details of the technique. *Anesth Analg* 6:81–82, 1927.
5. Accardo NJ, Adriani J. Brachial plexus block: A simplified technique using the axillary route. *South Med J* 42:420–923, 1949.
6. De Jong RH. Axillary block of the brachial plexus. *Anesthesiology* 22:215–225, 1961.
7. Eriksson E, Skarby HG. A simplified method of axillary block [Swedish]. *Nord Med* 68:1325, 1962.

8. Brand L, Pepper EM. A comparison of supraclavicular and axillary techniques for brachial plexus blocks. *Anesthesiology* 22:226–229, 1961.

9. Burnham PJ. Regional block of the great nerves of the upper arm. *Anesthesiology* 19:281–284, 1958.

10. Retzl G, Kapral S, Greher M, et al. Ultrasonic findings of the axillary part of the brachial plexus. *Anesth Analg* 92:1271–1275, 2001.

11. Thompson GE, Rorie DL. Functional anatomy of the brachial plexus sheaths. *Anesthesiology* 59:117–122, 1983.

12. Winnie AP, Radonjic R, Akkineni SR, et al. Factors influencing distribution of local anesthetic injected into the brachial plexus sheath. *Anesth Analg* 58:225–234, 1979.

13. Partridge BL, Katz J, Bernischke K. Functional anatomy of the brachial plexus sheath: Implications for anesthesia. *Anesthesiology* 66:743–747, 1987.

14. Klaastad O, Smedby O, Thompson GE, et al. Distribution of local anaesthetic in axillary brachial plexus block: A clinical and magnetic resonance imaging study. *Anesthesiology* 96:1315–1324, 2002.

15. Pignotti MS, Messeri A, Calamandrei M, et al. Percutaneous catheterization of the newborn: Control of pain and easy insertion with brachial plexus block. *Acta Biomed L'Ateneo Parmense* 71:641–645, 2000.

16. Koscielniak-Nielsen ZJ, Rotboll-Nielsen P, Rassmussen H. Patient's experience with multiple stimulation axillary block for fast-track ambulatory hand surgery. *Acta Anaesth Scand* 46:789–793, 2002.

17. Marhofer P, Greher M, Kapral S. Ultrasound guidance in regional anaesthesia. *Br J Anaesth* 94:7–17, 2004.

18. Denny NM, Harrop-Griffiths W. Location, location, location! Ultrasound imaging in regional anesthesia. *Br J Anaesth* 94:1–3, 2004.

19. Lavoie J, Martin R, Tetrault JP, et al. Axillary plexus block using a peripheral nerve stimulator: Single or multiple injections. *Can J Anaesth* 39:583–586, 1992.

20. Inberg P, Annila I, Annila P. Double injection method using peripheral nerve stimulator is superior to single injection in axillary plexus block. *Reg Anesth Pain Med* 24:509–513, 1999.

21. Hickey R, Hoffman J, Tingle L, et al. Comparison of the clinical efficacy of three perivascular techniques for axillary brachial plexus block. *Reg Anesth Pain Med* 18: 335–338, 1983.

22. Sia S, Lepri A, Ponzecchi P. Axillary brachial plexus block using peripheral nerve stimulator: A comparison between double- and triple-injection techniques. *Reg Anesth Pain Med* 26:499–503, 2001.

23. Koscielniak-Nielsen ZJ, Rotball Nielsen P, Sorensen T, et al. Low dose axillary block by targeted injections of the terminal nerves. *Can J Anaesth* 46:658–664, 1999.

24. Carre P, Joly A, Cluziel Field B, et al. Axillary block in children: Single or multiple injection? *Paediatric Anaesthesia* 10:35–39, 2000.

25. Vester-Andersen T, Eriksen C, Christiansen C. Perivascular axillary block III: Blockade following 40 mL of 0.5%, 1%, or 1.5% mepivacaine with adrenaline. *Acta Anaesth Scand* 28:95–98, 1984.

26. Harrop-Griffiths W. Peripheral nerve catheter techniques. *Anaesth Intens Care Med* 4:124, 2004.

27. Cheney FW, Domino KB, Caplan RA, et al. Nerve injury associated with anaesthesia: A closed claims analysis. *Anesthesiology* 90:1062–1069, 1999.

28. Stan TC, Krantz MA, Solomon DL, et al. The incidence of neurovascular complications following axillary brachial plexus block, using transarterial approach. *Reg Anesth Pain Med* 20:486–492, 1995.

29. Carles M, Pulchini A, Macchi P, et al. An evaluation of the brachial plexus block at the humeral canal using a nerve stimulator (1417 patients): Rhe efficacy, safety, and predictive criteria of failure. *Anesth Analg* 92:194–198, 2001.

30. Auroy Y, Benhamou D, Bargues L, et al. Major complications of regional anesthesia in France. *Anesthesiology* 97:1274–1280, 2002.

31. Hebl JR, Horlocker TT, Sorenson EJ, et al. Regional anesthesia does not increase the risk of postoperative neuropathy in patients undergoing ulnar nerve transposition. *Anesth Analg* 93:1606–1611, 2001.

32. Perris TM, Watt JM. The road to success: A review of 1000 axillary brachial plexus blocks. *Anaesthesia* 58:1220–1224, 2003.

CHAPTER 26

Femoral Nerve Block

FRANCIS V. SALINAS

▶ INTRODUCTION

Femoral nerve block is the most widely used and successful peripheral nerve block for the lower extremities. It can be used as the sole anesthetic for superficial and deep soft tissue procedures in the mid- to lower anterior thigh region (such as muscle biopsy or patellar tendon repair). However, owing to the multiplicity and divergence of the lumbosacral plexus, major orthopaedic surgical procedures involving the lower extremity (hip joint, femur, knee joint, and ankle joint) almost always require simultaneous blockade of the obturator, lateral femoral cutaneous, and sciatic nerves to provide complete unilateral lower extremity anesthesia.

There has been a desire to achieve simultaneous blockade of all three major branches of the lumbar plexus (femoral, lateral femoral cutaneous, and obturator nerves) with a single-injection technique. Although the posterior paravertebral approach to the lumbar plexus (psoas compartment block) has been shown to consistently block all three nerves, clinical and radiographic studies have shown that anterior approaches to the lumbar plexus (inguinal paravascular three-in-one block or the fascia iliaca compartment block) block only the femoral and lateral femoral cutaneous nerves consistently.[1] Despite the obvious "anatomic advantage" of the psoas compartment block, there is an increased potential for serious complications (local anesthetic toxicity, unintended high central neuraxial blockade, and retroperitoneal hematoma). Clinical studies have demonstrated that a femoral nerve block is the key to providing effective analgesia after major knee surgery.[2,3]

▶ INDICATIONS

Although femoral nerve blocks have been shown to provide effective postoperative analgesia after major hip and femur surgery, their most useful and widely utilized clinical application has been for major knee surgery (Table 26-1). Single-injection femoral nerve blocks have been consistently shown to provide excellent analgesia for 12 to 24 h after total knee arthroplasty or knee ligament reconstruction.[4,5] The increasing use of continuous peripheral nerve blocks has greatly increased the flexibility and indications for femoral nerve blocks by extending the duration of site-specific postoperative analgesia for several days after surgery. Significant improvements in postoperative analgesia, quality of recovery, and functional recovery after total knee arthroplasty has been associated with the use of continuous femoral nerve blocks.[6,7] Additionally, the increased risk of spinal/epidural hematoma associated with central neuraxial techniques in the setting of systemic anticoagulation has decreased the applicability of continuous lumbar epidural analgesia after major knee surgery. The important role of continuous femoral block in major knee surgery is therefore increasingly realized.

▶ FEMORAL NERVE BLOCK ANATOMY

Gross Anatomy

The femoral nerve is the largest terminal branch of the lumbar plexus and originates in the dorsal divisions of the primary ventral rami of the second, third, and fourth lumbar nerve roots. The lumbar plexus is formed by the

▶ **TABLE 26-1.** INDICATIONS FOR FEMORAL NERVE BLOCK

Single-injection and continuous femoral nerve blocks
Surgery of anterior thigh (skin graft and muscle biopsy)
Patellar fractures, patellar realignment, and quadriceps muscle tendon surgery
Preoperative analgesia for femoral neck fractures
Postoperative analgesia after major knee surgery (cruciate ligament reconstruction, total knee
  arthroplasty)

Femoral nerve block with sciatic and/or obturator nerve block
Arthroscopic knee procedures (diagnostic, meniscus resection/repair)
Total knee arthroplasty
Open or arthroscopic major knee ligament reconstruction
Open reduction/internal fixation femoral shaft fractures
Proximal and distal femoral osteotomy
Thigh tourniquet analgesia

anastomosis of the ventral rami of the first four lumbar spinal nerves (Table 26-2). The ventral rami descend laterally into the posterior part of the psoas major muscle, which is situated anterior to the lumbar transverse processes. The three main branches of the lumbar plexus are all contained within the substance of the psoas muscle in a medial-to-lateral distribution. The obturator nerve is situated most medially within the psoas, the lateral femoral cutaneous nerve most laterally, and the femoral nerve between the two other nerves. The femoral nerve descends through the posterior fibers of the psoas muscle and emerges from the posterolateral border of the muscle at the junction of the muscle's upper two-thirds and lower third. After emerging from the psoas muscle, the femoral nerve descends in the groove between the psoas and the iliacus, deep to the iliacus muscle fascia (Fig. 26-1). It then continues inferiorly deep to the inguinal ligament and passes into the thigh within the femoral triangle.

At the level of the inguinal ligament, the femoral nerve lies anterior to the iliopsoas muscle and slightly lateral to the femoral artery (Fig. 26-1). At the level of the inguinal crease (a naturally occurring skin fold distal to the inguinal ligament and parallel to it), the femoral nerve is adjacent and posterolateral to the femoral artery (Fig. 26-1). Additionally, the femoral nerve is wider and located more superficially at the level of the inguinal crease than at the level of the inguinal ligament.[8] Within the femoral triangle, the femoral sheath is located medially to the femoral nerve, contains the femoral vessels and femoral canal, and lies in a fascial plane between the fascia lata and the fascia iliaca (Fig. 26-1). Although the femoral nerve is located immediately laterally to the femoral sheath, it is contained within its own fascial place, deep to both the fascia lata and the fascia iliaca (Fig. 26-1), anatomically separating it from the femoral vessels.

After passing under the inguinal ligament, the femoral nerve divides into anterior (superficial) and pos-

terior (deep) branches (Table 26-3). The anterior division supplies cutaneous branches to the anterior (intermediate cutaneous branch) and medial (medial cutaneous branch) aspects of the thigh as well as a muscular branch to the sartorius muscle. The posterior division supplies muscular branches to the four parts of the quadriceps muscle. The branch to the rectus femoris muscle enters the proximal posterior surface of the muscle and also supplies articular innervation to the anterolateral portion of the hip joint. The saphenous nerve is the terminal cutaneous branch of the posterior division and supplies cutaneous innervation to the medial aspect of the distal thigh, knee, and lower leg as distal as beyond the medial malleolus. The three muscular branches to the vastus muscles and a branch from the saphenous nerve provide the femoral contribution to the articular innervation of the knee joint. The branch from the saphenous nerve supplies the anteromedial part of the knee joint, and a branch from the vastus medialis supplies the medial aspect. A branch from the vastus intermedius supplies the suprapatellar aspect of the knee joint, and a branch from the vastus lateralis supplies the anterolateral aspect of the joint. The sciatic nerve (posterior and anterolateral aspect) and posterior division of the obturator nerve (posteromedial aspect) supply the remainder of the articular innervation to the knee joint (Table 26-2).

Functional Neuroanatomy

Knowledge of the peripheral sensory distribution of the femoral nerve to the skin, muscles, bones, and joints of the lower extremity allows the anesthesiologist to understand the proper application of a femoral nerve block for surgical anesthesia and postoperative analgesia (Table 26-2). Knowledge of the functional neuroanatomy of the terminal branches of the lumbosacral plexus also helps the anesthesiologist not only to understand the limitations of a femoral nerve block but also to choose

▶ TABLE 26-2. LUMBAR-SACRAL PLEXUS NEUROANATOMY

Lumbar Plexus Branches	Origin	Sensory Innervation	Motor Innervation
Femoral nerve	Dorsal divisions of primary ventral rami of L2-L4	**Dermatomes:** anteromedial thigh and medial lower leg **Myotomes:** quadriceps femoris, pectineus, and sartorius **Osteotomes:** anterolateral length of femur, patella, superomedial tibial plateau, and medial aspects of tibia **Articular:** hip joint, knee joint and ankle joint (saphenous br.)	Quadriceps femoris (rectus femoris, vastus medialis, vastus lateralis, vastus intermedius), pectineus, sartorius, and iliacus muscles
Lateral femoral cutaneous nerve	Dorsal divisions of primary ventral rami of L2-L3	**Dermatomes:** anterolateral thigh Myotomes: none Osteotomes: none	None
Obturator nerve	Ventral divisions of primary ventral rami of L2-L4	**Dermatomes:** posteromedial and posterior lower thigh, absent in up to 57% of patients. **Myotomes:** Adductor muscles (longus, brevis, and magnus), abductor longus, and gracilis muscles **Osteotomes:** medial length of femur **Articular:** hip and knee joint	Adductor muscles (longus, brevis, and magnus), abductor longus, and gracilis muscles
Sacral plexus branches			
Sciatic nerve (tibial and common peroneal nerves)	Ventral divisions (tibial) of primary ventral rami of L4-S3 Dorsal divisions (common peroneal) of primary ventral rami of L4-S2	**Dermatomes:** entire lower leg and foot, except for saphenous distribution (medial aspect) of femoral nerve **Myotomes:** Posterior compartment of thigh and all the muscles of the lower leg and foot **Osteotomes:** posterior femur, tibia, fibula, and entire foot **Articular:** hip, knee, and ankle joint	Posterior thigh muscles (adductor magnus, biceps femoris, semitendinosus, semimembranosus) and all the muscles of the lower leg and foot
Posterior femoral cutaneous nerve	Dorsal division (S1-S2) and ventral divisions (S2-S3) of primary ventral rami of S1-S3	**Dermatomes:** posterior thigh and popliteal fossa **Myotomes:** none **Osteotomes:** none	None

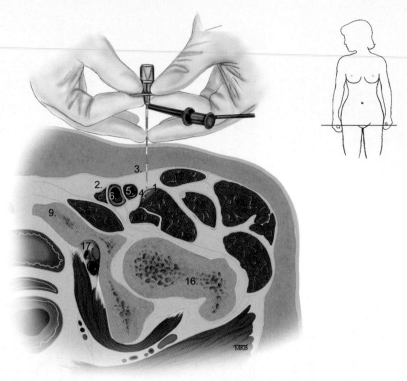

1. Fascia iliaca
2. Femoral sheath
3. Fascia lata
4. Femoral nerve
5. Femoral artery
6. Femoral vein
7. Lymphatics in femoral canal
8. Pectinius muscle
9. Pubic tubercle
10. Psoas muscle
11. Iliacus muscle
12. Sartorius muscle

13. Rectus femoris muscle
14. Tensor fascia lata muscle
15. Gluteus medius muscle
16. Head of femur
17. Obturator vein, artery, and nerve

Figure 26-1. Cross-sectional anatomy of the femoral nerve.

▶ **TABLE 26-3.** FEMORAL NERVE BRANCHES

Main femoral nerve trunk
  Muscular branch to pectineus

Anterior (superficial) division
  Intermediate (middle) cutaneous nerve of the thigh
  Medial cutaneous nerve of the thigh
  Muscular branch to the sartorius

Posterior (deep) division
  Saphenous nerve (to the medial lower leg)
  Muscular branches to quadriceps femoris muscles
   (rectus femoris, vastus medialis, vastus lateralis,
   and vastus intermedius)
  Articular branches to hip joint capsule
   (from rectus femoris)
  Articular branches to knee joint (from three
   vasti muscles and a branch from saphenous nerve)

the appropriate complementary peripheral nerve blocks for specific surgical procedures. The cutaneous distribution of the femoral nerve has been described in the previous paragraph (Fig. 26-2).

The myotomes (sensory nerve supply to the muscles) of the femoral nerve are the quadriceps femoris, sartorius, and pectineus muscles. It is important to note that the peripheral nerve supply of the bones is closely linked with the myotomes, as the majority of skeletal innervation (osteotomes) is derived from nerve branches that have penetrated the periosteum from the attached muscles. Thus, the femoral nerve supplies sensory innervation to the entire anterolateral portion of the femur, the patella, and the anteromedial aspect of the tibial plateau. The obturator nerve supplies sensory innervation to the medial aspect of the femur (where the medial compartment muscles of the thigh attach). The sciatic nerve

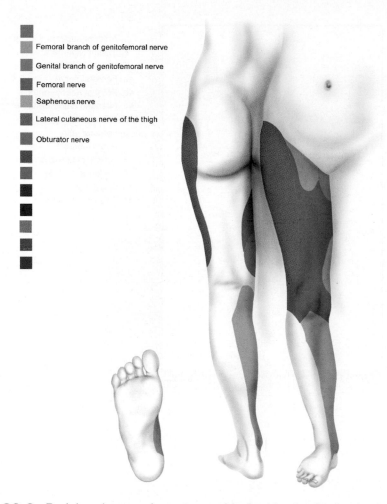

Femoral branch of genitofemoral nerve

Genital branch of genitofemoral nerve

Femoral nerve

Saphenous nerve

Lateral cutaneous nerve of the thigh

Obturator nerve

Figure 26-2. Peripheral nerve dermatomes blocked by the femoral nerve block.

supplies sensory innervation to the posterior aspect of the femoral shaft, most of the tibia, the fibula, and foot; the peripheral sciatic nerve myotomes include the posterior hamstring muscles of the thigh and all of the muscles of the lower leg.

Surface and Applied Anatomy

The pertinent surface landmarks for a femoral nerve block are the anterior superior iliac spine, pubic tubercle, inguinal ligament, inguinal crease, and femoral artery pulsation (Fig. 26-3). These surface landmarks are the basis for the femoral nerve block, inguinal paravascular three-in-one lumbar plexus block, and fascia iliaca compartment block. Although these three techniques have been described as "unique approaches" to a femoral nerve block, anatomically they are similar and based on the clinical goal of injecting local anesthetic near the femoral nerve within the fascial plane deep to the fascia iliaca (Fig. 26-1).

A peripheral nerve stimulator (PNS)–guided femoral nerve block is based on locating the posterior division of the femoral nerve deep to the iliacus muscle fascia, as evidenced by eliciting quadriceps muscular contractions resulting in cephalad movement of the patella. Based on anatomic dissections and sonographic studies, the femoral nerve is more easily located at the inguinal crease, where it is more superficial, wider, and separated from the femoral artery.[8] The muscular branch to the sartorius muscle arises in common with the intermediate cutaneous branch, both of which are superficial to the fascia iliaca. Thus, PNS-elicited contraction of the sartorius muscle (contraction of the medial aspect of the leg, without cephalad movement of the patella) indicates that the stimulating needle is located in a tissue plane superficial to the posterior division of the femoral nerve, and injection of local anesthetic would not block the posterior division.

In the fascia iliaca compartment block, a short-bevel needle is introduced just below the junction of the medial two-thirds and lateral third of the inguinal ligament. Rather than PNS-guided placement, the blunt needle is slowly advanced while feeling for a "double loss of resistance," as the needle passes through the fascia lata initially and then through the fascia iliaca.[3] The fascia iliaca compartment

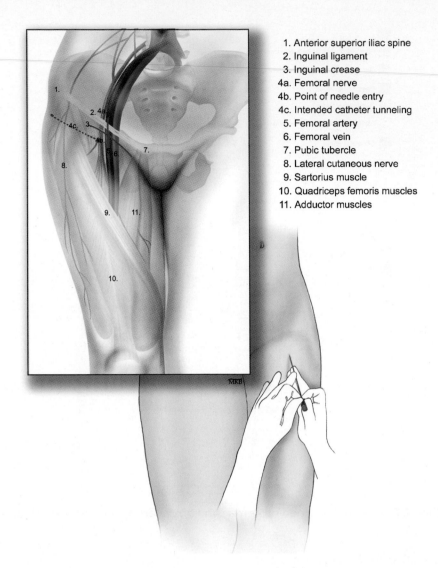

1. Anterior superior iliac spine
2. Inguinal ligament
3. Inguinal crease
4a. Femoral nerve
4b. Point of needle entry
4c. Intended catheter tunneling
5. Femoral artery
6. Femoral vein
7. Pubic tubercle
8. Lateral cutaneous nerve
9. Sartorius muscle
10. Quadriceps femoris muscles
11. Adductor muscles

Figure 26-3. Surface anatomy and positioning for the femoral nerve block.

block is based on the premise that a sufficiently large volume of local anesthetic injected deep to the fascia iliaca will spread within this fascial plane toward the proximal branches of the lumbar plexus and provide simultaneous block of the femoral, lateral femoral cutaneous, and obturator nerve (three-in-one block).[3] In the inguinal paravascular block, the needle insertion site is 2 to 3 cm lateral to the femoral artery pulsation immediately below the inguinal ligament and PNS-guided localization of the femoral nerve is sought.

After proper localization of the femoral nerve, local anesthetic is injected while firm digital pressure is simultaneously applied just distal to the needle so that a sufficient amount of local anesthetic would theoretically spread cephalad under the fascia iliaca toward the proximal branches of the lumbar plexus. However, clinical and imaging studies have consistently demonstrated that diffusion of local anesthetic toward the obturator nerve

(which emerges from the posteromedial border of the psoas muscle) is exceptional.[3,9] Thus, both the fascia iliaca compartment block and the three-in-one block consistently block only the femoral and lateral femoral cutaneous nerve. From a clinical standpoint, a femoral nerve block is most consistently successful when penetration of both fascial planes is appreciated during the PNS-guided localization of quadriceps muscular contractions.

▶ BLOCK TECHNIQUE

Patient Preparation, Position, and Timing of Block

For a single-injection femoral nerve block or placement of a catheter for continuous block, the patient is supine with both legs extended, with the leg to be blocked in slight abduction and at zero degree of frontal rotation or in slight external rotation (Fig. 26-3). In obese patients, two techniques can be useful to facilitate location of both the inguinal crease and femoral artery pulsation: a pillow can be placed underneath the hips and an assistant can constantly retract the overhanging abdominal pannus. A clear fenestrated sterile drape offers ideal access to the inguinal region, providing the ability to observe for PNS-elicited muscular responses clearly.

The choice of a single-injection or continuous femoral nerve block is based on requirements for surgical anesthesia and postoperative analgesia. Single-injection femoral nerve block, like most other single-injection nerve blocks, has limited utility in the management of acute postoperative pain. A femoral nerve block before surgery is required if it is to be used as the primary anesthetic technique or in combination with a general anesthetic. The advantages of a femoral nerve block (continuous or single-injection) before surgery is that it precedes the application of the heavy bandages and braces that are often placed after major knee or femoral surgery (which can impair ability to position the patient properly and visualize muscular contractions) and the presence of an analgesic block on emerging from a general anesthetic. The concern that a single-injection femoral nerve block done before surgery will not provide effective postoperative analgesia for long enough has been minimized by the use of continuous femoral blocks. The preoperative placement of femoral nerve catheters before major knee surgery allows analgesic treatment immediately after surgery or even intraoperatively. Either practice facilitates a more efficient and rapid recovery in the recovery room.

Single-Injection Femoral Nerve Block

PNS-Guided Technique

It is useful to mark the surface landmarks for a femoral nerve block (Fig. 26-3). The primary surface landmarks are the inguinal crease and the femoral artery pulsation.[8] After sterile skin preparation and draping, the skin and subcutaneous tissue of the initial puncture site is infiltrated with 1% lidocaine. The infiltration should be shallow (so as not to partially block the femoral nerve) and in a line extending superolaterally just below the inguinal crease to allow for a more lateral needle reinsertion when required. A 22-gauge 50-mm short-bevel insulated stimulating needle is inserted 1 cm lateral to the femoral artery pulsation, approximately 1 cm below the inguinal crease and slowly advanced at a 45- to 60-degree angle to the skin in a cephalad direction along a sagittal plane. The PNS is initially set to deliver 1.5 mA at a frequency of 2 Hz and pulse duration of 100 to 300 μs.

As the stimulating needle is advanced, the proper motor response is upward movement of the patella due to the elicited muscular contractions of the quadriceps femoris muscles (QFM). The penetration of the fascia lata and fascia iliaca is often obvious if a "B"-beveled needle is used. In adult patients, the average needle depth needed to localize the posterior division of the femoral nerve is 2 to 4 cm, but it may be deeper in obese patients. After initial stimulation of the QFM is obtained, the current output from the PNS is gradually decreased until muscle contractions (patellar movement) are still observed at ≤0.5 mA. After initial localization of the femoral nerve, only small changes in needle position are required to maintain muscle contractions at a current output ≤0.5 mA. Additionally, knowledge that the needle has penetrated both the fascia lata and fascia iliaca is important to ensure that local anesthetic will be injected below the fascia iliaca within the tissue plane containing the femoral nerve.

If the initial needle pass fails to elicit a QFM response, the needle tip is withdrawn to the skin and redirected in systematic fashion by observing whether there are no muscular responses or muscular responses other than quadriceps contractions (Table 26-4). The most common initial muscular response is that of the sartorius muscle, which will cause contraction of the medial aspect of the thigh without upward movement of the patella. If sartorius muscle contractions are accepted for placement, the femoral nerve block will invariably fail because local anesthetic will not reach the posterior division of the femoral nerve. After obtaining optimal needle position, the needle is held steady and aspirated to detect possible intravascular placement. An initial test dose of local anesthetic is injected, which should immediately abolish the elicited muscular response. The disappearance of muscle contractions after injection of local anesthetic ("Raj test") was originally thought to be due to physical displacement of the nerve away from the needle (or catheter) tip. However, recent work has demonstrated that the injection of any current-conducting solution (local anesthetic or saline) expands the conductive area surrounding the needle tip, thereby reducing the current density at the target nerve/needle interface ("Tsui test").[10] The Tsui test is a fundamental requirement for a successful PNS-guided femoral nerve block. If the muscle contractions persist after injection local anesthetic, it may indicate that the femoral nerve is separated from the tip of the stimulating needle by fascial layers that can conduct electrical current easily but will prevent local anesthetic from reaching the femoral nerve. After a negative aspiration test for blood, and a positive Tsui test, 20 to 35 mL of local anesthetic is slowly injected in 3- to 5-mL increments.

Continuous Femoral Nerve Block

Needle Placement

The anatomic approach and technique for localizing the femoral nerve for continuous femoral nerve block is very similar to the single-injection technique except that

▶ TABLE 26-4. INTERPRETATION OF PNS-ELICITED MOTOR/MUSCULAR RESPONSES

Elicited Response	Clinical-Anatomic Correlation	Corrective Action
Quadriceps femoris (QFM) contractions with upward movement of patella. Contractions disappear with local anesthetic injection.	Needle (catheter) is close to posterior division of femoral nerve, deep to the fascia iliaca.	None. Incrementally inject local anesthetic bolus or begin local anesthetic infusion.
QFM contractions with upward movement of patella. Contractions do not disappear with local anesthetic injection.	Needle (catheter) is close to posterior division of femoral nerve, but may be either superficial to fascia iliaca or intravascular.	Advance needle slightly, feeling for needle passage through fascia iliaca. Carefully repeat local anesthetic injection.
Sartorius muscle contraction (contraction of medial thigh without upward movement of patella).	Needle (catheter) is stimulating anterior division of femoral nerve, and is superficial to posterior division.	Initially advance needle 1–3 mm directly posterior. If no response, then withdraw slightly and redirect needle posterolaterally.
No response after 5 cm insertion depth.	Needle is inserted either too medially or too laterally to femoral nerve. In obese patients, may require use of longer stimulating needle.	Withdraw needle tip to just below the skin and redirect needle laterally first (and then medially if required) in 10- to 15-degree increments and advance needle. Consider longer needle in obese patients.
Local muscle twitches	Direct stimulation of iliopsoas or pectineus muscle and needle is inserted either too deep or too cephalad.	Withdraw needle tip to just below the skin and repeat needle advancement.
Blood	Vascular puncture of femoral artery and needle tip is inserted too medially (initial needle insertion site too medial or needle angle too medial during advancement).	Withdraw needle and assess for formation of hematoma. Local compression for 2–5 min. Reassess landmarks and repeat attempts to elicit muscle responses. Carefully interpret muscular responses, as the presence of blood may disperse current density at needle tip/nerve interface. Consider fascia iliaca compartment technique.
QFM contraction elicited with stimulating needle, but contractions disappear, decrease in intensity, or change in character (change to sartorius muscle contraction) with catheter advancement.	Stimulating catheter tip has migrated away from femoral nerve a distance greater than initial needle tip location. Needle tip may be very close to posterior division of femoral nerve, but still superficial to fascia iliaca.	Pull catheter back so tip is inside needle shaft. Change catheter direction with systematic changes in needle rotation, needle angulation, or needle depth and repeat catheter advancement.

the goal now is to place an indwelling catheter 3 to 5 cm along the femoral nerve below the fascia iliaca. Specialized equipment for continuous peripheral nerve blocks allows a catheter to be inserted through the stimulating needle after the femoral nerve has been properly localized (Table 26-5). For the continuous femoral nerve block technique, the skin infiltration is extended 6 to 10 cm superolaterally just below the inguinal crease to allow for subsequent subcutaneous tunneling of the catheter. A 17-gauge insulated Tuohy stimulating needle and a specialized stimulating catheter are used to facilitate proper placement of the indwelling catheter. The larger-gauge needle significantly improves the ability to feel needle passage through the fascial layers, and the stimulating catheter confirms that the catheter tip remains close to the femoral nerve during catheter advancement. The bevel of the Tuohy needle should initially face directly cephalad so as to facilitate catheter movement along the long axis of the femoral nerve.

Catheter Placement

After QFM contractions have been obtained at ≤0.5 mA via the Tuohy needle, the PNS is connected to the proximal end of the stimulating catheter. The stimulating catheter is inserted into the needle and advanced to its tip. At this point there should be no change in the previously observed QFM contractions. The catheter is now advanced 3 to 5 cm beyond the needle tip. The elicited muscular contractions should remain unchanged during the entire period of catheter advancement. If the QFM ceases to contract during catheter advancement, it indicates that the catheter tip has migrated away from the femoral nerve a distance greater than initial needle placement. If this occurs, the catheter should be carefully withdrawn into the stimulating needle. The course of the catheter can be changed systematically by rotating the needle or by changing its angle or depth (Table 26-4). These adjustments are continued until QFM contractions remain unchanged throughout catheter advancement. The nature of the elicited muscular response can provide clues to the type of needle readjustment needed. For example, a change from quadriceps to sartorius muscle contractions should prompt a small change in needle angulation or possibly a slight increase in needle depth to facilitate catheter advancement under the fascia iliaca.

Catheter Fixation

Once the femoral catheter is properly placed, it must be secured to prevent dislodgment during the patient's recovery period. Numerous methods (suturing the catheter, sterile adhesive dressings, and 2-octyl cyanoacrylate glue) have been used with varying degrees of success. One of the most effective methods to secure catheters is simply to tunnel the catheters 6 to 10 cm subcutaneously superolaterally below and parallel to the inguinal crease. In our experience, tunneling has significantly decreased premature or accidental dislodgment. Subcutaneous tunneling of femoral catheters may also decrease the possibility of catheter-related infections. A prospective study has shown a 57 percent bacterial colonization rate and a 1.5 percent incidence of bacteremia related to the presence of indwelling femoral perineural catheters. Although tunneling of femoral perineural catheters has not yet been proven to decrease the rate of infection, the use of tunneled catheters is associated with a threefold decrease in infection related to femoral vascular catheters.[11]

► SELECTION OF LOCAL ANESTHETIC

The choice of local anesthetic for single-injection femoral nerve blocks should be based on the desired onset time, duration of action of surgical anesthesia, surgical requirements for muscle relaxation, duration of postoperative analgesia, and the potential for systemic toxicity. For

TABLE 26-5. REQUIRED EQUIPMENT FOR FEMORAL NERVE BLOCK

Equipment	Single-Injection Femoral Nerve Block	Continuous Femoral Nerve Block
Pulse oximetry, noninvasive blood pressure	X	X
Resuscitative equipment and medications	X	X
Skin marker	X	X
Povidone-iodine or chlorhexidine solution	X	X
Block tray (transparent fenestrated drape)	X	X
Peripheral nerve stimulator	X	X
22-gauge, 50- (100) mm, insulated needle	X	
17-gauge, 50- (90) mm insulated Tuohy needle		X
19-gauge, 90-cm stimulating catheter		X
Transparent adhesive dressings		X
Connection tubing and infusion pump		X

single-injection femoral nerve blocks, 30 to 35 mL of bupivacaine (0.25 to 0.5%) or ropivacaine (0.375 to 0.75%) will have an onset time of 15 to 30 min, provide 5 to 10 h of surgical anesthesia, and will ensure 12 to 24 h of effective postoperative analgesia. Mepivacaine 2% (25 to 30 mL) is an excellent choice for ambulatory femoral nerve blocks when extended postoperative analgesia is not required. It provides rapid onset of surgical anesthesia (10 to 15 min), rapid resolution of motor block at the knee (3 to 4 h), and an intermediate duration of postoperative analgesia (5 to 8 h). Epinephrine (2.5 μg/mL) should be added to all local anesthetic solutions to help detect inadvertent intravascular injection and decrease systemic local anesthetic levels when a large volume is given as a single injection. The choice of a local anesthetic solution for continuous femoral nerve blocks is based on balancing effective analgesia and minimizing undesirable degrees of QFM motor block. In our experience, bupivacaine (0.125%) or ropivacaine (0.2%) will provide effective analgesia at a continuous infusion rate of 4 to 6 mL/h. Continuous infusions, patient-controlled boluses, and continuous infusion with patient-controlled supplemental boluses are all equally effective, providing the femoral catheter is placed and maintained close to the femoral nerve.

▶ POTENTIAL PROBLEMS AND COMPLICATIONS

As with all single-injection peripheral nerve blocks, the reported complications include peripheral nerve injury, bleeding with hematoma formation, infection, and systemic local anesthetic toxicity. The true incidence of nerve injury associated with femoral nerve block is unknown, but in a recent large prospective series, the incidence of significant femoral nerve injury was only 0.03 percent.[12] In the most recent closed claims analysis of injuries associated with regional anesthesia in the 1980s and 1990s from the American Society of Anesthesiologists, femoral nerve block was associated with permanent nerve injury in 1 percent of all peripheral nerve block claims.[13] During the performance of PNS-guided femoral nerve blocks, patients should not be heavily sedated and paresthesia should not be sought. Although the use of PNS for peripheral nerve blocks has yet been proven to be associated with a lower incidence of peripheral nerve injury, another large prospective survey reported that all cases of peripheral nerve injury were associated with paresthesia during needle placement or local anesthetic injection.[14] In the only reported series to date of adverse effects associated with continuous femoral nerve blocks, there was only one instance of long-term femoral nerve neuropathy in 211 cases.[15]

An indwelling catheter in the groin area always poses the risk of catheter-related infection. Strict aseptic technique is therefore essential in performing continuous femoral nerve blocks, and the catheter site should be inspected daily for early signs of infection. As noted previously, subcutaneous tunneling of femoral catheters not only decreases catheter dislodgement but also may decrease catheter-related infections. Systemic local anesthetic toxicity is always a possibility when large volumes of these drugs are injected. However, clinically significant systemic toxic reactions due to unintentional intravascular injection are extremely rare in properly performed femoral nerve blocks. Important steps to minimize toxic effects include using the minimum effective concentration and volume of local anesthetic, aspiration tests for blood before injection, incremental injection (3 to 5 mL) while monitoring for early signs of central nervous system toxicity, the use of epinephrine (as a pharmacologic indicator of intravascular injection and to decrease peak local anesthetic plasma levels), and the use of less potent long-acting amide local anesthetic agents.

▶ SPECIAL CONSIDERATIONS AND PRACTICAL POINTS

Choice of Needle and Catheter Systems

The use of nonstimulating catheters for continuous femoral nerve block has been associated with up to a 15 to 25 percent failure rate for secondary block. In other words, when the initial block (30 to 35 mL of concentrated local anesthetic injected before catheter placement) has resolved, the continuous analgesic infusion via the catheter will fail to provide analgesia owing to incorrect placement of the catheter. Clinical and radiographic studies have consistently demonstrated that the course of continuous anterior lumbar plexus/femoral catheters is unpredictable and that the success of femoral analgesia decreases to 25 percent within 24 to 48 h.[2,3,16] In a prospective randomized double-blind study, continuous femoral nerve block that utilized stimulating catheter-guided placement was associated with a higher success rate (100 versus 85 percent) and a significantly greater depth of nerve block compared to cases in which a nonstimulating catheter was used.[17] In our clinical experience, the use of stimulating catheters for continuous femoral nerve blocks has decreased our failure rate for secondary analgesic infusions to less than 3 percent. The ability to place the catheter tip close to the nerve and confirm its position allows low continuous infusion rates (4 to 6 mL/h of bupivacaine 0.125% or ropivacaine 0.2%) to provide effective analgesia, without requiring supplemental local anesthetic boluses.

Practical Management of Continuous Femoral Nerve Block

The use of continuous femoral nerve block has greatly improved the quality of recovery after total knee arthroplasty. Effective continuous femoral analgesia significantly improves rest and dynamic analgesia, decreases the need for opioids and thus reduces their side effects of nausea, vomiting, and sedation. Incomplete analgesia during effective continuous femoral nerve block after total knee arthroplasty is usually in the posterior aspect of the knee and is primarily due to pain in the sensory distribution area of the either obturator and or sciatic nerve. This pain is usually short-lived and is effectively managed with a combination of systemic opioids and nonsteroidal anti-inflammatory agents. Occasionally, patients (and physical therapists) will note excessive weakness during the course of active postoperative rehabilitation, which may contribute to accidental falls. Patients should therefore always be warned about the possibility of quadriceps weakness when attempting to stand and walk. Simply turning the infusion off for several hours and/or decreasing the continuous infusion rate will correct this minor problem. In our current practice, femoral catheters are removed 24 h before discharge (usually the morning of the second postoperative day).

REFERENCES

1. Parkinson SK, Mueller JB, Little WL, et al. Extent of blockade with various approaches to the lumbar plexus. *Anesth Analg* 68:243–248, 1989.
2. Capdevila X, Biboulet P, Morau D, et al. Continuous three-in-one block for postoperative analgesia: Where do the catheters go? *Anesth Analg* 94:1001–1006, 2002.
3. Capdevila X, Biboulet P, Rubenovitch J, et al. Comparison of the three-in-one and fascia iliaca compartment blocks in adults: Clinical and radiographic analysis. *Anesth Analg* 86:1039–1044, 1998.
4. Allen HW, Liu SS, Ware PD, et al. Peripheral nerve blocks improve analgesia after total knee replacement surgery. *Anesth Analg* 87:93–97, 1998.
5. Ng HP, Cheong KF, Lim A, et al. Intraoperative single-shot "3-in-1" femoral nerve block with ropivacaine 0.25%, ropivacaine 0.5% or bupivacaine 0.25% provides comparable 48-hr analgesia after unilateral total knee replacement. *Can J Anesth* 48:1102–1108, 2001.
6. Capdevila X, Barthelet Y, Biboulet P, et al. Effects of perioperative analgesic technique on the surgical outcome and duration of rehabilitation after major knee surgery. *Anesthesiology* 91:8–15, 1999.
7. Singelyn FJ, Deyaert M, Joris D, et al. Effects of intravenous patient-controlled analgesia with morphine, continuous epidural analgesia, and continuous three-in-one block on postoperative pain and knee rehabilitation after total knee arthroplasty. *Anesth Analg* 87:88–92, 1998.
8. Vloka JD, Drobnik L, Ernest A, et al. Anatomical landmarks for femoral nerve block: A comparison of four needle insertion sites. *Anesth Analg* 89:1467–1470, 1999.
9. Marhofer P, Nasel C, Sitzwohl C, et al. Magnetic resonance imaging of the distribution of local anesthetic during the three-in-one block. *Anesth Analg* 90:119–124, 2000.
10. Tsui BCH, Wagner A, Finucane B. Electrophysiological effect of injectates on peripheral nerve stimulation. *Reg Anesth Pain Med* 29:189–193, 2004.
11. Timsit JF, Bruneel F, Cheval C, et al. Use of tunneled femoral catheters to prevent catheter-related infection: A randomized, controlled trial. *Ann Intern Med* 130:729–735, 1999.
12. Auroy Y, Benhamou D, Bargues L, et al. Major complications of regional anesthesia in France: The SOS regional anesthesia hotline service. *Anesthesiology* 97:1274–1280, 2002.
13. Lee LA, Posner KL, Domino KB, et al. Injuries associated with regional anesthesia in the 1980s and 1990s: A closed claims analysis. *Anesthesiology* 101:143–152, 2004.
14. Auroy Y, Narchi P, Messiah A, et al. Serious complications related to regional anesthesia: Results of a prospective survey in France. *Anesthesiology* 87:479–486, 1997.
15. Cuvillon P, Ripart J, Lalourcey L, et al. The continuous femoral nerve block catheter for postoperative analgesia: Bacterial colonization, infectious rates, and adverse affects. *Anesth Analg* 93:1045–1049, 2001.
16. Ganapathy S, Wasserman RA, Watson JT, et al. Modified continuous femoral three-in-one block for postoperative pain after total knee arthroplasty. *Anesth Analg* 89:1197–1202, 1999.
17. Salinas FV, Neal JM, Sueda LA, et al. Prospective comparison of continuous femoral nerve block with nonstimulating catheter placement versus stimulating catheter-guided perineural placement in volunteers. *Reg Anesth Pain Med* 29:212–220, 2004.

CHAPTER 27

Sciatic Nerve Blocks

Carlo D. Franco / Steven C. Borene

▶ INTRODUCTION

The sciatic nerve is the largest peripheral nerve in the body, measuring almost 2 cm across at its origin. Despite its size and very constant relationship to the pelvic bone, it has been commonly considered a difficult nerve to block.

When the sciatic nerve is approached proximally at the buttock area, the block provides anesthesia in the areas supplied by its two main components, the tibial and common peroneal nerves, and of the posterior femoral cutaneous nerve, the latter a branch of the sacral plexus (S1, S2, and S3). For surgery below the knee, any approach to the sciatic nerve is adequate but usually requires the addition of a saphenous nerve block. The sciatic nerve contributes, directly or indirectly, to the sensory innervation of the hip, knee, and ankle joints.

The sites at which the nerve can be blocked can be grouped into gluteal (buttock), subgluteal, and popliteal.

▶ PATIENT SELECTION

Sciatic nerve block combined with saphenous nerve block provides anesthesia of the lower extremity below the knee. Surgery to the lateral side of the tibia, fibula, lateral ankle and foot, Achilles' tendon, and other soft tissues below the knee calls for sciatic nerve block. All the major joints of the lower extremity, however, get their nerve supply from the sciatic as well as the femoral and obturator nerves.

Applied Anatomy

Proximal Sciatic Nerve

The sciatic nerve originates from the ventral rami of L4-S3, which make out the lumbosacral trunk and the sacral plexus (Fig. 27-1). The anterior branches of the ventral rami form the tibial or medial component of the sciatic nerve, while its lateral component, or common peroneal nerve, originates from the posterior branches of the ventral rami of L4-S2. The sciatic nerve forms in the pelvis on the anterior surface of the piriformis muscle and enters the buttock along with this muscle through the greater sciatic foramen. In up to 90 percent of people, the tibial and peroneal components form a single nerve structure surrounded by a common sheath. In approximately 10 percent of people, the tibial nerve passes by itself below the piriformis muscle, while the common peroneal nerve passes through and rarely above this muscle.[1]

Regardless of the arrangement, both components become physically contiguous immediately below the piriformis muscle (Fig. 27-1). They run together surrounded by a common sheath until they reach the popliteal fossa where they finally diverge from each other. Despite their close proximity, the two nerve components do not mix their fibers. On its course in the buttocks, the sciatic nerve is covered by thick connective tissue, which is a continuation of the fascia lata into the buttocks, and more superficially by the gluteus maximus muscle.

Despite the large number of nerve branches found in the buttock, the sciatic nerve itself gives off only one branch here, that to the hamstring muscles at the level of the ischial tuberosity. The fibers in the sciatic nerve that supply the hamstring muscles occupy the most medial part of its tibial component and can easily be separated from the rest of the nerve by dissection.

The proximal trajectory of the sciatic nerve in the buttock is curved, with its concavity facing inferiorly and medially until it clears the ischial tuberosity. After reaching the lateral aspect of this prominence, it turns inferiorly to run vertically down toward the thigh. Therefore it is the

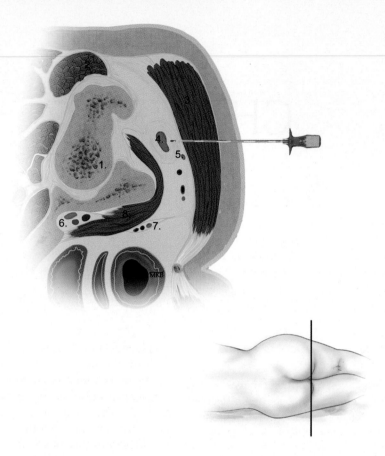

1. Hip joint
2. Gluteus medius muscle
3. Gluteus maximus muscle
4. Sciatic nerve
5. Posterior cutaneous nerve of the thigh
6. Obturator vein, artery, and nerve
7. Pudendal vein, artery, and nerve
8. Obturator internus muscle

Figure 27-1. Cross section of the thigh at the subgluteal level.

position of the ischial tuberosity that determines how far from the midline the nerve travels in the buttock. Anthropometric studies have demonstrated that the adult human pelvis is surprisingly similar in size in males and females.[2] Although the female birth canal is wider than the inner pelvis of males, the male bones are thicker; thus the bicrestal diameter or total width of the pelvis is similar in both sexes. The characteristically different contour of male and female pelvises is due to different hormone-dependent fat deposition around the pelvis in both sexes and not to bony differences. As a result, the sciatic nerve of adults is at a fixed distance from the midline, but its relative position in the buttock changes (e.g., it seems eccentrically located in the buttock of a lean person and centrally located in people of average weight, while it seems increasingly closer to the midline with increasing body weight).

Other structures that pass through the greater sciatic foramen are the superior and inferior gluteal nerves and vessels, the pudendal nerve and vessels, the posterior femoral cutaneous nerve, and some other muscular branches. The pudendal nerve has a short trajectory in the buttock, several centimeters medial to the sciatic nerve, before it exits through the lesser sciatic foramen, deep to the sacrotuberous ligament. The superior and inferior gluteal nerves supply the gluteus muscles of the buttock. The posterior femoral cutaneous nerve enters the buttock below the piriformis muscle just posterior and somewhat medial to the sciatic nerve. During most of its trajectory in the gluteal region, this cutaneous nerve has an intimate contact with the posterior aspect of the sciatic nerve, running within its sheath. As the nerves approach the subgluteal fold, the posterior femoral cutaneous nerve abandons the sheath to eventually perforate the fascia lata and become the cutaneous nerve of the inferior part of the buttock and posterior thigh.

In the Thigh

The sciatic nerve enters the thigh first under the gluteus maximus and then under the long head of biceps. It provides several muscular branches at different levels in the thigh that innervate the hamstring muscles. These fibers arise from the medial side of the nerve. The only branch that arises from its lateral side is the branch to the short head of the biceps femoris muscle. The trajectory of the sciatic nerve in the thigh in general follows the direction of the femur; that is, it becomes slightly closer to the midline as it descends into the popliteal fossa. Its final position with respect to the midline, however, contrary to the situation in the buttock, is influenced by the variable accumulation of fat in the inner thigh.

In the Popliteal Fossa

The two components of the sciatic nerve eventually diverge from each other in the vicinity of the apex of the popliteal fossa. The tibial nerve continues almost vertically down while the common peroneal nerve swings laterally to run alongside the biceps femoris muscle. The thick sheath that surrounded the two components of the nerve from the buttocks to the lower thigh merges with the adipose tissue that fills the popliteal fossa. In fact, immediately below the actual separation of the branches, connective tissue and fat can be seen interposing between them, establishing a barrier to the diffusion of local anesthetic between one branch and the other. The sciatic nerve in the popliteal fossa runs slightly lateral to the midpoint between the biceps and semitendinosus tendons (Fig. 27-2). The nerve is also lateral and more superficial to the popliteal vein, while the popliteal artery is medial to the vein.

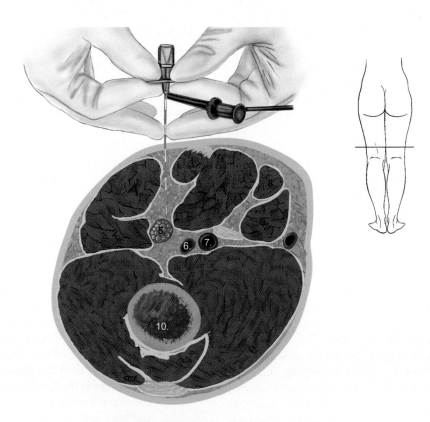

1. Long head of biceps femoris muscle
2. Short head of biceps femoris muscle
3. Semitendinosus muscle
4. Semimembranosus muscle
5. Sciatic nerve
6. Popliteal vein
7. Popliteal artery
8. Gracilis muscle
9. Sartorius muscle
10. Femur

Figure 27-2. Cross section of the thigh approximately 10 cm proximal of the crease behind the knee.

Approaches to Blocking the Sciatic Nerve

Several approaches to block the sciatic nerve have been described, some of which are presented here.

Gluteal Approaches to the Sciatic Nerve

Classic Approach

In 1922 Labat described an approach to the sciatic nerve using the greater trochanter and posterosuperior iliac spine as the main landmarks. In 1974 Winnie et al.[3] modified this approach by adding a line from the sacral hiatus to the greater trochanter. Labat's approach and Winnie's modification together are usually referred to as the "classic" approach.

Patient Position

The patient is placed in the lateral position slightly rotated forward. The dependent leg is extended while the one to be blocked is flexed at the hip and at the knee (Sims position).

Needle Insertion and Technique

The posterosuperior iliac spine is identified by palpation, and so is the highest point of the greater trochanter. A line is drawn between these two prominences. A second line (Winnie's modification) is drawn between the sacral hiatus and the greater trochanter. The iliac spine–trochanter line is bisected and a perpendicular line is traced caudally from this midpoint until the sacral hiatus–trochanter line is intersected. This is the point where the needle is inserted.

The needle is inserted perpendicular to the skin in all planes. While the needle goes through the skin and subcutaneous tissue, no muscle twitch is visible. When the needle reaches the gluteus maximus muscle, a motor response confined to the buttock may become visible. The more superficial fibers of the gluteus muscle are more diagonal (toward the iliotibial tract), while the deeper fibers are somewhat more horizontal. Because of this different arrangement of muscle fibers, it is frequently observed that as the needle progresses through the gluteus maximus muscle, the buttock muscle contracts with visible movements down and lateral toward the upper thigh, followed by a more localized motor twitch of the buttock. When the needle pierces the deep aspect of the muscle, this motor response disappears. If the needle–nerve stimulator combination fails to identify the nerve, the needle is withdrawn and reinserted up and down along the perpendicular line described above.

Special Considerations

1. This anatomic approach is accurate in locating the sciatic nerve in the buttock at the point where this nerve appears below the piriformis muscle. However, its success depends on the precise location of buried landmarks. Any soft tissue lateral to the greater trochanter would lengthen the line between the posterior iliac spine and greater trochanter, making its midpoint too lateral. It is therefore crucial to estimate the position of the posterior projection of the greater trochanter correctly and not its lateral projection.

2. The posterosuperior iliac spine and the greater trochanter are not located on the same horizontal plane, as is sometimes shown. Instead, the line joining these bony landmarks forms approximately a 45-degree angle with the horizontal, the greater trochanter being higher.

Franco's Approach

A new and simplified approach has recently been introduced.[4] This approach does not rely on the identification of any bony landmarks but is based on the concept that the bony pelvis is similar in all adults of both sexes and that the posterior projection of the ischial tuberosity, despite its different anterior angulation in males and females, is located at approximately the same distance from the midline. Dissections of the adult human pelvis show that the sciatic nerve, after reaching the upper part of the ischial tuberosity, runs vertically down at about 10 cm from the midline in both male and female adults. This technique uses the intergluteal sulcus (cleft between the buttocks) to determine the patient's midline.

Patient Position

This technique can be performed in the prone or lateral position. If the patient is placed in the lateral position, the preferred method, the patient's hips and knees are flexed.

Needle Insertion and Technique

The insertion point is marked at 10 cm from the midline (intergluteal sulcus) at any point in the gluteal region because the sciatic nerve runs parallel to the midline for almost its entire course in the buttock. The distance, however, is shorter lateral to the uppermost part of the intergluteal sulcus. This is the level at which the nerve exits the pelvis, describing a wide curve over the ischial tuberosity before running vertically in the buttock. The needle is then inserted directly parallel to the midline. The rest of the technique is similar to the classic one. Needle repositioning when necessary is accomplished by a slight lateral or medial correction of the angle of insertion of the needle, using the same original insertion point in the skin.

Special Considerations

1. We now realize that the sciatic nerve's position in the adult buttock depends on the position of the

ischial tuberosity and that its distance from the midline is therefore fixed and not related to body weight.

2. Because the 10-cm measurement should reflect the linear distance between the midline and the outer side of the ischial tuberosity, a straight measurement from the midline is performed, disregarding the patient's individual contour.

3. In some cases, when the patient is placed on lateral decubitus, the midline "sags." It is then useful to notice that because the upper end of the intergluteal sulcus attaches to the sacrum, it is unaffected by gravity and can be used to estimate the true midline.

Subgluteal Approach

The subgluteal is a popular approach for single-injection blocks as well as for catheter insertion. Many techniques have been described. In 2001 di Benedetto[5] described a variation of the subgluteal block, which is described here.

Patient Position

The patient is placed in the lateral decubitus position, with the leg to be blocked uppermost and rolled forward and the hip and knee flexed. The dependent leg is extended (Sims position) (Fig. 27-3).

Needle Insertion and Technique

A line is drawn between the greater trochanter and the ischial tuberosity. The midpoint between these two points is identified. A perpendicular line from this point is drawn caudally for 4 cm, and this is the point of needle insertion (Fig. 27-3).

The needle is directed perpendicularly to the skin for single-injection blocks or approximately at a 45-degree angle if a continuous block with a catheter is planned.

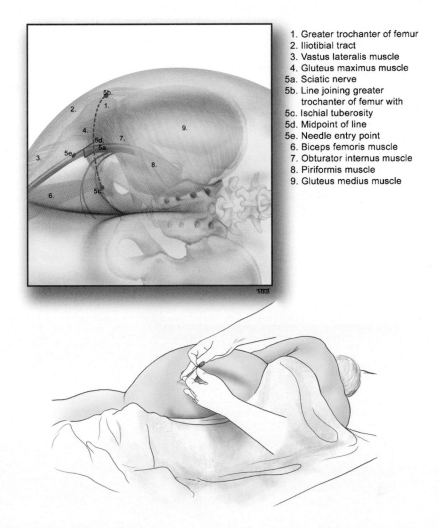

1. Greater trochanter of femur
2. Iliotibial tract
3. Vastus lateralis muscle
4. Gluteus maximus muscle
5a. Sciatic nerve
5b. Line joining greater trochanter of femur with
5c. Ischial tuberosity
5d. Midpoint of line
5e. Needle entry point
6. Biceps femoris muscle
7. Obturator internus muscle
8. Piriformis muscle
9. Gluteus medius muscle

Figure 27-3. Surface anatomy and positioning for the subgluteal approach to the sciatic nerve block.

Repositioning when necessary is either lateral or medial along the subgluteal fold. If a catheter is placed for continuous sciatic nerve block, it can be directed proximally or distally, depending on the planned positioning of the tourniquet.

Special Considerations

1. The subgluteal fold is formed by attachment of the deep layers of the skin into the fascia lata and does not correspond with the inferior border of the gluteus maximus muscle. The lower border of this muscle crosses the subgluteal fold obliquely as it travels down and lateral to insert in the iliotibial tract. Therefore in the subgluteal approach the needle passes through the gluteus maximus muscle, although it encounters a thinner layer of adipose tissue than in the buttock.
2. This approach may not involve the posterior femoral cutaneous nerve, which at this point is posterior to the sciatic nerve but already outside its sheath.

Popliteal or Distal Approaches to the Sciatic Nerve

This block is performed high enough above the crease behind the knee joint to block the nerve before its two main components diverge[6] but low enough to be in the area where the sciatic nerve is not covered by muscles.

Popliteal Block, Posterior Approach

Every description of a popliteal nerve block is based on identifying the muscular boundaries of the popliteal fossa. Defining these boundaries invariably introduces some subjectivity and increases the difficulty of the technique. Instead, we prefer to identify the tendons of the biceps femoris and semitendinosus muscles at the popliteal crease, eliminating the need to identify the more proximal trajectory of these muscles.

Patient Position

The patient is positioned prone with the foot moving freely and the knee in a neutral position, not internally or externally rotated (Fig. 27-4).

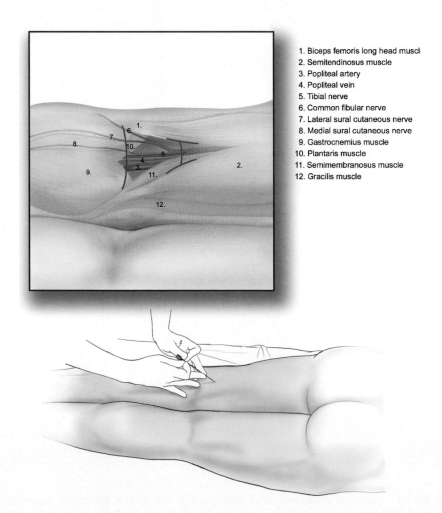

1. Biceps femoris long head muscl
2. Semitendinosus muscle
3. Popliteal artery
4. Popliteal vein
5. Tibial nerve
6. Common fibular nerve
7. Lateral sural cutaneous nerve
8. Medial sural cutaneous nerve
9. Gastrocnemius muscle
10. Plantaris muscle
11. Semimembranosus muscle
12. Gracilis muscle

Figure 27-4. Surface anatomy and positioning for the popliteal approach to the sciatic nerve block.

Needle Insertion and Technique

The patient is asked to flex the knee, making visible the tendons of biceps femoris muscle (lateral) and semitendinosus muscle (medial). The presence of these two tendons at the crease is marked (Fig. 27-4) and the midpoint between these two tendons at the crease is found. The point of needle entrance is located at 7 to 9 cm above this midpoint.

The needle is directed approximately 45 degrees proximally and advanced through the adipose tissue in the popliteal fossa before reaching the sciatic nerve. Because the midpoint of the nerve is slightly lateral to the midpoint between the tendons, the needle tends to come in contact with its tibial component or to miss the nerve on its medial side, which will require a slight lateral redirection. Contact with the femur indicates that the needle has penetrated too far.

Special Considerations

1. The neutral position of the knee on the table cannot be assessed reliably by the position of the foot. Instead, the patella must be palpated for this purpose.
2. The distance between the biceps and semitendinosus tendons at the popliteal crease in adults is about 6 to 9 cm.
3. The needle is advanced proximally for two reasons. First, it allows the needle to make contact with the sciatic nerve at a higher level than the skin puncture would be. This increases the chances of nerve block proximal to where the two branches diverge yet still avoids a path through muscle. The second reason is that it may promote proximal spread of the local anesthetic.
4. Because the nerve sheath at this level merges with the popliteal adipose tissue, a larger volume of local anesthetic is required than at more proximal levels.

Popliteal Block, Lateral Approach

Many patients who cannot be placed in the prone position can benefit from a sciatic nerve block performed from a lateral approach.

Patient Position

The patient is positioned supine with the knee slightly flexed and a pillow under the leg to be blocked.

Needle Insertion and Technique

The level of the popliteal crease is marked laterally. The groove between the biceps femoris and vastus lateralis muscles on the thigh is identified. A point on the skin in this groove approximately 10 cm above the popliteal crease marks the point where the needle is inserted.

The needle is advanced at a 10-degree posterior angle. If the leg is not flexed at the knee, contact can be made with the femur, which marks the approximate depth at which the nerve can be expected. After contact with the femur, aiming the needle at an angle of 30 degrees posterior should bring the needle tip in contact with the sciatic nerve. A localized twitch of the biceps femoris muscle may be elicited before reaching the sciatic nerve. If the needle fails to reach the sciatic nerve, it is redirected in a posterior direction.

Special Considerations

1. In contrast to the posterior approach, the operator cannot avoid passing the needle through muscle. There is accordingly no advantage to inserting the needle any less than 10 cm from the crease, and higher insertion makes proximal angulation unnecessary.
2. Although the needle penetrates the skin between the biceps femoris and vastus lateralis muscles, it has to be directed through the biceps femoris muscle (posterior) in order to reach the sciatic nerve lying medial to it. If the needle were to be directed parallel to the bed, it would come close to the plane of the popliteal vein (not the femur as frequently suggested), missing the sciatic nerve anterior and the femur posterior.
3. The projection of the sciatic nerve on the anterior thigh corresponds approximately to the level of the midpoint of the patella. This point can therefore be marked on the anterior thigh, as an indicator of depth, before performing the block. This would avoid the need to direct the needle toward the femur to obtain similar information.
4. A blanket roll can be place under a large thigh to compress the soft tissues behind the femur, thus reducing the area to be searched.

The Different Motor Responses Elicited from the Sciatic Nerve with a Nerve Stimulator and Their Significance

Any of the approaches described above, when performed with the aid of a nerve stimulator, produces muscle responses, which result from the action of different muscles.[7,8] The following is an interpretation of the muscles twitches that are possible during a sciatic nerve block at different levels:

1. Buttock motor response: This is caused by contraction of the gluteus maximus muscle due to direct muscle stimulation at relatively high current settings. It indicates that the nerve stimulator is functional and that the tip of the needle is still shallow to the nerve. This is not an acceptable motor response.

2. Posterior thigh motor response: This is caused by contraction of the hamstring muscles (usually the biceps femoris muscle), which could be due to stimulation of the most medial part of the sciatic nerve or direct hamstring muscle stimulation. The needle should be repositioned slightly laterally.

3. Foot dorsiflexion: This is caused by contraction of the tibialis anterior and/or extensor digitorum longus muscles and/or extensor hallucis longus muscle due to stimulation of the deep peroneal nerve. This is an acceptable response.

4. Foot plantarflexion: This is caused by contraction of the gastrocnemius and soleus muscles and/or flexor digitorum longus and/or flexor hallucis longus muscles and tibialis posterior muscle due to stimulation of the tibial nerve. This is an acceptable response.

5. Foot inversion: This is caused by contraction of the tibialis anterior muscle due to stimulation of the fibers to the deep peroneal nerve. The tibialis posterior muscle (innervated by the tibial nerve)

also causes weak foot inversion, but its main action is adduction of the foot. This is an acceptable response.

6. Foot eversion: This is caused by contraction of the peroneus longus and brevis muscles by stimulating fibers of the superficial peroneal nerve. This is an acceptable twitch.

The neurotomes covered by the sciatic block are depicted in Fig. 27-5.

Catheter Techniques

A variety of lower extremity operations can be performed successfully under a sciatic block. A catheter kept in place for 1 to 7 days prolongs the analgesia block into the postoperative period until the pain becomes manageable with oral analgesics. All the techniques described above are also used for catheter placement. The subgluteal approach is the most suitable. Detailed catheter placement technique and methods of securing the catheter are described elsewhere in this volume.

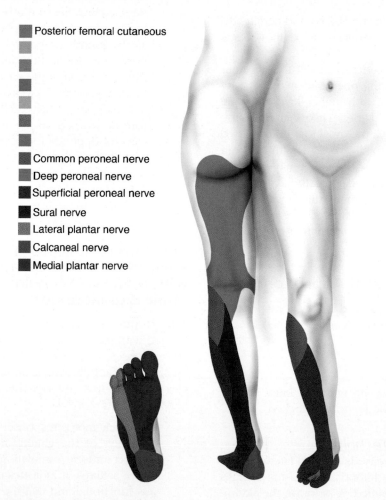

Posterior femoral cutaneous

Common peroneal nerve
Deep peroneal nerve
Superficial peroneal nerve
Sural nerve
Lateral plantar nerve
Calcaneal nerve
Medial plantar nerve

Figure 27-5 (Plate 4). Peripheral nerve dermatomes blocked by the sciatic nerve block.

Pharmacologic Choice

Sciatic nerve block lasts longer than other peripheral nerve blocks. Therefore, when it is used as the main anesthetic for a surgical procedure (e.g., foot and ankle surgery, Achilles' tendon repair, etc.), we prefer to use an intermediate-acting agent like mepivacaine. For example, 30 mL of a 1.5% solution provides about 3 h of anesthesia and 4 to 5 h of analgesia. Epinephrine (1:200,000) and 2 mL of 8.4% sodium bicarbonate for every 20 mL of local anesthetic solution can be added. The addition of epinephrine prolongs the anesthesia to about 4 to 5 h and the analgesia to 5 to 7 h. The same concentration and volume of lidocaine can be used. If more prolonged anesthesia is desired, 30 mL of 0.625% levobupivacaine, ropivacaine, or bupivacaine (equal volumes of 0.5 and 0.75%) can be used. The onset of complete anesthesia with mepivacaine takes approximately 15 to 20 min; for the longer acting agents, it is between 20 and 40 min.

Potential Problems and Final Considerations

1. When the needle needs to be moved closer to the nerve with a nerve stimulator technique, the first step is to continue to move it in the original direction (usually deeper). If moving the needle by 1 mm makes the response stronger, the nerve is in fact deeper than the tip of the needle. Sometimes, when the needle has approached the nerve tangentially on one of its sides, thrusting the needle deeper makes the twitch weaker. In this case the needle is withdrawn and redirected laterally if the original twitch was a tibial nerve response or medially if the twitch was a peroneal nerve response.

2. If a muscle twitch is still strong at low output (less than 0.4 mA), it is necessary to determine the current at which it would disappear, because the needle could be in the nerve. If the current is less than 0.2 mA, intraneural placement must be suspected and the needle withdrawn somewhat.

REFERENCES

1. Hollinshead WH. *Anatomy for Surgeons. The Back and Limbs*, 3d ed. Philadelphia: Harper & Row, 1982.
2. Hall J, Froster-Iskenius U, Allanton J. *Handbook of Normal Physical Measurements*. Oxford, UK: Oxford University Press, 1989.
3. Winnie A, Ramamurthy S, Durrani Z, et al. Plexus blocks for lower extremity surgery. *Anesth Rev* 1:11–16,1974.
4. Franco CD. Posterior approach to the sciatic nerve in adults: Is euclidean geometry still necessary? *Anesthesiology* 98:723–728, 2003.
5. Di Benedetto P, Bertini L, Casati A, et al. A new posterior approach to the sciatic nerve block: A prospective randomized comparison with the classic posterior approach. *Anesth Analg* 93:1040–1044, 2001.
6. Hadzic A, Vloka JD. *Peripheral Nerve Blocks. Principles and Practice*. New York: McGraw-Hill, 2004.
7. Hoppenfeld S. *Orthopaedic Neurology. A Diagnostic Guide to Neurological Levels*. Philadelphia: Lippincott Williams & Wilkins, 1997.
8. Sunderland S. The sciatic nerve and its tibial and common peroneal divisions. Anatomical and physiological features, in Sunderland S (ed): *Nerves and Nerve Injuries*, 2d ed. Edinburgh: Churchill Livingstone, 1978.

CHAPTER 28

Ankle Block

Theresa Rickelman / André P. Boezaart

▶ INTRODUCTION

The ankle block is very widely used for anesthesia of the distal foot or for postoperative analgesia.[1] It is regarded as a "basic" block[2] but is probably the most commonly failed block of all the peripheral nerve blocks, for two main reasons:

1. The fascial layers and the relative position of the five nerves to the fascial layers around the ankle are not widely understood.[1,2]
2. Not all five nerves are always blocked—in ignorance or disregard of the fact that the areas of sensory nerve supply of the foot overlap, and that this overlap is not consistent.

Patient Selection

The most common indication for an ankle block is surgery of the diabetic foot. The other widely used indication is postoperative pain of bunion surgery and surgery for rheumatoid arthritis. Ankle block can be used for most distal foot surgery, but it is not suitable for ankle surgery. An ankle tourniquet is usually tolerated well by patients with minimal sedation. An ankle block is useful for fragile patients who are unable to withstand general anesthesia or are unable to have epidural or spinal anesthesia. The presence of anticoagulation is not a contraindication for ankle block.

It can be painful to place an ankle block, and liberal skin infiltration with a fast-acting local anesthetic agent such as lidocaine without epinephrine, injected slowly and with a fine needle, is advised. With the exception of the posterior tibial nerve, the nerves to the foot are all sensory nerves, so there is no problem of accidentally blocking a nerve with skin infiltration. Ankle blocks are frequently done in a heavily sedated or even anesthetized patient.

▶ APPLIED ANATOMY

Gross Anatomy

All the nerves that supply the bones of the foot originate from all the lumbar and most of the sacral roots. Selective nerve blocks around the ankle therefore almost always lead to some degree of failure. Because there is great variation of the dermatomal nerve supply of the foot, it is prudent to block all five nerves around the ankle joint for every foot operation except perhaps for the most superficial skin surgery. In these cases, local field blocks could be a better choice.

The medial aspect of the foot and the medial part of the ankle joint receive their sensory supply from the saphenous nerve, which is the terminal branch of the femoral nerve (Fig. 28-1).[3] The deep peroneal nerve supplies the area between the first and second toes, while most of the dorsal aspect of the foot gets its sensory nerve supply from the superficial peroneal nerve. Both these nerves originate from the common peroneal nerve.[3] (See Chap. 12.)

The lateral aspect of the foot is supplied by the lateral dorsal cutaneous and lateral calcaneal branches of the sural nerve, which in turn originate from the tibial nerve in the popliteal fossa (Fig. 28-1). The medial and posterior aspects of the heel receive their sensory nerve supply from the medial calcaneal branch of the tibial nerve.

It is important for a successful ankle block to realize that there are three nerves that are superficial to the fascia, which is represented by a purple line in Fig. 28-2 and

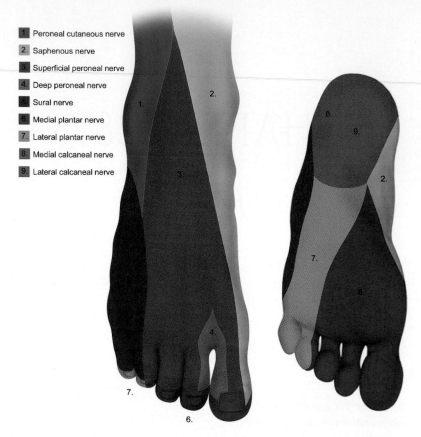

Figure 28-1. Dermatomes of the peripheral nerves of the foot.

1. Superficial peroneal nerve
2. Deep peroneal nerve
3. Saphenous nerve
4. Posterior tibial nerve
5. Sural nerve

6. Achilles tendon
7. Fascia layers
8. Extensor hallucis longus tendon
9. Anterior tibialis tendon

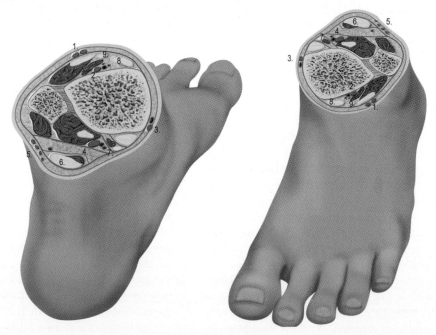

Figure 28-2. Cross section of the ankle. The purple lines represent the fascial layers. Note the intricate array of fascial layers surrounding the posterior tibial nerve.

is indicated by the arrows. These nerves are (A) the superficial peroneal, (C) saphenous, and (E) sural nerves. Note that the names of all three of these nerves start with the letter "S."

Deep to this fascia and between the tendons of the hallucis longus (I) and tibial (H) muscles is the deep peroneal nerve. In close proximity to the tibia as well as posterior and adjacent to the tibial artery and vein, in a complex array of fascial compartments, is the tibial nerve (G) (Fig. 28-2). The tibial nerve is a motor nerve, which makes its identification with a stimulating needle and nerve stimulator relatively easy. Because local anesthetic agents do not cross fascial layers readily, it is important to place the needle in the same fascial compartment as the nerve.[4] The method, described in many older textbooks, of approaching the tibial nerve from posterior until the bone of the tibia is encountered and then withdrawing the needle slightly, is outdated; this is a possibly important reason why many ankle blocks fail.[1] The tibial nerve is important, since it supplies approximately all of the sole of the foot[5] (Fig. 28-1).

It is important to remember that the addition of epinephrine to the local anesthetic agent is absolutely contraindicated in doing an ankle block, since this can seriously threaten the integrity of the blood supply to the foot. It can be seen in Fig. 28-3 that the main blood supply to the foot (i.e., the dorsal pedal artery and the posterior tibial artery) is situated in close proximity to the tibial nerve (G) and the deep peroneal nerve (B).

Functional Neuroanatomy

A nerve stimulator can be used to identify the posterior tibial nerve at the ankle. When the nerve is stimulated, plantar flexion movements of the toes will be observed.

1. Great saphenous vein
2. Dorsal venous arch
3. Small saphenous vein
4. Superficial peroneal nerve
5. Saphenous nerve
6. Deep peroneal nerve
7. Peroneal artery
8. Sural nerve
9. Posterior tibial vein
10. Posterior tibial artery
11. Posterior tibial nerve
12. Dorsal pedis artery

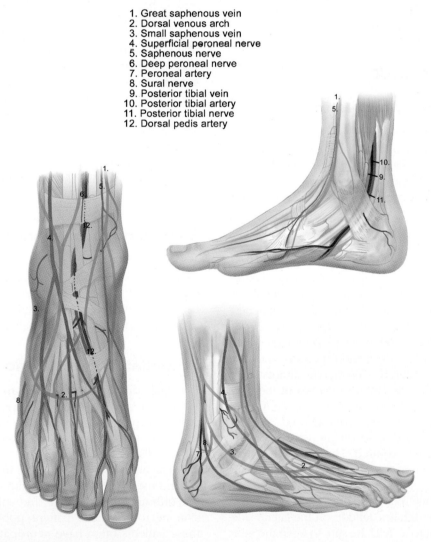

Figure 28-3. Surface anatomy of the ankle. Note the retinacula and areas where nerves are in confined spaces.

Surface Anatomy (Landmarks)

The posterior tibial artery can usually be palpated behind the medial malleolus (Fig. 28-3). The tibial nerve is just posterior to the artery. If the artery cannot be palpated, the surface landmark of the nerve, which is usually halfway between the medial malleolus and the Achilles' tendon, can be used.[6]

The sural nerve is in the subcutaneous area superficial to the fascia, immediately posterior to the lateral malleolus.[6] The area forms a "valley" and, with this block, this valley is converted to a "hill" (Robert Koorn, MD, personal communication). (Figs. 28-2 and 28-3).

It is important to avoid injecting in or through the retinaculum joining the two malleoli (Figure 28-3); the ankle block should be done above this retinaculum. Palpation of the area between the tendons of the tibial and extensor hallucis longus muscles can identify the deep peroneal nerve, while the superficial peroneal nerve is situated in the area lateral to these tendons.[4] The saphenous nerve is next to and immediately anterior to the saphenous vein on the anterior aspect of the medial malleolus[6] (Fig. 28-3).

▶ BLOCK TECHNIQUE

Patient Positioning and Timing

The patient is placed in the supine position and the foot raised 6 in. by placing a pillow under the calf. Ankle block is often done after the induction of general anesthesia to provide postoperative analgesia. The duration of the block is relatively long, and blocks lasting up to 36 h have been recorded.

Single-Injection Ankle Block

The skin and subcutaneous tissue in the area of the tibial nerve is infiltrated with 1 to 2% lidocaine, taking care not to penetrate the fascia with the fine needle at this stage. A 22-gauge 2-in. stimulating needle attached to a nerve stimulator set at a current output of 1 to 2 mA, 2 Hz, and a pulse width of 100 to 300 μs is used to locate the posterior tibial nerve. Toe flexion indicates that the nerve has been encountered. The nerve stimulator is now turned down until brisk motor twitches of the toes can still be seen at a current output of 0.3 to 0.5 mA. This may not be possible in diabetic patients and patients with Charcot-Marie-Tooth disease owing to neuropathy. Higher currents are often required. The motor response will immediately cease upon injection of local anesthetic agent.

The foot is internally rotated and the "valley" from the lateral malleolus to the Achilles' tendon on the lateral side of the ankle is turned into a "hill." Be sure to keep the needle superficial to the fascia and be sure that a skin wheal is observed when the sural nerve is blocked. This is a purely sensory nerve and it does not matter if this skin infiltration affects the nerve. The main dose of the local anesthetic agent is now injected subcutaneously and superficial to the fascia, again observing the skin wheal.

Taking care to remain proximal to the retinaculum that joins the medial and lateral malleoli, the tendons of the anterior tibial muscle and extensor of the big toe are palpated. Extension (or dorsiflexion) of the big toe makes the tendon easy to palpate. Lidocaine is injected all the way down to the tibial bone between these two tendons. The same needle entry site is used and the lateral subcutaneous area toward the fibula is injected with lidocaine, and the area around the saphenous vein is anesthetized.

A 25-gauge needle attached to a syringe with local anesthetic agent is inserted between the tendons of the anterior tibial muscle and the extensor hallucis longus until it encounters the tibia. It is then slightly withdrawn and 3 to 7 mL of local anesthetic agent is injected. Without leaving the skin, the needle is now directed laterally between the skin and fascial layer toward the fibula. Note the skin wheal that is raised during injection, which indicates that the injection is subcutaneous yet superficial to the fascia. Intradermal injection, like injection deep to the fascia, will lead to failed block.

Direct the needle medially and subcutaneously toward the anterior aspect of the medial malleolus and observe the skin wheal while injecting on the saphenous nerve, subcutaneously and superficial to the fascia, around the saphenous vein. Take care not to puncture the saphenous vein.

Selection of Local Anesthetic Agent

Most local anesthetic agents have been used for this block.[1,2,4] We use 0.5 to 0.75% ropivacaine or 0.5% bupivacaine. Usually 5 to 7 mL is all that is required to block each nerve. It is emphasized that epinephrine should not be used with the local anesthetic agent.

Potential Problems and Complications

Potential complications of the ankle block include persistent paresthesia and skin necrosis. Injury can occur from hydrostatic pressures secondary to high-volume injections. Overall, this is a very safe and effective block for any distal foot surgery.

Practitioners should keep in mind that the skin around the ankle of patients with diabetes and rheumatoid arthritis is often fragile, and ankle blocks can lead to skin necrosis in this patient population. Furthermore, these patients often have neuropathy, which may cause the block to be mistakenly judged successful.

REFERENCES

1. Brown DL. *Atlas of Regional Anesthesia*, 2d ed. Philadelphia: Saunders, 1999:131–133.
2. Hadzic A, Vloka JD. *Peripheral Nerve Blocks.* New York: McGraw-Hill, 2004:317–330.
3. Sarrafian SK. *Anatomy of the Foot and Ankle: Descriptive, Topographic, Functional*, 2d ed. Philadelphia: Lippincott, 1993:385–389.
4. Meier G, Büttner J. *Atlas der Peripheren Regionalenästesie.* Stuttgart: Thieme, 2004:203–214.
5. Sarrafian SK. *Anatomy of the Foot and Ankle: Descriptive, Topographic, Functional*, 2d ed. Philadelphia: Lippincott Company, 1993:383–385.
6. Sarrafian SK. *Anatomy of the Foot and Ankle: Descriptive, Topographic, Functional*, 2d ed. Philadelphia: Lippincott, 1993:391–473.

CHAPTER 29

Lumbar Paravertebral (Psoas Compartment) Block

XAVIER CAPDEVILA/MARIE-JOSÉE NADEAU

► INTRODUCTION

The lumbar paravertebral or psoas compartment block is a lumbar plexus block. This is the most reliable regional anesthesia technique for blocking major branches of the lumbar plexus. Major surgical procedures of the hip and knee are the most common indications for this block. A catheter can be inserted to provide prolonged analgesia. Because it is a deep technique, near the neuraxis, many precautions should be taken. Major adverse events have been described after the performance of this block. Epidural block is the most frequent complication, but among the most dangerous complications are total spinal anesthesia and systemic toxicity. It is therefore important to select patients carefully, with good indications. When possible, a femoral block should be preferred to a lumbar paravertebral approach. Moreover, only experienced anesthesiologists should perform the lumbar paravertebral block. A methodical approach to the technique and a sound knowledge of anatomy are essential to perform the block safely and successfully.

History of the Block

Winnie et al. renewed interest in lower extremity blocks in 1973 with the description of the "3 in 1" block.[1] A year later, in 1974, they described the "combined lumbosacral plexus block,[2] stating that with a large volume of local anesthetic (40 mL), both the lumbar and the sacral plexus could be blocked by a paravertebral approach. Subsequent studies demonstrated the failure of this technique to anesthetize the sacral plexus completely.[3-7] Two years after Winnie,

Chayen et al. described a second approach to the lumbar plexus: the "psoas compartment block."[8] The two techniques are similar. They are performed at the L4-5 interspace with different surface anatomy landmarks. In 1993, Hanna et al. proposed another more cephalad approach at the L2-3 interspace.[9] This technique had the theoretical advantage of being performed centrally to the anterior primary rami forming the lumbar plexus. However, L4-5 approaches are more popular since the report by Aida et al.[10] of two renal subcapsular hematomas that occurred after the block was performed at L2-3. In 2002, Capdevila et al.[6] proposed different surface anatomy landmarks for Winnie's block in order to reduce adverse events and increase block success. The groups of Ben-David,[11] Vagadhia,[12] and Pandin[7] described catheter techniques. These techniques are variations of the Winnie and Chayen approaches. Ultrasound assistance has been proposed recently by Kirchmair et al.[13-14] to learning the block techniques and lessen complications.

Winnie's, Chayen's, and Hanna's groups used loss-of-resistance and paresthesia to localize the plexus. Advances in nerve stimulation and insulated needle technology have improved the technique, and nerve stimulation is actually the localization method of choice.[5]

► ANATOMY

Applied and Functional Anatomy

In the literature the lumbar plexus localization is still a controversial issue. Some authors, like Winnie et al.,[2]

located the plexus between the psoas and quadratus lumborum muscles. Recent studies of the plexus place the nerve branches within the psoas muscle[6,8,15] between its anterior and posterior masses (Fig. 29-1). The plexus is formed by the first three and the greater part of the fourth lumbar ventral rami. A contribution of the twelfth thoracic nerve is common. When the L1, L2, L3, and L4 ventral rami leave the intervertebral foramina, they become embedded in the psoas muscle, anterior to the transverse processes. At the L4-5 level, contrary to what is frequently published, lumbar plexus branches are still medial, close to the transverse processes (Fig. 29-2). The distance from the lumbar plexus to the skin varies with body mass index (BMI)[6,13] and gender.[6,15] In one study, the distances varied from 57 to 93 mm in women and 61 to 101 mm in men.[6] Insertion of a needle to greater depths than these could result in a retroperitoneal puncture.

The first three and the greater part of the fourth lumbar ventral rami split into anterior and posterior divisions within the psoas muscle. These divisions join to form the individual branches of the lumbar plexus. The superior branches are the iliohypogastric, ilioinguinal, and genitofemoral nerves. Caudal to these three nerves are the three major branches: laterally, the femoral cutaneous nerve; centrally, the femoral nerve; and medially, the obturator nerve. Farny et al.[15] demonstrated variations in the localization of the three main branches of the plexus within the psoas muscle. The obturator nerve was the more variable one. In two of their four cadavers, the nerve was in a fold different from the fold enclosing the femoral and the lateral femoral cutaneous nerve. The smaller part of the fourth lumbar ventral rami joins the fifth rami to form the lumbosacral trunk, the upper portion of the sacral plexus.

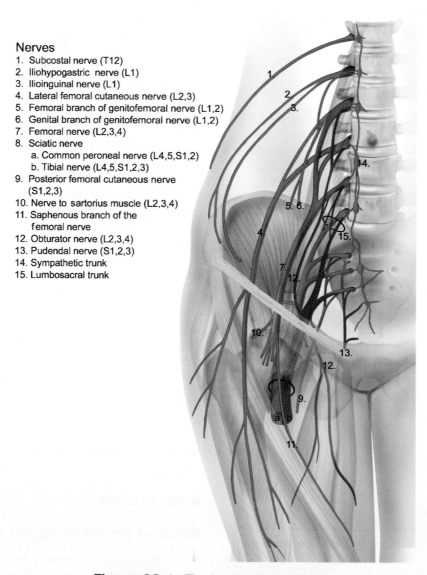

Nerves
1. Subcostal nerve (T12)
2. Iliohypogastric nerve (L1)
3. Ilioinguinal nerve (L1)
4. Lateral femoral cutaneous nerve (L2,3)
5. Femoral branch of genitofemoral nerve (L1,2)
6. Genital branch of genitofemoral nerve (L1,2)
7. Femoral nerve (L2,3,4)
8. Sciatic nerve
   a. Common peroneal nerve (L4,5,S1,2)
   b. Tibial nerve (L4,5,S1,2,3)
9. Posterior femoral cutaneous nerve (S1,2,3)
10. Nerve to sartorius muscle (L2,3,4)
11. Saphenous branch of the femoral nerve
12. Obturator nerve (L2,3,4)
13. Pudendal nerve (S1,2,3)
14. Sympathetic trunk
15. Lumbosacral trunk

Figure 29-1. The lumbosacral plexus.

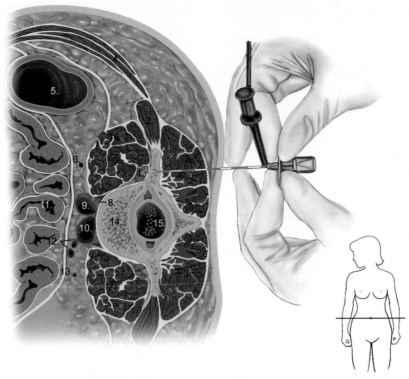

1. Lumbar plexus (ventral rami of
   L2-L4 becoming femoral and
   obturator nerves and L4 part of
   lumbosacral trunk)
2. Quadratus lumborum muscle
3. Erector spinae muscle
4. External and internal oblique muscles
   and transversus abdominis muscle
5. Ascending colon
6. Right ureter
7. Psoas major muscles
8. Sympathetic trunk

9. Inferior vena cava
10. Aortic bifurcation, common iliac arteries
11. Loops of small intestine
12. Inferior mesenteric artery and vein
13. Left ureter
14. Body of L4 vertebra
15. Cauda equina
16. Genitofemoral nerve

Figure 29-2. Cross section through the L4 vertebra area.

The iliohypogastric nerve is the more cephalad branch of the lumbar plexus originating from the superior division of the first lumbar ventral rami (often with a contribution from the twelfth thoracic nerve). It passes through the transverse abdominis muscle to supply motor fibers to the abdominal muscles and sensitive fibers to the suprapubic and superolateral hip regions.

The ilioinguinal nerve also arises from the superior division of the first lumbar ventral rami. It runs slightly caudal to the iliohypogastric nerve. It passes in the inguinal canal to supply sensitive fibers to the upper and medial parts of the thigh.

The genitofemoral nerve is the union of the inferior division of the first lumbar ventral rami and the small superior division of L2 ventral rami. It crosses the psoas muscle obliquely, emerges at its medial border, and runs down between the psoas muscle and the peritoneum, close to the vertebral column. It innervates the cremaster muscle and the skin over the femoral triangle, scrotum/labium major, and mons pubis.

The lateral femoral cutaneous nerve is formed from the dorsal divisions of the L2 and L3 ventral rami. It leaves the lateral part of the psoas at L4 level[15] and passes under the lateral part of the inguinal ligament to supply the skin of the lateral part of the thigh.

The femoral nerve is the largest branch of the lumbar plexus. It is the union of the large dorsal divisions of the L2, L3, and L4 ventral rami. It emerges from the posterolateral border of the psoas muscle at the junction of the muscle's upper two-thirds and lower third.[15] It then runs caudally in the groove between the psoas and iliacus muscles, behind the fascia iliaca, and continues on below the inguinal ligament, lateral to the inguinal artery, where it divides into numerous branches. At this point, it is covered by two fascial layers, the fascia iliaca and fascia lata (Fig. 26-1). The fascia iliaca covers the psoas and iliacus muscles from the iliac crest to the inguinal ligament. This fascia is continuous with the fascia covering the front of the quadratus lumborum muscle. The fascia iliaca and a portion of the psoas muscle separate the femoral nerve from the femoral vessels. The fascia lata is the deep fascia of the thigh. It is attached to the inguinal ligament and the iliac crest. The femoral nerve provides sensory and motor innervation to the anterior thigh, anterior part of the knee, and hip joints. A branch of the femoral nerve becomes the saphenous nerve, which gives sensory innervation to the skin over the medial aspect of the leg to the first metatarsal.

The obturator nerve is formed from the smaller anterior divisions of the L2, L3, and L4 ventral rami. It leaves the psoas at its internal and posterior border between L5 and S1.[15] At this point, the fascia iliaca and the psoas muscle separate the obturator nerve from the femoral nerve. The anterior branch innervates the adductors brevis and longus, pectineus, and gracilis muscles. It sometimes gives sensory innervation to the medial or posterior aspect of the knee. Bouaziz et al. demonstrated that cutaneous distribution of the obturator nerve is highly variable and frequently absent.[16] After an isolated obturator nerve block, it was shown that 57 percent of their patients had no cutaneous distribution of this nerve, 23 percent had an area of hypoesthesia at the superior part of the popliteal fossa, and 20 percent had a sensory deficit at the medial aspect of the thigh.

Figure 29-3 illustrates the innervation by peripheral nerves of the lower extremity. A good knowledge of these distributions is important for the performance of adequate regional anesthesia. Complete anesthesia of the lower extremity is possible with combined block of the lumbar and sacral plexus. For surgery in a proximal area of the thigh, a block of the subcostal nerve (from the twelfth thoracic nerve) might be necessary.

Surface Anatomy

The iliac crest is the ridge of pelvic bones. A line drawn between the highest points of both iliac crests generally passes over the spinous process of the fourth lumbar vertebra. This is Tuffier's line.

The posterosuperior iliac spine (PSIS) is the bony prominence at the posterior end of the iliac crest. It is just

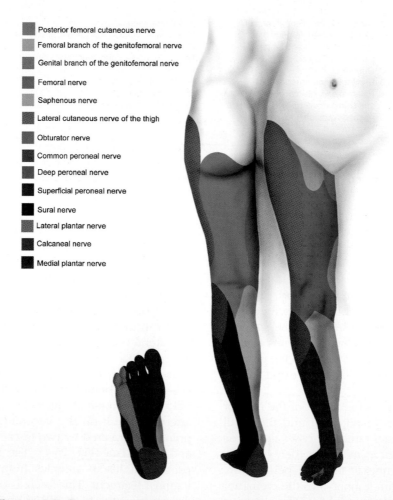

Posterior femoral cutaneous nerve
Femoral branch of the genitofemoral nerve
Genital branch of the genitofemoral nerve
Femoral nerve
Saphenous nerve
Lateral cutaneous nerve of the thigh
Obturator nerve
Common peroneal nerve
Deep peroneal nerve
Superficial peroneal nerve
Sural nerve
Lateral plantar nerve
Calcaneal nerve
Medial plantar nerve

Figure 29-3. Lower extremity dermatomes of the peripheral nerves.

caudal to the skin depression visible close to the midline; it is above buttocks on both sides and can be palpated easily by following the iliac crest to its posterior end.

▶ PATIENT SELECTION

Diffusion Space and Extent of Blockade

To select an adequate block for a patient, the anesthesiologist must know exactly the anesthetic extent of the block chosen compared with other blocks. Two different approaches are available for lumbar plexus anesthesia: the inguinal paravascular 3-in-1 block and the lumbar paravertebral block. Each approach has specific advantages; which one is chosen depends on block extension, possible complications, and patient considerations. The approach with the better risk/benefit balance must be chosen.

An injection site corresponds to a common distribution pattern: the diffusion space. It depends on the surrounding fatty and connective tissues. Fascial layers constitute a frequent barrier to local anesthetic diffusion. Each injection site in a diffusion area corresponds to a preferential distribution of local anesthetics toward less resistant regions. The diffusion space concept were utilized by Winnie when he described his 3-in-1 block.[1] Unfortunately this technique could not consistently block the superior branches of the lumbar plexus (the iliohypogastric, ilioinguinal, and genitofemoral nerves)[17] or the obturator nerve. The obturator nerve is anesthetized in 4 to 10 percent of such cases. Anatomic factors explain this: the obturator nerve is separated from the femoral nerve at the inguinal level by the fascia iliaca and the psoas muscle. Diffusion of local anesthetic agent across these barriers is unlikely. Consequently, to block the obturator nerve, local anesthetics must spread up to the lumbar plexus, as Winnie hypothesized in his description of the inguinal paravascular approach. The diffusion space available in performing an inguinal approach is very broad under the fascia iliaca, at the surface of the psoas and iliacus muscles. Cephalic spread of local anesthetics above L4 is uncommon, and it does not seem to be greatly influenced by injected volumes. After injection of 30 mL of local anesthetics with 5 mL of contrast media using the inguinal paravascular approach, a front-view x-ray revealed a spread in the plexus area in 8,3 percent of cases.[18] With the insertion of a catheter 16 to 20 cm below the fascia iliaca, results were slightly better.[19] Twenty-three percent of catheters reached the lumbar plexus area and in 91 percent of these achieved a block of the three main nerves (lateral femoral cutaneous, femoral, and obturator nerves). In this study, a block of the three main nerves was observed in 27, 52, and 91 percent of cases, depending whether the tips of the catheters were situated in an external, internal, or lumbar position, respectively. Based on these results, for a "complete block" of the lumbar plexus, another block technique should be chosen.

In performing a lumbar paravertebral block, the injection is most frequently within the psoas muscle.[6,7] In this situation, the diffusion space corresponds to the psoas compartment bordered medially by the attachments of the psoas muscle to the vertebral bodies and the transverse processes, anterolaterally by the psoas muscle's fascia, and posteriorly by the quadratus lumborum muscle's fascia. Occasionally (in approximately 20 to 25 percent of cases), the tip of the needle is situated between the psoas and quadratus lumborum muscles.[6,7] When this happens, the distribution of local anesthetic distribution is similar to the lumbar plexus distribution, attained in 8 to 25 percent of cases with the inguinal paravascular approach.[6,18,19] Blockade of the obturator and accessory (iliohypogastric, ilioinguinal, and genitofemoral) nerves is observed more often with the psoas compartment distribution.[7] In a study of lumbar paravertebral blocks, complete anesthesia of the lumbar plexus (three main and accessory branches) was observed in 64 percent of patients with psoas compartment distribution compared to 14 percent in the group with a distribution under the fascia iliaca.[7] In the group with distribution of local anesthetic under the fascia iliaca, dermatome anesthesia of the first sacral root was noted in 43 percent of patients.[7] The lumbar paravertebral technique achieved lateral femoral cutaneous nerve block in 85 to 100 percent of cases,[3,6,7,17,20,21] femoral nerve block in 95 to 100 percent,[3,6,7,17,20,21] and obturator nerve block in 90 to 100 percent.[3,6,7,21] One study reported an obturator nerve block in only 63 percent of cases following a lumbar paravertebral technique using Winnie's approach.[20] The sacral plexus is rarely blocked by the lumbar paravertebral technique.[3–7] A partial blockade of the lumbosacral trunk is sometimes noted.[3–7] A sciatic nerve block should be added to anesthetize the whole lower limb.[4,7,8]

Compared to the anterior inguinal paravascular approach, the posterior lumbar paravertebral technique provides a more reliable and extensive block of all branches of the lumbar plexus.[3,17,20,21] Undoubtedly the obturator nerve is more regularly blocked.[3,20,21] Also, the proximal thigh, innervated by superior branches of the lumbar plexus (iliohypogastric, ilioinguinal, and genitofemoral nerves), is more consistently anesthetized.[17]

Clinical Indications

The lumbar paravertebral block has been used in many clinical situations. As a single-injection technique, it was used in combination with a sciatic nerve block for surgery of the entire lower limb. Catheter techniques have been used for postoperative analgesia after major knee and hip surgery. In each situation, the balance between risks and benefits must be carefully evaluated before choosing the anesthetic technique. The relatively high incidence of complications reported with the lumbar paravertebral block (more than 1 major adverse event for 400 blocks in one report[22]) should be taken into consideration.

Surgery below the Knee

Lumbar paravertebral block is not indicated for surgery below the knee. Since the only lumbar plexus branch involved below the knee is the saphenous nerve, it can be blocked with an inguinal femoral block or a more distal approach.

Surgery of the Knee

SINGLE-INJECTION TECHNIQUE

For knee surgery, both the femoral and the obturator nerves must be anesthetized. The lumbar paravertebral block permits anesthesia of these two nerves with a single injection. Alternatively, they can be blocked separately. Since the description of a superficial approach to the obturator nerve in the inguinal region,[23] the combination of this block with an inguinal femoral block may be associated with a lower risk of complications. Jankowski et al.[24] compared lumbar paravertebral block with spinal and general anesthesia for outpatient knee arthroscopy. They found significantly less postoperative pain and better patient satisfaction with spinal and lumbar paravertebral block anesthesia. No difference was noted between regional techniques. Time to meet hospital discharge criteria was not different between the three groups.

CONTINUOUS CATHETER TECHNIQUE

An opioid-free analgesic combined with a continuous lumbar paravertebral block has been described in cases of total knee arthroplasty.[5] However, in a recent study, the continuous lumbar paravertebral block did not show any advantages over the continuous femoral nerve block after total knee replacement.[21] Since the anterior approach poses less risk of complications, it should be preferred over the posterior one. Some exceptions may be discussed. Continuous lumbar paravertebral block can be useful in major knee operations like prosthesis replacement or oncologic surgery.

Surgery above the Knee

SINGLE-INJECTION TECHNIQUE

For hip fracture in the elderly, the single-injection technique was associated with significantly less ephedrine consumption compared to single-injection spinal anesthesia.[25] There was no difference in arterial blood pressure measurements between groups.[25] In surgical correction of fractured femoral neck, White and Chappell[26] obtained greater

hemodynamic stability using a lumbar plexus block combined with light general anesthesia compared with spinal anesthesia combined with light general anesthesia or with general anesthesia only. Stevens et al.[27] reported a decrease in blood loss when a lumbar paravertebral plexus block was combined with general anesthesia for total hip arthroplasty compared with general anesthesia alone, but arterial blood pressure was significantly lower in the first group. There is no study yet that has compared lumbar paravertebral block with continuous spinal anesthesia; but in our clinical experience, hemodynamic stability is comparable. In the elderly, complication risks are probably fewer with continuous spinal anesthesia, since headache after dural puncture is less frequent in this population. Further research is needed.

The literature on the subject indicates that single-injection lumbar paravertebral block for postoperative analgesia of primary total-hip arthroplasty has not proven useful. One study compared intravenous patient-controlled analgesia (PCA) with morphine, single injection of femoral nerve, and single-injection lumbar paravertebral block.[17] Morphine consumption per hour, as "rescue analgesia," was lower in the lumbar block group for the first 4 h only.

After that, morphine consumption per hour was equivalent and low in the three groups. There was no difference in respiratory rate or in frequency of nausea, vomiting, or pruritus among the three groups. Souron et al.[28] obtained better analgesia after primary hip arthroplasty with intrathecal morphine (0.1 mg) than with single-injection lumbar paravertebral block. The lumbar block group had higher pain scores on the visual analog scale (VAS) and 15-fold higher morphine requirements. The incidence of pruritus, nausea, and vomiting was not different between the two groups. The incidence of urinary retention was higher in the spinal group (37 versus 11.5 percent). The results of these two studies may be explained by the fact that primary hip arthroplasty is not as painful as knee surgery; therefore regional anesthesia techniques are not routinely indicated.

Lumbar paravertebral blocks have been used for the management of chronic hip pain.[29] Because of their relatively short duration of action, many blocks must be performed. Other techniques should be tried first and the lumbar paravertebral block used only when usual treatments have failed.

CONTINUOUS CATHETER TECHNIQUE

Continuous lumbar paravertebral block is effective for postoperative analgesia after hip surgery, especially revision hip arthroplasty.[4,6,30] Primary hip replacement does not require long-term nerve block. There are, however, only a few studies comparing this technique with other available techniques. Türker et al. compared continuous lumbar paravertebral block with epidural block for analgesia in partial hip replacement surgery.[30] Analgesia was similar for the two groups, but there were fewer side effects in the lumbar block group. Perioperatively, the epidural group showed a greater decrease in blood pressure and required more ephedrine. Orthostatic hypotension, urinary retention, nausea, and vomiting were also significantly more frequent in the epidural group. It can be concluded that continuous lumbar paravertebral block is a better choice than epidural block in providing analgesia after partial hip surgery.

Is a continuous lumbar paravertebral block better than PCA with morphine? The question is still unanswered, but single-injection technique did not show any advantages over PCA with morphine.[17] This is probably so because all the studies done compared the block with morphine following primary hip replacement, which does not require much analgesia. The discouraging results of a single-injection block after primary hip arthroplasty lead us to suppose that continuous techniques are not a good choice for postoperative analgesia in this kind of surgery. As with knee surgery (see "Continuous Catheter Technique," under "Surgery of the Knee," above), continuous lumbar paravertebral block should be restricted to major hip operations such as revision hip replacement with a prosthesis.

Contraindications

The usual contraindications to nerve blocks apply to lumbar paravertebral block. There are also specific contraindications to this block. These general and specific absolute contraindications are as follows[23]:

> Patient refusal
> Infection in the puncture region
> Abnormal coagulation or anticoagulation medication
> Local anesthetic contraindication
> Vertebral and meningeal infectious syndromes
> Lumbar vertebral trauma
> Significant scoliosis

The lumbar paravertebral block is a deep technique near the neuraxis. In case of vascular puncture, compression is not possible. Cases of retroperitoneal hematoma with anemia[31] and plexopathy[32] have been described after the use of enoxaparin. Precautions are the same as those taken with neuraxial blocks.[31] There are few recommendations for the use of peripheral block and anticoagulation. For the lumbar paravertebral block, the recommendations of the American Society of Regional Anesthesia on Neuraxial Anesthesia and Anticoagulation[33] are good to use.[5]

Other situations represent relative contraindications.[23] In these cases, the benefit/risk ratio should be assessed before selecting the anesthetic or analgesia technique. Other available techniques should be considered. These relative contraindications are as follows:

> Sepsis
> Anxious or agitated patient
> Psychiatric illness
> Diabetic neuropathy
> Neurologic lesion in the lumbar plexus region

▶ PERFORMANCE OF THE BLOCK

Sedation

Mild sedation of the patient is acceptable and may be preferable in certain situations. Heavy sedation should probably be avoided, since patient cooperation may be essential for safe performance of the block. The anesthesiologist should continuously communicate with the patient to detect early signs of intravascular or neuraxial injection.

Patient Positioning

The patient is placed in a lateral decubitus position with the operative extremity uppermost (Fig. 29-4). Some have suggested placing the patient with the operative side dependent in order to diminish chances of epidural diffusion.[5,24] To date, there is no published study on this subject. Knees and hips are flexed for patient stabilization. The anesthesiologist takes a position similar to the one for performing an epidural block. An assistant is positioned in front of the patient. One of his hands is on the thorax, to support the patient, and the other is between the patient's knees, with the hand's palm on the knee to be blocked. This second hand is used to identify the muscle contractions obtained with neurostimulation.

Needle Placement

Surface Landmarks and Puncture Site
With the patient in the lateral position, surface landmarks are identified and marked[6] (Fig. 27-6).

> Step 1: A first line is drawn between the most cephalad points of the iliac crests (Tuffier's line). This line most often passes at the level of the L3-4 interspace.
> Step 2: A second line, perpendicular to the first, is drawn over the lumbar spinous processes.
> Step 3: Marks are made on the L3, L4, and L5 spinous processes.
> Step 4: The PSIS is localized and a third line, parallel to the second and passing through the PSIS, is drawn.
> Step 5: The distance between the second and third lines is divided in three equal parts.

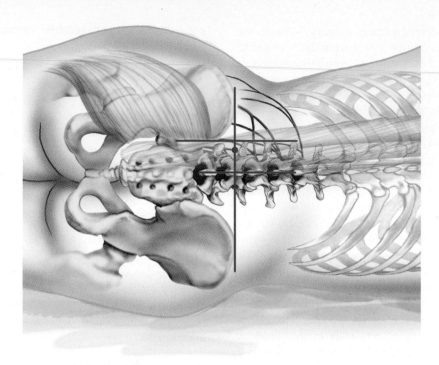

Figure 29-4. Surface anatomy and positioning for lumbar plexus block.

The puncture site is lateral to the spinous process of L4, approximately 1 cm cephalad to Tuffier's line (first line drawn in step 1), at the junction of the lateral third and medial two-thirds of the distance measured in step 5.[6]

These landmarks are slightly more medial than those in the initial technique described by Winnie et al.[2] They were modified after a radiologic demonstration that the initial landmarks were too lateral compared to the plexus[6] (Fig. 29-4). If these classic landmarks were used, the needle would have to be directed medially to encounter the lumbar plexus,[2,6] thereby increasing the risks of epidural or spinal anesthesia. With the new landmarks, the needle is not and should not be directed medially.[6]

Puncture Procedure

For safety and success, a puncture procedure was suggested.[23] Under aseptic conditions, the needle is introduced at the puncture site strictly perpendicular to the skin. It is important to keep a strict anteroposterior needle trajectory. After puncturing the skin, a nerve stimulator, is set at 2 mA with impulse width of 0.1 to 0.3 ms at a frequency of 1 to 2 Hz. The needle is slowly pushed through the muscles and not inserted more than 8 cm. Beyond this depth (see "Applied and Functional Anatomy," above), there is a high risk of retroperitoneal puncture. During this procedure, the needle can take many paths (Fig. 29-2).

Path 1 is ideal. The needle is advanced until it encounters the transverse (costiform) process of L4. The needle depth is noted. Then the needle is withdrawn slightly and angled 5 degrees caudad to pass under the costiform process. It is now slowly advanced until a motor response in the quadriceps muscles is observed. The needle should not be pushed more than 2 cm further than the distance noted after contact with the costiform process. If the lumbar plexus is not localized after 2 cm, the needle is withdrawn, reoriented 5 degrees cephalad to the costiform process, and advanced again, but not more than 2 cm.

In path 2, the needle stimulation produces contractions of the sacrolumbar muscles. The needle is advanced until the contractions disappear. The puncture depth is then noted. The needle should not be advanced more than 3 cm further. The following three situations could develop:

Path 2a: The costiform process is encountered and path 1 is followed.

Path 2b: The lumbar plexus is localized with a contraction of the quadriceps muscles.

Path 2c: The needle is advanced 3 cm further after the sacrolumbar muscle contractions disappear without costiform process contact or lumbar plexus identification. The needle should be withdrawn into subcutaneous tissues and reoriented 5 degrees more cephalad or caudad to try to localize the costiform process. Surface landmarks should be verified.

Path 3 is the situation where contact with the costiform process or contraction of the sacrolumbar muscles is not obtained before lumbar plexus localization at a maximal depth of 6 to 8 cm.

In Path 4, insertion of the needle does not produce any muscle contraction or contact with the costiform process. In this situation, the needle should not be inserted more than 6 to 8 cm, even in an obese patient. After 6 to 8 cm, the needle must be withdrawn into subcutaneous tissues and reoriented 5 degrees more cephalad or caudad in order to locate the costiform process. If this fails, landmarks should be checked and the puncture site moved 0.5 cm caudad or cephalad.

Ultrasound Guidance

Some authors have suggested ultrasound guidance [13,14,34] to reduce complication rates and teach nerve block techniques. However, there is no evidence to date that ultrasound guidance offers any advantages. Ultrasound apparatus is expensive and cumbersome to use, and additional research is required to prove its usefulness.

Motor Responses due to Nerve Stimulation

During the procedure, many types of motor responses can be obtained. All of them should be correctly interpreted to ensure block success.

Normal Motor Response

These motor responses are usually obtained during the puncture procedure:

> Sacrolumbar muscles contractions. These are normal during the procedure. Such contractions are due to direct muscle stimulation and are felt around the tip of the needle. They are a useful indication for the procedure (see "Puncture Procedure," above).
>
> Quadriceps muscle contractions with patellar movement. These correspond to femoral nerve stimulation and are the desired response. Isolated quadriceps muscle contraction with patellar movement is the only acceptable final response, which indicates that the local anesthetic agent can be injected. Other responses help to orient the needle but should not be viewed as indications for anesthetic agent injection.

Abnormal Motor Responses

The following motor responses are not desired; when they are encountered, they should be used for proper needle reorientation:

> Contractions of adductor muscles. These reflect obturator nerve or nerve root stimulation and indicate that the puncture is too medial. The needle should be withdrawn into subcutaneous tissues and reoriented 5 degrees laterally.
>
> Contractions of adductor muscles in combination with quadriceps muscles and patellar ascension. These could be due to nerve root stimulation. To avoid neuraxial anesthesia, the needle is pulled under the skin and reoriented 5 degrees laterally.
>
> Contractions of muscles under the knee. All movements of the feet and toes are caused by stimulation of a branch of the sacral plexus. This could represent stimulation of the sciatic nerve, indicating a puncture that is too caudad, or it could stem from stimulation of the lumbosacral trunk, indicating a puncture that is too medial. In the latter situation, the risk of epidural injection is very high.[35] When contractions of the leg muscles are obtained, the needle should be redirected 5 degrees laterally and more cephalad after being withdrawn below the skin.
>
> Contractions of the psoas muscle. In this case, hip flexion is observed. It is direct muscle stimulation, and the lumbar plexus is close by. The femoral nerve will probably be found after reorientation of the needle 5 degrees more cephalad or caudad. Needle depth should be verified to make sure that it is not inserted more than 6 to 8 cm.

After many unsuccessful attempts, surface landmarks should be verified. In no circumstance should the needle be inserted in a medial direction.

Pharmacologic Choice

There is no dose-range study available in the literature. The optimal volume and solution for lumbar paravertebral block is not precise. Recent publications have advocated, for the initial bolus, 0.4 to 0.8 mL/kg [4–6,17,26] or, more frequently, a 30- to 35-mL fixed volume.[7,20,21,25,28,30] The local anesthetic of choice is 0.5% ropivacaine, which is used more and more. According to the latest studies, ropivacaine shows less neurologic and cardiac toxicity than bupivacaine[37] and is a better choice than the latter (see Chaps. 18 and 21). A concentration of 0.5% is sufficient to obtain an adequate block and poses fewer risks of toxicity than a 0.75% concentration. For shorter block duration, 1.5% mepivacaine can be used. However, even with safer local anesthetics, toxicity is always a risk and care must be taken at all times. For safety, utilization of a test dose with epinephrine should be injected before bolus injection. The literature on continuous infusion solutions for lumbar paravertebral block is scanty. Recently, Capdevila et al.[6] and Kaloul et al.[21] have used 0.2% ropivacaine at rates of 0.15 mL/kg/h and 12 mL/h, respectively. Alternatively, Türker et al.[30] have advocated 0.125% bupivacaine with 2μg/mL fentanyl at a rate of 10 mL/h, in addition to a 5-mL bolus

PCA with a lockout time of 30 min. Based on the available literature and our clinical experience, we suggest the following protocols:

For anesthesia:

20 to 30 mL of 0.5% ropivacaine or 1.5% mepivacaine

For analgesia:

Continuous infusion: 0.2% ropivacaine at a rate of 10 mL/h

Perineural PCA: 0.2% ropivacaine at a rate of 5 mL/h with a 5-mL bolus permitted each 30 min

Single-Injection Technique

For the single-injection technique, a 10- to 12-cm insulated, short-beveled 24- or 22-gauge needle is utilized. After obtaining minimal stimulation intensity between 0.3 and 0.5 mA for stimulation duration of 0.1 ms, a careful aspiration is made followed by a test dose with a local anesthetic containing epinephrine. The test dose may allow the physician to detect intravascular or intrathecal injection. However, a false-negative aspiration and test dose response is possible. For this reason and to be on the safe side, when negative aspiration (no blood or cerebrospinal fluid) and test dose (no tachycardia or spinal block) is observed, the local anesthetic bolus is injected in 5-mL increments. We suggest waiting about 60 s and making an aspiration test before injecting each increment while monitoring for possible occurrence of toxic effects or neuraxial anesthesia (spinal or epidural).

Continuous Catheter Technique

For catheter insertion, strict sterile technique is mandatory. A continuous catheter kit with an insulated 10- or 11-cm end is used. It is preferable to insert the final catheter through a blunt needle rather than through another catheter[23] because the latter is soft and more easily displaced than a needle. Stimulating catheters are available and can help to position the catheter correctly. After correct needle placement, the space is dilated with 10 mL of normal saline solution and the catheter threaded 5 cm into the space. It is safer to inject local anesthetics through the catheter because the injection can be more easily given in increments. Before local anesthetic injections, it is preferable to verify correct catheter placement with a radiograph after injection of 10 mL of a contrast medium.[36] During infusion, the block level should be closely monitored for possible epidural diffusion. In this situation, a bilateral block will be noted. See Chap. 21 for further information about infusion strategy and catheter monitoring and Chap. 20 for the stimulating catheter technique, which may provide better results with fewer complications.

▶ POTENTIAL PROBLEMS

The lumbar paravertebral block is an advanced anesthesia technique in which many problems can occur. Inexperience in performing the block is a risk factor in the occurrence of complications.[38] In France, Auroy et al.[22] published a retrospective study on complications of regional anesthesia in 394 lumbar paravertebral blocks. Among the complications were 1 cardiac arrest, 2 respiratory failures, 1 seizure, and 1 death. Macaire et al.[38] performed a retrospective study of 4319 blocks performed by 42 teams in the United States, Canada, France, Belgium, and Switzerland. The teams reported 1 to 10 percent of epidural diffusions. Other complications included 25 cases of spinal anesthesia (11 with total spinal anesthesia and 1 death), 13 intravascular injections (with 3 seizures and 1 reanimated cardiac arrest), 4 delayed toxic reactions, and 13 wrong catheter paths.

Epidural Spread

Epidural spread is the most frequent problem, with a reported incidence varying from 1 to 16 percent.[3,6,17,20,27,38] In one study, epidural spread was more frequent with the approach at the L3 level compared to the L5 level.[3] Dalens et al.[35] reported 88 percent of epidural anesthesia cases with lumbar paravertebral block when performed by Chayen's technique. In all Dalens's cases, a motor response of the lumbosacral trunk was probably elicited, indicating a too medial position of the needle. Epidural catheter localization is also possible.[36,38] Catheter opacification is helpful in detecting this radiographically.[36]

Block Failure

The lumbar paravertebral block is a reliable block. The reported failure rate when neurostimulation for locating the lumbar plexus is used is around 5 to 7 percent.[25,38] In a partial failure situation, an anterior block of the nonanesthetized nerve (lateral femoral cutaneous, femoral, or obturator nerve) can be done.[23] Maximum doses of local anesthetics should then be considered.

Subarachnoid Injection

Subarachnoid injection is a dangerous complication when a lumbar paravertebral block is being performed. In the retrospective study of Macaire et al.,[38] use of a test dose allowed the detection of 11 of the 25 spinal injections observed. In the same study, 11 cases of total spinal anesthesia were reported, with one associated death. There are two case reports of total spinal anesthesia in the literature. In the first, the injection was done after the observation of a myotonic response of the adductor muscles.[39] In the second report, the continuous block was performed under general anesthesia with Chayen's technique.[40] In these two cases, patients were resuscitated without sequelae. A case of subarachnoid placement of a catheter without initial aspiration of cerebrospinal fluid (CSF) has also been described.[34] Subarachnoid injection can probably be prevented to a large extent by using large-bore, relatively blunt needles such as Tuohy needles.

Local Anesthetic Drug Toxicity

Intravascular injection of a local anesthetic can rapidly lead to seizures,[37,38,41,42] cardiac arrest,[37,38,41] and eventually death. An adequately performed test dose helped to detect 7 out of 13 intravascular injections in one study.[38] However, false-negative results are possible,[42] more so if the patient is elderly or treated with beta-adrenergic antagonists. A negative test dose does not preclude a fractioned injection. The persistence of a myotonic response with neurostimulation after the injection of 1 mL of normal saline or local anesthetic should alert the anesthesiologist to a possible intravascular injection. Deep sedation can mask the initial symptoms of systemic local anesthetic absorption.[42] Radiology can detect intravascular catheter placement.[38]

Delayed reactions can also occur.[38] They are mainly associated with the absorption of large doses of local anesthetic. Continuous infusion may also be involved. This highlights the importance of patient surveillance after performing a block and during catheter maintenance.

Incorrect Catheter Placement

In addition to epidural and intravascular catheter placement,[36,38] many other incorrect positions have been described. Catheter tips have been located in the abdominal cavity,[6,38] the retroperitoneal cavity,[6] the L4-5 intervertebral disk,[6] the subarachnoid space[34,40] and the paravertebral space.[38] For this reason we suggest a radiologic control after each lumbar paravertebral catheter placement before a local anesthetic is injected. Incorrect catheter placement is highly unlikely with a stimulating catheter.

Hematoma

Lumbar paravertebral blocks are best avoided in patients treated with anticoagulants (see "Patient Selection" and "Contraindications," above). Renal subcapsular hematomas have been described after the the performance of lumbar paravertebral blocks at the L3 level.[10] The inferior renal pole is dangerously close at this level. An approach at the L4 level is safer.[10]

Neuropathy

Direct nerve injury is rare with the lumbar paravertebral block. Macaire et al.[38] reported two cases of neuropathy out of a total of 4319 blocks, one neuropathy of the lateral femoral cutaneous nerve and one of the femoral nerves, but both patients had a favorable outcome. A case of femoral nerve injury has recently been published.[43] There are also three case reports of plexopathy associated with psoas compartment hematomas.[31,32]

Injections should probably not be made if a motor response is obtained with a current intensity less than 0.3 mA. In this situation, the needle should be pulled back to attain a minimal stimulation intensity between 0.3 and 0.5 mA. Injection should be stopped if it is painful. When a neurologic deficit is noted, the continuous infusion should be stopped. If the deficit persists for more than the expected duration of action of the local anesthetic, radiologic tests should be done rapidly to rule out a possible hematoma.

Other Complications

An infection is always possible. A strict aseptic technique should be used to lessen infection risks, even more so for catheter insertion.

Lumbar paravertebral block results in unilateral sympathectomy. Patients may develop hemodynamic instability. Furthermore, a bilateral sympathectomy is possible in the case of an epidural spread. Every patient should be monitored during and after the performance of a lumbar paravertebral block in the same manner as those receiving an epidural block.

REFERENCES

1. Winnie AP, Ramamurthy S, Durrani Z. The inguinal paravascular technique of lumbar plexus anesthesia: The "3 in 1" block. *Anesth Analg* 52:989–996, 1973.
2. Winnie AP, Ramamurthy S, Durrani Z, et al. Plexus blocks for lower extremity surgery: New answers to old problems. *Anesth Rev* 1:1–6, 1974.
3. Parkinson SK, Mueller JB, Little WL, et al. Extent of blockade with various approaches to the lumbar plexus. *Anesth Analg* 68:243–248, 1989.
4. Chudinov A, Berkenstadt H, Salai M, et al. Continuous psoas compartment block for anesthesia and perioperative analgesia in patients with hip fractures. *Reg Anesth Pain Med* 24:563–568, 1999.
5. Horlocker TT, Hebl JR, Kinney MAO, et al. Opioid-free analgesia following the total knee arthroplasty: A multimodal approach using continuous lumbar plexus (psoas compartment) block, acetaminophen, and ketorolac. *Reg Anesth Pain Med* 27:105–108, 2002.
6. Capdevila X, Macaire P, Dadure C, et al. Continuous psoas compartment block for postoperative analgesia after total hip arthroplasty: New landmarks, technical guidelines, and clinical evaluation. *Anesth Analg* 94:1606–1613, 2002.
7. Pandin PC, Vandesteene A, Hollander AA. Lumbar plexus posterior approach: A catheter placement description using electrical nerve stimulation. *Anesth Analg* 95:1428–1431, 2002.

8. Chayen D, Nathan H, Chayen M. The psoas compartment block. *Anesthesiology* 45:95–99, 1976.

9. Hanna MH, Peat SJ, D'Costa F. Lumbar plexus block: An anatomical study. *Anaesthesia* 48:675–678, 1993.

10. Aida S, Takahashi H, Shimoji K. Renal subcapsular hematoma after lumbar plexus block. *Anesthesiology* 84:452–455, 1996.

11. Ben-David B, Lee E, Croitoru M. Psoas block for surgical repair of hip fracture: A case report and description of a catheter technique. *Anesth Analg* 71:298–301, 1990.

12. Vaghadia H, Kapnoudhis P, Jenkins LC, et al. Continuous lumbosacral block using a Tuohy needle and catheter technique. *Can J Anaesth* 39:75–78, 1992.

13. Kirchmair L, Entner T, Wissel J, et al. A study of the anatomy for ultrasound-guided posterior lumbar plexus block. *Anesth Analg* 93:477–481, 2001.

14. Kirchmair L, Entner T, Kapral S, et al. Ultrasound guidance for the psoas compartment block: An imaging study. *Anesth Analg* 94:706–710, 2002.

15. Farny J, Drolet P, Girard M. Anatomy of the posterior approach to the lumbar plexus block. *Can J Anaesth* 41:480–485, 1994.

16. Bouaziz H, Vial F, Jochum D, et al. An evaluation of the cutaneous distribution after obturator nerve block. *Anesth Analg* 94:445–449, 2002.

17. Biboulet P, Morau D, Aubas P, et al. Postoperative analgesia after total-hip arthroplasty: Comparison of intravenous patient-controlled analgesia with morphine and single injection of femoral nerve or psoas compartment block. A prospective, randomized, double-blind study. *Reg Anesth Pain Med* 29:102–109, 2004.

18. Capdevila X, Biboulet P, Bouregba M, et al. Comparison of the three-in-one and the fascia iliaca compartment blocks in adults: Clinical and radiographic analysis. *Anesth Analg* 86:1039–1044, 1998.

19. Capdevila X, Biboulet P, Morau D, et al. Continuous three-in-one block for postoperative pain after lower limb orthopedic surgery: Where do the catheters go? *Anesth Analg* 94:1001–1006, 2002.

20. Tokat O, Türker YG, Uckunkaya N, et al. A clinical comparison of psoas compartment and inguinal paravascular blocks combined with sciatic nerve block. *J Intern Med Res* 30:161–167, 2002.

21. Kaloul I, Guay J, Côté C, et al. The posterior lumbar plexus (psoas compartment) block and the three-in-one femoral nerve block provide similar postoperative analgesia after total knee replacement. *Reg Anesth Pain Med* 51:45–51, 2004.

22. Auroy Y, Benhamou D, Bargues L, et al. Major complications of regional anesthesia in France: The SOS regional anesthesia hotline service. *Anesthesiology* 97:1274–1280, 2002.

23. Gaertner E, Al Nasser B, Choquet O, et al (eds). *Regional Anesthesia: Peripheral Nerve Blockade in Adults.* Paris, France: Arnette, 2004.

24. Jankowski CJ, Hebl JR, Stuart MJ, et al. A comparison of psoas compartment block and spinal and general anesthesia for outpatient knee arthroscopy. *Anesth Analg* 97:1003–1009, 2003.

25. De Visme V, Picart F, Le Jouan R, et al. Combined lumbar and sacral plexus block compared with plain bupivacaine spinal anesthesia for hip fractures in the elderly. *Reg Anesth Pain Med* 25:158–162, 2000.

26. White IWC, Chappell WA. Anesthesia for surgical correction of fractured femoral neck: A comparison of three techniques. *Anaesthesia* 35:1107–1110, 1980.

27. Stevens RD, Van Gessel E, Flory N, et al. Lumbar plexus block reduces pain and blood loss associated with total hip arthroplasty. *Anesthesiology* 93:115–121, 2000.

28. Souron V, Delaunay L, Schifrine P. Intrathecal morphine provides better postoperative analgesia than psoas compartment block after primary hip arthroplasty. *Reg Anesth Pain Med* 50:574–579, 2003.

29. Goroszeniuk T, di Vadi PP. Repeated psoas compartment blocks for the management of long-standing hip pain. *Reg Anesth Pain Med* 26:376–378, 2001.

30. Türker G, Uçkunkaya N, Yavasçaoglu B, et al. Comparison of the catheter-technique psoas compartment block and the epidural block for analgesia in partial hip replacement surgery. *Acta Anaesthesiol Scand* 47:30–36, 2003.

31. Weller RS, Gerancher JC, Crews JC, et al. Extensive retroperitoneal hematoma without neurologic deficit in two patients who underwent lumbar plexus block and were later anticoagulated. *Anesthesiology* 98:581–585, 2003.

32. Klein SM, D'Ercole F, Greengrasss RA, et al. Enoxaparin associated with psoas hematoma and lumbar plexopathy after lumbar plexus block. *Anesthesiology* 87:1576–1579, 1997.

33. Horlocker TT, Wedel DJ, Benzon H, et al. Regional anesthesia in the anticoagulated patient: Defining the risks. *Reg Anesth Pain Med* 2(Suppl 1):1–11, 2004.

34. Litz RJ, Vicent O, Wiessner D, et al. Misplacement of a psoas compartment catheter in the subarachnoid space. *Reg Anesth Pain Med* 29:60–64, 2004.

35. Dalens B, Tanguy A, Vanneuville G. Lumbar plexus block in children: A comparison of two procedures in 50 patients. *Anesth Analg* 67:750–758, 1988.

36. De Biasi P, Lupescu R, Burgun G, et al. Continuous lumbar plexus block: Use of radiography to determine catheter tip location. *Reg Anesth Pain Med* 28:135–139, 2003.

37. Huet O, Eyrolle LJ, Mazoit JX, et al. Cardiac arrest after injection of ropivacaine for posterior lumbar plexus blockade. *Anesthesiology* 99:1451–1453, 2003.

38. Macaire P, Gaertner E, Choquet O. Le bloc du plexus lombaire est-il dangereux?, in *Évaluation et traitement de la douleur.* SFAR 2002. Paris: Elsevier et SFAR Ed, 2002:37–50.

39. Gentili M, Aveline C, Bonnet F. Rachianesthésie totale après bloc du plexus lombaire par voie postérieure. *Ann Fr Anesth Reanim* 17:740–742, 1998.

40. Pousman RM, Mansoor Z, Sciard D. Total spinal anesthetic after continuous posterior lumbar plexus block. *Anesthesiology* 98:1281–1282, 2003.

41. Pham-Dang C, Beaumont S, Floch H, et al. AmLident aigu toxique après bloc du plexus lombaire à la bupivacaine. *Ann Fr Anesth Reanim* 19:356–359, 2000.

42. Breslin DS, Martin G, Macleod DB, et al. Central nervous system toxicity following the administration of the levobupivacaine for lumbar plexus block: A report of two cases. *Reg Anesth Pain Med* 28:144–147, 2003.

43. Al-Nasser B, Palacios JL. Femoral nerve injury complicating continuous psoas compartment block. *Reg Anesth Pain Med* 29:361–363, 2004.

CHAPTER 30

Continuous Spinal and Epidural Anesthesia

MILTON RAFF

▶ INTRODUCTION

Neuraxial anesthesia is an accepted method of providing anesthesia for a myriad of surgical procedures, either as part of a balanced anesthetic technique or as the sole method of anesthesia. Neuraxial techniques have evolved from a single-injection spinal injection through the development of the single-injection epidural injection to the present-day use of indwelling catheters. This has led to an increase in the applications of neuraxial anesthesia, as the block can now provide longer periods of anesthesia. The same indwelling catheter may now also be used in the postoperative phase to facilitate analgesia. Many studies have shown the benefits of neuraxial anesthesia in terms of postoperative morbidity when compared with general anesthesia alone.

When applied specifically to orthopaedic surgery, it is evident that neuraxial anesthesia will reduce the incidence of deep venous thrombosis (DVT) and pulmonary embolus (PE), and it will also reduce surgical blood loss, renal failure, myocardial infarction, and postoperative pulmonary complications. Based on these findings, we can safely state that the practice of neuraxial anesthesia and analgesia is essential for the orthopaedic anesthesiologist.

Spinal anesthesia has been practiced for 100 years. The evolution of this anesthetic technique encompasses the development of local anesthetic agents and spinal needles needed to identify the subarachnoid space and to administer the anesthetic agent. Further engineering developments have enabled the placement of subarachnoid catheters for prolonged delivery of the anesthetic

agents. The practice of epidural anesthesia began in the early 1900s, but the greatest strides in its development started in 1940.

The injection of a local anesthetic solution into the subarachnoid space has been incorrectly described as spinal anesthesia, spinal or subarachnoid analgesia, and spinal or subarachnoid block. The correct term is *subarachnoid anesthesia*, since the agent is injected into the subarachnoid space and produces anesthesia, not analgesia. The addition of analgesic agents to the local anesthetic will alter the properties of the mixture, so that the term *subarachnoid analgesia* has evolved. Similarly, one can differentiate between epidural anesthesia and epidural analgesia.

▶ HISTORY

The first reported use of a local anesthetic was that of Koller in 1884; he applied cocaine topically to the eye, producing anesthesia of the cornea and conjunctiva. A short time thereafter, in 1885, cocaine was used to produce regional anesthesia when Halstead used it to block the brachial plexus. In the same year, Corning, a neurologist, used cocaine to perform an intervertebral block in dogs and then in patients. It is not clear whether these injections were made into the epidural or the subarachnoid space. Quincke described a reliable method for performing lumbar punctures in 1891, but it was only in 1899 that Bier, using Quincke's technique, injected cocaine into the subarachnoid space to produce operative anesthesia.

This is the first description of spinal anesthesia. The technique was then used in France by Tuffier and in the United States by Matas and Tait. General acceptance of this technique was, however, prevented by the high incidence of side effects such as tremors, hyperreflexia, headaches, and muscle pains.

The introduction of procaine in 1904 by Einhorn, and its subsequent use in 1905 by Braun, initiated a new phase in the development of subarachnoid anesthesia. The technique now became widely used. In 1907, Barker added glucose to the procaine to make the solution hyperbaric and the level of anesthesia controllable. Jones, in 1930, introduced dibucaine, while tetracaine was synthesized in 1931.

Dean performed the first continuous spinal anesthesia (CSA) by leaving the spinal needle in place during the operation. Lemmon in 1940 and Tuohy in 1945 published the first reports of CSA. Tuohy inserted a no. 4 urethral catheter via a 15-guage needle. The major problem associated with this technique was the occurrence of "postdural puncture headache (PDPH)." In 1989, Hurley and Lambert, introduced microcatheters to try and decrease the incidence of these headaches.

Epidural anesthesia originated when Kreis used cocaine at the L4-5 level to alleviate pain in childbirth. Marx, in 1900, reported on "lumbar cocainization." In 1901, Cathelin described the caudal injection of fluids whereby the height of the fluid column could be determined by the speed of injection and the volume of the injectate. In 1909, Stoeckel described his experience of caudal injection in the management of labor. Several authors then described the technique using different volumes and concentrations of procaine. Lawen was the first to describe surgery of the perineum and lower extremity using procaine and bicarbonate salts. Anesthesia endured for $1\frac{1}{2}$ h.

The technique of continuous anesthesia in obstetrics was first described by Edwards and Hingson in 1940. They used metycaine in saline as their agent of choice. In order to prolong the duration of anesthesia, catheters were introduced by Manalan in 1942. The epidural technique then developed rapidly as the catheters, needles, and agents used for anesthesia improved.

► PATIENT SELECTION

Neuraxial anesthesia in orthopaedic surgery is usually selected for surgery involving the lower extremity. It serves as a frequent adjunct to general anesthesia when it is used to provide both intraoperative and postoperative analgesia as well as a degree of protection against venous and pulmonary thromboembolism. In major orthopaedic procedures it has also been shown to reduce blood loss and to diminish the frequency of postoperative pulmonary complications as well as improving the quality of postoperative analgesia. Neuraxial anesthesia is a popular anesthetic technique for both knee and hip arthroplasty, where it may be combined with general anesthesia. High-risk patients will also benefit from the use of neuraxial anesthesia.

► CONTRAINDICATIONS TO NEURAXIAL ANESTHESIA

Sepsis: Local sepsis in the area where the needle or catheter is to be inserted or systemic sepsis are reasons to avoid neuraxial blockade.

Clotting abnormalities: A relative platelet deficiency or prolongation of the normal indices of hemostasis constitutes an absolute contraindication to spinal or epidural anesthesia. The role of anticoagulants is discussed in more detail later in this chapter.

Allergy to the anesthetic agent.

Refusal by the patient to undergo the procedure.

► ANATOMY

The Vertebral Column

Vertebrae

The spinal column consists of 33 vertebrae. There are 7 cervical, 12 thoracic, 5 lumbar, 5 sacral (fused), and 4 coccygeal vertebrae. There are 4 curves, the cervical and lumbar being convex anteriorly while the thoracic and sacral are convex posteriorly.

All vertebrae have a common structure. This consists of an anterior vertebral body and an arch of bone posteriorly that surrounds the spinal canal. This arch comprises two pedicles anteriorly and two laminae posteriorly. The transverse processes are situated at the junction of the pedicles and the laminae. The laminae meet at the spinous process (Fig. 30-1).

There is a variation in the caudal angulation of these spinous processes. In most cases they are almost horizontal but steeply angulated in the thoracic region. The direction of insertion of the epidural or spinal needle will differ according to the level of insertion, as this direction will be determined by the anatomy of the vertebral spine at that level. It is the angulation of the spinous process that affects the epidural needle and catheter placement rather than the various anatomic curves of the spinal column.

The lumbar curve plays a role in subarachnoid anesthesia because it is at this level at which the spinal needle or catheter is inserted and the local anesthetic solution injected. The lumbar curve will therefore have an influence on the spread of the local anesthetic solution. In the supine patient, the high point of the lumbar curve is at L5, while the low point of the sacral curve is at S2.

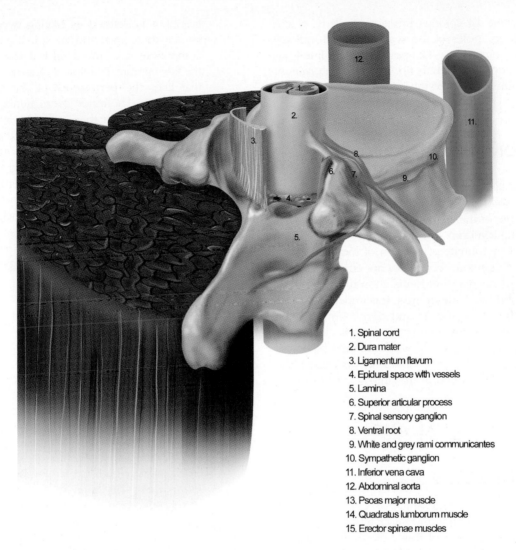

1. Spinal cord
2. Dura mater
3. Ligamentum flavum
4. Epidural space with vessels
5. Lamina
6. Superior articular process
7. Spinal sensory ganglion
8. Ventral root
9. White and grey rami communicantes
10. Sympathetic ganglion
11. Inferior vena cava
12. Abdominal aorta
13. Psoas major muscle
14. Quadratus lumborum muscle
15. Erector spinae muscles

Figure 30-1. Anatomy of the epidural and subarachnoid space.

Ligaments

1. The supraspinous ligament is a strong structure connecting the apices of the spinous processes. It is present from the sacrum to C7 and then continues upward to the external occipital protuberance as the ligamentum nuchae. The thickness of this ligament varies; it is thickest and broadest in the lumbar region.
2. The interspinous ligament is a thin membranous structure connecting the adjacent spinous processes. It blends posteriorly with the supraspinous ligaments and anteriorly with the ligamentum flavum. The interspinous ligament is also thickest in the lumbar region.
3. The ligamentum flavum gets its name from the fact that it consists of yellow elastic fibers. These fibers connect the adjacent laminae. Laterally the ligament begins at the root of the articular process and extends medially and posteriorly to the junction of the lamina and the spinous process. The two components fuse at this point, thus covering the entire interlaminar space. This ligament is readily palpable with an epidural or spinal needle.
4. The longitudinal ligaments (anterior and posterior) bind the vertebral bodies together.

▶ SURFACE ANATOMY

The spinous processes may be palpated in the midline as bony prominences running from the base of the skull to the gluteal cleft. A line joining the iliac crests will approximate the position of the L4 spinous process. Similarly, a line joining the inferior poles of the scapula would indicate the level of T7 spine, while L2 approximates a line joining the lateral ends of the 12th rib. The most prominent bony point in the midline at the base of the neck is the spinous process of C7 (vertebra prominens).

▶ FUNCTIONAL ANATOMY

The level of anesthesia attained by spinal or epidural anesthesia is determined by several factors. The level of insertion of the needle or the cannula will influence the height of the block. The level can also be affected by the volume of injectate and by the rate of infusion of local anesthetic solution when continuous techniques are employed.

The level of needle insertion is chosen according to the area of neural blockade desired. It is imperative to be familiar with the nerve supply and dermatomes of the limbs in order to perform adequate neural blockade. For lower limb and hip surgery, this would require blockade of up to the L1 level, but it can obviously be lower if the site of surgery is more distal in the limb.

▶ THE SPINAL CANAL AND ITS CONTENTS

The Epidural Space

Identification of the epidural space is essential for the placement of both epidural and subarachnoid catheters as well as for the injection of bolus medication into the epidural space.

This space extends from the foramen magnum to the sacral hiatus and surrounds the spinal meninges. It is bounded anteriorly by the posterior longitudinal ligament, laterally by the pedicles of the vertebrae and the intervertebral foramina, and posteriorly by the ligamentum flavum and the anterior surfaces of the laminae. The space can be envisaged as a continuous ring surrounding the cerebrospinal fluid (CSF), but in reality the shape is somewhat eccentric. The narrowest part is found anteriorly, since the dura and the anterior surface of the vertebral canal are in close proximity. The widest space is posterior. Its size varies at different vertebral levels from 1.5 mm at C5 to 5 or 6 mm at L2. In addition to the nerve roots traversing it, the epidural space contains fat, lymphatic vessels, arteries, areolar tissue, and the venous plexus of Batson.

The Spinal Meninges

1. *Dura mater:* The dura mater is the outermost layer of the meninges. Of note is the fact that the fibers of this layer run longitudinally. It is a continuous layer but is defined as having two components, namely the cranial and the spinal dura. The cranial component lines the skull but also folds to form the falx cerebri. The spinal dura has an outer layer that lines the periosteum of the vertebral canal (endosteal). The inner layer (meningeal) serves as the spinal dura or theca. This layer attaches superiorly to the circumference of the foramen magnum while caudally it ends at S2. At this level it is pierced by the filum terminale (the terminal end of the pia mater). The filum extends from the distal tip of the spinal cord to fuse with the periosteum of the coccyx and serves as an anchor to the cord and the dura. The spinal dura also extends laterally, providing a very thin covering to the spinal nerve roots. It eventually terminates as connective tissue around the nerve roots.

2. *Arachnoid mater:* The middle of the three meningeal coverings is known as the arachnoid mater. This is a nonvascular layer. It is interesting to note that there is a capillary interval or potential space between the arachnoid and the dura known as the subdural space. This potential space contains a lubricating fluid that moistens the surfaces of the opposing membranes, but it does not communicate directly with the subarachnoid space. The space terminates at S2. An unintentional injection of local anesthetic into this space can result in an excessively high nerve blockade.

3. *Pia mater:* This layer is a vascular membrane closely investing the spinal cord and brain. The space between the arachnoid and the pia is known as the subarachnoid space. It contains CSF, spinal nerves, blood vessels, and the trabeculae that span the space in a web-like fashion.

The Spinal Cord

The spinal cord begins at the foramen magnum, at which point it is in continuity with the medulla oblongata. In the adult, the cord terminates as the conus medullaris at the lower border of L1; in the neonate, it ends at L3. The 31 pairs of spinal nerves are attached to the cord by two roots.

The five lumbar and five sacral nerve roots project beyond the end of the cord as the cauda equina. Only a thin layer of the pia mater covers these nerves. For this reason it has been suggested that the nerves forming the cauda equina are particularly susceptible to the effects of local anesthetic solutions injected into this region.

This space is filled by the cerebrospinal fluid. It is bounded internally by the pia mater and externally by the arachnoid mater. It also contains the arachnoid trabeculae that form an extensive web within the space.

Cerebrospinal Fluid

The CSF is clear, colorless ultrafiltrate of blood plasma. It is found in the subarachnoid space and in the ventricles of the brain, where it is produced by the choroid plexus in the ventricular walls. There is total continuity between the CSF in the subarachnoid space and that in the ventricles. The total CSF volume in an adult is 100 to 150 mL, of which 25 mL is found in the subarachnoid space. The composition of the CSF is described in Table 30-1.

The detection of CSF in the subarachnoid cannula indicates the endpoint for catheter insertion in continuous subarachnoid anesthesia. It also serves to confirm correct positioning of a spinal needle for single bolus injection into the CSF.

Spinal Arteries

The blood supply of the spinal cord is provided by spinal branches of the aorta and the subclavian and iliac arteries as well as by the arteries of the brain. These arteries supply "feeder" vessels to the spinal cord. The spinal arteries traverse the intervertebral foramina and the epidural space, entering the subarachnoid space in the region of the dural cuff of the spinal nerve roots. They then enter the spinal cord. These arteries mainly supply the spinal nerve roots.

The posteroinferior cerebellar arteries and anterior spinal artery supply the actual cord. The posteroinferior cerebellar arteries descend, supplying penetrating vessels to the posterior part of the cord. The anterior spinal artery is formed by the confluence of the terminal branches of each vertebral artery. It supplies blood to the periphery of the cord and to parts of the anterior cord.

It is important to note that the largest feeder vessel, known as the radicularis magna (artery of Adamkiewicz), supplies the anterior spinal artery in the lumbar area of the cord. It is mostly found on the left side (in 78 percent of instances), entering the canal by a single intervertebral foramen. It is consistently found between T8 and L3. Damage to this vessel by a spinal or epidural needle may cause severe ischemia of the lumbar region of the cord, with all the disastrous sequelae.

▶ TECHNIQUES FOR CONTINUOUS NEURAXIAL ANESTHESIA

Equipment

These procedures should be performed in a sterile environment with strict attention to aseptic technique. Each of the techniques has its own requirements.

Continuous Spinal Anesthesia

This technique requires a needle to "find" the epidural space and a second needle to enter the subarachnoid space. An indwelling subarachnoid catheter must then be inserted via the needle so that it may remain in the subarachnoid space. The most commonly used needle for detecting the epidural space is a simple Tuohy needle. A syringe used to detect the "loss of resistance" of the epidural space is usually supplied, as is a microfilter and connection device to join the catheter and the filter. The subarachnoid needles vary in design and the subarachnoid catheter is passed either through or over this needle.

In 1996, a unique device was developed whereby the catheter is sited over the needle used to perforate the dura, the "catheter over needle." This entire needle-catheter unit is passed through a modified Tuohy needle. This needle does not have a blunt curve on its distal end. It has been modified to end as a straight bevel. A multicenter trial using this device revealed low incidences of dural tap and postdural puncture headache, and there were no neurologic sequelae. These results led to the marketing of the Spinocath (B. Braun, Melsuneen, Germany).

The Spinocath system consists of the following:

1. An 18-gauge by 88-mm epidural needle with beveled tip.
2. Catheter Luer lock screw connector.
3. An 0.2-m epidural filter with a priming volume of 0.5 mL.
4. Perifix loss-of-resistance (LOR) syringe 10-mL Luer slip.
5. An over-the-needle spinal catheter system.

   Spinocath 22-gauge, consisting of a Quinke 27-gauge spinal needle (OD 0.42 mm) connected to a braided pull wire and a 720-mm 22-gauge catheter (OD 0.85 mm) having a priming volume of 0.1 mL.

   Spinocath 24-gauge, consisting of a Quinke 29-gauge spinal needle (OD 0.35 mm) connected

▶ **TABLE 30-1.** COMPOSITION OF CEREBROSPINAL FLUID

pH	7.27–7.37
Sodium	133–145 meq/L
Chloride	15–20 meq/L
Proteins	23–38 mg/dl
Calcium	2–3 meq/L
Magnesium	2.0–2.5 meq/L
Phosphorus	1.6 meq/L
HCO_3^-	23 meq/L
PCO_2	48 mmHg
Specific gravity	1.003–1.009
Volume	100–150 mLs
CSF pressure	60–80 mmH$_2$O (horizontal)

to a braided pull wire and a 720-mm 24-gauge catheter (OD 0.71 mm) having a priming volume of 0.1 mL.

6. Red "spinal" sticker.

Single-Bolus Spinal Anesthesia

Several spinal needles are commercially available. The major difference in these needles is the shape of the needle tip. The newer needles have a "pencil point" and are of a much narrower gauge. Commercial variations of this type of needle include the Quincke and Sprotte needles. These pencil points do not cut the dural fibers as opposed to the older "beveled tips" that cut a hole in the dura. It is this hole that cause leaking of CSF and has been deemed responsible for the post-dural puncture headache. This issue is dealt with in more detail elsewhere in this chapter. The needles are supplied in kit form containing the spinal needle, a Trochar, and a short introducer. Needles vary from a 24- to a 29-gauge.

Epidural Anesthesia

A large number of epidural "kits" are available, each with its own specific properties. The commonly supplied components are as follows:

1. A Tuohy needle. This type of needle has replaced the older beveled-tip needle. The tip of the Tuohy needle has a gentle curve that will guide a catheter in the designated direction.
2. The epidural catheter. These catheters vary in their construction and composition.
3. A "loss-of-resistance" device. This resembles an ordinary syringe but is constructed to facilitate the loss of resistance encountered on entering the epidural space.
4. A microfilter.
5. A connecting device facilitating the connection of the epidural catheter to the filter.

Patient Monitoring

Every patient undergoing a surgical procedure must be monitored for the standard physiologic functions. When surgery is to be performed employing a neuraxial block as the sole form of anesthesia, one must accept that the block may fail, necessitating general anesthesia, and that physiologic functions may alter directly as a result of the block. All patients must therefore be monitored for pulse rate, pulse oximetry, blood oxygen saturation, and blood pressure. Every patient must have a functional intravenous access line.

The operating room must be equipped with an operating table that can be tilted and all standard resuscitation drugs must be readily available, as should a full range of airways, endotracheal tubes, laryngoscopes, and any other equipment necessary for the maintenance of an airway.

Position of the Patient

The patient may sit upright or be placed in the lateral decubitus position. The position is often dictated by the patient's condition, in that a patient with a fractured neck of femur would find it uncomfortable to sit upright or to lie on the side of the fracture. The training and experience of the physician may also determine patient positioning. The patient should be placed as close to the edge of the table as possible so that he or she is near the anesthesiologist.

Whatever the choice of the patient's position, it is essential that the spine be flexed so as to widen the interlaminar spaces. To achieve this in the lateral decubitus position, the hips and knees should be flexed and the chin placed on the chest, the neck being supported by a pillow. When the patient is in the upright position, the head should be flexed and the spine extended, with the feet supported on a footstool. Whatever the chosen position, an assistant should be present to ensure the patient's comfort and stability.

Of equal importance is the position in which the patient is placed after injection of the local anesthetic. This is critical after spinal blockade. If the patient is to be placed in the supine or prone position, the baricity of the local anesthetic plays little role. If, on the other hand, a unilateral block is to be performed, the baricity of the anesthetic and positioning are of paramount importance. Position plays a lesser role after performing an epidural block.

Techniques

Strict aseptic techniques are to be observed. In certain countries it is mandatory to obtain a signed consent form specific for an anesthetic procedure. It remains the duty of the anesthesiologist to check all anesthetic equipment, monitors, and drugs that may become necessary during the block or subsequent surgical procedure.

An intravenous access line must be established in all cases, preferably using a large-bore intravenous cannula. Intravenous fluid should be commenced. All baseline physiologic variables must be measured and noted.

The patient is positioned with all the appropriate monitors attached. The anesthesiologist must do a surgical scrub and don the appropriate clothing. In performing a spinal or continuous spinal block, the patient's lumbosacral area is cleaned with a non-alcohol-containing solution (alcohol has been shown to ablate nerve tissue). The appropriate area for the selected epidural site must be similarly cleaned. The patient is then covered with surgical drapes, leaving the sterile area exposed.

The area selected for insertion of the spinal indwelling cannula should be distal to the termination of the spinal cord, which is below the conus medullaris at L1. This will ensure that the cord is not directly damaged by the spinal or the epidural needle. The most common areas used for continuous subarachnoid anesthesia are the L3-4 and L4-5 spinous interspaces. Similarly, these spaces are the most common site selected for epidural insertion for lower extremity orthopaedic surgery. A single–injection spinal needle will, for similar reasons, also be inserted at this level.

A skin wheal is raised using 1 or 2% lidocaine and a small-gauge needle (27 gauge). Deeper tissue infiltration may now be performed using a larger and longer needle.

After waiting a few minutes for the local anesthesia to take effect, the epidural needle is inserted. The introducer must be left inside the epidural needle during penetration of the skin and subcutaneous tissue to ensure that tissue does not block it. The epidural space is located by the "loss of resistance" technique. The loss of resistance is noticed when the epidural space is penetrated while maintaining pressure on the plunger of the syringe or is determined by the "hanging drop" method described by Doglotti. The reason for this loss of resistance is that the two outer layers of the dura, the dura mater and the arachnoid mater, come into close proximity to each other owing to a negative pressure generated in the thorax. Doglotti observed a negative pressure in the thoracic region that diminished as the sacral region was approached. Penetration of the epidural space by the epidural needle would cause the two layers to separate, with the subsequent sensation of a "loss of resistance." Specialized syringes have been constructed for this purpose. They are almost frictionless and offer minimal resistance to pressure exerted on the plunger, similar to that shown by a piston system. (If these syringes are not available, a glass syringe may be substituted.) It is still debated whether the syringe should be filled with air or 0.9% saline. This choice depends purely on one's of preference. Several authors have stated that air injected into the epidural space may be responsible for a "patchy" block, as the presence of the air bubble may prevent local anesthetic from reaching that area. Although the epidural needle supplied for the combined spinal epidural (CSE) technique is straight, it gives the same "gritty" feel as a Tuohy needle when penetrating the ligamentum flavum.

The layers penetrated from the surface to the epidural space using the midline approach are skin, subcutaneous fat, supraspinous and interspinous ligaments, connective tissue, ligamentum flavum, and the dura mater.

It is at this point that the techniques differ. With CSE, once the epidural space has been identified, the insertion of the subarachnoid cannula becomes specialized. The epidural needle is held in place and the spinal catheter system passed through it. While the epidural needle is held in position with one hand, the Spinocath is inserted with the other hand. The Spinocath should be held firmly between the thumb and the second and third fingers at the point where the needle is welded to the pull wire. With gentle insertion of the Spinocath, a slight resistance will be encountered (the dura mater). A "pop" will be felt as the needle of the Spinocath pierces the dura mater. At this point a small amount of CSF may be noted in the catheter. This is due to the presence of a side hole in the needle that allows CSF to enter the catheter.

Once the needle is in the subarachnoid space, the catheter must be advanced over the needle into the subarachnoid space. Since the tip of the catheter is tapered, this should be fairly easy. The catheter is advanced over the needle with one hand while the pull wire is fully extended and retracted with the other hand. Correct positioning of the subarachnoid catheter is confirmed by the easy flow of CSF from the catheter. This is a very specific endpoint indicator, and if no CSF can be drawn from the catheter, it is probably incorrectly positioned. Once correctly placed, the catheter is retracted to the determined length.

The epidural technique differs in that once the epidural space has been identified, the epidural catheter is simply passed through the needle. Slight resistance may be encountered, but if this resistance is excessive, the cannulation should be stopped and the epidural needle reinserted afresh. The catheter should pass freely into the epidural space. It should be advanced 3 to 5 cm beyond the needle tip. This can be approximated, as all of the commercially available catheters have visible surface markings indicating distance from the distal tip.

If blood flows freely from the epidural catheter, it should be withdrawn, since the blood may indicate cannulation of an epidural vessel. Injection of local anesthetic under these conditions may lead to cardiac and neurologic complications and must not be done under any circumstances. Do not simply withdraw the catheter through the needle, as this could lead to shearing of the catheter, so that a piece of the catheter could be left in the epidural space. The catheter should be withdrawn as a unit together with the Tuohy needle. A similar situation may also occur with a spinal catheter.

Clear fluid flowing from an inserted epidural needle or catheter would indicate dural puncture. The situation must then be reappraised and the epidural anesthesia must either be abandoned or continued as a spinal anesthetic with the necessary precautions. There will be an associated high incidence of postdural puncture headache.

The catheter systems are closed by the firm attachment of the microfilter and connector. A sterile dressing should be placed over the skin puncture site and the rest of the catheter should be firmly taped in place. If prolonged catheterization is anticipated, then it may be necessary to tunnel the catheter subcutaneously at the skin puncture site to prevent sepsis and catheter colonization.

The single-spinal-injection technique does not require the use of the loss of resistance (LOR) syringe. The spinal needle is simply advanced until the backflow of CSF is noted. The finer-gauge spinal needles are inserted through an introducer because they are too fine to penetrate the ligamentum flavum and will usually bend if strong tissue resistance is encountered. Once placed through the introducer, the trocar may be removed; the needle is then advanced until the CSF is detected. The desired local anesthetic is then injected. Similar restraints and conditions to as those outlined for CSA apply for the single-injection block.

The patient should now be placed in the selected position (supine or lateral decubitus). The level of anesthesia required and volume of anesthetic agent will be determined by the surgical procedure and the height of the desired block. Before injection into the CSF or the epidural space, the system should be primed by filling the microfilter and the catheter with the chosen local anesthetic. This requires about 0.6 to 1.5 mL of local anesthetic, depending on the kit being used.

A unilateral spinal block performed in the lateral decubitus position will require a smaller volume of local anesthetic. This process is also made easier by using a hyperbaric solution. Start with 1 mL and adjust the volume of anesthetic to the desired sensory level by injecting 0.5-mL increments. The onset of anesthesia will take longer when small volumes are used. In the supine patient, the onset of spinal anesthesia is rapid. Inject 1.5 mL of local anesthetic and further smaller volumes until the desired level of anesthesia is obtained.

With surgery of long duration or when the CSA is to be prolonged into the postoperative phase, an infusion of the anesthetic agent is started. The flow rate should be 0.5 to 1.0 mL/h. When bupivacaine is used, it should be diluted to 0.25%. The addition of opioids to increase the block duration and density is discussed later in the chapter.

▶ PHARMACOLOGY

Of the various agents that have been injected into the CSF and the epidural space, the first were local anesthetics and the sole aim was to achieve anesthesia. More recently, additives such as vasoconstrictors, analgesics, N-methyl-D-aspartate (NMDA) agonists, and neostigmine have been used to prolong the duration of anesthesia and analgesia

and to increase the intensity of the motor and sensory blockade. Both spinal and epidural techniques make use of similar agents. The drug-regulating authorities in certain countries limit the use of some of the agents.

▶ DRUGS (SEE TABLES 30-2 AND 30-3)

The local anesthetics most often used are lidocaine, bupivacaine, procaine, tetracaine (amethocaine), ropivacaine, and levobupivacaine.

Lidocaine
Lidocaine is widely available. It has a rapid onset of action (2 to 5 min) and its effect will last for up to 90 min. Lidocaine is commercially available in a variety of preparations depending on the supplier and the country. The preparations most frequently used are 1.5, 2, and 5% solutions. These solutions may contain additives such as 7.5% dextrose, which renders the solution "heavy" and thus specific for spinal use, as well as adrenaline (epinephrine), which prolongs the duration of anesthesia. The lidocaine dose depends on the type of surgery to be performed and on the site of surgery.

A controversy arose when case reports of cauda equina syndrome after spinal lidocaine use were published. It was proposed that a relatively high concentration of local anesthetic solution was neurotoxic. Further studies demonstrated that 5% lidocaine, when placed directly on myelinated or unmyelinated nerve fibers, caused irreversible conduction loss. The use of such high concentrations of lidocaine (5%) has been questioned, when lower concentrations of the same drug have been shown to be equally effective and significantly safer. Similar considerations apply to the tonicity of the local anesthetic, since there is evidence that tonicity may play a role in neurotoxicity. The entire picture has been further complicated by the role of spinal catheters in neural damage. (See further on.)

Bupivacaine
Bupivacaine produces anesthesia within 8 min. The duration of anesthesia is longer than with lidocaine, lasting from 2 to 4 h. Spinal bupivacaine is supplied as a 0.5

▶ **TABLE 30-2.** DRUGS USED IN SPINAL ANESTHESIA

Drug	Dose (mg) To L4	Dose (mg) To T10	To T4	Plain	Duration (min) with 0.2 mg Adrenaline
Lignocaine	25–50	50–75	75–100	60–70	60–70
Bupivacaine	10–15	15–20	20	90–110	90–110
Procaine	50–75	100–150	150–200	40–55	60–75
Tetracaine	4–6	6–10	12–16	60–90	120–180

▶ **TABLE 30-3.** CLINICAL EFFECTS OF LOCAL ANESTHETICS COMMONLY USED FOR EPIDURAL ANESTHESIA

Drug	Time Spread to four Segments (min) ±1 SD	Time to Two-Segment Regression (min) ± 2 SD	"Top-up" Time following Initial Dose
Lidocaine 2%	15 ± 5	100 ± 40	60
Prilocaine 2–3%	15 ± 4	100 ± 40	60
Chloroprocaine 2–3%	12 ± 5	60 ± 15	45
Mepivacaine 2%	15 ± 5	120 ± 150	60
Bupivacaine 0.5–0.75%	18 ± 10	200 ± 80	120
Ropivacaine 0.75–1%	20 ± 8	177 ± 49	120
Levobupivacaine 0.5–1%	20 ± 8	180 ± 50	120
Etidocaine 1–1.5%	10± 5	200 ± 80	120

or 0.75% solution, and it too may contain additives such as adrenaline and dextrose. The volumes of the ampules vary from 5 to 20 mL. The plain agent supplied as a 0.5% solution is in reality lighter than CSF (although it may be treated as equally dense), whereas the dextrose additive makes the solution hyperbaric.

Procaine

Procaine is not freely available worldwide. It causes anesthesia within 5 min and lasts up to 1 h. It is supplied as a 10% aqueous solution but is usually diluted with CSF to form a 5% solution that is isobaric with CSF. Dextrose may be added to form a hyperbaric solution. It is important to note that procaine should not be used in a concentration exceeding 5%. The suggested dosage varies from 50 to 200 mg.

Tetracaine

Tetracaine is supplied in two forms, one containing 20 mg of crystals, the other a 1% aqueous solution. It too is not freely available in all countries. Dextrose may be added to make the solution hyperbaric, water to make the solution hypobaric. The onset of anesthesia occurs from 5 min, and it will last up to 4 h.

Ropivacaine

Ropivacaine is the S-enantiomer of a chain-shortened homolog of bupivacaine. It is associated with less A-fiber depression than bupivacaine with equal C-fiber suppression. This agent is reported to be less arrhythmogenic than bupivacaine and causes fewer central nervous system (CNS) symptoms. It is an effective long-acting local anesthetic. Ropivacaine is supplied commercially as 0.2, 0.75, and 1 solutions.

Levobupivacaine

Levobupivacaine is the most recently developed agent and it is simply the L-isomer of bupivacaine. This molecule has been isolated because it causes less arrhythmias

and CNS symptoms than bupivacaine, which is a racemic mixture of L- and D-forms. It has a similar onset and duration of action as bupivacaine.

Additives

Vasoconstrictors

These agents have been used in neuraxial anesthesia for many years. There was an initial fear that the vasoconstrictors in spinal anesthetic solutions might lead to neurologic complications. There are conflicting animal studies concerning the possible effects on spinal blood flow when vasoconstrictors are added to the anesthetic spinal solution, but controlled human clinical trials have yielded no data indicating deleterious effects.

The most commonly used vasoconstrictor to prolong the duration of neuraxial anesthesia is epinephrine. The recommended dose for this purpose is 0.2 to 0.5 mg (0.2 to 0.5 mL of 1:1000 adrenaline). Phenylephrine may be used at a dose of 0.5 to 5 mg (0.05 to 0.5 mL of a 1% solution).

The doses of vasoconstrictors used vary widely, but there is no discernible relationship between the dose of vasoconstrictor and the extent to which anesthesia is prolonged. This may be ascribed to the failure to take into account the age of the patient, the amount of local anesthetic used, and the level of anesthesia.

The duration of anesthesia has been defined as the time required for the maximum level of sensory anesthesia to decrease by a certain number of spinal segments. Studies indicate that the effect of adrenaline or phenylephrine on the duration of spinal anesthesia depends on the local anesthetic used. The addition of these two agents to lidocaine and bupivacaine produced no clinically significant prolongation of anesthesia as determined by two-segment regression. This was not the case with tetracaine. When epinephrine was added to tetracaine, there was a significant dose-dependent prolongation of the duration of anesthesia. The reasons for this difference between different local anesthetics are unknown.

Clonidine

The addition of 150 mg of clonidine to isobaric bupivacaine will prolong the sensory and motor anesthesia of the subarachnoid block. In addition, the block will apparently cause less hypotension.

Dextrose

Dextrose is often added to an anesthetic agent solution to alter the baricity of the solution. The manufacturers may add the dextrose, in which case the product is supplied as a "spinal solution"; or the user can add it. The addition of dextrose will make the solution "heavy."

Water or Normal Saline

When water or saline is added to the anesthetic agent, the solution will become "light" in relation to the CSF.

▶ SPREAD OF ANESTHETIC SOLUTIONS THE CSF

Many factors may determine the spread of an anesthetic solution within the CSF (Table 30-4).

Baricity

Baricity of the anesthetic solution, or its density relative to the density of the CSF, is the single most important factor determining the spread of an anesthetic solution within the CSF. Additives rendering the solution hyperbaric or hypobaric relative to the CSF may alter the baricity of the anesthetic solution (its density relative to that of CSF).

The baricity of a spinal anesthetic solution is the ratio obtained by dividing the density of the anesthetic solution by the density of the CSF at 37°C. The aim in changing the baricity of local anesthetic solutions is to make their spread in the CSF predictable. For example,

a hypobaric solution will rise within the CSF while a hyperbaric solution will sink (Table 30-5).

Concentration

It is almost impossible to determine the individual contribution of concentration, dose, and volume of local anesthetic, since a change in one variable directly affects the other two. It was only after all other factors affecting distribution were controlled that any conclusion could be drawn. It has been demonstrated that the total dose of bupivacaine is more important than the volume or concentration in determining the spreading of the anesthetic solution. These conclusions have been strongly supported in other studies. There is no evidence that the concentration of the local anesthetic alone has any clinically discernible influence on the anesthetic effect.

Site of Injection

The intervertebral spaces most often chosen for continuous subarachnoid block are the lumbar spaces, since one does not wish damage to the spinal cord by a direct needlestick. A hyperbaric solution will thus move to the apex of the lumbosacral area when a patient is horizontal and supine.

Anatomy of the Spinal Column

Pronounced kyphosis will decrease the cephalad spread of the anesthetic agent.

Patient Height

Height will not play a role in the spread of the local anesthetic unless the patient is extremely tall.

▶ **TABLE 30-4.** FACTORS AFFECTING THE DISTRIBUTION OF LOCAL ANESTHETIC SOLUTIONS WITHIN THE CSF

Proven Effects	No Effects
Baricity of local anesthetic	Patient weight
Site of injection	CSF composition
Anatomy of spinal column	CSF circulation
Patient height	Diffusion in CSF
Needle angulation	Vasoconstrictors
CSF volume	Direction of needle bevel
Dose of local anesthetic	Rate of injection
Volume of local anesthetic	Barbotage
Position of patient during injection	Coughing
Position of patient after injection	Age
	Gender

▶ **TABLE 30-5.** PHYSICAL CHARACTERISTICS OF SPINAL ANESTHETIC SOLUTIONS AT 37°C

	Density	Baricity
Water	0.9934	0.9931
CSF	1.0003	1.0000
Lidocaine		
2% in water (isobaric)	1.0003	1.0003
5% in 7.5% dextrose (hyperbaric)	1.0265	1.0265
Bupivacaine		
0.5% in water (isobaric)	0.9993	0.9990
0.5% in 8% dextrose (hyperbaric)	1.0210	1.0207
Procaine		
2.5% in water (hypobaric)	0.9983	0.9983
Tetracaine		
0.33% in water (hypobaric)	0.9980	0.9977
1.0% in water	1.0003	1.0000
0.5% in 50% CSF	0.9998	0.9995
0.5% in half normal saline	1.0000	0.9997
0.5% in 5% dextrose (hyperbaric)	1.0136	1.0133

Direction of the Injecting Needle/Cannula

If the needle or cannula is pointing in a cephalad direction, the distribution of hyperbaric solutions will be slightly more cephalad if the patient is in a horizontal lateral position. It follows that if the catheter is inserted in a caudal direction, the effects of a hyperbaric local anesthetic solution will be more caudal than expected.

Volume of CSF

This factor plays a fairly significant role in the distribution of drug. Any chronic increase in intraabdominal pressure may cause the development of collateral veins that will pass through the lumbar epidural space. The net effect of this is that the dura will impinge on the subarachnoid space, causing a reduction in the volume of CSF in the lumbar area. Normal doses of local anesthetic solutions can therefore result in a higher than expected block in many cases.

Position of the Patient

If a hypobaric solution is used with the patient in a head-up position, the local anesthetic will spread in a cephalad direction, but it will spread caudally if the patient is placed head-down. Conversely, a hyperbaric solution will "sink" caudally with the patient in the head-up position and will "sink" in a cephalad direction with the patient in the head-down position.

▶ SPREAD OF SOLUTION WITHIN THE EPIDURAL SPACE

The height of the block attained is determined by the volume of fluid injected into the epidural space, by the site of the epidural needle insertion, or the position of the tip of the epidural catheter. Most of the factors that determine the spread of local anesthetic in subarachnoid injection play no role at all in epidural injection. It is generally accepted that a volume of $1\frac{1}{2}$ to 2 mL of local anesthetic will block one spinal segment.

In the case of spinal stenosis, one must be aware that the block achieved may be higher than expected because the volume of the epidural space may be significantly reduced. Similarly, if the epidural needle or catheter has been placed in the subarachnoid space, the spread of local anesthetic will be dramatically higher than expected.

▶ COMPLICATIONS AND TECHNICAL PROBLEMS OF CSA, SPINAL, AND EPIDURAL ANESTHESIA

Hypotension

The degree of hypotension will vary with the number of spinal segments that are blocked. The problem is compounded by the degree of sympathetic blockade, and this will vary according to the level of the blockade. Some drop in blood pressure is always noted with neuraxial anesthetic techniques. Therefore all patients must have venous access lines and all resuscitation facilities must be available when these blocks are being performed.

Kinking and Knotting

Kinking and knotting of the catheter and dislodgment of connectors are typical problems encountered while one is still learning the technique. With experience, these problems will occur less frequently.

Breakage of the Catheter during Removal

The patient should be placed in the "spinal/epidural position" so that the interspinous space is at its widest. This will ensure that the catheter is not "clamped" between the vertebrae, thus preventing its removal.

Postdural Puncture Headache

One of the major complications of CSA is postdural puncture headache. This was considered a major setback to the use of the technique. The causes of this phenomenon were thought to be inadvertent puncture of the dura by the large-bore Tuohy needle and by leakage of CSF around the subarachnoid catheter in the "needle-over-catheter" technique. In this technique, a needle punctures the dura and a catheter passed through the needle into the subarachnoid space. The needle is then withdrawn over the catheter. The needle hole in the dura is wider than the catheter, so that CSF is able to leak out around the catheter. This problem has been overcome by the "catheter-through-needle" method. A comparison of the incidence of postdural puncture headache between CSA and single-injection spinal anesthesia is difficult owing to the wide variation in the reported incidence of this complication, the lack of control of variables, and the small size of many of the studies. The highest incidence reported is 22.2%, whereas a more acceptable incidence of 3.5% has been reported. Perforation of the dura by an epidural needle or catheter will have similar consequences.

Cauda Equina Syndrome

The symptoms of the cauda equina syndrome are urinary and fecal incontinence, sensory loss in the perineal area, and motor weakness in the legs.

It was noted that the incidence of the cauda equina syndrome increased when subarachnoid catheters were introduced in place of single-injection spinal blocks. Several reasons were proposed for this, including high concentrations of anesthetic agent, admixture of the agent in the CSF, and direct damage to the nerves themselves. This led to an FDA ban on microcatheters. It is now accepted that the most likely cause of the syndrome is maldistribution of the local anesthetic solution (5% lidocaine) that has been slowly injected through a small-end-hole catheter.

The following recommendations can be made to prevent cauda equina syndrome:

1. Insert a multiorifice catheter.
2. Direct the catheter cephalad.
3. Inject the lowest effective concentration of the local anesthetic. Lidocaine (2%) and bupivacaine (0.5%) are the recommended agents and concentrations.
4. If a given dose does not produce the expected block then accept failure and abandon the procedure.

Using the above recommendations, the reported incidence of the cauda equina syndrome decreased, which led to FDA approval of the microcatheter technique.

Infection

This is a rare problem. Meticulous sterility must be maintained during catheter insertion. Connections should not be opened in the ward and bacterial filters must be used for all bolus/infusions.

Fistulas

A spinal cutaneous fistula has been described.

Time

Both CSA and epidural anesthesia are generally considered to be time-consuming procedures. This disadvantage is mostly due to inexperience and diminishes as experience is gained.

Subdural or Intravascular Catheterization

Despite a negative blood aspiration test, the catheter may be intravascular. The catheter may also be in the subdural space despite the apparent free flow of CSF. The doses of local anesthetic used for CSA are, however, much lower than those used for epidural anesthesia and usually too small to produce clinically serious complications such as systemic toxicity or high blocks.

Nerve Trauma

In addition to the cauda equina syndrome, adhesive arachnoiditis and other permanent neurologic complications have been described, but these are rare. A high incidence of paresthesia due to spinal catheters (22.9 percent) was found to be associated with difficulty in inserting the catheter. A recent specific study of neurologic complications has revealed a very low incidence of permanent neurologic damage. The frequency of this type of injury is much less with epidural anesthesia.

Method Failure

"Failure" may refer to inadequate anesthesia despite correct catheter placement or failure to place a subarachnoid catheter correctly. The reported incidence of inadequate anesthesia when catheters were correctly positioned varies between 0 and 11 percent in different series. Difficulty in placing the catheter can be ascribed to many of the factors discussed above, but catheter size appears to be the most important. One must not, however, conclude that larger catheters produce better anesthesia than smaller ones. Failure using variable-sized catheters has an incidence ranging up to 29.2 percent.

▶ BENEFITS OF CONTINUOUS SPINAL ANESTHESIA

1. Spinal anesthesia has a rapid onset.
2. Small amounts of anesthetic agent are required.
3. The desired level of anesthesia can easily be acquired by continuous adjustment of the anesthetic agent.
4. The duration of the anesthesia can be extended by infusion of drug during long operations.
5. Anesthesia can be extended to provide postoperative analgesia.
6. The recovery period is short.

▶ ADVANTAGES OF CSA OVER CONTINUOUS EPIDURAL TECHNIQUES

1. CSA has a more rapid onset.
2. The presence of CSF in the catheter serves as confirmation of correct catheter placement.
3. The neural blockade is more dense.
4. The volume of anesthetic agent used for CSA is 10 to 15 times less than that used for continuous epidural anesthesia. This reduces the risk of systemic toxicity.
5. The recovery period is shorter with CSA than with epidural anesthesia.

▶ ADVANTAGES OF CSA OVER THE COMBINED SPINAL EPIDURAL TECHNIQUE (CSE)

1. The presence of CSF in the catheter indicates correct placement and gives CSA a positive endpoint.
2. CSA allows continuous and better control by spinal top-ups, which gives better reproducibility.

3. The level of anesthesia can be adjusted when using CSA even in a unilateral block.
4. The insertion is by a straightforward "all in one" technique.

▶ POSTOPERATIVE ANALGESIA FOLLOWING CSA

The presence of the indwelling catheter during surgery makes the technique ideal for use in the postoperative phase. It is possible to infuse a pure local anesthetic solution, an opioid solution, or a combination of both into the subarachnoid space, or to use the same combination of agents as a single dose bolus. This will facilitate varying degrees of sensory and motor blockade, depending on the agent used, its concentration, and the flow rate.

▶ OPIOIDS

The opioids most commonly used are morphine, fentanyl, and sufentanil, the effects of which have been well studied. The common side effects seen with opioid use apply to these agents regardless of their route of injection. These include respiratory depression, generalized itching, nausea and vomiting, urinary retention, and constipation/decreased bowel motility. Since only small amounts of these agents are used in subarachnoid blockade, the frequency of these side effects is reduced. Respiratory depression remains the biggest danger because the agents have direct access to the respiratory center.

A bolus of 100 μg morphine is injected into the CSF via the subarachnoid catheter and a further 200 μg of morphine is added to the 24-h local anesthetic infusion solution. This is equivalent to 8.3 μg/h morphine as an infusion.

When fentanyl is used, a 1-mL bolus containing 20 to 50 μg is injected. The onset of analgesia will be within 5 min and will last from 2 to 5 hours. The suggested infusion rate for fentanyl is 0.2 μg/kg/h.

The same agents are used for epidural infusion.

▶ LOCAL ANESTHETICS

Ropivacaine and levobupivacaine are not yet approved for subarachnoid use.

Typical infusion rates for spinal analgesia are 10 mL/24 h of a plain 0.25% bupivacaine solution. If breakthrough pain is experienced, a single 1.0-mL bolus of plain 0.25% bupivacaine can be injected via the subarachnoid catheter.

Epidural infusions have been extensively used. Typical flow rates vary from 6 to 10 mL/h. The agents may be diluted. This is done in an effort to spare the motor nerve fibers while blocking the pain-conducting fibers. This has the advantage of allowing early ambulation while also ensuring good anesthesia.

▶ CONTROVERSIES

Spinal Microcatheters versus Macrocatheters

The maldistributon of local anesthetic has been partially attributed to the fact that the catheters used were 28-gauge microcatheters. Subsequent studies have determined the neurotoxic effects of the local anesthetic and other contributing factors such as catheter size, tip configuration, tip position, injection rate, and injection velocity.

Catheter diameter is a variable that may be implicated in maldistribution. Maldistribution has even been reported with a 3.5-Fr gauge and with open-end and side-port catheters. To identify risk solely on the basis of the diameter of the catheter would therefore be unjustified. Since the role of local anesthetic toxicity has been determined and because there are commercially available catheters with multiple openings and different gauges, the incidence of cauda equina syndrome has markedly decreased.

▶ NEURAXIAL ANESTHESIA AND ANTICOAGULANTS (See also Chap. 4)

Neuraxial bleeding has received much attention because an increasing number of patients are receiving low-molecular-weight heparin (LMWH) to prevent perioperative thromboembolism (Chap. 4). Reports of an increased incidence of epidural hematomas and subsequent paraplegias made further study and analysis of the problem essential. It became clear that this complication was rare in Europe and that clinicians in the United States used not only higher doses of anticoagulants than their European colleagues but also administered them at more frequent intervals. This resulted in a consensus conference in 1998. It should be stated that most of the data pertain to epidural anesthesia and inferences are drawn for spinal catheter insertion. Because CSA requires the insertion of an epidural needle and subarachnoid placement of a catheter, there are two penetrations that can damage an epidural vessel and cause hematoma formation.

It is mandatory that all patients who have had some form of neuraxial blockade be monitored for the occurrence of a spinal hematoma. Important signs to be noted are a slow regression of the motor and/or sensory block, back pain, difficulty in urination, and reccurrence of a sensory/motor deficit after complete regression of the block. When a spinal hematoma is suspected, aggressive diagnostic and therapeutic steps become mandatory. This includes an MRI scan and neurosurgery within 6 h.

SUGGESTED FURTHER READING

Cord S, Mollmann M. Continuous intrathecal versus continuous epidural analgesia with bupicavacaine. *Br J Anaesth* Suppl 1, 1998.

Culling RD. Incidence of postdural puncture headache after continuous spinal anesthesia. *Anesthesiology* 71:A723, 1989.

Denny N, Masters R, Pearson D, et al. Postdural puncture headache after continuous spinal anaesthesia. *Anesth Analg* 66:791, 1987.

Horlocker TT, Wedel DJ. Anticoagulation and neuraxial block: Historical perspective anesthetic implications, and risk management. *Reg Anesth Pain Med* 23:199, 1998.

Horlocker TT, Wedel DJ, Schroder DR. Preoperative antiplatelet therapy does not increase the risk of spinal haematoma associated with regional anesthesia. *Anesth Analg* 80:303, 1995.

Hurley RJ, Lambe DH. Continuous spinal anesthesia with a microcatheter technique: Preliminary experience. *Anesth Analg* 70:97, 1990.

Lambert DH, Hurley DJ. Cauda equina syndrome and continuous spinal anesthesia. *Anesth Analg* 72:817, 1991.

Mollman M, Cord S, Mayweg S, et al. Spinocath. A new approach to continuous spinal anesthesia: Preliminary results of a multicenter trial. *Int Monit Regional Anaesth* 74, 1996.

Mollman M, Cord S, Mayweg S, et al. The risk of permanent neurologic sequelae after continuous spinal anaesthesia. *Reg Anesth Pain Med* 24(Suppl 1):22, 1999.

Norris MC. Patient variables and the subarachnoid spread of hyperbaric bupivacaine in the term parturient. *Anesthesiology* 72:478, 1990.

Rigler ML, Drasnes K, Kiejcie TC. Cauda equina syndrome after continuous spinal anesthesia. *Anesthesia* 72:275, 1991.

Standl T, Eckest S, Schultze am, Esch J. Micro catheter continuous spinal anesthesia in the postoperative period: A prospective study of its effectiveness and complications. *Eur J Anesth* 12:273, 1995.

Stienstra R, Greene NM. Factors affecting the subarachnoid spread of local anesthetic solutions. *Reg Anesth* 16:1, 1991.

CHAPTER 31

Regional Anesthesia for Pediatric Orthopaedic Surgery

SANTHANAM SURESH/ADRIAN T. BÖSENBERG

► INTRODUCTION

Regional anesthesia is commonly used as an adjunct to general anesthesia and plays a key role in the multimodal approach to perioperative pain management in children. Its use in pediatric orthopaedic surgery is gaining in popularity[1,2] despite concerns from some orthopaedic surgeons that the profound analgesia offered may mask ischemic pain of compartment syndromes.

The worldwide trend toward more day-case surgery and the associated advantages offered has increased the use of regional anesthetic techniques. Furthermore, the advent of more complex and innovative surgical procedures in children has improved outcome but also led to more invasive surgery and consequently more pain in the postoperative period. These factors have provided the impetus for the development of continuous peripheral nerve block techniques that target the site of surgery in both children[1] and adolescents.

The practice of peripheral nerve blockade continues to improve with the development of age-appropriate equipment and the introduction of safer long-acting local anesthetic agents such as ropivacaine and levobupivacaine. Although caudal blockade remains the most popular and frequently used block in infants and small children, the safety of peripheral nerve blocks has been established in large-scale prospective studies in children.[3] Peripheral nerve blocks have consequently been recommended, rather than central neuraxial techniques, where appropriate.[3] The majority of peripheral nerve blocks are performed in the operating room by experienced anesthesiologists,

but there are several blocks, such as femoral nerve or digital block, that may be done in the emergency room or even the intensive care unit.

The purpose of this chapter is to outline some methods used to identify and block individual nerves and to consider regional anesthetic techniques that can be used for surgical procedures of the upper and lower limbs in children. The choice of technique may be dictated by the pathology, the extent of surgery, the child's body habitus, and the presence of contractures. The differences between adults and children are highlighted, together with techniques to improve the success of blocks.

► METHODS TO IMPROVE THE ACCURACY OF PERIPHERAL NERVE BLOCKS

Peripheral nerve blocks, particularly in young children, can be difficult. Anatomic landmarks are poorly defined and vary according to the stage of the child's development, particularly in those with limb defects. The successful placement of peripheral nerve blocks requires an awareness of these differences, knowledge of developmental anatomy, and an understanding of the equipment used. For most of the blocks presented in this chapter, the use of an insulated needle and peripheral nerve stimulator is recommended although successful blocks may also be achieved with noninsulated needles.[4]

Given the difficulty in obtaining cooperation, particularly in young infants, most children are sedated or under general anesthesia when nerve blocks are performed. Caution must therefore be exercised while placing the blocks, since paresthesias and pain cannot be elicited.

Nerve Stimulator

A number of basic principles need to be emphasized regarding the use of a nerve stimulator (see Chap. 19). In order to locate a peripheral nerve or plexus accurately, neuromuscular blocking agents should be withheld until after completion of the nerve block. The proper functioning of the nerve stimulator, according to the manufacturer's recommendations, should be understood before it is used.[5] With the many peripheral nerve stimulators currently on the market, it is best to familiarize oneself thoroughly with one particular model and to stick with it.[5]

The *negative* electrode should be attached to the *needle* and the *positive* electrode attached to the *patient* with a standard electrocardiographic (ECG) skin attachment. Once the appropriate landmarks have been determined or "surface mapped" and the peripheral nerve stimulator initially set at 1 to 1.5 mA, 100 to 300 μs. and 1 to 2 Hz, the needle should be advanced through the skin and underlying tissue planes until appropriate distal muscle contractions are elicited. The current output should then be decreased and the needle moved until a brisk motor response is elicited with the least amount of current; i.e., 0.3 to 0.5 mA. The appropriate dose of local anesthetic should be injected at this point. If the needle is correctly placed, the muscle contractions will immediately cease, indicating that a successful block is likely. Failure to elicit this response requires the needle to be repositioned before repeating the process. At this stage of our knowledge we believe that the local anesthetic should not be injected if intense muscle contractions are elicited at <0.2 mA or if there is resistance to injection. Both events suggest that the tip of the needle may be intraneural and that the nerve may be damaged by further injection.

Newer techniques for improving the success of peripheral nerve blocks include surface nerve mapping[6] and ultrasonography,[7,8] because both techniques are particularly useful in small children, who are considered to be a group at greater risk for complications or failure.

Surface Nerve Mapping

This is a modification of the standard nerve stimulator technique.[6] The path of a superficial peripheral nerve or plexus can be traced before skin penetration by stimulating the motor component of the nerve transcutaneously. The nerve stimulator's output is set at 2 to 5 mA at 1 to 2 Hz and the negative electrode is used as the mapping electrode. The current required varies and depends on the depth of the nerve and the moistness of the overlying skin. The point at which the appropriate muscle responses are strongest is marked and used as the landmark for that specific nerve block.

Direct muscle stimulation is finer and more localized and should be recognized as a "false positive" response. Excessive pressure applied over the nerve may inhibit the response. The nerve-mapping technique may be used for various approaches to the brachial plexus as well as for axillary, musculocutaneous, ulnar, median, and radial nerve blocks of the upper limb and femoral, sciatic, and popliteal nerve blocks in the lower limb. Surface nerve mapping is particularly useful when classic anatomic landmarks are absent or difficult to define; for example, in children with arthrogryposis or those with major congenital limb defects.

Ultrasound Imaging

Ultrasound is becoming an important adjunct to regional anesthesia.[8] Ultrasonography is noninvasive, relatively inexpensive, being used to improve the accuracy of local anesthetic placement. Technological advances have allowed the development of small portable ultrasound equipment that can be taken into the operating theater. Finally, the technique is easily taught.

There are a number of reasons why ultrasonography may be of greater value in pediatric regional anesthesia. In the sedated or anesthetized child, direct visualization of the nerve or neuraxial structures, vessels, tendons, and bones and placement of the local anesthetic is possible. Since, in children, most peripheral nerves lie within range of portable ultrasound probes, good definition can be achieved. Using real-time imaging, ultrasound can verify correct needle and local anesthetic placement around the nerve and reduce the risk of intraneural or intravascular injection. The position of continuous catheters can also be confirmed.

Proponents of ultrasound guidance claim earlier onset times, improved quality and duration of block with smaller volumes of local anesthetic, and fewer complications in children.[8] To date the use of ultrasound in pediatric regional anesthesia is limited but gaining in popularity, particularly in Europe.[8]

► REGIONAL ANESTHESIA FOR THE UPPER EXTREMITY

The motor and sensory innervation of the whole upper extremity is supplied by the brachial plexus with the exception of part of the shoulder, which is innervated by the cervical plexus, and the sensory innervation to the medial aspect of the upper arm, which is supplied by the intercostobrachial nerve, a branch of the second intercostal nerve.

Anatomy of the Brachial Plexus

The anterior primary rami of C5-8 and the bulk of T1 form the brachial plexus (Fig. 23-1). These five roots emerge from the intervertebral foramina to lie between the scalenus anterior and scalenus medius muscles (which attach to the anterior and posterior tubercles of the transverse process of the cervical vertebrae, respectively).

The fascia from these muscles encloses the plexus in a sheath that extends laterally into the axilla. A single injection of local anesthetic within this sheath produces complete plexus blockade by blocking the trunks (supraclavicular approaches) or the cords (infraclavicular approaches). As the five spinal roots pass between the scalene muscles, they unite to form three trunks: upper C5-6, middle C7, and lower C8-T1 (Fig. 23-4). Emerging from the interscalene groove, the three trunks pass downward and laterally to lie posterolaterally to the subclavian artery as it cross the upper surface of the first rib. The subclavian artery is not as easily palpable above the clavicle in children as it is in adults. At the lateral border of the first rib, each trunk divides into anterior and posterior divisions, which then join to form the three cords, named according to their relationship to the axillary artery: lateral, medial, and posterior. These cords then divide into the nerves of the brachial plexus: musculocutaneous, ulnar, median, and radial (see Chaps. 23 and 24).

Many anatomic landmarks used in adults may be difficult to find in children of different ages, particularly if they are sedated or under anesthesia.[6] The younger the child is, the poorer the definition of the muscular landmarks. The interscalene groove is difficult to delineate because the scalenus muscles are poorly developed. The subclavian artery is seldom palpable in the supraclavicular region in infants and preadolescent children.

The brachial plexus can be blocked at various levels.[9] The choice of a particular technique is based on the planned surgical procedure, the experience of the anesthesiologist, the presence of contractures, and the potential benefits for the patient, which may include placing a catheter for continuous infusions.

The infraclavicular and the axillary approaches are considered safer and easier for the placement and fixation of an indwelling catheter for continuous peripheral nerve blocks. Although the use of the interscalene approach has been reported for shoulder surgery and for elbow surgery in children,[9] it should be used with caution in children because of the increased risk of intravascular or intrathecal injection or temporary phrenic nerve palsy.

Axillary Approach to the Brachial Plexus

The axillary block is the most popular approach in children.[9–12] It is relatively safe and provides good analgesia for surgery of the forearm and hand. The primary advantages of this block are its easy placement and low risk of complications. Its main limitations are incomplete block of the shoulder and lateral aspect of the forearm onto the thenar eminence (sensory distribution of the musculocutaneous nerve). It may be used for a variety of procedures on the forearm (particularly on the medial aspect) and hand, such as open reduction with internal fixation of a forearm fracture or the repair of congenital anomalies (syndactyly) of the hand (see Chap. 15),[12] vascular insufficiency, finger reimplantation, or closed reduction of forearm fractures (see Chap. 16).[11]

Axillary Perivascular Approach
The patient is positioned supine with the arm abducted 90 degrees, elbow flexed, and hand behind the head. The landmarks are the pectoralis major and coracobrachialis muscles and the axillary artery. Surface nerve mapping, ultrasound, or a nerve stimulator may be used to aid in the correct placement of the block. The dose of local anesthetic is 0.2 to 0.3 mL/kg 0.25 to 0.5% bupivacaine, ropivacaine, or levobupivacaine. Lower concentrations will reduce the degree of motor block if required.

TECHNIQUE
Palpate the axillary artery in the tissues overlying the humerus at the junction of the lower border of pectoralis major and coracobrachialis muscles or as high as possible in the axilla. The nerve stimulator output is set at 1 mA. An insulated needle should be introduced immediately superior to the axillary arterial pulsation at a 45- to 60-degree angle to the skin and directed parallel to the artery[13] or toward the midpoint of the clavicle. Muscle twitches are usually elicited in the areas of median or radial nerve distribution (rarely in the ulnar nerve) as the plexus sheath is penetrated. The output of the nerve stimulator should then be gradually reduced to approximately 0.3 to 0.4 mA while the muscle twitch is maintained by adjusting the position of the needle as needed. Local anesthetic solution can then be injected.

Alternatively, a nerve stimulator set at 3 to 5 mA can be used to map the median, radial, and or musculocutaneous nerve transcutaneously in the axilla on either side of the arterial pulsation. An insulated needle should be inserted at the point where the stimulator causes maximum muscle twitches.

Multiple injection techniques have been described in both adults and children. There is little advantage to multiple injections in children[10] because the loose fascial attachments allow the even spread of the anesthetic. A single-injection can provide adequate blockade of the brachial plexus.

As the local anesthetic solution fills the sheath, a longitudinal swelling may become visible beneath the skin, but it should disappear quickly as the solution spreads proximally. Distal pressure may be applied during and immediately following injection, while the arm should be adducted to release the pressure from the head of the humerus from the fossa in order to facilitate the proximal spread of the solution and facilitate blockade of the musculocutaneous nerve.

The musculocutaneous nerve may be blocked separately to provide reliable analgesia for procedures that involve the lateral forearm (lateral cutaneous nerve of forearm). This should be done by advancing a needle introduced perpendicularly to the skin, just above the axillary artery pulsation, into the coracobrachialis muscle until forearm flexion is elicited by using a nerve stimulator. Then 0.5 to 1 mL of local anesthetic solution should be injected just deep to the fascia.

When long-term pain relief or relief of chronic pain is required, a catheter can be introduced into the axilla for the continuous infusion of a local anesthetic. The immobilization, fixation, and dressing of these catheters are rather difficult in the axilla, but this may be overcome by tunneling the catheter medially onto the chest or laterally over the deltoid area. After the initial block dose, an infusion rate of 0.2 to 0.4 mg/kg/h should be adequate.

COMPLICATIONS

Complications of axillary block are rare but include hematoma from accidental vascular puncture. If the artery is inadvertently punctured, pressure should be applied for at least 5 min to avoid possible vascular insufficiency due to compressive hematoma formation.

Transarterial Approach

The transarterial approach, traditionally used in adults,[14-16] is not popular for children but is included here for completeness. Proponents of this approach claim greater success with posterior cord (musculocutaneous) blockade. Among the reasons for avoiding the transarterial approach in children is the fact that most soft tissue surgery of the upper extremity (e.g., syndactyly, reimplants) is vascular in nature; hence it is important to avoid vascular insufficiency caused by vessel spasm or hematoma formation.

The risk of toxicity is also high in children, and even relatively small volumes may produce toxic effects. The detection of intravascular injection and toxicity under general anesthesia is difficult but may be detected by transient changes in the heart rate or ECG.[17] These include changes in the amplitude of T waves or ST segments when using a local anesthetic solution containing epinephrine (usually 1:200,000).

Infraclavicular Approach

The patient's position is supine with a pillow under the shoulder, the head turned to the opposite side, and the upper arm abducted alongside the body. The elbow is flexed to 90 degrees with the forearm placed on the abdomen. The landmarks are the lower border of the clavicle, coracoid process of the scapula, and axillary artery as it emerges beneath the clavicle. A nerve stimulator, surface mapping, and ultrasound can aid correct placing.

The dose of local anesthetic can be 0.2 to 0.3 mL/kg 0.5% bupivacaine, 0.5% ropivacaine, or 0.5% levobupivacaine. Lower concentrations may reduce the degree of motor block.

TECHNIQUE

Safety considerations have steered practitioners away from the supraclavicular approach in order to reduce the risk of pneumothorax. A number of infraclavicular approaches have been described.[18-20] With the child correctly positioned, the clavicle is divided visually into three parts. A mark should be made at the point where the arterial pulsation is felt as it emerges below the clavicle or where any distal flexion or pronation is "mapped" with a nerve stimulator. An insulated needle should be inserted infraclavicularly at the junction of the middle and lateral thirds of the clavicle and directed toward this mark. The needle passes lateral to the cupola of the lung and has little chance of encountering the lung along its course. Pronation or flexion at the elbow should be sought. Once the nerve is located, the nerve stimulator's current should be reduced to 0.2 to 0.3 mA.

Alternatively, the needle can be inserted at the midpoint of the lower border of the clavicle at a 45- to 60-degree angle and directed toward the axilla in the same manner until distal muscle twitches are elicited.

A vertical infraclavicular approach using the coracoid process as a landmark has been described in children.[18,20] The site of puncture is 1 to 2 cm caudal and 0.5 to 1 cm medial to the coracoid process in the lower part of the deltopectoral groove. An insulated needle should be inserted perpendicular to the skin until distal muscle twitches are elicited. The brachial plexus may be difficult to locate in some patients, and an ultrasound-guided approach has been recommended.[21] Proponents of this technique claim more effective sensory and motor block than with the axillary approach.[20,21]

When long-term pain relief or relief of chronic pain is necessary, a catheter for continuous infusion of a local anesthetic solution can be used. Immobilization and fixation of these catheters to the chest is easier than in the axilla, and tunneling is seldom required.

Supraclavicular Approach

The patient's position is supine, with a pillow under the shoulders, the arm extended alongside the body, and the head turned to the opposite side.

The landmarks are the midpoint of the clavicle, the transverse process of C6 (Chassaignac's tubercle), the posterior border of the sternocleidomastoid muscle, and the cricoid cartilage.

Surface nerve mapping, nerve stimulator, or ultrasound will aid placement.

The dose of local anesthetic may be 0.2 to 0.3 mL/kg of 0.5% bupivacaine, 0.5% ropivacaine, or 0.5% levobupivacaine; lower concentrations may reduce the degree of motor block.

TECHNIQUE

Although the reported incidence of pneumothorax in children is low,[22] the fear of this complication remains high among most pediatric practitioners. The supraclavicular approach is indicated for all upper extremity surgery, but particularly so if the shoulder is involved. With the patient correctly positioned, the components of the brachial plexus become more superficial and are easily palpable in most children. The site of puncture should be at the junction of the middle third and the lower third of a line joining Chassaignac's tubercle to the midpoint of the clavicle[22] (if Chassaignac's tubercle cannot be palpated, a line extending from the cricoid cartilage to posterior border of sternocleidomastoid should suffice).

Alternatively, an insulated needle can be inserted perpendicular to the skin at the stimulation site where the strongest distal muscle contractions (usually flexion or extension at the elbow) can be evoked or simply over the point where the brachial plexus can be palpated subcutaneously with the patient in the supine position.

The success rate is high, but complications caused by faulty technique include pneumothorax, vascular puncture, Horner's syndrome, and phrenic nerve palsy.[9] Nerve damage is possible with injudicious injection against resistance, but the possibility of surgical damage should always be excluded.

When long-term pain relief or relief of chronic pain is necessary, a catheter for the continuous infusion of a local anesthetic solution can be inserted.[23] Immobilization and fixation of the catheter can be achieved by tunneling subcutaneously to the chest or shoulder.

Blocks at the Elbow

A single nerve or combination of nerves can be blocked at the elbow to provide analgesia distally. These blocks are particularly useful for pain relief after operations on the forearm or hand without the risks associated with brachial plexus blocks. Four nerves—the median, radial, ulnar, and musculocutaneous nerves—can be located at the elbow. These can be found by surface mapping, using a nerve stimulator capable of generating about 5 mA, as described previously. Once the surface landmark has been mapped, the nerve can be located and blocked using a nerve stimulator and a sheathed needle, thus avoiding multiple skin punctures and reducing the risk of nerve injury.

Median Nerve

The patient's position is supine with the arm extended and the elbow slightly flexed to accentuate the tendons of the biceps and the brachioradialis. The landmarks are the cubital fossa, brachial artery, and biceps tendon. Surface nerve mapping, ultrasound, or a nerve stimulator can aid placement of the block. The median nerve in the cubital fossa is located medial to the brachial artery and the biceps tendon beneath the deep fascia.

After the median nerve has been located, an insulated needle should be inserted medial to the pulsation of the brachial artery. Pronation of the arm with opposition of the fingers is noted when the median nerve is stimulated. The anesthetic dose is 1 to 2 mL of 0.25 to 0.5% bupivacaine, ropivacaine, or levobupivacaine. The indications for this block are surgery on the volar aspect of the forearm and the palmar portion of the hand. Potential complications include hematoma, paresthesias, and intravascular injection.

Ulnar Nerve

The patient's position is supine, with the elbow flexed 90 degrees, the arm on the chest, and the hand on the opposite shoulder. The landmark is the olecranon groove, and surface mapping, ultrasound, or nerve stimulator aids placement.

The ulnar nerve lies in the groove posterior to the medial condyle of the humerus midway between the olecranon and the medial epicondyle. The anesthetic dose is 1 to 2 mL of 0.25 to 0.5% bupivacaine, ropivacaine, or levobupivacaine. Indications for this block are surgery in the ulnar distribution of the hand, including the medial aspect of the hand and fingers. The ulnar nerve can easily be blocked at the olecranon groove. A small volume of 0.25% bupivacaine with 1:200,000 epinephrine is injected into the area. Complications are nerve injury and compression of the nerve if an excessive volume of local anesthesia solution is used. Note that the nerve is in a confined space here, and this approach should be used with caution.

Radial Nerve

The patient's position is supine with the elbow slightly flexed. Landmarks are the biceps tendon and lateral condyle of the humerus. Surface nerve mapping, ultrasound, and the use of a nerve stimulator can aid correct placement. The anesthetic dose is 1 to 2 mL of 0.25 to 0.5% bupivacaine, ropivacaine, or levobupivacaine. The lateral condyle of the humerus and the tendon of the biceps muscle should be identified. The radial nerve lies adjacent to the condyle, lateral to the biceps tendon. With the arm slightly flexed at the elbow, the radial nerve can be stimulated with a mapping probe. Movement of the thumb confirms the location of the radial nerve, and a small volume of local anesthetic can be injected at that point.

Musculocutaneous Nerve

The patient's arm is either extended or on the abdomen and the landmark is the lateral condyle of the humerus. Surface nerve mapping, ultrasound, or a nerve stimulator can confirm this. The anesthetic dose is 1 to 2 mL of 0.25 to 0.5% bupivacaine, ropivacaine, or levobupivacaine. The musculocutaneous nerve courses superficially along the lateral aspect of the forearm and can easily be blocked in this location. A superficial ring of local anesthetic injections (0.1 mL/kg) at the distal end of the lateral condyle of the humerus, along the pronator teres muscle, should block the musculocutaneous nerve. The nerve can be mapped along most of its course.

Wrist Blocks

Analgesia for children undergoing minor surgical procedures of the hand or fingers can be provided by an appropriate nerve block at the wrist. The nerves that can be blocked at this level are the median, ulnar, and radial nerves. Small volumes of local anesthetic (1 to 2 mL) can provide good analgesia for several hours.

Median Nerve

The hand is pronated and the palmaris longus tendon and the volar aspect of the wrist are used as landmarks. Surface nerve mapping aids placement of the block.

An anesthetic dose of 0.5 to 1 mL of 0.25 to 0.5% bupivacaine, ropivacaine, or levobupivacaine is used.

The median nerve is the major nerve supplying the hand; most surgical operations of the hand will therefore require a median nerve block at least.

The median nerve is located in a fascial sheath between the palmaris longus tendon and the flexor carpi radialis. Surface nerve mapping with a nerve-stimulating electrode at this point will elicit opposition of the thumb. A bursa that communicates with the neurovascular bundle is located at the ulnar aspect of the palmaris longus tendon. The median nerve can be blocked by injecting local anesthetic into this bursa.

Complications such as carpal tunnel syndrome or injury to the median nerve are rare and can be avoided by using the above technique or restricting the volume of local anesthetic used.

Radial Nerve

The hand is supinated. The landmarks are the anatomic "snuffbox," styloid process, and radial artery. The anesthetic dose is 1 to 2 mL of 0.25 to 0.5% bupivacaine, ropivacaine, or levobupivacaine.

The radial nerve at the wrist is purely sensory; thus nerve mapping is not possible here. Just above the styloid process, the radial nerve divides into two branches, one supplying the dorsum of the hand and the other supplying the thenar eminence and 1.5 fingers.

The nerve is superficial proximal to the anatomic snuffbox. A wheal of local anesthetic solution should be injected subcutaneously, starting lateral to the radial artery on the lateral aspect of the wrist, using a fine (27-gauge) needle.

Ulnar Nerve

The hand is supinated. The landmarks are the flexor carpi ulnaris tendon and the ulnar artery. Surface nerve mapping and the use of a nerve stimulator aid placement.

The anesthetic dose is 1 to 2 mL of 0.25 to 0.5% bupivacaine, ropivacaine, or levobupivacaine.

The ulnar nerve is located in the palmar sheath immediately lateral to the flexor carpi ulnaris tendon but medial to the ulnar artery. Surface nerve mapping with a stimulator at this point will elicit flexion of the little finger. Using a fine needle, 1 to 2 mL of local anesthetic can be injected into the area to provide analgesia for surgery on the ulnar aspect of the hand and the medial 1.5 fingers.

► REGIONAL ANESTHESIA FOR THE LOWER EXTREMITY

Most lower extremity operations can be performed with a caudal block, the most common block used in children. Some children, particular those of school age, find the altered sensation and bilateral weakness associated with neuraxial blocks disturbing. Peripheral nerve blocks are more specific, can be confined to the site of surgery, and have a longer duration of analgesia.[24–26] They also avoid the side effects of neuraxial blockade (bilateral motor weakness, urinary retention). For quick discharge, peripheral nerve blocks are therefore better than caudal or other neuraxial blocks.

Anatomy of the Lumbar and Sacral Plexus

The motor and sensory innervation of the lower extremity is supplied by the lumbar plexus and the sacral plexus and is more complex than that of the upper extremity (see also Chap. 29). The lumbar plexus is derived from the anterior primary rami of the lumbar nerves from L1 to L4 with a variable contribution from T12 and L5. It is located anterior to the transverse processes of the lumbar vertebrae within the psoas major muscle. The psoas compartment is bordered posteriorly by quadratus lumborum and anteriorly by psoas major muscles. The femoral nerve, lateral cutaneous nerve of the thigh, and obturator nerve are branches of the lumbar plexus and supply the majority of the upper leg, including the thigh and its lateral aspect (Fig. 31-1). The saphenous nerve, the largest sensory branch of the femoral nerve, provides sensory innervation to the medial aspect of the leg below the knee and to the foot.

The sacral plexus is derived from the anterior primary rami of L5, and S1 to S3 with contributions from L4 and S4. The plexus lies anterior to the piriformis muscle behind the pelvic fascia on the posterior wall of the pelvic cavity. The sciatic nerve, the largest nerve of the body, is derived from the sacral plexus and supplies the knee, the leg, and most of the foot except for the medial aspect supplied by the saphenous nerve. A proximal branch of the sciatic nerve, the posterior cutaneous nerve of the thigh, supplies the posterior aspect of the thigh and the hamstring muscles.

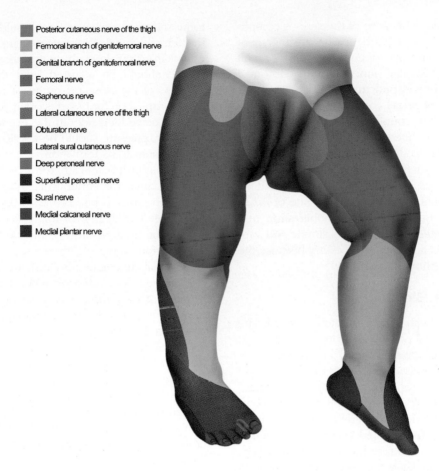

- Posterior cutaneous nerve of the thigh
- Femoral branch of genitofemoral nerve
- Genital branch of genitofemoral nerve
- Femoral nerve
- Saphenous nerve
- Lateral cutaneous nerve of the thigh
- Obturator nerve
- Lateral sural cutaneous nerve
- Deep peroneal nerve
- Superficial peroneal nerve
- Sural nerve
- Medial calcaneal nerve
- Medial plantar nerve

FIGURE 31-1. Lower extremity dermatomes of the peripheral nerves in the infant.

Psoas Compartment Block

The patient is placed in the lateral position with the hips and knees flexed. The landmarks are the posterosuperior iliac spine, intercristal (Touffier's) line, and spinous process L4.

A nerve stimulator and ultrasound aid placement of the block.

The anesthetic dose is 0.5 mL/kg of 0.25 to 0.5% bupivacaine, ropivacaine, or levobupivacaine.

The lumbar plexus can be blocked in the psoas compartment within the psoas muscle at the level of the transverse process of L4. It provides a unilateral block of the thigh or hip for congenital dislocation of hip, thigh for open reduction and internal fixation of femoral fractures, or knee surgery.

TECHNIQUE

Several approaches that rely on bone contact with the transverse process of L4 have been described in adults. In children, the transverse process is not fully developed, and using it as a guide places the needle far too medially and increases the risk of spinal anesthesia sec-

ondary to puncture of the dural cuff on the spinal roots or retrograde epidural spread to the opposite side.

The approach that should be used in children is a modification of Winnie's approach.[27] With the child in a lateral position, an insulated needle should be inserted perpendicularly to the skin, where a line drawn from the posterior superior iliac spine parallel to the spinous processes of the vertebrae crosses the intercristal (Touffier's) line. The needle should be advanced through the posterior lumbar fascia, paraspinous muscles, anterior lumbar fascia, quadratus lumborum, and into the psoas muscle. Passage through these fascial layers may be detected by distinct "pops" when a short-beveled needle is used. With a nerve stimulator, quadriceps muscle twitches in the ipsilateral thigh will confirm stimulation of the lumbar plexus. If hamstring contractions are observed, the needle should be directed more laterally; if hamstring and quadriceps contractions are observed simultaneously, the needle should be directed more cephalad to isolate the lumbar plexus rather than the sacral plexus.

The depth from the skin to the lumbar plexus is approximately the same distance as the posterior superior iliac spine is to the intercristal line.[28] The depth of the needle is emphasized because of the serious complications associated with wayward needle advancement into the peritoneum or retropritoneum, which may result in renal hematoma, vascular puncture (retroperitoneal hematoma), or even bowel puncture.

Ultrasound-guided psoas compartment blockade is possible[8] but is limited to younger children. In older children, the definition obtained with portable ultrasound units is inadequate for accurate placement.

If long-term pain relief is required, a catheter can be inserted for continuous infusion of a local anesthetic solution. After the initial block, an infusion rate of 0.2 to 0.4 mg/kg/h should be adequate. Immobilization and fixation of these catheters on the back is simple and subcutaneous tunneling is not usually necessary because the large muscle mass anchors the catheter.

Femoral Nerve Block

The position is supine with the foot rotated outward. The landmarks are the femoral pulse and the inguinal ligament. Surface nerve mapping, ultrasound, and a nerve stimulator aid placement. The anesthetic dose is 0.2 to 0.3 mL/kg of 0.25 to 0.5% bupivacaine, ropivacaine, or levobupivacaine.

The femoral nerve blocks is probably the most common peripheral nerve block performed in children, its most useful application being for fractured femurs,[24,29,30] where it provides for painless transport, radiographic examination, and application of splints. There are several large studies on the use of femoral nerve blocks, alone or in combination with sciatic nerve or lateral cutaneous nerve of thigh block, for postoperative analgesia in lower limb surgery. For surgical procedures on the knee, the femoral nerve block is best used in combination with a sciatic nerve block.[24,31]

Technique

The femoral nerve may be blocked where it emerges from below the inguinal ligament in the femoral canal lateral to the femoral artery in the femoral triangle. The use of a nerve stimulator can make femoral nerve block more successful, but the block can be done without it; e.g., for an unsedated child with a femoral fracture, so that pain caused by muscle contraction can be avoided.

With the child supine and the foot rotated outward, a short-bevel or insulated needle should be inserted approximately 0.5 to 1 cm lateral to the femoral artery pulsation and approximately 0.5 to 1 cm below the inguinal ligament. This distance will vary according to the size of the child; it is therefore better to map the course of the femoral nerve before inserting the needle.[6]

The nerve lies beneath the fascia lata and fascia iliaca, and often two distinct "pops" are felt when a needle pierces these layers. Contraction of the quadriceps, a "patellar kick," confirms femoral nerve stimulation and should not be confused with direct stimulation of the sartorius muscle. Local anesthetic should be easy to inject into the femoral canal. Resistance to injection suggests intraneural injection; in such an instance the position of the needle should be adjusted until the resistance is lost. Because of the close proximity of femoral vessels, intermittent aspiration for blood is obligatory before and during femoral nerve blockade. In the event of a femoral arterial puncture, pressure should be applied for at least 5 min to prevent hematoma formation.

An appropriate catheter can be inserted into the femoral canal for continuous infusion. After the initial block, an infusion rate of 0.2 to 0.4 mg/kg/h should be adequate. The degree of analgesia obtained is dependent on the final position of the catheter. Immobilization and fixation of these catheters on the thigh is relatively simple, but subcutaneous tunneling may be necessary to reduce the risk of infection when long-term pain relief is required. Psoas abscess is a rare but serious complication associated with femoral nerve catheters that to date has been described only in adults.[32]

A "3 in 1" block is essentially a femoral nerve block that attempts to anesthetize the femoral nerve, lateral cutaneous nerve of the thigh, and obturator nerves with one injection. This is done by promoting retrograde spread of the local anesthetic within the femoral sheath up to the lumbar plexus by applying digital pressure distal to the injection site and increasing the volume of the local anesthetic. The 3-in-1 block has been shown to anesthetize the femoral nerve 100 percent of the time, but it is only 20 percent effective in blocking all three nerves.[33] To do this more reliably, a fascia iliaca or lumbar plexus block should be employed.

Lateral Femoral Cutaneous Nerve of the Thigh

The patient is in the supine position. The landmarks are the anterosuperior iliac spine and the inguinal ligament. Ultrasound aids the placement of the block. The anesthetic dose is 1 to 3 mL of 0.25 to 0.5% bupivacaine, ropivacaine, or levobupivacaine.

The lateral cutaneous nerve of the thigh is derived from the lumbar plexus (L2-L3) and is purely sensory, supplying the anterolateral aspect of the thigh for a variable distance down to the knee. The nerve descends over the iliacus muscle just below the pelvic rim in an aponeurotic canal formed in the fascia lata and enters the thigh close to the anterosuperior iliac spine behind the inguinal ligament. In the thigh, it crosses or passes through the tendinous origin of the sartorius muscle. It divides into anterior and posterior branches.

Blockade of this nerve provides analgesia for plating of the femur, plate removal, drainage of femoral osteitis, harvesting of skin grafts, or obtaining muscle biopsies.

TECHNIQUE

A point 1 to 2 cm below and medial to the origin of the inguinal ligament at the anterosuperior iliac spine is identified. A blunt needle should be inserted perpendicular to the skin until a "pop" is felt as the fascia lata is penetrated and a second "pop" is felt when the fascia iliaca is entered. If bone contact is made, the needle should be withdrawn and redirected. Correct placement of the needle can also be determined with loss of resistance, which is noted when the fascia iliaca compartment is entered. Alternatively, withdraw and redirect the needle laterally and advance deep to the fascia lata in a fan-like manner, or direct the needle laterally in order to make bone contact and deposit the local anesthetic just medial to the anterosuperior iliac spine.

Fascia Iliaca Compartment Block

The patient is in the supine position. The landmarks are the anterosuperior iliac spine, the inguinal ligament, and the pubic tubercle. Ultrasound aids placement of the block.

The anesthetic dose is 0.5 to 1 mL/kg of 0.25 to 0.5% bupivacaine, ropivacaine, or levobupivacaine.

A fascia iliaca compartment block in children was originally described by Dalens.[33] It is more effective in blocking the femoral nerve, lateral cutaneous nerve of the thigh, and the obturator nerves than the 3-in-1 block, with a reported success rate of 90 percent, compared to 20 percent for the 3-in-1 block.[33] It is particularly useful for any surgery on the lower extremity above the knee and for femoral shaft fractures.

The aim of a fascia iliaca compartment block is to deliver local anesthetic deep to the fascia iliaca and superficial to the iliacus muscle, where the three nerves of the lumbar plexus emerge from the psoas muscle.

With the child in the supine position and the thigh slightly abducted and externally rotated, a line should be drawn from the pubic tubercle to the anterosuperior iliac spine along the inguinal ligament. A short beveled needle should be inserted perpendicular to the skin 0.5 to 1 cm below the junction of the lateral and middle thirds of this line. Two "pops" are felt as the needle pierces the fascia lata and then the fascia iliaca. A slight loss of resistance may be detected if light pressure is held on the plunger of the syringe. After a negative aspiration test for blood, local anesthetic (0.5 to 1 mL/kg) may be injected. Because the aim is to block all three nerves with one injection, larger volumes of local anesthetic solution are required with this block than with many others. Massaging the area in an upward direction facilitates the upward spread of local anesthetic. A nerve stimulator is of no benefit, since there is no motor nerve that can be directly stimulated at the point of entry.

No significant complications have been described in association with a fascia iliaca compartment block if the needle remains inferior to the inguinal ligament and away from the femoral vessels. Some investigators have shown particularly high blood levels of local anesthetic after a fascia iliaca compartment block, which could be explained by the large surface area available for absorption.

Continuous infusions have been used for femoral lengthening procedures, internal fixation of femoral fractures, and amputations. The degree of analgesia obtained is dependent on the final position of the catheter. After the initial block, an infusion rate of 0.2 to 0.4 mg/kg/h should be adequate. Immobilization and fixation of these catheters on the thigh is simple.

Obturator Nerve

An isolated obturator nerve block is seldom performed to provide analgesia for orthopaedic surgery in children. However, the obturator nerve may be included with the lateral femoral cutaneous nerve and the femoral nerve in a 3-in-1 nerve block.[33] The obturator nerve (L2-L4) supplies the motor innervation to the adductors of the leg and sensory innervation to the medial portion of the lower thigh and knee joint. Blockade of this nerve can be considered for pain management after adductor tendon releases in children with spastic cerebral palsy.

Sciatic Nerve Block

The sciatic nerve leaves the posterior pelvis through the greater sciatic foramen and the piriformis muscle into the buttock and descends down the midline of the back of the leg to the apex of the popliteal fossa. The sciatic nerve lies midway between the greater trochanter and the ischial tuberosity at the gluteal cleft, where it is palpable in most young children.[4] It divides into the common peroneal and tibial nerves within the popliteal fossa in the majority of children.[34]

The sciatic nerve can be blocked using several different approaches at the hip[35-37] (anterior, posterior and lateral) or in the popliteal fossa.[34] In children, the posterior approach is more popular than in adults because their smaller limbs are easily lifted. The chosen approach ultimately determines the distribution of motor and sensory blockade. Block of the sciatic nerve at the gluteal level provides anesthesia of the posterior aspect of the thigh (posterior cutaneous nerve of thigh) and leg below the knee but excludes the medial aspect of the lower half of the leg, the medial malleolus, and the medial aspect of the foot.

Sciatic nerve block is suitable for all surgical procedures involving the posterior aspect of the leg, especially below the knee—for example, in lengthening of the Achilles' tendon and clubfoot repair as well as major foot arthrodesis.[4] Sciatic nerve block may need to be supplemented with other blocks, depending on the type of surgery; this would, for example, be the case with knee surgery or tibial osteotomies.

The different approaches to the sciatic nerve in children are described below.

Posterior Approach to the Sciatic Nerve

The patient's position is laterally recumbent with the hip and knee flexed. Landmarks are the coccyx, greater trochanter, and ischial tuberosity. A nerve stimulator aids in placement of the block. The anesthetic dose is 0.2 to 0.3 mL of 0.25 to 0.5% bupivacaine, ropivacaine, or levobupivacaine.

TECHNIQUE

A modified posterior approach to the sciatic nerve is easy to use and poses a low risk of complications. With the child in the lateral position, the side to be blocked should be uppermost, with the leg flexed at the hip and knee (modified Sims position); a line is then drawn from the tip of the coccyx to the greater trochanter of the femur. An insulated needle is inserted at the midpoint of this line and directed toward the ischial tuberosity. Nerve mapping is not possible, but a nerve stimulator, set at 0.3 to 0.4 mA, will elicit distal motor responses in the leg, foot, or both (plantar- or dorsiflexion, inversion or eversion) and will confirm stimulation of the sciatic nerve (which supplies all the muscles below the knee). Careful aspiration should be performed before injection of local anesthetic to avoid the risk of intravascular injection.

Infragluteal Approach to the Sciatic Nerve

The patient is in the supine or lateral decubitus position with the hip flexed and the knee extended.

Landmarks are the greater trochanter, ischial tuberosity, gluteal crease, and biceps femoris muscle. A nerve stimulator and ultrasound aid in placement of the block.

The anesthetic dose is 0.2 to 0.3 mL of 0.25 to 0.5% bupivacaine, ropivacaine, or levobupivacaine.

TECHNIQUE

Raj[37] described an approach that is particularly useful in children.[4] With the hip flexed and knee extended, the sciatic nerve can be approached posteriorly by inserting a needle perpendicular to the skin at a point midway between the ischial tuberosity and greater trochanter on the gluteal crease. With exaggerated hip flexion, the glutei may be flattened, so that the sciatic nerve becomes relatively superficial even in some obese children. The greater trochanter is not easily defined in non-weight-bearing children, but the sciatic nerve may be palpable in the groove lateral to the biceps femoris muscle in children.

An alternative approach that can also be applied in children has recently been described.[36] The surface landmarks are the gluteal crease and the lateral border of the biceps femoris muscle. An insulated needle is inserted at an angle of 70 to 80 degrees 1 cm distal to the gluteal crease along the lateral border of the biceps femoris muscle. The needle should be directed cephalad with an anterior orientation in the parasagittal plane.[36] Plantarflexion, inversion, or dorsiflexion at 0.3 to 0.4 mA confirms sciatic nerve stimulation. If bone contact is made before a motor response is elicited, the needle should be withdrawn and redirected. The posterior cutaneous nerve of the thigh can be missed, since it may separate more proximally in the thigh.

Posterior Midthigh Approach to the Sciatic Nerve

The patient's position is supine, with the hip flexed and the knee flexed or extended.

Landmarks are the ischial tuberosity and the head of the fibula. Surface nerve mapping, ultrasound, and a nerve stimulator aid in placement of the block.

The anesthetic dose is 0.2 to 0.3 mL/kg of 0.25 to 0.5% bupivacaine, ropivacaine, or levobupivacaine.

TECHNIQUE

An insulated needle is inserted perpendicular to the skin at the midpoint of a line drawn from the head of the fibula to the ischial tuberosity in the posterior thigh. The nerve is surrounded by the hamstring muscles at this point, and this compartment can be detected using a loss of resistance technique as the needle tip emerges from the deep surface of the biceps femoris.[38] A more accurate location of the nerve may be obtained by a distal motor response in the ankle or foot or simply the big toe (plantarflexion, inversion, eversion, or dorsiflexion). The posterior cutaneous nerve of the thigh is missed at this level.

Lateral Approach to the Sciatic Nerve at the Thigh

The patient's position is prone, lateral, or supine. A nerve stimulator aids placement of the block. The anesthetic dose is 0.2 mL/kg of 0.25 to 0.5% bupivacaine, ropivacaine, or levobupivacaine.

TECHNIQUE

An insulated needle is inserted 0.5 to 1 cm below the greater trochanter and advanced toward the posterior border of the femur. With this approach, the broadest aspect of the nerve is targeted. If bone contact is made, the needle can be "walked off" the femur posteriorly or withdrawn and redirected until muscle twitches are elicited in the lower leg or foot. Continuous catheters have been placed using this technique, but their fixation is difficult unless the leg is immobilized.

Sciatic Nerve Block at the Popliteal Fossa

The patient's position is prone, lateral, or supine. The landmark is the apex of the popliteal fossa. Surface nerve mapping, ultrasound, and a nerve stimulator aid in placement of the block. The anesthetic dose is 1 to 2 mL of 0.25 to 0.5% bupivacaine, ropivacaine, or levobupivacaine.

The sciatic nerve may be blocked where it courses through the popliteal fossa behind the knee for operations on the distal lower extremity.[38–40] The boundaries of the popliteal fossa are formed by the semimembranosus and semitendinosus tendons medially, the biceps femoris tendon laterally, and the popliteal crease between the femoral condyles inferiorly.

Near the popliteal fossa, the sciatic nerve divides into two branches: the common peroneal and the posterior tibial nerves. The exact location of this division varies, but in the majority of children it is within the popliteal fossa.[34,41] The common peroneal nerve then runs laterally medial to the biceps femoris tendon before passing over the lateral head of the gastrocnemius muscle and around the head of the fibula. The posterior tibial nerve extends down the midline of the posterior aspect of the lower leg in close proximity but superficially to the popliteal artery within the popliteal fossa.

Although the nerves branch, there is a common epineural sheath that envelops both the posterior tibial and the common peroneal nerves.[40] For this reason a high rate of success can be achieved even when the motor response of only one branch is elicited. Stimulation of the common peroneal nerve will cause dorsiflexion and eversion of the foot, while stimulation of the posterior tibial nerve will elicit inversion and plantarflexion of the foot. (Internal nerve; i.e., posterior tibial nerve results in inversion of the foot; external nerve; i.e., common peroneal nerve results in eversion of the foot.) The nerves are superficial enough to be "surface mapped" individually, particularly in young infants.

Various landmarks have been described for the insertion of the needle. Konrad and Johr base their point of insertion on the weight of the child. For each 10 kg body weight, the needle insertion is moved 1 cm further above the popliteal crease just lateral to the midline.[34] Alternatively, an insulated needle may be inserted midway between the intercondylar line and the apex of the popliteal fossa to block the posterior tibial nerve and then directed laterally at the same level to block the common peroneal nerve. In small children, the block can also be performed with the patient lying supine by elevating the limb; in older children, this can be done by resting the foot on the operator's shoulders while accessing the popliteal fossa.

More recently, ultrasonography has been utilized to determine the exact location of the bifurcation.[41] With this information, the nerves can be blocked individually below the bifurcation or simultaneously above the bifurcation of the sciatic nerve.[24] Surface mapping may be used in thin children to achieve similar results. Complications are rare, but care should be taken to avoid intravascular injection (the popliteal artery lies deep to the nerves in the popliteal fossa).

Lateral Approach to Sciatic Nerve at the Knee

The patient's position is supine. The landmark is the biceps femoris tendon. A nerve stimulator aids in placement of the block.

The anesthetic dose is 0.1 mL/kg of 0.25 to 0.5% bupivacaine, ropivacaine, or levobupivacaine.

TECHNIQUE

A lateral approach to the popliteal fossa, originally described in adults,[25] has recently been described in children.[42] The advantage of this approach is that it can be performed on a supine patient. The biceps femoris tendon is identified on the posterolateral aspect of the knee. A point 4 to 6 cm above the crease of the popliteal fossa is identified. An insulated needle is then inserted anterior to the biceps femoris tendon until it contacts the shaft of the femur. At this point, the needle is gently walked off the femur posteriorly and, using a nerve stimulator, is slowly inserted until a motor response is elicited with a current of 0.3 to 0.4 mA. Dorsiflexion or plantarflexion along with eversion is desirable. Careful aspiration for blood should be carried out to avoid intravascular injection.

Anterior Approach to the Sciatic Nerve

The patient's position is supine. The landmarks are the anterosuperior iliac spine, pubic tubercle, and greater trochanter. A nerve stimulator aids in placement of the block. The anesthetic dose is 0.1 to 0.2 mL of 0.25 to 0.5% bupivacaine, ropivacaine, or levobupivacaine.

TECHNIQUE

The anterior approach is less commonly used but has the advantage that the patient need not be turned.[43] The need for only one sterile area is a further advantage when this approach is combined with a femoral or saphenous nerve block for lower limb surgery.

A line drawn from the pubic tubercle to the anterosuperior iliac spine (inguinal ligament) is divided into thirds. A perpendicular line is then drawn from the junction of the inner and middle thirds onto a line drawn parallel to the inguinal ligament through the greater trochanter. Using a nerve stimulator, an insulated needle is inserted perpendicular to the skin until contact is made with the femur of the femur. The needle is then "walked off" the lesser trochanter posteriorly and advanced about 1 cm or until distal motor responses are elicited. A loss of resistance can also be detected as the needle passes through the posterior aspect of the adductor magnus muscle.[43]

Saphenous Nerve Block

The patient is supine and the landmarks are the femoral artery, sartorius muscle, and inguinal ligament. A nerve stimulator and ultrasound are used to aid in placement of the block.

The anesthetic dose is 0.1 to 0.2 mL/kg of 0.25 to 0.5% bupivacaine, ropivacaine, or levobupivacaine.

TECHNIQUE

The saphenous nerve runs along the medial aspect of the thigh just lateral to and within the same fascial sheath as the motor nerve supplying the vastus medialis. The main indication for blocking this nerve is to complement a sciatic nerve block for surgery on the medial aspect of the lower limb or foot.

The nerve to the vastus medialis muscle can be located using a nerve stimulator. With the child in the supine position, an insulated needle is inserted perpendicularly to the skin 0.5 cm lateral to the point where the femoral artery crosses the medial border of the sartorius muscle in the anterior thigh. Muscle twitches of the sartorius muscle confirm the close proximity to the saphenous nerve at this level. The distance from the inguinal ligament (3 to 5 cm) varies with age, as does the depth of the nerve (0.5 to 3 cm). An advantage of this block over a femoral block is that motor activity in the remainder of the quadriceps is spared.

The saphenous nerve is a purely sensory nerve at the knee. It is therefore difficult to identify it with a nerve stimulator, making blockade at this level unreliable. At the level of the tibial plateau, the saphenous nerve perforates the fascia lata between the sartorius and gracilis muscles, where it lies subcutaneously in close proximity to the long saphenous vein.

A deep linear subcutaneous infiltration below and behind the insertion of the sartorius tendon (medial surface of tibia) is performed where the nerve lies in a shallow gutter immediately in front of the upper part of the medial head of the gastrocnemius muscle. Intermittent aspiration tests for blood will reduce the risk of injection into the long saphenous vein.

Ankle Block

The patient's position is supine or prone. The landmarks are the medial and lateral malleolus, extensor hallucis longus tendon, Achilles' tendon, and dorsalis pedis pulse.

The anesthetic dose is 0.1 mL/kg of 0.25 to 0.5% bupivacaine, ropivacaine, or levobupivacaine.

An ankle block can be used for procedures confined to the foot, including distal phalangeal amputations, foreign-body removal, and simple reconstructive surgery including syndactyly or polydactyly repair. The peripheral nerves blocked at this level are the terminal branches of both the sciatic (posterior tibial, superficial peroneal, deep peroneal, and sural nerves) and femoral (saphenous) nerves. There is considerable variation in the branching and sensory distribution of these nerves, and for this reason block of all five nerves is advocated.

An ankle block is relatively easy to perform by injecting local anesthetic solution subcutaneously in a ring-like fashion at the ankle. It is important to avoid using local anesthetics that contain epinephrine, since the end arteries in the foot may be compromised. Each nerve should be blocked separately for best results (Figs. 28-1 to 28-3 and Fig. 31-1).

1. The tibial nerve innervates the sole of the foot and medial aspect of the heel and is located between the medial malleolus and the calcaneum deep to the flexor retinaculum immediately posterior to the posterior tibial artery. Local anesthetic injected through a needle inserted posteriorly and medially to the Achilles' tendon and directed toward the pulsation of the artery should block the tibial nerve.
2. The superficial peroneal nerve supplies the dorsum of the foot. A subcutaneous injection across the dorsum of the foot between the lateral malleolus and the extensor hallucis longus tendon will block the nerve. Sometimes it is useful to perform this block with a 25-gauge spinal needle, since the entire block can be achieved by using one needle puncture.
3. The deep peroneal nerve innervates the first web space between the first and the second toe. A needle is passed medial to the extensor hallucis longus tendon along the pulsation of the anterior tibial artery until contact with the tibia is made. The needle should then be withdrawn a few millimeters and the local anesthetic solution injected.
4. The sural nerve innervates the lateral aspect of the foot. A needle is introduced posteriorly and laterally to the Achilles' tendon between the lateral malleolus and the calcaneum until contact with the calcaneum is made. The needle is then withdrawn a few millimeters and the local anesthetic solution injected.
5. The saphenous nerve innervates the medial aspect of the ankle and foot and lies in close proximity to the saphenous vein. It is located on the medial side of the dorsum of the foot anterior

to the medial malleolus. A subcutaneous injection of local anesthetic from the medial malleolus along the anterior aspect of the ankle toward the saphenous vein using a fine needle will effectively block the nerve.

▶ METHODS FOR PROLONGING DURATION OF NERVE BLOCKS

Continuous Peripheral Nerve Blocks

Catheters for continuous peripheral nerve blocks have not been readily available for use in children until recently (see also Chap. 20). A variety of improvised methods, some of which formed the basis for the development of the modern "designer" catheters, were used. As the appropriate equipment has become available, an increasing number of reports of their use for continuous postoperative pain management or therapeutic care have been published.[19,23,30,44–50]

The main indications for continuous blocks have been for children who undergo procedures, or have procedures that are associated with significant or prolonged postoperative pain[44]; or to improve peripheral perfusion in microvascular surgery or in vasospastic disorders involving the limbs. In selected cases, patient-controlled analgesia is also feasible. Continuous infusions have also been used to provide analgesia and to allow physical therapy in chronic regional pain syndromes. Blood levels reached during continuous brachial plexus infusions are less than those attained during continuous epidural analgesia.

For the lower extremity, the main indication has been the management of femoral fracture[30,45] or major trauma. Catheters have also been placed in the lumbar plexus (psoas compartment)[46] or fascia iliaca compartments[47] to provide unilateral analgesia of the hip or thigh. The psoas compartment block provides a more reliable block of all three nerves of the lumbar plexus. Fixation of the catheters for continuous use is considered easier on the lower extremity, particularly for psoas compartment blocks.

Ideally, a commercially available kit should be used, since it allows a nerve stimulator to identify the correct nerve sheath before placement of the catheter. Several manufacturers now provide insulated Tuohy needles of "child friendly" length through which an appropriate sized catheter can be passed. Research on the role of stimulating versus nonstimulating catheters for continuous peripheral nerve blocks is continuing.

Instead of stimulating catheters, one could improvise with a modification of the Seldinger technique. With this technique, the nerve to be blocked is stimulated via a guidewire passed through a needle or intravenous cannula. The needle is then removed and a catheter placed over the wire or threaded through the cannula. These improvised methods are very reliable for accurate catheter placement; radiographic confirmation may be required.

The dosage recommended for continuous infusions after an initial bolus dose are 0.1 to 0.2 mL/kg/h of either bupivacaine or levobupivacaine (0.125 to 0.25%) or ropivacaine (0.15 to 0.2%). The lower rates are generally used for upper extremity catheters and the higher rates for lower extremity plexus analgesia. The infusion rate may be adjusted as needed up to the maximum recommended rates of 0.2 mg/kg/h for infants less than 6 months of age and 0.4 mg/kg/h in children older than 6 months.[48] Disposable infusion pumps, which may be programmed to deliver local anesthetic based on a child's weight, are currently available and may offer an option for pain control in outpatients in the future.[49]

To date the reported incidence of complications has been low. They include catheter-induced infection, particularly in immunocompromised patients, as well as hematoma formation, catheter breakage, or knot formation on removal.

Additives and Adjuvants

Additives are used to prolong the duration of analgesia and improve safety by reducing the dose of local anesthetic required. By reducing the concentration, some of the unwanted side effects, such as motor blockade, can be eliminated.

A variety of additives has been studied in adults; these include opiates (morphine, fentanyl, sufentanil, buprenorphine) ketamine, neostigmine, ketorolac, hyaluronidase, and clonidine. One of the advantages of regional anesthesia is the low incidence of nausea and vomiting, but this advantage is lost with some additives without any convincing evidence that they enhance analgesia in acute pain.

Clonidine (0.5 to 1 mL/kg) may have a peripherally mediated effect. It seems to be effective in prolonging the duration of the shorter-acting agents (e.g., mepivacaine after single-injection peripheral nerve blocks) but is less effective when used with bupivacaine or ropivacaine. Research in this area is ongoing, as the clinical efficacy of peripheral clonidine remains unresolved. Studies in children are limited.[51]

▶ CAUDAL BLOCK

Caudal anesthesia is the most useful technique in children for operations below the umbilicus.[52–55] Its popularity stems from its simplicity, safety, and efficacy in all pediatric age groups, and it is extensively used in conjunction with light general anesthesia for postoperative pain relief for orthopaedic procedures on the lower extremities.

Anatomy

The sacral hiatus is formed as a result of failure of fusion of the fifth sacral vertebral arches. The remnants of the arch are represented by two prominences, the sacral cornua, on either side of the hiatus. The sacral cornua are approximately 0.5 to 1 cm apart, depending on the age of the child. The sacral hiatus extends from the sacral cornu to the fused arch of the fourth sacral vertebra. The sacrococcygeal membrane covers the sacral hiatus, separating the caudal space from the subcutaneous tissue. In some individuals, the fourth and even the third sacral vertebral arch may not be fused.

The sacral bones are not completely ossified in neonates and infants. The cortex of the sacral bones is wafer-thin and the risk of interosseus injection is high, particularly in this age group. Ossification of the sacrum starts in the teens and is complete by the end of the second decade. As a result, a sacrointervertebral block can be performed in young children, and this is a useful alternative when the caudal approach is not possible.

There is considerable variation in the sacral hiatal anatomy, mainly due to incomplete posterior fusion of the sacral vertebrae and ossification that starts at about age 7. However, a few important surface landmarks need to be identified to enhance the success of the block in both normal and abnormal sacra. The sacral hiatus lies at the apex of an equilateral triangle that has the line drawn between the posterior superior iliac spines as its base. Furthermore a line drawn from the patella through the greater trochanter with the hips flexed will transect a line drawn down the vertebral column at the sacral hiatus. This landmark is useful when the sacral cornua are covered by adipose tissue and difficult to identify, particularly toddlers and prepubertal children.

The distance between dural sac and the sacral hiatus is extremely variable. The dural sac ends at S3-S4 in newborns and is usually situated at S2 in adults. Individual variation occurs and the dural sac may even extend down into the caudal canal in 1 to 2 percent of the population.

The caudal space contains the cauda equina (sacral nerves), blood vessels, lymphatics, fat, and connective tissue. The consistency of the fat and connective tissue varies with age; the connective tissue is loose and the fat less gelatinous in infants and small children.

Technique

Caudal block is performed in the lateral decubitus position with both knees drawn up. The prone or knee-chest position has also been described but is usually reserved for small infants and neonates. The sacral hiatus and cornua are identified by palpation and feel similar to a metacarpal interspace. Under sterile conditions, a short beveled needle held gently between the thumb and index finger is introduced at approximately 30 to 45 degrees to the skin (i.e., with the bevel parallel to the skin) at the sacral hiatus and advanced until it pierces the sacrococcygeal ligament. This can be detected by a distinct "give" as it enters the caudal epidural space and may be confirmed by loss of resistance. Changing the angle and advancing the needle as described in adults is unnecessary. This maneuver would simply increase the risk of dural puncture or a bloody tap without improving the success of the block.

Styletted needles are considered mandatory in some institutions to reduce the risk of an epidermal inclusion cyst, which may be caused by introducing a skin plug into the epidural space. Others prefer to use an intravenous cannula.

Penetration of the sacrococcygeal membrane just above the sacral cornua is associated with a lower incidence of bloody tap. The caudal space at this point is deeper than below the cornua, where it narrows significantly and makes identification of the narrower space difficult. An approach that is too low is one of the commonest reasons for failure.

Failure to obtain loss of resistance after the sacrococcygeal ligament has been penetrated may indicate that the bevel is lying directly up against the anterior wall of the caudal space. This may be overcome by simply rotating the needle through 180 degrees.

Once the needle position is confirmed and aspiration for blood and CSF has been negative, the appropriate volume of local anesthetic can be injected. Confirming the correct placement of the caudal needle with the "whoosh test," whereby the injection of air into the epidural space is confirmed by auscultation, is potentially dangerous (air embolus) and should be avoided.

A test dose has been advocated to detect the possibility of intravascular injection. The standard test dose contains 0.5 to 1 µg/kg epinephrine and is defined as an increase in heart rate (10 to 20 beats per minute) or systolic blood pressure (10 percent) following intravenous injection in awake patients. The reliability of the test dose is reduced under general anesthesia and varies under different anesthetic conditions.

The use of epinephrine-containing solutions as a test dose in children under anesthesia may, but does not always, produce an increase in heart rate when injected intravascularly.[58-61] Atropine administered prior to the test dose improves reliability. Halothane, sevoflurane, and isoflurane attenuate the tachycardic response to epinephrine. Atropine administered prior to test dose may improve the sensitivity under halothane anesthesia.

Careful observation of the electrocardiogram (ECG), particularly an increase in T-wave amplitude, ST-segment elevation, or any other arrhythmia, is more sensitive in detecting an intravascular injection of bupivacaine with epinephrine.[62]

Dosage

The most commonly used drugs for caudal block are bupivacaine,[52,53,55] lignocaine,[56] and more recently ropivacaine[57] and levobupivacaine.[63] The most practical formula is that suggested by Armitage: 0.5 mL/kg of local anesthetic for sacrolumbar dermatomes, 1 mL/kg for lumbar thoracic dermatomes (subumbilical), and 1.25 mL/kg for midthoracic dermatomes (upper abdominal), respectively.[64]

The duration of analgesia is dependent on the drug and dose administered, the age of the patient, the site of surgery, and whether epinephrine is used. Bupivacaine 0.125 to 0.25% and ropivacaine 0.2% are effective for 4 to 6 h of analgesia. Increasing the concentration does not offer any additional advantage but may increase the incidence of motor blockade and urinary retention.[65,66]

Adjuvants

Various agents have been added to prolong the analgesic effect of the local anesthetics or to reduce the side effects during caudal block. *Opiates* (morphine, fentanyl, sufentanil) are effective but unwanted side effects (pruritus, nausea and vomiting, and respiratory depression) have limited their use in the day care setting and prompted the search for alternatives. Clonidine, an alpha$_2$-adrenoreceptor agonist, has been shown to be effective.[67,68] No significant hypotension and minimal sedation is apparent when the dose is limited to 1 to 2 µg/kg. Ketamine, an NMDA receptor antagonist, is also effective in prolonging the duration of analgesia; 0.5 to 1 mg/kg has been used with minimal side effects.

Continuous Caudal Block

Continuous caudal catheter techniques are also used to prolong the duration of analgesia.[69] Several kits are now marketed for caudal catheter placement. Essentially all that is required is an intravenous cannula, which is introduced through the sacrococcygeal ligament and into the caudal space; an epidural catheter can pass through this cannula to facilitate the continuous infusion of local anesthetic agents.[9] The catheter need only be introduced a short distance for surgery on the lower extremities. Because of its proximity to the anus, care must be taken to protect the catheter site from fecal contamination. To reduce the risk of contamination or infection, the catheter should be removed after 48 to 72 h or if the dressings become soiled.

Complications

These are uncommon but are usually caused by misplacement of the needle. Systemic toxicity may manifest as arrhythmia, cardiovascular collapse, or convulsions following accidental intravascular or sacral interosseous injections. The incidence of bloody tap (2 to 10 percent)

varies with experience, the age of the patient, and the equipment used.

Urinary retention and delayed micturition are related not only to the duration of preoperative starvation but also to the concentration of the local anesthetic solution. The incidence is negligible when 0.25% bupivacaine or 0.2% ropivacaine or lower concentrations are used. Motor blockade and inability to walk is also concentration-dependent.

Total spinal anesthesia may occur following an undetected dural puncture. Supportive management until the return of diaphragmatic function and spontaneous respiration should be instituted. Nerve injury and neurologic defects have been reported but are extremely uncommon following caudal blockade. Intrapelvic injections have also been reported but should not occur.

▶ CONCLUSION

There are a variety of reasons why regional anesthesia, particularly peripheral nerve blocks, is advantageous for children who undergo elective or emergency orthopaedic surgery. Regional anesthesia provides good pain relief without the need for additional analgesia in both healthy children as well as those with compromised respiratory function or increased sensitivity to opiates (muscle disorders, mucopolysaccharidoses, cerebral palsy, kyphoscoliosis). The reduction of unwanted side effects such as nausea and vomiting can aid in the "fast tracking" (early discharge) of day-stay patients and improve the quality of care of hospitalized patients.

As better techniques are developed, the utilization of peripheral nerve blocks in children should gradually increase. Surface nerve mapping and more recently portable ultrasound are promising developments. These should encourage skilled practitioners to improve their success rates and inexperienced practitioners to develop their skills.

Further development of continuous peripheral nerve blocks will enhance patient comfort for longer into the postoperative period. Their use in children to date has been confined to special circumstances. It is too early to judge the risk-benefit ratio, but it seems likely that they will find a place, particularly in children with associated diseases.

REFERENCES

1. Suresh S, Wheeler M. Practical pediatric regional anesthesia. *Anesthesiol Clin North Am* 20:83–113, 2002.
2. Ross AK, Eck JB, Tobias JD. Pediatric regional anesthesia: Beyond the caudal. *Anesth Analg* 91:16, 2000.
3. Giaufre E, Dalens B, Gombert A. Epidemiology and morbidity of regional anesthesia in children: A one-year

prospective survey of the French-language society of pediatric anesthesiologists. *Anesth Analg* 83:904–912, 1996.

4. Bösenberg AT. Lower limb blocks in children using unsheathed needles and a nerve stimulator. *Anaesthesia* 50(3):206–210, 1995.

5. Hadzic A. Peripheral nerve stimulators: Cracking the code—one at a time. *Reg Anesth Pain Med* 29(3):185–188, 2004.

6. Bosenberg AT, Raw R, Boezaart AP. Surface mapping of peripheral nerves in children with a nerve stimulator. *Paediatr Anaesth* 12:398–403, 2002.

7. Chan V. Advances in regional anaesthesia and pain management. *Can J Anaesth* 45:R49–R63, 1998.

8. Marhofer P, Greher M, Kapral S. Ultrasound guidance in regional anaesthesia. *Br J Anaesth* 94:7–17, 2005.

9. Tobias JD. Brachial plexus anaesthesia in children. *Pediatr Anesth* 11:265, 2001.

10. Carre P, Joly A, Field BC, et al. Axillary block in children: Single or multiple injection? *Pediatr Aaesth* 10:35–39, 2000.

11. Cramer KE, Glasson S, Mencio G, et al. Reduction of forearm fractures in children using axillary block anesthesia. *J Orthop Trauma* 9:407–410, 1995.

12. Altintas F, Bozkurt P, Ipek N, et al. The efficacy of pre-versus postsurgical axillary block on postoperative pain in paediatric patients. *Pediatr Anesth* 10:23–28, 2000.

13. Fisher WJ, Bingham RM, Hall R. Axillary brachial plexus blocks for perioperative analgesia in 250 children. *Pediatr Anesth* 9:435–458, 1999.

14. Pere P, Pitkanen M, Tuominen M, et al. Clinical and radiological comparison of perivascular and transarterial techniques of axillary brachial plexus block. *Br J Anaesth* 70:276–279, 1993.

15. Aantaa R, Kirvela O, Lahdenpera A, et al. Transarterial brachial plexus anesthesia for hand surgery: A retrospective analysis of 346 cases. *J Clin Anesth* 6:189–192, 1994.

16. Hepp M, King R. Transarterial technique is significantly slower than the peripheral nerve stimulator technique in achieving successful block. *Reg Anesth Pain Med* 25:660–661, 2000.

17. Freid EB, Bailey AG, Valley RD. Electrocardiographic and hemodynamic changes associated with unintentional intravascular injection of bupivacaine with epinephrine in infants. *Anesthesiology* 79:394–398, 1993.

18. Kilka HG, Geiger P, Mehrkens HH. Infraclavicular vertical brachial plexus blockade. A new method for anesthesia of the upper extremity. An anatomical and clinical study. *Anaesthesist* 44:339–344, 1995.

19. Dadure C, Raux O, Troncin R, et al. Continuous infraclavicular brachial plexus block for acute pain management in children. *Anesth Analg* 97:691–393, 2003.

20. Fleischman E, Marhofer P, Greher M, et al. Brachial plexus anaesthesia in children: Lateral infraclavicular vs axillary approach. *Pediatr Aaesth* 13:103–108, 2003.

21. Marhofer P, Sitzwohl C, Greher M, et al. Ultrasound guidance for infraclavicular brachial plexus anaesthesia in children. *Anaesthesia* 59:642–646, 2004.

22. Dalens B, Vanneuville G, Tanguy A. A new parascalene approach to the brachial plexus in children: Comparison with the supraclavicular approach. *Anesth Analg* 66:1264–1271, 1987.

23. Lehtipalo S, Koskinen LO, Johansson G, et al. Continuous interscalene brachial plexus block for postoperative analgesia following shoulder surgery. *Acta Anaesthesiol Scand* 43:258–264, 1999.

24. Tobias JD. Regional anesthesia of the lower extremity in infants and children. *Pediatr Anesth* 13:152–163, 2003.

25. McLeod DH, Wong DH, Claridge RJ, et al. Lateral popliteal sciatic nerve block compared with subcutaneous infiltration for analgesia following foot surgery. *Can J Anaesth* 41:673–676, 1994.

26. Tobias JD, Mencio GA. Popliteal fossa block for postoperative analgesia after foot surgery in infants and children. *J Pediatr Orthop* 19:511–514, 1999.

27. Dalens B, Tanguy A, Vanneuville G. Lumbar plexus block in children: A comparison of two procedures in 50 patients. *Anesth Analg* 67:750–758, 1988.

28. Bösenberg A, Cronje L. Psoas compartment block in children (abstr). *5th European Paediatric Anaesthesia Congress*, Helsinki, Finland, 2001.

29. Ronchi L, Rosenbaum D, Athouel A, et al. Femoral nerve blockade in children using bupivacaine. *Anesthesiology* 70:622–624, 1989.

30. Tobias JD. Continuous femoral nerve block to provide analgesia following femur fracture in a pediatric ICU population. *Anesth Intens Care* 22:616–618, 1994.

31. Reuben SS, Sklar J. Pain management in patients who undergo outpatient arthroscopic surgery of the knee. *J Bone Joint Surg Am* 82-A:1754–1766, 2000.

32. Adam F, Jaziri S, Chauvin J. Psoas abscess complicating femoral nerve block catheter. *Anesthesiology* 99:230–231, 2003.

33. Dalens B, Vanneuville G, Tanguy A. Comparison of the fascia iliaca compartment block with the 3-in-1 block in children. *Anesth Analg* 69:705–713, 1989.

34. Konrad C, Johr M. Blockade of the sciatic nerve in the popliteal fossa: A system for standardization in children. *Anesth Analg* 87:1256–1258, 1998.

35. Dalens B, Tanguy A, Vanneuville G. Sciatic nerve blocks in children: Comparison of the posterior, anterior, and lateral approaches in 180 pediatric patients. *Anesth Analg* 70:131–137, 1990.

36. Sukhani R, Candido KD, Doty R, et al. Infragluteal-parabiceps sciatic nerve block: An evaluation of a novel approach using a single-injection technique. *Anesth Analg* 96:868–873, 2003.

37. Raj PP, Parks RI, Watson TD, et al. A new single-position supine approach to sciatic-femoral nerve block. *Anesth Analg* 54:489–494, 1975.

38. Kempthorne PM, Brown TCK. Nerve blocks around the knee in children. *Anaesth Intens Care* 12:14–17, 1984.

39. Tobias JD, Mencio GA. Popliteal fossa block for postoperative analgesia after foot surgery in infants and children. *J Pediatr Orthop* 19:511, 1999.

40. Vloka JD, Hadzik A, Lesser JB, et al. A common epineural sheath for the nerves in the popliteal fossa and its possible implications for sciatic nerve block. *Anesth Analg* 84:387–390, 1997.

41. Schwemmer U, Markus CK, Greim CA, et al. Sonographic imaging of the sciatic nerve and its division in the popliteal fossa in children. *Pediatr Anesth* 14:1005–1008, 2004.

42. terRahe CT, Suresh S. Popliteal fossa block: Lateral approach to the sciatic nerve. *Tech Reg Anesth Pain Mgt* 6:141–143, 2002.

43. McNicol LR. Sciatic nerve block for children. Sciatic nerve block by the anterior approach for postoperative pain relief. *Anaesthesia* 40:410–414, 1985.

44. Diwan R, Lakshmi V, Shah T, et al. Continuous axillary block for upper limb surgery in a patient with epidermolysis bullosa simplex. *Pediatr Anesth* 11:603–606, 2001.

45. Johnson CM. Continuous femoral nerve blockade for analgesia in children with femoral fractures. *Anesth Intens Care* 22:281–283, 1994.

46. Sciard D, Matuszczak M, Gebhard R, et al. Continuous posterior lumbar plexus block for acute postoperative pain control in young children. *Anesthesiology* 95:1521–1523, 2001.

47. Paut O, Sallabery M, Schreiber-Deturmeny E, et al. Continuous fascia iliaca compartment block in children: A prospective evaluation of plasma bupivacaine concentrations, pain scores, and side effects. *Anesth Analg* 92:1159, 2001.

48. Berde CB. Toxicity of local anesthetics in infants and children. *J Pediatr* 122(Pt 2):S14–S20, 1993.

49. Dadure C, Raux O, Gaudard P, et al. Continuous psoas compartment blocks after major orthopedic surgery in children: A prospective computed tomographic scan and clinical studies. *Anesth Analg* 98:623–628, 2004.

50. Dadure C, Pirat P, Raux O, et al. Perioperative continuous peripheral nerve blocks with disposable infusion pumps in children: A prospective descriptive study. *Anesth Analg* 97:687–690, 2003.

51. Ivani G, Conio A, De Negri P, et al. Spinal versus peripheral effects of adjunct clonidine: Comparison of the analgesic effect of a ropivacaine-clondine mixture when administered as a caudal or ilioinguinal-iliohypogastric nerve blockade for inguinal surgery in children. *Pediatr Anesth* 12:680–684, 2002.

52. Dalens B, Hasnaoui A. Caudal anesthesia in pediatric surgery. *Anesth Analg* 68:83–89, 1989.

53. Broadman LM, Hannalah RS, Norden RS, McGill WA. "Kiddie caudals" experience with 1154 consecutive cases without complications. *Anesth Analg* 66:818, 1987.

54. Schulte-Steinberg O, Rahlfs VW. Spread of extradural analgesia following caudal injection in children: A statistical study. *Br J Anaesth* 1027–1034, 1977.

55. Brown TCK, Schulte-Steinberg O. Neural blockade for pediatric surgery, in Cousins MJ, Bridenbaugh PO (eds): *Neural Blockade in Clinical Anaesthesia and Management Of Pain,* 2d ed. Philadelphia: Lippincott, 1980:676.

56. Takasaki M, Dohi S, Kawabata Y, Takayashi T. Dosage of lidocaine for caudal anaesthesia in infants and children. *Anesthesiology* 47:527–529, 1977.

57. Bosenberg A, Thomas J. The efficacy of caudal ropivacaine 1, 2 and 3 mg.kg for postoperative analgesia in children. *Paediatr Anaesth* 12:53–58, 2002.

58. Desparmet J, Mateo J, Ecoffey C, Mazoit X. Efficacy of an epidural test dose in children anesthetised with halothane. *Anesthesiology* 72:249–251, 1990.

59. Tanaka M, Nishikawa T. Simulation of an epidural test dose with intravenous epinephrine in sevoflurane-anesthetised children. *Anesth Analg* 86:952–957, 1998.

60. Kozek-Langnecker S, Chiari A, Semsroth M. Simulation of an epidural test dose with intravenous isoproterenol in awake and halothane-anesthetized children. *Anesth Analg* 85:277–280, 1996.

61. Kozek-Langnecker SA, Marhofer P, Krenn CG, et al. Simulation of an epidural test dose with intravenous isoproterenol in sevoflurane and halothane anesthetized children. *Anesth Analg* 87:549–552, 1998.

62. Fisher QA, Shaffner DH, Yaster M. Detection of intravascular injection of regional anaesthetics in children. *Can J Anaesth* 44:592–598, 1997.

63. Ivani G, De Negri P, Lonnqvist PA, et al. A comparison of three different concentrations of levobupivacaine for caudal block in children. *Anesth Analg* 97:368–371, 2003.

64. Armitage EN. Regional anaesthesia, in Sumner E, Hatch DJ (eds): *Textbook of Pediatric Anaesthesia Practice.* London: Saunders, 1989:221.

65. Gunter JB, Dunn CM, Bennie JB, et al. Optimum concentration of bupivacaine for combined caudal-general anaesthesia in children. *Anesthesiology* 75:57–61, 1991.

66. Wolf AR, Valley RD, Fear DW, et al. Bupivacaine for caudal analgesia in infants and children. The optimal effective concentration. *Anesthesiology* 69:102–106, 1988.

67. Constant I, Gall O, Gouyet L, et al. Addition of clonidine or fentanyl to local anaesthetics prolongs the duration of surgical analgesia after single shot caudal block in children. *Br J Anaesth* 80:294–298, 1998.

68. Breschan C, Krumpholz R, Likar R, et al. Can a dose of 2 microg.kg(-1) caudal clonidine cause respiratory depression in neonates? *Paediatr Anaesth* 9:81–83, 1999.

69. Bosenberg AT, Bland BA, Schulte-Steinberg O, et al. Thoracic epidural anesthesia via caudal route in infants. *Anesthesiology* 69:265–269, 1988.

CHAPTER 32

Nerve Injuries

BASEM HAMID/LISA ZUCCHERELLI

▶ INTRODUCTION

This chapter focuses on nerve injuries associated with orthopaedic anesthesia, including peripheral nerve injuries due to orthopaedic trauma and those occurring in the perioperative period, such as complications of regional anesthesia and other factors.

Anatomy

Skeletal muscle innervation arises from the anterior horn cells via the motor fibers forming the ventral motor root. Sensation arises from stimuli of pain, thermal, tactile, and stretch receptors, which are transmitted to the cell bodies in the dorsal root ganglion (DRG) and through the dorsal sensory root to the posterior horn of the spinal cord. The union of the ventral motor root and the dorsal sensory root immediately adjacent to the DRG forms the spinal nerve. Each of the 31 mixed spinal nerves (8 cervical, 12 thoracic, 5 lumbar, 5 sacral, and 1 coccygeal) exits the spine through its respective foramen and divides into a dorsal ramus, which supplies the back, and a ventral ramus, which supplies the limbs and ventrolateral part of the body wall. The anterior primary rami of all the cervical, the first thoracic, and all the lumbosacral nerves join in the formation of the plexuses. Several peripheral nerves emerge from a plexus. Each nerve may contain fibers from several spinal nerves. Dermatomes, myotomes, and osteotomes refer respectively to the skin, muscle, and bone areas supplied by a single spinal root.[1-3] The anatomy of autonomic nerves is not discussed in this chapter.

Microscopic Anatomy

Each nerve consists of nerve fibers, or axons, which are direct extensions of their anterior horn (motor) or DRG (sensory) cells; they are myelinated or unmyelinated. In the unmyelinated fibers, a single Schwann cell envelops several axons (Fig. 32-1). In the myelinated fibers, the Schwann cells form by rotation a multilaminated structure that encloses a single axon within a myelin sheath. The myelin sheath is divided into segments, each about 1 mm long, by small gaps where myelin is absent; these are called the nodes of Ranvier. The axon with its Schwann cell and myelin sheath is surrounded by a layer of connective tissue called the *endoneurium*, which surrounds a number of Schwann cell sheaths to form a fascicle. A denser layer of connective tissue, called the *perineurium*, surrounds each fascicle. The entire group of fascicles with their surrounding perineurium is encased in dense areolar connective tissue, called the *epineurium*, to form a mixed spinal or peripheral nerve. The epineurium contains variable quantities of fat, which may play a protective role by cushioning the fascicles against compression. Loss of epineurial fat, which can be due to generalized wasting, appears to be a predisposing factor in pressure palsies. The *mesoneurium*, a loose connective tissue, extends from the epineurium to the surrounding tissues.

Nerve fibers are divided into three types according to their diameters, conduction velocities, and physiologic characteristics. A fibers (Aα, Aβ, and Aγ) are large and myelinated, have fast conduction, and conduct various motor and sensory impulses. They are most susceptible to injury by mechanical pressure or lack of oxygen. B fibers are smaller myelinated fibers, which have slower conduction and serve autonomic functions. C fibers are the smallest and slowest, are unmyelinated, and transmit pain and autonomic signals (Fig. 32-1).[1-3]

Blood Supply

Vasa nervorum enter the epineurium through the mesoneurium and provide a unique protective blood supply

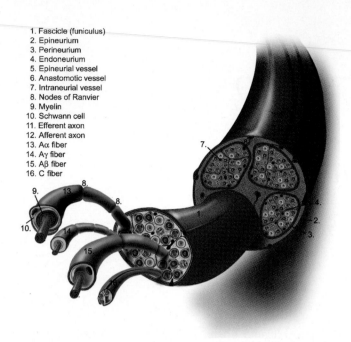

1. Fascicle (funiculus)
2. Epineurium
3. Perineurium
4. Endoneurium
5. Epineurial vessel
6. Anastomotic vessel
7. Intraneurial vessel
8. Nodes of Ranvier
9. Myelin
10. Schwann cell
11. Efferent axon
12. Afferent axon
13. Aα fiber
14. Aγ fiber
15. Aβ fiber
16. C fiber

Figure 32-1. Schematic morphology of a peripheral nerve.

via an extrinsic system of epineurial vessels and an intrinsic system of longitudinal microvessels within the fascicular endoneurium (Fig. 32-1). Extensive anastomoses interconnect the two systems and make the nerve resistant to ischemia. Functional or structural injury occurs only when there is widespread vascular damage.[1,3,4]

Etiology and Epidemiology

Nerve injuries can result from various acute or chronic causes, such as metabolic diseases, collagen disorders, vasculitides, hereditary neuropathies, neoplasms, infections, endogenous or exogenous toxins, and thermal, chemical, or mechanical trauma.[1,2] In this chapter, only causes related to perioperative orthopaedic surgery are considered.

The exact incidence of peripheral nerve injuries in the perioperative period is uncertain. However, peripheral nerve injury is commonly associated with gunshot wounds, where spontaneous recovery is expected in most instances.[4] Bone or joint injury is associated with a 40 percent incidence of peripheral nerve lesions.[2] Although most primary injuries of peripheral nerves result from the same initial force that injures a joint or bone, they are occasionally caused by displaced bone fragments, stretching, or manipulation. Secondary nerve injuries result from infection, scar and callus formation, or vascular complications, such as hematoma, arteriovenous fistula, ischemia, or aneurysm.[2]

The relationship between nerve damage and regional anesthesia is controversial. In many instances it is impossible to establish a definitive cause, since numerous causative mechanisms may be involved. In 1999, the American Society of Anesthesiology (ASA) Closed Claims Analysis reviewed the available data and found an incidence of nerve damage of 16 percent out of a total of 4183 claims.[5] Ulnar neuropathies accounted for 28 percent of the total nerve injury claims; brachial plexus, 20 percent; lumbosacral nerve roots, 16 percent; spinal cord, 13 percent; and claims involving other or multiple nerves, 21 percent. The injuries were bilateral in 14 percent of ulnar and 12 percent of brachial plexus claims. Ulnar and brachial plexus injuries were associated with regional anesthesia in 15 and 25 percent of cases, respectively, whereas injuries to the spinal cord and lumbosacral nerve root were associated with regional anesthesia in 58 and 92 percent, respectively. These figures underscore the relatively low incidence of peripheral nerve injuries associated with regional anesthesia. A definitive causative mechanism relating to the technique or drug injected during performance of a regional block was impossible to identify in most instances, but other factors associated with brachial plexus injuries included positioning of the patient's head and arms, sustained neck extension, and the use of shoulder braces.

A prospective survey in France evaluated the incidence of serious complications related to regional anesthesia in a total of 103,730 cases, including 21,278 peripheral nerve blocks.[6] Only four peripheral nerve and four root injuries were reported. In all injuries, needle placement was associated with either paresthesia during insertion or pain on injection. In all cases, the postoperative deficit had the same topography as the associated paresthesia. The authors concluded that direct trauma from the needle and local anesthetic neurotoxicity were responsible for the majority of neurologic complications. From reports in the current literature, it appears that the incidence of severe nerve injury after peripheral blocks is very low.[6] However, clinically important persistent dysesthesia after peripheral blockade is not rare at all. Dysesthesia lasting more than 1 week has been estimated to occur in between 1 and 5 percent of cases, but there is disparity in the reported incidence (0.04 to 32 percent).[6,7]

Pathophysiology

Degeneration and Regeneration

Primary damage to peripheral nerves may involve any of their four components: the cell body and its axon (neuronal or axonal neuropathy), the Schwann cell sheath (demyelinating neuropathy), the supporting tissue, or the vascular supply.[8]

When axonal injury is the result of a focal lesion, such as trauma or ischemia, the distal portion of the fiber undergoes secondary or *wallerian degeneration*, in which it is broken down by macrophages within hours to a few days.[1,4] The proximal portion might undergo a similar primary degeneration, depending on the degree of the neuronal insult.[2] Regeneration of peripheral nerve axons does occur, albeit slowly, on the order of 1 to 2 mm/day. This process is apparently limited by the rate of the slow component of axonal transport—the movement of tubulin, actin, and intermediate filaments. In spite of its slow pace, axonal regeneration accounts for some of the potential for functional recovery after injury. Regrowth may be complicated by discontinuity between the proximal and distal portions of the nerve sheath as well as by the misalignment of individual fascicles. Even in the absence of correctly positioned distal segments, axons may continue to grow, resulting in a mass of tangled axonal processes known as a traumatic neuroma (pseudoneuroma or amputation neuroma).[4]

Apoptosis

Apoptosis is a programmed form of cell death designed to eliminate unwanted host cells during various physiologic and pathologic processes. This is done through activation of a coordinated, internally controlled series of events affected by a dedicated set of gene products.[4]

Peripheral nerve injury has been shown to induce neuronal apoptosis in the DRG, the dorsal horn, and the anterior horn.[9–12] Skeletal muscle atrophy induced by denervation is also associated with apoptosis.[13] Data suggest that local anesthetic neurotoxicity and myotoxicity involve activation of apoptotic pathways.[14,15]

Apoptosis can further complicate the neural injury and induce neuronal sensitization and loss of inhibitory systems, which may play a role in neuropathic pain.[10]

Classification of Nerve Injury

An elaborate classification, which is practical, readily applicable, and has a prognostic value, was described by Sunderland.[16] In this classification, five degrees of injury are recognized and arranged in order of increasing severity from one to five.

First-degree injury is the physiologic interruption of axonal conduction without physical damage. No wallerian degeneration occurs and a complete recovery can be expected in a few days. The loss of function is variable and usually the motor deficits are more profound than the sensory. This has been referred to as *neuropraxia* in other classifications (Seddon's classification).[17]

In *second-degree* injury, there is disruption of the axon and wallerian degeneration occurs distal to the site of injury. The integrity of the endoneurial tube (Schwann cell) is maintained, thus providing a perfect anatomic guide for regeneration. There is complete loss of function, which improves slowly with regeneration of the nerve. A good functional recovery is usually achieved. This degree corresponds to *axonotmesis* in Seddon's classifications.

In *third-degree* injury, the axons and endoneurial tubes are disrupted but the perineurium is preserved. There is disorganization within the fascicles involving the endoneurial connective tissue. In most instances, loss of function is more complete and prolonged than in second-degree injury and complete recovery is not expected.

In *fourth-degree* injury, the perineurium is also disrupted, but the continuity of the nerve is maintained by some of the epineurium and possibly some of the perineurium. The prognosis for return of useful function is poor without surgery.

In *fifth-degree* injury, the nerve trunk is completely severed. These injuries occur only in open wounds. Without surgery, the possibility of any significant functional recovery is remote.[1,2,16]

Mechanism of Injury

Nerve lacerations can result from common injuries such as sharp bone fragments in fracture cases. Avulsions occur when tension is exerted on a peripheral nerve, often as the result of a force applied to one of the limbs.[3] Anesthetized patients are particularly prone to such injuries because they are insensible to postural insults that would normally not be tolerated and their muscle tone is reduced by anesthesia or abolished if muscle relaxants are used.[1]

Nerve injuries associated with regional anesthesia may be due to the following mechanisms:

Chemical injury: Excessive concentration of local anesthetic, or other toxic drug.

Physical trauma: Intraneural injection, direct damage by the needle tip or catheter.

Ischemia: Vasoconstrictors, pressure-related effects of high-volume injections, damage to nerve microvasculature, and pressure caused by intra- and extraneuronal hematoma. Nerves located in confined spaces, such as the ulnar sulcus and neuroforamina of the vertebrae, are especially prone to ischemia.

With regard to needle trauma, herniation of nerve fibers through perineural gaps—with accompanying hemorrhage, edema, axonal degeneration, and ultimately demyelination—may explain the substantial number of cases of nerve injury with delayed onset (up to 2 to 3 weeks). Surgical trauma and traction or pressure injuries due to positioning; postoperative factors such as ischemia due to tight casts and dressings must also be considered. Another factor is perioperative infection.[18–20]

Hemorrhagic complications can occur after virtually any regional anesthetic technique and can result in neural injury. The risk of hemorrhagic complications in patients who undergo peripheral blocks while receiving anticoagulants is not well defined. Single-injection and continuous peripheral blocks may be suitable alternatives to neuraxial techniques in these patients. In considering a peripheral block for such patients, benefits and risks should be carefully assessed, taking into account the compressibility of the needle insertion site and the vascular structure.[19] Nerves situated in confined spaces are especially vulnerable.

The Mechanisms of Injury Due to Peripheral Nerve Blockade

NERVE INJURY FROM NEEDLE AND CATHETER PLACEMENT

Direct trauma by a needle or catheter can result in neural injury, which classically evolves from a phase of microhematoma, extraneural or intraneural inflammation and edema, to cellular proliferation and scar formation. This process provides a plausible explanation for the commonly observed delay between injury and the appearance of clinical manifestations.[19,20] Although the elicitation of a paresthesia in regional anesthesia may indicate direct needle trauma and a risk of persistent paresthesia, there are no clinical studies that prove or refute this idea.[19,21] Theoretically, localization of neural structures with a nerve stimulator would allow a high success rate without increasing the risk of neurologic complications, but this has not been objectively evaluated. There is accordingly no compelling evidence to endorse a single technique as superior with respect to success rate or incidence of complications. Fortunately, with or without a nerve stimulator, nerve injuries are very rare after peripheral blocks.[19,22]

Needle gauge and bevel shape may influence the degree of nerve injury. A short bevel needle may be less likely to cause injury, since nerve fascicles tend to slide away from the advancing needle tip. If the nerve is impaled, however, a short bevel will cause more damage than a long bevel needle.[20] The degree of injury also varies with the orientation of the bevel in laboratory studies: with the bevel parallel to the direction of nerve fibers, less severe damage occurred than when the bevel was at right angles.[20] Despite controversy, a majority of anesthesiologists favor a short bevel, because tissue planes and fascia may be easier to identify than with a long bevel.[22]

The risk of neurologic complications resulting from peripheral catheters remains undefined but appears to be similar to that of single-injection nerve blocks.[23,24] While difficulty with catheter insertion may cause puncture of blood vessels, tissue trauma, and bleeding, significant complications are uncommon and permanent sequelae are rare.[7,19,25]

INFLUENCE OF TECHNIQUE ON NERVE INJURY

Blocking of a nerve or plexus requires that a certain amount of local anesthetic be injected as close to as long a section of nerve as possible. Regional anesthesia involves the predominantly "blind" insertion of a needle at a point determined by detailed knowledge of surface anatomy, with endpoints determined by indicators such as of loss of resistance or fascial "clicks." Paresthesia elicited in the distribution of the nerve to be blocked, or electrically induced muscle twitches, indicate proximity to a nerve. It is the essentially blind nature of the technique that causes complications such as nerve injury, which has prompted some authors to investigate ultrasound- or x-ray guided techniques as suitable alternatives.

Although the paresthesia technique implies direct needle-nerve contact whereas a nerve stimulator technique theoretically avoids such contact, recent studies have questioned this idea.[29,30] The distance between needles and nerves indicated by paresthesia and other techniques is a complex matter. A muscle twitch is not always elicited despite a definite paresthesia in the distribution of the nerve being sought.[26,27] In addition, nerve-needle contact alone does not imply that fascicle penetration has occurred[28] or that nerve injury is inevitable, since the majority of paresthesias elicited daily by dentists, nurses, and doctors during injections are of no clinical consequence. Nevertheless, pain or dysesthesia caused by an injection has been linked by many studies to perioperative nerve dysfunction. Similarly, serious nerve injuries have been reported with the use of a nerve stimulator technique.[29,30]

The experience of the operator plays an important role in the incidence of complications with any technique, including general anesthesia, but this remains a poorly studied area in regional anesthesia.

LOCAL ANESTHETIC (LA) TOXICITY

All local anesthetics are potentially neurotoxic. However, their application in clinically recommended concentrations around a nerve causes no detectable nerve injury because of protection afforded by the myelin sheath, whereas intrafascicular injection is associated with considerable axonal degeneration and intraneural hemorrhage.[7] The neurotoxicity of LAs varies and depends on their concentration, dose, pKa, lipid solubility, protein binding, and potency.[19,25,31] The intraneural injection of LA in combination with epinephrine can cause significant nerve injury,[7,32–34] although the topical application of epinephrine appears to be safe. Carbonation may further increase neurotoxicity,[35] and a concurrent injury, ischemia, or disease may predispose to neurotoxic injury. Lidocaine and tetracaine appear to be more neurotoxic than bupivacaine at recommended concentrations, while preservatives in LA solutions may also be neurotoxic when injected intraneurally.[36] There is no clinical evidence that prolonged blockade or persistent bathing of a nerve with LA in clinically recommended concentrations, as in continuous nerve block, predisposes to neurotoxic injury, although this is theoretically possible.[19,31] Toxicity of local anesthetics also applies to muscle, where it causes focal necrosis with regeneration occurring over several weeks.[7,37–39] This myotoxicity is increased by the addition of epinephrine to the LA.[40]

NEURAL ISCHEMIA

Peripheral nerves have a dual protective blood supply, as explained above (Fig. 32-1). Medullary or neural ischemia appears to result from a reduced oxygen supply and depends mainly on the perfusion pressure and factors that modify it. Any reduction of nerve blood flow may result in neural ischemia. Intraneural injections of volumes as small as 50 to 100 µL may generate intraneural pressures that exceed capillary perfusion pressure for as long as 10 min and thus cause neural ischemia. Epineural blood flow also responds to adrenergic stimuli. Local anesthetic agent solutions containing epinephrine may theoretically produce peripheral nerve ischemia via vasoconstriction of the vasa nervorum, especially in patients with microvascular disease.[18,19,22,41–42]

TOURNIQUET INJURY

Nerve lesions can occur after compression for 2 h at a pressure of 350 mmHg. This can be attributed to force applied to nerve trunks at the edge of the tourniquet or to neural hypoxia. Although injury starts at the myelin invaginations at the nodes of Ranvier, higher pressures can induce further axonal degeneration. The injury is typically a neuropraxia and the prognosis is generally favorable, with symptoms resolving within 6 to 12 months. This injury is often misdiagnosed as a complication of regional block.[22,43] One technique in orthopaedic surgery should be specifically discouraged: that is, to place a tourniquet around the thigh of a patient with the knee flexed and then, after inflating the cuff, straightening the leg. This fixates the sciatic nerve to the femur and causes extreme traction on the nerve.

INFECTIOUS COMPLICATIONS

Infection can complicate any regional technique. The infectious source can be contaminated equipment or medication or an endogenous source in the patient that spreads to the site of needle or catheter insertion. Indwelling catheters may be colonized from a superficial site and serve as a wick that spreads infection from the skin to the neural sheath. Contamination with *Streptococcus viridans* from the operator's buccal mucosa has also been described.[19]

PERIOPERATIVE POSITIONING

The main mechanisms involve direct or indirect compression or traction. Elongation or prolonged stretching are especially conducive to brachial plexus injuries. Compression between bone and a hard surface is more often the mechanism responsible for ulnar and common peroneal nerve neuropathy. Severe injuries are, however, infrequent (less than 1 percent).[22,44]

PATIENTS AT INCREASED RISK FOR NERVE INJURY

Nerve damage may be caused by physical, chemical, or ischemic mechanisms, alone or in combination. A particularly dangerous combination is that of compression and ischemia. The "double crush" concept[19,44,45] proposes that nerve damage caused by needle placement or local anesthetic toxicity may be worsened by an additional patient factor or surgical injury. A detailed preoperative history and examination may reveal an existing neurologic lesion or a patient at risk for such a lesion (e.g., one with diabetes mellitus). In such situation, a nerve block should be carefully considered. Other patients at increased risk of perioperative neurologic injury include those with progressive neurologic disorders, since their symptoms may coincidentally worsen after performance of a regional block. While a nerve block may not be absolutely contraindicated, the patient should be informed about possible progression of an underlying disease process; then, if the block is still indicated or requested, specific consent should be obtained. In such situations, the use of dilute or less potent local anesthetic should be considered to reduce the risk of neurotoxicity.

There are some locations where the nerves or plexuses are in confined spaces and therefore potentially vulnerable to ischemic injury. It may be prudent to be cautious when doing peripheral nerve blocks in these areas. Areas where caution should be exercised include the following:

1. The neuroforamina where the brachial plexus exits the spine
2. The area where the brachial plexus crosses the first rib in the narrow space between the first rib and the clavicle
3. The ulnar nerve behind the elbow where the nerve lies in the sulcus ulnaris
4. The median nerve as it passes through the carpal tunnel
5. The common peroneal nerve as it courses around the head of the fibula

Areas where nerves are particularly at risk in the postoperative period and where special attention should be paid to the placement of casts and slings are the radial nerve as it curls around the humerus (Fig. 32-2); the ulnar nerve behind the elbow (Fig. 32-3); and the common peroneal nerve at the head of the fibula (Fig. 32-4). These nerves are very commonly injured if they are subjected to pressure during continuous nerve block.

PERFORMING BLOCKS IN ANESTHETIZED PATIENTS

Performance of regional anesthesia in anesthetized patients has become accepted in children but is controversial in adult patients. There is no compelling evidence that regional anesthesia is unsafe in anesthetized patients. However, there appears to be a relationship

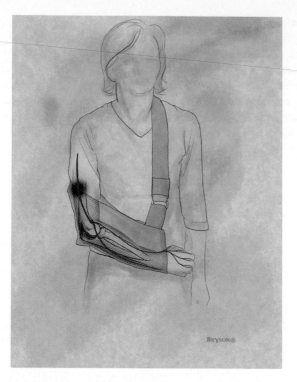

Figure 32-2. Ill-fitting slings can injure the insensate radial nerve where it curls around the shaft of the humerus.

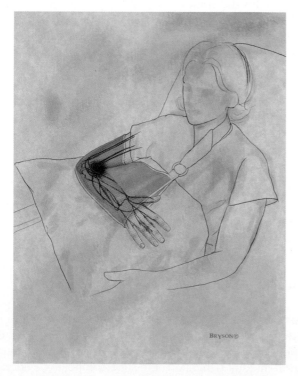

Figure 32-3. If not protected, the insensate ulnar nerve is prone to pressure injury.

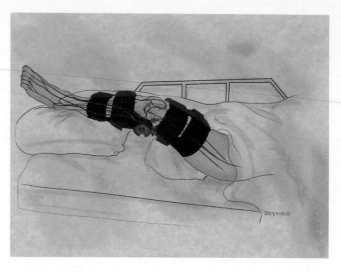

Figure 32-4. Ill-fitting braces can injure the insensate common peroneal nerve as it curls around the fibular head.

between painful paresthesia experienced during injection and postblock nerve dysfunction.[20] If an awake patient complains of severe pain or discomfort, the operator should discontinue probing and withdraw the needle or change its direction. One advantage of placing a block in an unanesthetized patient is that the operator can note whether or not paresthesia was elicited, in what distribution, and the presence or absence of pain on injection. However, there are many instances in which it may be advantageous to perform blocks in anesthetized or heavily sedated patients; for example, in mentally challenged patients, very anxious patients, and patients being treated for painful conditions such as fractures. If the operator relies on complaints of pain to provide warning of a possible intraneural injection, it is probably inappropriate to use a test dose containing local anesthetic agents, since this will numb the nerve and give false-negative feedback. For this reason, we recommend the use of normal saline (with 1:400,000 epinephrine as a marker for intravascular injection) as a test dose. Each patient and surgical situation should, however, be evaluated and treated individually.

Clinical Evaluation Of Possible Nerve Injury

Injuries to peripheral nerves cause various symptoms and signs that correspond to the regions supplied by each particular nerve. An accurate diagnosis of nerve injury therefore requires thorough knowledge of individual nerves.[46] If regional anesthesia is planned, the importance of a thorough baseline neurologic examination with meticulous documentation of deficits cannot be overemphasized, especially in patients with suspected preexisting nerve injury. A neurologic consultation should be obtained promptly whenever a neurologic complication is suspected in the perioperative period.

Sensory Disturbances

If a nerve is severed, complete sensory loss is found exclusively in the area supplied by it. This is called the *autonomous* zone. An intermediate zone supplied by the adjacent sensory nerves surrounds it. The autonomous plus intermediate zones together constitute the *maximal* zone. In general, the area where light touch sense is lost is greater than the area where a pinprick cannot be sensed. If the injury is partial, paresthesia may be present in the distribution area of the affected nerve with varying degrees of sensory disturbance. Sensory modalities are affected in order of decreasing frequency as follows: proprioception, touch, temperature and pain.[2,46]

Sensory testing is performed on the area outlined by the patient. Light touch perception is tested by using a soft object, such as cotton swab, working from the insensitive toward the sensitive area. If the abnormal area is hypersensitive, the direction is reversed. A continuous line delineates the area. A disposable sharp object, such as a toothpick, tests superficial pain. It is also important to test two-point discrimination, proprioception (joint position sense), and deep pressure sense.[47]

Motor Disturbances

The muscle or muscle groups supplied by the injured nerve will exhibit variable degrees of motor loss. The involved muscles may become hypotonic or atonic, with decreased resistance to passive motion.[2,47]

The strength of suspected muscles is examined individually in relation to the movement of a single joint and is graded according to the following scale:

5 Normal
4 Weak but able to move against gravity and resistance
3 Able to move against gravity but not resistance
2 Able to move joint if gravity is eliminated
1 Flicker or trace of muscle contraction
0 No perceptible muscle contraction

Owing to the large range of muscle strength graded 4 to 5, grades 4−, 4, and 4+, may be used to indicate movement against slight, moderate, and strong resistance respectively.[47,48]

Muscle Stretch Reflex Disturbances

As a consequence of sensorimotor loss, the muscle stretch reflex subserved by each damaged nerve is decreased or absent. Reflex activity can be completely abolished even in partial injuries and is therefore not a reliable guide to the severity of the injury. The following roots subserve the following commonly evaluated reflexes: biceps and brachioradialis, C5-C6; triceps reflex, C7-C8; knee jerk, L3-L4; and ankle jerk, S1-S2. In examining

reflexes, asymmetry is the most important factor to evaluate. Reflexes should be elicited by percussing the tendons on both sides with the same force and with the two limbs in similar positions.[2,47–49]

Autonomic Disturbances

The area supplied by the injured nerve becomes anhydrotic if the injury is complete. If the injury is incomplete, sweating may be excessive. Vasodilatation occurs in complete lesions in the early phase and the affected area is warm and well perfused. After 2 to 3 weeks, however, the affected area becomes cooler. Subsequently, the skin may become thin, inelastic, and scaly. The nails may become curved and both nail and hair growth may be retarded in the affected area. Because sensation is lost in the affected area, it becomes susceptible to injury, and ulcers may develop.[2,46]

Diagnostic Tests

Electrophysiologic studies (EPSs) remain the main diagnostic tool in nerve injuries. They not only provide an objective method for describing the injury but also help to differentiate between axonal and demyelinating lesions and indicate whether lesions are acute or chronic. In addition, they help to determine the severity of an injury, to identify the pattern of recovery, and offer a more accurate prognosis. Although abnormalities may not be detected within 2 to 3 weeks of injury, it is always advisable to obtain baseline EPS if injury is suspected so as to rule out any preexisting pathology. Failure to detect small and unmyelinated fiber injuries with conventional studies and lack of experience with EPS can limit the value of these studies. A complete study consists of nerve conduction studies (NCSs) and electromyography (EMG).[50,51]

Nerve Conduction Studies

Nerve conduction studies evaluate the function of motor and sensory nerves by recording certain variables, such as amplitude and conduction velocity, of a generated electrical impulse in different areas along peripheral nerves. The F-wave studies are especially useful for investigating proximal lesions. Nerve conduction velocities are typically normal or near normal in axonal degeneration. However, the amplitude is often decreased because of a reduction in the number of functioning axons. Demyelinating lesions reduce conduction velocity; if severe enough, they can cause failure of impulse transmission, resulting in conduction block.[50–53]

Electromyography

Electromyography records the activity of motor units by means of a needle electrode. Nerve injury can result in spontaneous activity, manifest as sharp waves and fibrillations. These findings appear acutely within 2 to 3 weeks of nerve injury and indicate an active axonal degeneration.

Within 3 months, as regeneration and sprouting of axons begin, "polyphasic" motor unit potentials can be recorded. This signifies the chronicity of the injury and continues until reinnervation and recovery is complete. The EMG may, however, never return to normal.[1,2,50,51,54]

Imaging

Imaging studies, including computed tomography (CT) and magnetic resonance imaging (MRI), are useful for evaluating nerve injuries when certain processes are suspected, such as infection, inflammation, hematoma, or other structural causes of nerve damage.[19]

Specific Nerve Injuries

Nerve injuries in the perioperative period are often multifactorial, and it may be difficult to assign a single cause. The distribution, time of onset, severity, and clinical course of nerve injuries resulting from regional anesthesia will depend on the factors that have caused them. In general, paresthesia and hypoalgesia suggest the involvement of small-diameter nerve fibers and indicate injury by local anesthetic or extra- or intraneural hematoma or edema. The symptoms and signs are therefore usually sensory rather than motor and typically appear within 24 h of regional anesthesia. The onset can, however, be delayed by days or weeks in some cases.

Gross motor loss following regional anesthesia usually indicates an additional mechanism of injury, such as tissue reaction, scar formation, or ongoing mechanical or chemical trauma, especially if the onset is late.[19,55] The anesthesiologist must be familiar with common nerve injuries encountered in orthopaedic surgery and their possible etiology in order to differentiate between complications of anesthesia and other causes. Major nerve injuries are discussed here.

The Brachial Plexus

The brachial plexus is formed from the anterior (ventral) rami of the segments C5, C6, C7, C8, and T1. It is divided from proximal to distal into roots, trunks, divisions, cords, and branches (Fig. 23-1). The plexus epineurium is a continuation of the epidural tissue and the dura becomes its perineurium.

Trauma in general is the most frequent cause of injury and may occur as a penetrating or a closed injury (traction, avulsion, compression, or stretch). Motorcycle accidents are a common cause of brachial plexus injury in civilian life. Common associated injuries include fractures of the proximal humerus, scapula, ribs, clavicle, transverse process of the cervical vertebrae, and dislocation of the shoulder, the acromioclavicular and sternoclavicular joints. The brachial plexus is the most susceptible of all nerve groups to injury from positioning during anesthesia, perhaps because of its long mobile course between its two points of fixation, the

paravertebral fascia proximally and the axillary fascia distally, and its proximity to a number of freely movable bony structures.[1,2,44] Stretching of nerve fibers, rather than compression, is the main cause of injury.[44] However, shoulder braces used in certain procedures may cause direct compression or stretching of the plexus (Figs. 32-2 and 32-3). Upper plexus lesions (C5, C6, and C7 occur with full arm abduction, whereas lower plexus lesions (C7, C8, and T1) occur primarily when the arm is close to the side.[46,55–57]

TOTAL PLEXUS PARALYSIS

This rare syndrome is usually due to severe trauma (often a fall from a moving vehicle) and is characterized by complete paralysis of the arm and rapid atrophy of the muscles. There is complete anesthesia of the arm distal to a line extending obliquely from the tip of the shoulder down the medial aspect of the arm halfway to the elbow. The entire upper extremity is areflexic.[46,55]

UPPER PLEXUS PARALYSIS (ERB-DUCHENNE TYPE)

This condition results from damage to the fifth and sixth cervical roots or the upper trunk of the brachial plexus. It is a common deficit and is usually due to forceful lateral flexion of the head, but it may also be due to pressure on the shoulder (e.g., knapsack paralysis, firearm recoil).[58] The muscles supplied by the C5-6 roots are weak or paralyzed and atrophic. These include the deltoid, biceps, brachioradialis, and brachialis muscles and occasionally also the supraspinatus, infraspinatus, and subscapularis muscles. The position of the arm is characteristic: the limb is internally rotated and adducted and the forearm is extended and pronated, the palm thus facing out and backward. This is the "policeman's tip" or "porter's tip" position. Sensation is usually intact. The biceps and brachioradialis reflexes are depressed or absent.[46,55]

MIDDLE PLEXUS PARALYSIS

Lesions of the middle trunk are rare but occasionally result from trauma. The seventh cervical fibers to the radial nerve are primarily involved; the extensors of the forearm, hand, and fingers are therefore paretic. Forearm flexion is spared. The triceps muscle reflex may be depressed or absent. Sensory deficit may occur over the extensor surface of the forearm and the radial aspect of the dorsum of the hand (Fig. 32-5).[46,55]

LOWER PLEXUS PARALYSIS (DEJERINE-KLUMPKE TYPE)

This condition follows injury to the eighth cervical and first thoracic roots of the lower trunk of the plexus. It is usually the result of trauma, particularly arm traction in the abducted position. All the muscles supplied by the eighth cervical and first thoracic roots are paretic and eventually become atrophic, causing weakness of wrist and finger

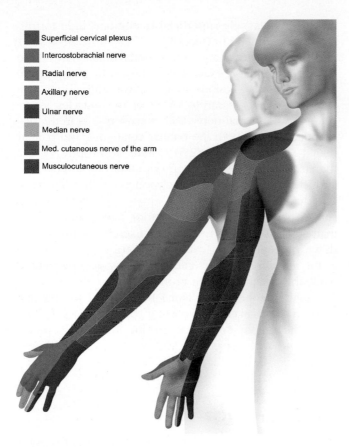

Superficial cervical plexus

Intercostobrachial nerve

Radial nerve

Axillary nerve

Ulnar nerve

Median nerve

Med. cutaneous nerve of the arm

Musculocutaneous nerve

Figure 32-5. Dermatomes of the nerves of the upper limb.

flexion and of the intrinsic hand muscles. A claw-hand deformity is often evident. Sensation may be intact or absent on the medial arm, medial forearm, and ulnar aspect of the hand (Fig. 32-5). The finger flexor reflex (C8-T1) is depressed or absent. When the first thoracic root is injured, an ipsilateral Horner's syndrome results.[46,55]

LESIONS OF THE LATERAL CORD
Lateral cord lesions are usually due to surgical or local trauma and result in paresis of the muscles innervated by the musculocutaneous nerve and lateral head of the median nerve. Thus there is paresis of the biceps, brachialis, and coracobrachialis (which control elbow flexion and forearm supination), and all muscles innervated by the median nerve except the intrinsic hand muscles. The biceps reflex is depressed or absent and sensory loss may occur on the lateral forearm (Fig. 32-5).[46,55]

LESIONS OF THE MEDIAL CORD
Lesions of the medial cord of the brachial plexus result in weakness of the hand flexor muscles innervated by the ulnar nerve. A sensory loss may occur on the medial arm and forearm (Fig. 32-5).[46,55]

LESIONS OF THE POSTERIOR CORD
Lesions of the posterior cord result in paresis of the muscles supplied by the subscapular nerve (teres major and subscapularis), thoracodorsal nerve (latissimus dorsi paresis), axillary (deltoid and teres minor), and radial nerve. A variable sensory loss may occur (Fig. 32-5).[46,55]

Dorsal Scapular Nerve (C4-C5)

A lesion of the dorsal scapular nerve (which supplies the rhomboid muscles) causes rotation of the scapula, so that its inferior angle is displaced laterally.

Long Thoracic Nerve (C5-C7)

The long thoracic nerve is rarely injured alone, most frequently by sharp or blunt trauma, from traction when the head is forced acutely away from the shoulder or when the shoulder is depressed, as in carrying heavy objects. Other causes include the placement of patients in the Trendelenburg position with shoulder braces, which compress the supraclavicular areas.[1] Athletic activity may also cause stretch injury. This nerve supplies the serratus muscle, which fixes and stabilizes the scapula against the chest wall; its functioning is tested by observing scapular winging (the vertebral border of the scapula stands away from the thorax, forming a "wing") while the patient pushes with extended arms against an immovable object, such as a wall.[46,55]

Suprascapular Nerve (C5-C6)

This nerve may be injured by penetrating trauma in the posterior triangle of the neck, trauma to the supraclavicular region, or in proximal upper brachial plexopathies. Entrapment lesions may occur in the suprascapular foramen or notch.[1] Supraspinatus paresis causes weakness of arm abduction, while infraspinatus paresis causes impaired external rotation at the shoulder joint. A lesion of the suprascapular nerve at the glenoid notch, causing isolated infraspinatus paresis and atrophy, may occur as a professional hazard in volleyball players.[46,55]

Subscapular Nerve (C5-C7)

Subscapular nerve palsies usually occur with posterior cord brachial plexus lesions. The arm is partially externally rotated, with some weakness of internal rotation.[46,55]

Axillary Nerve (C5-C6)

The axillary nerve is thought to be the nerve most vulnerable to traction injury of the brachial plexus because it is tethered to the deltoid muscle very close to the shoulder. Stretch injuries of the axillary nerve occur in approximately 5 percent of shoulder dislocations.[2] It is most often injured where it winds around the lateral aspect of the humerus in a relatively exposed position (e.g., in fracture or dislocation of the humerus and total shoulder arthroplasty). It may also be injured when the shoulder joint is dislocated or when the scapula is fractured. Lesions of the posterior cord of the brachial plexus affect this nerve and the radial nerve. In axillary nerve lesions, the deltoid muscle becomes atrophic, causing a flattening or concavity of the shoulder contour. Deltoid paralysis results in inability to abduct the arm. Teres minor paralysis is usually not demonstrable by clinical examination. An axillary cutaneous sensory defect is located on the outer aspect of the upper arm and is maximal over the deltoid attachment, the "sergeant's patch" (Fig. 32-5).[46,55]

Musculocutaneous Nerve (C5-C7)

This nerve is most commonly injured by shoulder surgery or penetrating injuries and occasionally by anterior dislocation of the shoulder or fractures of the humeral neck. The autonomous zone of the lateral cutaneous nerve of the forearm (a narrow band along the radial forearm) shows sensory loss in the case of musculocutaneous nerve lesions. The cutaneous sensory loss may extend from the elbow to the wrist and cover the entire lateral forearm from the dorsal to the ventral midline. Nerve damage may result from lesions of the lateral cord of the brachial plexus. Because the nerve is deep and is protected between the entry site into the coracobrachialis muscle and the elbow, lesions here are uncommon. A predominantly motor neuropathy may develop after strenuous exercise of the upper extremity, probably due to entrapment or stretching of the nerve where it passes through the coracobrachialis muscle in the upper arm. A purely sensory syndrome may result when the lateral cutaneous nerve of the forearm is damaged in the cubital fossa or forearm (Fig. 32-5). This sensory branch may be injured by compression, venipuncture, or cut-down procedures because it lies directly under the median cubital vein in the center of the cubital fossa. Typically, patients notice pain in the proximal forearm (often aggravated by elbow extension) and paresthesia along the radial aspect of the forearm. Lesions result in atrophy of the biceps and brachialis muscles and wasting of the ventral aspect of the upper arm. Loss of coracobrachialis muscle function is difficult to detect clinically. With biceps weakness, flexion of the elbow is weak (especially when the forearm is supine) and the biceps reflex is lost.[46,55]

Median Nerve (C6-T1)

The median nerve is injured in approximately 15 percent of combined skeletal and neural injuries of the arm. It is most commonly injured by dislocation of the elbow or secondarily in the carpal tunnel after injury of the wrist or distal forearm. Injuries often result from lacerations of the forearm or wrist. In the upper arm, the nerve can be injured by relatively superficial lacerations, tight tourniquets and humeral fractures.[1,2]

Immobilization and intravenous fluids may cause sufficient edema to exacerbate a preexisting carpal tunnel syndrome.[57] Lesions in the axilla and upper arm cause paresis or paralysis of all of the muscles innervated by the medial nerve with a sensory loss in the distribution area of both the palmar cutaneous and palmar digital branches (Fig. 32-5). There is atrophy of the thenar eminence, which predominantly affects the abductor pollicis brevis and opponens pollicis muscles. The hand takes on an abnormal appearance called simian hand or ape hand. Anterior interosseous nerve injury may be due to strenuous exercise, trauma, cut-down procedures (for catheterization), or venipuncture in the antecubital fossa. The nerve may also be injured while the patient is in the prone position.

Injury to the deep palmar branches of the median nerve in the distal carpal canal (e.g., by a palmar ganglion) or at the thenar eminence produces a purely motor syndrome with weakness and wasting of the thenar muscles.[46,55] Sensory loss would be over the palm of the hand (Fig. 32-5).

Ulnar Nerve (C7-T1)

The ulnar nerve is injured in about 30 percent of patients with combined skeletal and neural injury of the upper arm. This injury is most commonly associated with fractures around the medial humeral epicondyle, but it may also result from formation of a callus at the elbow.[2] The nerve is most commonly injured in the distal forearm and wrist by gunshot wounds, lacerations, fractures, or dislocations. Ulnar neuropathy is a common complication of malpositioning during anesthesia or postoperatively, especially if continuous nerve blocks are used (Fig. 32-3).

When the ulnar nerve is injured above the elbow, the hypothenar eminence and interossei muscles atrophy and give the hand a "claw hand" appearance. There is also paresis or paralysis of ulnarflexion. Paresthesia and sensory loss occur on the dorsal and palmar surfaces of the fifth and ulnar half of the fourth finger and the ulnar portion of the hand to the wrist (Fig. 32-5).

The ulnar nerve is most commonly compressed at the elbow in the cubital tunnel, because this tunnel narrows during movement, especially as the elbow is flexed. Nerve entrapment is due to thickening of the aponeurotic arch (the humeroulnar aponeurotic arcade) between the two heads of the flexor carpi ulnaris or bulging of the medial collateral ligament of the elbow joint (floor to the cubital tunnel). The nerve may also become entrapped by a ganglion cyst of the elbow, by dense fibrous bands bridged directly between the medial epicondyle and the olecranon proximal to the cubital tunnel proper, by an accessory anconeus epitrochlearis muscle, or at its point of exit from the flexor carpi ulnaris muscle distally by a thickened muscular septum between the flexor carpi ulnaris and the flexor digitorum profundus. The ulnar nerve at the elbow is also subject to external trauma, especially during coma or general anesthesia or when the arm is anesthetized following continuous or single-injection nerve block.[46,55]

Ulnar nerve compression at the wrist or hand is most frequently caused by a ganglion from one of the carpal joints followed by occupational neuritis, laceration, ulnar artery disease, or carpal bone fracture.[46,55,57,59] Sensory loss involves the medial aspect of the hand (Fig. 32-5).

Radial Nerve (C5-C8)

The radial nerve is one of the most commonly injured nerves. Up to 14 percent of humeral shaft fractures are complicated by injury of this nerve. Conversely 33 percent of radial nerve injuries are associated with fractures of the middle third of the humerus, 50 percent with fracture of the distal third of the humerus, 7 percent with supracondylar fractures of the humerus, and 7 percent with dislocation of the radial head at the elbow. Gunshot wounds are the second most common cause of injury to the radial nerve. Other causes include lacerations of the arm and proximal forearm, needle injuries and prolonged local pressure,[1,2] and poorly fitted slings (Fig. 32-2) Lesions of this nerve in the axilla can be due to crutches or from the pitching motion used in competitive softball ("windmill pitcher's" neuropathy). The hands are in flexion (wrist drop); there is wasting of the dorsal aspect of the arm (triceps) and muscle mass on the posterior surface of the forearm. There is paresis or paralysis of extension of the elbow, extension of the wrist, supination of the forearm, extension of all five metacarpophalangeal joints, and extension and abduction of the interphalangeal joint of the thumb. Paresthesia and sensory loss occur on the entire extensor surface of the arm and forearm and on the back of the hand and dorsum of the first four fingers (Fig. 32-5). There is also hyporeflexia or areflexia of the triceps (C6-C8) and radial (C5) reflexes.[46,55]

Lesions at the spiral groove of the humerus are usually due to humeral fractures or compressive lesions.[46,60] The radial nerve may also be entrapped by a musculotendinous arch of the lateral head of the triceps muscle or damaged after repetitive arm exercise when a sudden forceful contraction and stretch of the arm muscles result in a delayed radial nerve palsy of the upper arm.[61,62] Soldiers may develop radial nerve palsies at the lateral border of the humerus after shooting training because of their persistent kneeling position during practice. The windmill pitching motion used in competitive softball may also injure the nerve at the spiral groove.[62] These patients have the same manifestations seen in axillary injuries except that sensation of the extensor aspect of the arm is spared because this nerve usually arises high in the axilla.

Sensation on the extensor aspect of the forearm may or may not be spared (Fig. 32-5), depending on the site of origin of this nerve from the radial nerve proper, and the triceps muscle is spared because the branches which supply this muscle have a more proximal origin.

Lesions at the distal groove and distal to the site of origin of the brachioradialis and extensor carpi radialis longus muscles (before the bifurcation of the nerve) cause symptoms similar to those seen in a spiral groove lesion except that these muscles are spared, and sensation on the extensor surface of the forearm is more likely to be spared. The posterior interosseous nerve (deep motor branch of the radial nerve) may be injured or entrapped at the elbow. Some of the causes include lacerations and gunshot wounds, closed injuries due to fractures of the proximal radius or both radius and ulna, chronic repeated trauma related to stressful supination and pronation, iatrogenic injury due to radial head resection or secondary to tumor removal, and compression from local masses.[46,63] When the posterior interosseous nerve is damaged at these locations, the supinator muscle and the superficial sensory branch of the radial nerve are often spared. These patients have difficulty in extending the metacarpophalangeal joints of all five fingers (drop-finger deformity), extending the wrist in an ulnar direction, and abducting the thumb.[46]

The Lumbosacral Plexus

The lumbosacral plexus is formed by the anterior (ventral) primary rami of the twelfth thoracic through fourth sacral levels (Fig. 29-1). The lumbosacral plexus is injured in less than 3 percent of pelvic fractures, but in 10 to 13 percent of posterior dislocations of the hip.[2] Other causes of lumbosacral plexus injury include retroperitoneal hemorrhage (e.g., due to anticoagulant therapy or hemophilia), psoas compartment abscess (e.g., from tuberculosis or pyogenic osteomyelitis), surgery (especially pelvic procedures), and inadvertent injections by heroin addicts.

LESIONS OF THE LUMBAR SEGMENTS

These lesions are usually incomplete; they are most often due to neoplasms, hemorrhage, or surgical injury. There is paresis and atrophy, predominantly in the motor distribution areas of the femoral and obturator nerves. This causes weakness of thigh flexion (iliopsoas), leg extension (quadriceps), thigh eversion (sartorius), and thigh adduction (adductor muscles). Sensation may be lost in the inguinal region and over the genitalia (innervated by the iliophyogastric, ilioinguinal, and genitofemoral nerves); on the lateral, anterior, and medial thigh (innervated by the lateral femoral cutaneous, femoral, and obturator nerves, respectively); and on the medial aspect of the lower leg (innervated by the saphenous nerve, a branch of the femoral nerve) (Figs. 29-3 and 31-1). The patellar reflex (femoral nerve) and cremasteric reflex (genitofemoral nerve) may be decreased or absent.[46,48]

LESIONS OF THE SACRAL PLEXUS

These lesions are frequently incomplete and are most commonly due to neoplasms or surgical trauma. If the entire sacral plexus is injured, a "flail foot" results owing to paralysis of the dorsiflexor and plantarflexor muscles of the foot. There is weakness of knee flexion (hamstring muscles), foot eversion (peronei nerves), foot inversion (tibialis anterior and posterior nerves), foot plantarflexion (gastrocnemius and soleus muscles), toe dorsiflexion (extensor muscles of toes), and toe plantarflexion (plantar flexor muscles of toes); all these muscles are in the sciatic distribution area. Paresis of abduction and internal rotation of the thigh (superior gluteal nerve palsy) and of hip extension (inferior gluteal nerve palsy) occurs. Sensation may be lost in the distribution areas of the sciatic nerve (Figs. 29-3 and 31-1). The Achilles' reflex (ankle jerk) may be decreased or absent because of sciatic nerve injury. Bladder or bowel control may be affected by injury to the pudendal nerve.[46,48]

Femoral Nerve (L2-L4)

The femoral nerve is often injured by penetrating wounds in the lower abdomen or by surgery. Femoral neuropathies may also result from hematoma formation or contusions associated with fractures.[1,2] Nerve injury has been reported after hip arthroplasty and may be due to various causes, such as trauma, bleeding, stretching, and encasement of the nerve in methylmethacrylate cement.[44] Lesions can also be caused by direct compression of the nerve during surgery (careless use of retractors). Hemorrhage into the iliopsoas muscle and subsequent compression or ischemia of the femoral nerve has also been reported perioperatively.[57]

A proximal lesion of the femoral nerve (at the lumbar plexus or within the pelvis) results in wasting of the musculature of the anterior part of the thigh. There is also weakness of hip flexion and inability to extend the leg at the knee joint (quadriceps femoris). With paralysis of the sartorius muscles, lateral thigh rotation may be impaired. Sensory loss, paresthesia, and occasionally pain affect the anteromedial thigh and inner leg as far as the ankle. The patellar reflex is depressed or absent.

Lesions at the inguinal ligament result in similar findings, but thigh flexion is spared because of the more proximal origin of the femoral nerve branches to the iliacus and psoas muscles. A purely motor syndrome (quadriceps atrophy and paresis) may result from lesions within the femoral triangle that affect the posterior division of the femoral nerve distal to the origin of the saphenous branch.[46] Sensory loss affects the anterior aspect of the thigh (Figs. 29-3 and 31-1).

Obturator Nerve (L2-L4)

Nerve damage may occur after hip surgery due to nerve traction or encasement of the nerve in a spur of methylmethacrylate cement.[64] Lesions of this nerve cause wasting of the muscles of the inner thigh, paresis of adduc-

tion, and a sensory disturbance that affects the medial aspect of the thigh (Figs. 29-3 and 31-1).[46]

Lateral Femoral Cutaneous Nerve (L2-L3)

Lesions of the lateral femoral cutaneous nerve cause paresthesia and insensitivity in its distribution area on the upper half of the lateral aspect of the thigh (meralgia paresthetica) (Figs. 29-3 and 31-1). This has been reported after iliac bone harvesting.[44,46]

Gluteal Nerves (L4-S2)

Lesions of the superior gluteal nerve result in weakness or paralysis of thigh abduction and medial rotation. On walking, the pelvis tilts toward the side of the unaffected raised leg. Isolated complete paralysis of the tensor fascia lata may develop after needle injuries sustained by intramuscular injection.[65] Inferior gluteal nerve injury causes weakness or paralysis of hip extension.

Sciatic Nerve (L4-S3)

Injury may result from gunshot wounds to the thigh or buttock, in fracture-dislocation of the hip, hip joint surgery (due to traction or from a projecting spur of methylmethacrylate), gluteal hemorrhage, or needle injuries from intramuscular injections. Motor fibers are more susceptible to injection injury than sensory fibers, and the peroneal division of the sciatic nerve is more severely injured because of its lateral position. Sciatic nerve lesions tend to affect the peroneal division more than the tibial division in about 75 percent of cases.[46,66,67]

High sciatic nerve lesions cause a flail foot because of the paralysis of foot dorsiflexors and plantarflexors. Muscle wasting affects the hamstrings and all the muscles below the knee. There is also weakness or paralysis of knee flexion (hamstring muscles), foot eversion (peronei muscles), foot inversion (tibialis anterior muscle), foot dorsiflexion (tibialis anterior and anterior leg musculature), foot plantarflexion (gastrocnemius and soleus muscles), toe dorsiflexion (extensor muscles of the toes), and toe plantarflexion (plantar flexor muscles of the toes). The Achilles' tendon reflex (S1-2), which reflects tibial nerve function, is absent or reduced. There are sensory changes (paresthesia and sensory loss) on the outer aspect of the leg and dorsum of the foot (common peroneal nerve distribution) and on the sole and inner aspect of the foot (tibial nerve) (Figs. 29-3 and 31-1). Loss of hair and changes in toenails and skin texture may occur in the leg below the knee.[54]

Tibial Nerve (L4-S3)

The tibial nerve may be injured in fractures of the proximal tibia and injuries of the ankle.[2] Lesions of the tibial nerve in the popliteal fossa result in weakness or paralysis of plantarflexion and inversion of the foot, plantarflexion of the toes, and movements of the intrinsic muscles of the foot. Sensory impairment is located on the sole and lateral border of the foot (Figs. 29-3 and 31-1). Lesions within the tarsal tunnel cause burning paresthesia in the sole of the foot and sensory loss that affects the skin of the sole and medial aspect of the heel. Lesions within the foot result in pain, paresthesia, and sensory loss in the distribution area of the individual nerve (e.g., the medial two-thirds of the sole of the foot in medial plantar nerve lesions).[46]

The Peroneal Nerve and Its Branches (L4-S1)

The common peroneal nerve is most often injured by trauma around the knee. Lesions at the fibular head are primarily traumatic (laceration, traction, or compression, especially by casts or knee splints following continuous sciatic nerve blocks or epidural blocks) (Fig. 32-4). Injuries may be caused by rupture of the fibular collateral ligament, fractures and dislocations of the head of the fibula, and even by crossing the legs.[2,58,69] Postoperative peroneal palsies occur especially after operations performed in the lateral decubitus position or when the outer aspect of the upper leg rests against a leg strap or metal brace.[46]

When both branches (deep and superficial) are affected, there is weakness or paralysis of toe and foot dorsiflexion as well as foot eversion, with a variable sensory disturbance (Figs. 29-3 and 31-1).

The anterior tibial (deep peroneal) nerve may be injured at the fibular head or more distally in the leg. This results in a motor deficit of toe and foot dorsiflexion, whereas sensory deficit is limited to the web of skin located between the first and second toes (Figs. 29-3 and 31-1).

Isolated deep peroneal nerve injury may complicate arthroscopic knee surgery.[69] This nerve may also be compressed at the ankle (anterior tarsal tunnel syndrome). The anterior tarsal tunnel syndrome results from distal deep peroneal compression beneath the inferior extensor retinaculum, which may be caused by ankle fractures, dislocations, sprains, ill-fitting footwear, posttraumatic fibrosis, synovitis, arthritis, or extreme ankle inversion.[70] This condition causes paresis and atrophy of the extensor digitorum brevis muscle alone. Lesions at this location may affect the terminal sensory branch to the skin web between the first and second toes. Isolated weakness or paralysis of the extensor hallucis longus muscle is a common complication of proximal tibial and fibular osteotomy, as the nerve supply to this muscle is at risk because of the proximity of the bone to the nerve's motor branches.[71] Distal peroneal neuropathy may occur due to nerve injury during needle aspiration of the ankle joint and ankle arthroscopy.

The superficial peroneal nerve may be affected in isolation by lesions at the fibular head or by others more distally in the leg. There is paresis and atrophy of the peronei muscles (foot eversion) and a sensory disturbance affecting the skin of the lateral distal portion of the lower leg and dorsum of the foot (Figs. 29-3 and 31-1). Iatrogenic neuropathy of the dorsal medial interosseous branch of the peroneal nerve has been attributed to venography (with needle insertion in the dorsum of the foot) and ankle arthroscopy.[38,72]

The Sural Nerve

Most sural nerve injuries are due to lacerations, trauma associated with fractures, Achilles' tendon reconstructive surgery, ankle arthroscopy, and stretch injuries due to sprains. Sural neuropathy presents with pain or paresthesia over the lateral ankle and border of the foot (Figs. 29-3 and 31-1).[38,73,74]

Prevention

Efforts to prevent perioperative neuropathies are debated, but no good data are available to support conclusions on these issues. However, certain measures and general recommendations have been adopted in an effort to minimize injury.

1. Decisions to perform any regional blockade should be taken judiciously, considering all risks and benefits, especially in patients with existing nerve disease or in anesthetized or heavily sedated patients who cannot complain of pain on needle insertion or injection.
2. Epinephrine should be used with caution, and reinjection of a partially blocked nerve should be done cautiously.
3. Good positioning and padding may help to reduce the risk of nerve injuries intraoperatively. In general, arm abduction should be limited to 90 degrees in supine patients. Arms should be positioned to decrease pressure on the postcondylar groove of the humerus (ulnar groove). When arms are tucked at the side, a neutral forearm position is recommended, whereas for arms abducted on arm boards, either supination or a neutral forearm position is acceptable. Prolonged pressure on the radial nerve in the spiral groove of the humerus, for example by ill-fitting arm slings, should be avoided. Extension of the elbow beyond a comfortable range may stretch the median nerve. Prolonged pressure on the peroneal nerve at the fibular head should be avoided. Of note, neither extension nor flexion of the hip has been proven to increase the risk of femoral neuropathy. Padded arm boards may decrease the risk of upper extremity neuropathy.

The use of axillary rolls in laterally positioned patients may decrease the risk of upper extremity neuropathies. Padding at the elbow and the fibular head may decrease the risk of upper and lower extremity neuropathies, respectively. Postoperatively, patients must be followed closely to detect injuries early and identify potentially treatable causes such as infection, hematoma, or tight dressings and casts.[19,22,57]

REFERENCES

1. Dyck PJ, Thomas PK, Griffin JW, et al. *Peripheral Neuropathy.* Philadelphia: Saunders, 1993.
2. Jobe MT, Martinez SF. Peripheral nerve injuries, in Canale ST (ed): *Campbell's Operative Orthopedics,* 10th ed. Philadelphia: Mosby, 2003.
3. Waxman SG. *Correlative Neuroanatomy.* Stamford, CT: Appleton & Lange, 1999.
4. Cotran R, Kumar V, Collins T. *Robbins Pathologic Basis of Disease.* Philadelphia: Saunders, 1999.
4. Foerster O. *Handbuch der Neurologie,* pt 2. Berlin: Springer, 1929.
5. Cheney FW, Domino KB, Caplan RA, Posner K. Nerve injury associated with anesthesia. A closed claims analysis. *Anesthesiology* 90:1062–1069, 1999.
6. Auroy Y, Narchi P, Messiah A, et al. Serious complications related to regional anesthesia. *Anesthesiology* 87:479–486, 1997.
7. Ben-David B. Complications of peripheral blockade. *Anesth Clin North Am* 20:695–707, 2002.
8. Noble J, Greene HL, Levison W, et al. *Textbook of Primary Care Medicine.* Philadelphia: Mosby, 2000.
9. Moore KA. Partial peripheral nerve injury promotes a selective loss of GABAergic inhibition in the superficial dorsal horn of the spinal cord. *J Neurosci* 22(15):6724–6731, 2002.
10. Zimmermann M. Pathobiology of neuropathic pain. *Eur J Pharmacol* 42:923–937, 2001.
11. Whiteside G, Doyle CA, Hunt SP, et al. Differential time course of neuronal and glial apoptosis in neonatal rat dorsal root ganglia after sciatic nerve axotomy. *Eur J Neurosci* 10:3400–3408, 1998.
12. Li L, Houenou LJ, Wu W, et al. Characterization of spinal motoneuron degeneration following different types of peripheral nerve injury in neonatal and adult mice. *J Comp Neurol* 29(396):158–168, 1998.
13. Jin H, Wu Z, Tian T, et al. Apoptosis in atrophic skeletal muscle induced by brachial plexus injury in rats. *J Trauma* 50:31–35, 2001.
14. Johnson ME, Uhl CB, Spittler KH, et al. Mitochondrial injury and caspase activation by the local anesthetic lidocaine. *Anesthesiology* 101(5):1184–1194, 2004.
15. Zink W, Seif C, Bohl JR, et al. The acute myotoxic effects of bupivacaine and ropivacaine after continuous peripheral nerve blockades. *Anesth Analg* 97:1173–1179, 2003.
16. Kondo, K, Tsubaki, T. Changing mortality pattern in motor neuron disease in Japan. *J Neurol Sci* 32:411, 1997.
17. Seddon HJ. Three types of nerve injury. *Brain* 66:237, 1943.
18. Liguori, G. Complications of regional anesthesia. Nerve injury and peripheral neural blockade. *J Neurosurg Anesthesiol* 16(1):84–86, 2004.
19. Horlocker TT. Neurologic complications of neuraxial and peripheral blockade. *Can J Anesth* 48:6, 2001.
20. Selander D, Dhuner K-G, Lundborg G. Peripheral nerve injury due to injection needles used for regional anaesthesia. *Acta Anaesth Scand* 21:182, 1977.
21. Selander D, Edshage S, Wolff T. Parasthesiae or no parasthesiae? *Acta Anesthesiol Scand* 23:27–33, 1979.
22. Borgeat A, Ekatodramis G. Nerve injury associated with regional anesthesia. *Curr Topics Med Chem* 1:199–203, 2001.
23. Bergman BD, Hebl JR, Kent J, et al. Neurological complications of 405 consecutive continuous axillary catheters. *Anesth Analg* 96:247–252, 2003.
24. Grant SA, Nielsen KC, Greengrass RA, et al. Continuous peripheral nerve block for ambulatory surgery. *Reg Anesth Pain Med* 26:209–214, 2001.
25. Myers RR, Heckman HM. Effects of local anesthesia on nerve blood flow: Studies using lidocaine with and without epinephrine. *Anesthesiology* 71:757–762, 1989.
26. Urmey WF, Stanton J. Inability to consistently elicit a motor response following sensory paresthesias during interscalene block administration. *Anesthesiology* 96:552–554, 2002.
27. Choyce A, Chen V, Middleton W, et al. What is the relationship between paresthesia and nerve stimulation for axillary brachial plexus block? *Reg Anesth Pain Med* 26:100–104, 2001.
28. Rice ASC, McMahon SB. Peripheral nerve injury caused by injection needles used in regional anesthesia: Influence of bevel configuration, studied in a rat model. *Br J Anesth* 69:433–438, 1992.
29. Benumof JL. Permanent loss of cervical spinal cord function associated with interscalene block performed under general anesthesia. *Anesthesiology* 93:1541–1544, 2000.
30. Passannante AN. Spinal anesthesia and permanent neurological deficit after interscalene block. *Anesth Analg* 82:873–874, 1996.
31. Hodgson PS, Neal JM, Pollock JE, Liu SS. The neurotoxicity of drugs given intrathecally (spinal). *Anesth Analg* 88:797–809, 1999.
32. Selander D, Brattsand R, Lundborg G, et al. Local anesthetics: Importance of mode of application, concentration, and adrenaline for the appearance of nerve lesions: An experimental study of axonal degeneration and barrier damage after intrafascicular injection or topical application of bupivacaine (Marcain). *Acta Anaesthesiol Scand* 23:127–136, 1979.
33. Selander D, Mansson LG, Karlsson L, et al. Adrenergic vasoconstriction in peripheral nerves of the rabbit. *Anesthesiology* 62:6–10, 1985.
34. Selander D. Neurotoxicity of local anesthetics: Animal data. *Reg Anesth* 18(suppl):461–468, 1993.
35. Gentili F, Hudson AR, Hunter D, et al. Nerve injection injury with local anesthetic agents: A light and electron microscopic, fluorescent microscopic, and horseradish peroxidase study. *Neurosurgery* 6:263–272, 1980.
36. Horlocker T. Neurologic complications of neuraxial and peripheral blockade. *Can I Anesth* 48:R1–R8, 2001.

37. Benoit PW, Belt WD. Some effects of local anesthetic agents on skeletal muscle. *Exp Neurol* 34:264–278, 1972.

38. Foster AH, Carslon BM. Myotoxicity of local anesthetics and regeneration of the damaged muscle fibers. *Anesth Analg* 59:727–736, 1980.

39. Komorowski TE, Shepard B, Okland S, et al. An electron microscopic study of local anesthetic–induced skeletal muscle fiber degeneration and regeneration in the monkey. *J Orthop Res* 8:4495–4503, 1990.

40. Yagiela JA, Benoit PW, Buoncristiani RD, et al. Comparison of myotoxic effects of lidocaine with epinephrine in rats and humans. *Anesth Analg* 60:471–480, 1981.

41. Selander D, Sjostrang J. Longitudinal spread of intraneurally injected local anesthetics. *Acta Anaesthesiol Scand* 22:622–634, 1978.

42. Kalichman MW, Calcutt NA. Local anesthetic–induced conduction block and nerve fiber injury in streptozotocin-diabetic rats. *Anesthesiology* 77:941–947, 1992.

43. Wedel DJ. Nerve blocks, in Miller RD (ed): *Miller's Anesthesia*, 6th ed. Philadelphia: Churchill Livingstone, 2004.

44. Dawson DM, Krarup C. Perioperative nerve lesions. *Arch Neurol* 46:1355–1360, 1989.

45. Upton ARM, McComas AJ. The double crush in nerve entrapment syndromes. *Lancet* 2:359–361, 1973.

46. Brazis PW, Masdeu JC, Biller J. *Localization in Clinical Neurology*. Philadelphia: Lippincott Williams & Wilkins, 2001.

47. *Aids to the Examination of the Peripheral Nervous System*. Edinburgh: Saunders, 2000.

48. Misulis KE. *Neurologic Localization and Diagnosis*. Boston: Butterworth-Heinemann, 1996.

49. Greenberg D, Aminoff M, Simon R. *Clinical Neurology*. New York: McGraw-Hill, 2002.

50. Misulis KE. *Essentials of Clinical Neurophysiology*. Boston, Butterworth-Heinemann, 1997.

51. Kimura J. *Electrodiagnosis in Diseases of Nerve and Muscle: Principles and Practice*. Philadelphia: Davis, 1989.

52. Victor M, Ropper AH, Adams RD. *Adams and Victor's Principles of Neurology*. New York: McGraw-Hill, 2001.

53. Merritts HH, Rowland LP. *Merritt's Neurology*. Philadelphia: Lippincott Williams & Wilkins, 2000.

54. Hogan Q, Hendrix L, Safwan J. Evaluation of neurologic injury after regional anesthesia, in Finucane BT (ed): *Complications of Regional Anesthesia*. New York: Churchill Livingstone, 1999.

55. Leffert RD. *Brachial Plexus Injuries*. New York: Churchill Livingstone, 1985.

56. Britt BA, Joy N, Mackey MB. Positioning trauma, in Orkin FK, Cooperman LH (eds): *Complications of Anesthesiology*. Philadelphia: Lippincott, 1983.

57. Warner MA. Perioperative neuropathies. *Mayo Clin Proc* 73:567–574, 1998.

58. Wanamaker WM. Firearm recoil palsy. *Arch Neurol* 31:208, 1974.

59. Shea JD, McClain EJ. Ulnar nerve compression syndromes at and below the wrist. *J Bone Joint Surg* 51:1095, 1969.

60. Brown WF, Watson BV. Acute retrohumeral radial neuropathies. *Muscle Nerve* 16:706, 1993.

61. Nakamichi K, Tachibana S. Radial nerve entrapment by the lateral head of the triceps. *J Hand Surg* 16:748, 1991.

62. Sinson G, Zager EL, Kline DG. Windmill pitcher's radial neuropathy. *Neurosurgery* 34:1087, 1994.

63. Wu KT, Jordan RR, Eckert C. Lipoma, a cause of paralysis of deep radial (posterior interosseous) nerve: Report of a case and review of the literature. *Surgery* 75:790, 1974.

64. Melamed NB, Satya-Murti S. Obturator neuropathy after total hip replacement. *Ann Neurol* 13:578, 1983.

65. Muller-Vahl H. Isolated complete paralysis of the tensor fascia lata muscle. *Eur Neurol* 24:289, 1985.

66. Bonney G. Iatrogenic injuries of nerves. *J Bone Joint Surg Br* 68:9, 1986.

67. Yuen EC, Olney RK, So YT. Sciatic neuropathy: Clinical and prognostic features in 73 patients. *Neurology* 44:1669, 1994.

68. Katirji MB, Wilbourn AJ. Common peroneal mononeuropathy. A clinical and electrophysiologic study of 116 lesions. *Neurology* 38:1723, 1988.

69. Esselman PC, Tomski MA, Robinson LR, et al. Selective deep peroneal nerve injury associated with arthroscopic knee surgery. *Muscle Nerve* 16:1188–1192, 1993.

70. Wibourn AJ. The anterior tarsal tunnel syndrome revisited. *Muscle Nerve* 15:1175, 1992.

71. Kirgis A, Albrecht S. Palsy of the deep peroneal nerve after proximal tibial osteotomy. *J Bone Joint Surg* 74A:1180, 1992.

72. Preston D, Logigian E. Iatrogenic needle–induced peroneal neuropathy in the foot. *Ann Intern Med* 109:921, 1988.

73. Reisin R, Pardal A, Ruggieri V, et al. Sural neuropathy due to external pressure: Report of three cases. *Neurology* 44:2408–2409, 1994.

74. Gross JA, Hamilton WJ, Swift TR. Isolated mechanical lesions of the sural nerve. *Muscle Nerve* 3:248, 1980.

CHAPTER 33

Bone Cement

STEVEN C. BORENE

▶ INTRODUCTION

When total hip arthroplasty was initially introduced into practice, it had the highest mortality rate of any noncardiac surgery. A considerable portion of the risk associated with this surgery has been attributed to methylmethacrylate (MMA) cement. Although the use of MMA for medical procedures—such as prosthetic middle ear ossicles, encapsulation of cerebral aneurysms, and prosthetic testicles—is long-standing, the large volume of MMA used and the fact that the curing process occurs primarily in vivo made hip arthroplasty a unique setting for this product. As surgeons and anesthesiologists gained experience with this method and learned how to anticipate the difficulties associated with it, the mortality rate of hip arthroplasty improved greatly.

Additionally, improved prosthetic joints make MMA necessary only in those patients in whom it is expected that the interface between the patient (bone) and the prosthesis will not tolerate the external stresses placed on them—for example, patients older than 70 years. However, even with its less frequent use, the implications of MMA use in patients demand that anesthesiologists have a full and complete understanding of its physiologic ramifications.

Another important aspect of bone cementing that requires attention is the setting in which cementing is done. Vertebroplasty and other uses of MMA not related to arthroplasty exhibit some of the physiologic challenges of MMA use. However, in looking at the effects of bone cement in the most significant orthopaedic uses, the effects of long bone reaming and prosthesis insertion cannot be overlooked. The rest of this chapter is therefore primarily devoted to the role of MMA in hip arthroplasty procedures in conjunction with the placement of prosthetic devices.

▶ CHEMICAL COMPOUND

MMA (more correctly polymethylmethacrylate), is a vinyl polymer formed by free-radical polymerization from the monomer MMA. This polymer is a strong, lightweight material, commonly seen as Plexiglas at hockey games or as large windows at aquariums. It is also utilized in acrylic latex paints and as a viscosity-reducing agent in oils and fluids. The strength and lightness of MMA and its ability to be shaped and molded also make it an ideal space-occupying, load-transferring material for distributing the forces of the various prosthetic components used in arthroplasty procedures.

methylmethacrylate   polymethylmethacrylate

MMA has been used in hip joint surgery for more than 40 years. It is not a glue, as is often thought, since it has no adhesive properties. Instead, it is bonded mechanically, not chemically, to cancellous bone through curing while in close contact with the bone. Although the use of MMA as a grout-like material for the replacement of joints, and more recently in vertebroplasty procedures, has increased the durability of these repairs, the use of this product has anesthetic implications. These implications are most evident in hip arthroplasty procedures, particularly because of the large amount of cement used in these cases.

The cement is supplied as two components, one a liquid and one a powder. The liquid contains MMA monomer with an accelerator (dimethylparatoluidine) included. The liquid also contains a retardant to prevent monomer polymerization during storage. The powdered polymer contains poly-MMA particles, a radiopaque component (barium sulfate or zirconium dioxide), and benzoyl peroxide to initiate the reaction. When mixed, the dimethylparatoluidine is activated by the benzyl peroxide in the powder. Dimethylparatoluidine is an aromatic tertiary amine that causes the benzyl peroxide to decompose rapidly, produces large amounts of free radicals, and catalyses the formation of the polymer. The curing process therefore occurs once all the products are mixed. Other additives may also be incorporated into the cement, including heat-stable antibiotics (gentamicin, tobramycin, erythromycin, vancomycin, or cephalosporin) or colorants, such as methylene blue or chlorophyll, to allow differentiation from bone during revision procedures. The powder and liquid components are mixed just before implantation, causing the liquid monomer to polymerize and form the final cement. To reduce the porosity of the cement, it is often mixed with a 500-mmHg vacuum or with the assistance of a centrifuge. Reducing the porosity improves the fatigue properties of the cement.

The exothermic polymerization reaction, known as curing, occurs over several minutes and is divided into time periods. The "dough" time begins at mixing of the liquid and powder and typically continues for 2 to 3 min, until the cement will no longer stick to unpowdered surgical gloves. The "working" time immediately follows dough time and continues for about 5 to 8 min, until the cement is too stiff to manipulate. These two times together make up the "setting" time of the cement. A decrease in room temperature increases the setting time by about 5 percent per degree centigrade. It is during the setting time that the cement is placed into close proximity to the patient's cancellous bone. Since the cement finishes curing in vivo in arthroplasty procedures, a unique physiologic response is attributed to it.

► PHYSIOLOGIC AND PHARMACOLOGIC EFFECTS OF METHYLMETHACRYLATE

The myriad of physiologic changes that are often attributed to MMA include both immediate and long-term effects. These effects include hypotension, pulmonary embolus, hemorrhage, hematoma, variations in cardiac conduction, myocardial infarction, cerebrovascular accident, deep and superficial wound infections, and thrombophlebitis in the period surrounding the placement of the bone cement. After placement of the bone cement, trochanteric separation, loosening or displacement of the prosthesis, heterotopic new bone formation, and trochanteric bursitis have been reported.

Of primary concern to the anesthesiologist are the immediate effects after the introduction of MMA into the body. The physiologic changes seen after implantation are variable in magnitude but qualitatively fairly consistent. These changes principally involve the cardiovascular and pulmonary systems, either directly or indirectly.

The main pharmacologic effect of the MMA monomer is as a direct vasodilator. This effect is typically seen in the first minute after application and can continue for as long as 10 min afterward. The amount of change in blood pressure is directly proportional to the patient's existing blood pressure, age, and blood loss. Conversely, euvolemic patients and those under epidural or spinal anesthesia exhibit less of a decrease in blood pressure, especially if blood pressure is not increased at the time of MMA insertion.

Another effect of the placement of cemented prostheses is a decrease of the patient's PaO_2. This is seen at its greatest magnitude in hip arthroplasty procedures with the insertion of the femoral prosthesis. It is thought that the drop in arterial oxygenation is primarily due to pulmonary embolism of MMA as well as fat, clots, air, and bone fragments. This drop can occur within the first minute after insertion of the prosthesis and continue for several minutes afterward. A decrease of 20 to 80 mmHg is typically seen. As expected, the decreasing arterial oxygenation causes an increase in pulmonary artery pressures.

Also seen with insertion of the prosthesis is a decrease in the total compliance of the lungs. This may occur as a result of airway constriction. Because of decreased compliance, end-inspiratory pressures increase. The increase in pulmonary end-inspiratory pressure may cause the increase in anatomic and alveolar dead space that is seen with prosthesis insertion.

In addition, it is important to recognize that when the net effects of MMA cement and emboli are combined, namely hypotension and pulmonary hypertension, reversal of the normal left-to-right atrial pressure gradient can occur. When this occurs in the presence of circulating emboli, especially if positive-pressure ventilation is being used, the patient is at risk for paradoxical embolic events.

Another interesting result of the use of MMA is the presence of specific tissue inflammatory mediators, particularly prostaglandin E2, interleukin-1, and tumor necrosis factor, which are seen at the cement-bone interface. In fact, a macrophage–giant cell reaction that is similar to a type IV hypersensitivity reaction is often found at the interface. The most common sequelae of this reaction appear to be early loosening of the prosthetic components (aseptic loosening). Of interest to the anesthesiologist, patients with this complication of arthroplasty may actually be manifesting a sign of allergy to the bone cement. There have been reports of allergic dermatitis to bone cement, particularly to the accelerant dimethylparatoluidine, in orthopaedic surgeons, dentists, and other operating-room personnel who have come into contact with the substance.

Other important issues to be aware of concern local tissue effects of the cement. Because of the heat produced by the exothermic polymerization reaction, local coagulation products may be ineffective.

▶ CEMENT IMPLANTATION SYNDROME

The most serious effect of the placement of MMA bone cement is the phenomenon known as cement implantation syndrome. This syndrome is a triad of systemic hypotension, pulmonary hypertension, and hypoxia at the time when a joint prosthesis is inserted. There have been many explanations for the syndrome, but it appears that a combination of MMA effects on vascular structures and pulmonary microembolism of fat and thromboplastic products or air are the culprits. It is essential that the anesthesiologist should understand this syndrome, since a vast number of case reports provide evidence of serious adverse events, including death, in patients with this syndrome.

As indicated, cement implantation syndrome is multifactorial, MMA being one of the main components. This cement is unusual among implanted materials in that it is created by a reaction in the operating room and in the patient. The significance of this reaction lies predominantly in the release of free, unpolymerized MMA monomer. This monomer is volatile, as people present in an operating room during its use well know. It can therefore easily be absorbed into the circulation, where it is either metabolized or excreted directly through the lungs. Intravascular MMA acts as a direct vasodilator, which partially explains the hypotensive episodes commonly seen between 1 and 10 min after its use.

During hip arthroplasty, MMA can enter the circulation and cause its potentially deleterious effects in two different ways. Just before the placement of the femoral prosthesis, the freshly reamed femoral shaft is filled with incompletely cured MMA. At this point, the volatile substance (monomer) can be absorbed directly into the circulation. Second, when the prosthesis is actually placed into the femoral canal, the bone cement, as well as air and fat, can be forced into the venous sinuses of the femur and thus cause venous emboli. Evidence supports the theory that the most important pathogenic factor for the development of embolism during arthroplasty is an increase in intramedullary pressure due to mechanical compression of the femoral canal

during insertion of a prosthesis. The heat generated by the implanted material during polymerization further increases the air pressure in the shaft, and air can then readily enter the bloodstream. Since the surgical approach determines much of the embolic risk of the procedure, it is of paramount importance that the anesthesiologist be involved in, or at least aware of, the chosen surgical plan. Surgical precautions are necessary to avoid or minimize cement implantation syndrome. The avoidance of excessive cement pressurization by venting of the shaft, utilization of a low-viscosity cement, meticulous high-pressure canal lavage, and the use of a venting hole are effective techniques to minimize intramedullary canal pressures and thus decrease emboli.

Despite all possible precautions, most practitioners caring for arthroplasty patients will undoubtedly observe the physiologic and pharmacologic effects of the implantation of bone cement. These effects vary in magnitude but are qualitatively consistent.

Pulmonary fat embolism has been strongly implicated as a main cause for the physiologic effects, and echocardiography studies have clearly shown emboli containing fat to be present during arthroplasty procedures. There are two theories to explain how fat emboli are formed. The first suggests that fat deposits in tissue and bone marrow are released into the circulation as a result of trauma. Supporting this theory is the finding that the medullary contents of the long bones embolize to the pulmonary circulation if intramedullary pressures are elevated. The second theory proposes that these emboli form as a result of changes in the physical state of lipids in the blood. The fact that pulmonary fat emboli are seen in nontraumatic inflammatory conditions, such as osteomyelitis, supports this theory. The issue may be more complicated, since there is no reason why the processes espoused by the two theories could not both play a role.

The treatment and prevention of hypotension and hypoxemia associated with the insertion of prostheses center around adequate hydration and oxygenation of all patients prior to the implantation procedure. These measures often reduce the severity of the above effects or reduce them to the level of clinical insignificance.

Treatment of Cement Implantation Syndrome

Anesthetic management of cement implantation syndrome necessitates supporting the cardiovascular system and treating a state of acute right heart failure. The first step includes administration of 100% inspired oxygen and aggressive volume support. Invasive hemodynamic monitoring should be instituted early, in view of the potential for severe pulmonary hypertension, impaired cardiac output, and to guide inotropic support. Early placement of a pulmonary artery catheter may be needed in order to utilize selective pulmonary vasodilators and assess the effects of high levels of positive end-expiratory pressure in extreme circumstances.

▶ CEMENTED VERSUS NONCEMENTED HIP ARTHROPLASTY

Background

In the past several years, improvements in prosthetic devices and surgical techniques have made hip arthroplasty a more durable and successful therapy (see Chap. 10). Another benefit of some of these advances is that not all hip arthroplasties require cementing. In fact, there is increasing evidence that, in selected patients, arthroplasty procedures may be performed without bone cement. Because of the close interaction between surgical technique and anesthetic management of the patient undergoing hip arthroplasty, it is important that the orthopaedic anesthesiologist should understand the issues involved in the surgical approach and advocate, in consultation with the surgeon, the best technique for a particular patient. The anesthesiologist must inform the surgeon of any specific concerns he or she has in regard to the use of bone cement and its physiologic effects. Likewise, only through an understanding of the concerns of the surgeon can the anesthesiologist best serve the patient's needs. To this end, we present some information on the immediate physiologic effects of arthroplasty procedures that utilize cement versus those that do not. This information does not weigh the advantages or disadvantages of bone cement on the long-term success of the procedure. That is the purview of the orthopaedic surgeon. It merely provides some information that must be considered in determining what the safest approach for a particular patient may be.

Parvizi and colleagues reported, in data obtained from a total joint registry, that sudden death occurred in 23 of 14,469 (0.16 percent) of patients undergoing primary total hip arthroplasties in which the femoral component was inserted with cement, but no deaths were reported during 15,411 primary hip arthroplasties performed without cement. Laupacis and colleagues compared the effects of cemented and noncemented arthroplasty on deep venous thrombosis and showed no difference between the two in the frequency of this effect. Pitto and colleagues demonstrated a lower risk of embolism with noncemented hip arthroplasty as well as procedures performed with a bone vacuuming technique when compared to a conventional cementing technique. Orsini et al. showed that the number of fat emboli and the severity of cardiorespiratory changes observed during total hip arthroplasty with cement were greater than those seen when cement was not used. Christie and colleagues showed that insertion of the femoral prosthesis with cement caused more severe and more prolonged embolic cascades than did insertion without cement. Ries et al. reported a 28 percent increase of intrapulmonary shunt when the femoral prosthesis was inserted with cement and no increase when it was placed without cement.

With an understanding of the physiologic and pharmacologic effects of MMA bone cement as well as the ability to anticipate those effects and knowledge of how to treat and avoid adverse outcomes, the orthopaedic anesthesiologist can better serve his or her patients as well as our orthopaedic colleagues.

SUGGESTED FURTHER READING

Brown DL, Parmley CL. Methylmethacrylate and atrioventricular conduction in dogs. *Acta Anaesth Scand* 28:77–80, 1984.

Byrick RJ. Cement implantation syndrome: A time limited embolic phenomenon. *Can J Anaesth* 44:107–111, 1997.

Charmley J. *Acrylic Cement in Orthopedic Surgery*. Edinburgh and London: Livingstone, 1970.

Duncan JAT. Intra-operative collapse or death related to the use of acrylic cement in hip surgery. *Anesthesia* 44:149–153, 1989.

Eskola A, Santavirta S, Konttinen YT, et al. Cementless revision of aggressive granulomatous lesions in hip replacements. *J Bone Joint Surg* 72B:212–216, 1990.

Fallon KM, Fuller JG, Morley-Forster P. Fat embolism and fatal cardiac arrest during hip arthroplasty with methylmethacrylate. *Can J Anaesth* 48:626–629, 2001.

Fries IB, Fisher AA, Salvati EA. Contact dermatitis in surgeons from methylmethacrylate bone cement. *J Bone Joint Surg* 57A:547–549, 1975.

Gresham GA, Kuczynski A, Rosborough D. Fatal fat embolism following replacement arthroplasty for transcervical fractures of femur. *Br Med J* Jun 12;2(762):617–619, 1971.

Haddad FS, Cobb AG, Bentley G, et al. Hypersensitivity in aseptic loosening of total hip replacements. *J Bone Joint Surg* 78B:546–549, 1996.

Horowitz SM, Doty SB, Lane JM, et al. Studies of the mechanism by which the mechanical failure of polymethylmethacrylate leads to bone resorption. *J Bone Joint Surg* 75A:802–813, 1993.

Hulman G. The pathogenesis of fat embolism. *J Pathol* 176:3–9, 1995.

Kallos T, Enis JE, Gollan F, et al. Intramedullary pressure and pulmonary embolism of femoral medullary contents in dogs during insertion of bone cement and a prosthesis. *J Bone Joint Surg* 56A:1363–1367, 1974.

Karlsson J, Wendling W, Chen D, et al. Methylmethacrylate monomer produces direct relaxation of vascular smooth muscle in vitro. *Acta Anaesth Scand* 39:685–689, 1995.

Kerstell J. Pathogenesis of post-traumatic fat embolism. *Am J Surg* 121:712–715, 1971.

Laupacis A, Rorabeck C, Bourne R, et al. The frequency of venous thrombosis in cemented and non-cemented hip arthroplasty. *J Bone Joint Surg* 78B:210–212, 1996.

Learned DW, Hantler CB. Lethal progression of heart block after prosthesis cementing with methylmethacrylate. *Anesthesiology* 77:1044–1046, 1992.

Logan SW. Death associated with disseminated intravascular coagulation after hip replacement. *Br J Anaesth* 80:853–855, 1998.

McBrien ME, Breslin DS, Atkinson S, et al. Use of methoxamine in the resuscitation of epinephrine-resistant electromechanical dissociation. *Anaesthesia* 56:1085–1089, 2001.

Mebius C, Hedenstierna G. Gas exchange and respiratory mechanics during hip arthroplasty. *Acta Anaesth Scand* 26:15–21, 1982.

Modig J, Busch S, Olerud S, et al. Arterial hypotension and hypoxemia during total hip replacement: The importance of thromboplastic products, fat embolism and acrylic monomers. *Acta Anaesth Scand* 19:28–43, 1975.

Orsini EC, Byrick RJ Mullen BM, et al. Cardiopulmonary function and pulmonary microemboli during arthroplasty using cemented or non-cemented components. The role of intramedullary pressure. *J Bone Joint Surg* 69A:822–832, 1987.

Parvizi J, Holiday AD, Ereth MH, et al. Sudden death during primary hip arthroplasty. Read at the 27th Open Scientific Meeting and the 5th Combined Open Meeting of the Hip Society and AAHKS, Anaheim, CA, February 7, 1999.

Pitto RP, Koessler M, Kuehle JW, et al. Comparison of fixation of the femoral component without cement and fixation with use of a bone-vacuum cementing technique for the prevention of fat embolism during total hip arthroplasty. *J Bone Joint Surg* 81A:831–843, 1999.

Wenda K, Degrief J, Runkel M, et al. Pathogenesis and prophylaxis of circulatory reactions during total hip replacement. *Arch Orthop Trauma Surg* 112:260–265, 1993.

Woo R, Minster GJ, Fitzgerald RH Jr, et al. Pulmonary fat embolism in revision hip arthroplasty. *Clin Orthop* 319:41–53, 1995.

Wozasek GE, Simon P, Redl H, et al. Intramedullary pressure changes and fat intravasation during intramedullary nailing: An experimental study in sheep. *Trauma* 36:202–207, 1994.

CHAPTER 34

Battlefield Orthopaedic Anesthesia

CHESTER C. BUCKENMAIER III

"What an infinite blessing."
Thomas "Stonewall" Jackson

Confederate surgeon Dr. Hunter Holmes McGuire anesthetized Lieutenant General Thomas J. "Stonewall" Jackson with chloroform prior to amputating his severely wounded left arm. Just before losing consciousness, General Jackson is quoted as having said, "What an infinite blessing." The "infinite blessing" of effective battlefield anesthesia is a vital component in the treatment of modern battlefield injury. In this chapter, the unique challenges of providing effective anesthesia and analgesia in orthopaedic surgery on the modern battlefield is discussed. The advantages and disadvantages of various anesthetic choices and the future of battlefield anesthesiology is also explored.

Military anesthesiology has both similarities to and vast differences from civilian anesthesiology as practiced in the modern industrialized world. Although the basic anesthetic principles for orthopaedic surgery are similar, whether it is practiced in a hospital building or in a combat support hospital tent, the factors that determine decisions regarding anesthesia can be very different on the battlefield. Patient and anesthesiologist preferences, procedure-specific issues, and costs are factors that affect such choices in civilian orthopaedic surgery. Civilian anesthesiologists also have the luxury of employing tremendous technological and medical resources on behalf of relatively few injured orthopaedic patients (following an automobile accident, for example), with little concern for the depletion of resources. In contrast, military anesthesiologists often face overwhelming numbers of casualties and are forced to make decisions with little technological support and limited resources rather than on the basis of medical preference. Essentially, the

military anesthesiologist must learn the art and science of providing effective anesthesia and analgesia under conditions that would be considered unacceptable and even dangerous in modern civilian practice.

The management of battlefield orthopaedic injuries and anesthesia has evolved, along with advancements in military weapons and tactics. Orthopaedic injuries during the Revolutionary War were frequently caused by pistol shots or musket balls. Management of these wounds was plagued by infection, and surgeons of the time spoke of "laudable" pus draining from wounds as a positive sign. Anesthesia was inconsistent at best, relying on "anesthetic" medications such as opium, wine, grog (rum), or vinegar when available. Frequent bloodletting, dietary restriction, and laxatives were acceptable treatments for war wounds and pain. Anesthesiology would not become established as a medical specialty for almost another century. Pain relief on the battlefield depended on the speed and dexterity with which surgeons of the time could operate. John Ranby, a physician describing the care of battlefield injuries in 1776, states "to act in all respects as if your are entirely unaffected by their groans and complaints, but at the same time behave with such caution as not to proceed rashly or cruelly, and be particularly careful to avoid unnecessary pain."[1] Concepts of pus drainage from wounds, fasciotomy for compartment syndrome, and early amputation to preserve life would improve the care of soldiers in the War of 1812 and the Indian Wars. Following William Morton's successful demonstration of anesthesia with ether in 1846, the first battlefield anesthetic was administered for bilateral amputation of the legs during the Mexican War in 1847. Many military physicians remained skeptical of the new discovery, and anesthesia and analgesia for soldiers remained rudimentary. The lack of adequate treatment for pain impeded further surgical development, since operations were reserved for only the direst of circumstances.

The introduction of anesthesia to American surgery in the late 1840s had a profound impact on Civil War surgery, where it was widely used to relieve operative pain and create conditions for more meticulous operations. Anesthesia was usually achieved with inhaled chloroform, ether, or a combination of the two.[2] Orthopaedic surgery for open fractures and severe soft tissue injury (common injuries with the introduction of high-velocity, conical bullets) was primarily amputation. Mortality from infection following wounding and surgery continued to claim many victims. The practice of bloodletting, diet restriction, and laxatives had mercifully been discarded by this time and good nutrition was recommended.

Orthopaedic care of war-wounded soldiers continued to develop through both World Wars and the Korean War as x-ray technology became available and aseptic surgery became common practice. The introduction of antibiotics and vascular surgery greatly enhanced the surgical management of orthopaedic injuries. These advances contributed much to reduce mortality following amputation (from 35 percent during the Civil War to 4 percent during the Vietnam War). Infection following amputation was also dramatically reduced, from approximately 75 percent of patients during World War I to almost zero in the Vietnam War.[3] Advances in civilian anesthesia equipment and drugs paralleled, and likely complemented, surgical advances during this period. American military anesthesia progressed more slowly, since equipment was scarce. Trained anesthesia personnel were rare in an American military system that lacked specialized physicians and nurses in anesthesia (and many other specialties) through World War II. The generally poor state of military anesthesia continued through the Korean War, but the lessons learned in this conflict and World War II caused the army to recognize the importance of anesthesia in military medicine, and a 3-year residency program in anesthesiology was finally instituted in 1954.[4] As graduate medical education programs in anesthesiology allowed the specialty to become independent from departments of surgery, the study of battlefield anesthesiology was improved and the problems with anesthesia in previous conflicts could be addressed.

When the Vietnam War started, military anesthesiologists and nurse anesthetists were vital components of the military medical team. It was during this conflict that the role of anesthesia on the battlefield began to expand beyond simply providing optimal operating conditions and surgical pain relief. Anesthesia personnel were now responsible for the resuscitation of the wounded individual and for correcting all abnormal physiologic and pharmacologic responses of the patient to surgery. Regional anesthesia (RA), as a supplement or alternative to general anesthesia (GA), was used extensively during the Vietnam War for the first time. Anesthesiologists appreciated the utility of RA in blocking extremities in stable patients for frequent debridement. Since RA could be performed in hospital holding areas, the debridement could be done with minimal surgical equipment outside the operating room and thus saved resources.[4]

The post-Vietnam evolution of orthopaedics and anesthesia on the battlefield has been typified by increasing capabilities pushed further forward toward the battle. This trend is partly due to the fact that rapid evacuation from the battlefield and early resuscitation have greatly improved the survival of wounded soldiers. Additionally, the increased demand for military medical participation in missions other then war has greatly influenced the capabilities of deployable medical units. The experience of the 212th Mobile Army Surgical Hospital (MASH) that was deployed from November 1992 until April 1993 to Zagreb, Croatia, to support the United Nations Protection Force is an example. In time of war and based on wartime doctrine, the 212th MASH would normally only hold patients for 72 h before their evacuation to the next level of care. In Zagreb, the holding period was extended to 30 days because of the multinational nature of the force being supported and the long distances involved in medical evacuation. This allowed for extensive orthopaedic surgery (internal fixation, open wound coverage, large joint arthroscopy) to be performed, but only with a significant expansion in the equipment inventory and size of the hospital (a physical therapy section was added).[5] This expansion came at a substantial cost to the unit's mobility and ease of logistical support.

Today, military medical units are being increasingly required to redefine themselves in response to the particular deployment situation in which they are engaged. American military medical planners can consistently depend on the inconsistency of world medical missions. As the lethality of modern weapons increases, so will the demand for more advanced orthopaedic care on the battlefield. More innovative and flexible anesthesia care will be required to support advanced orthopaedic procedures anytime, anywhere adequately. The complexities of the world after September, 11, 2001, will demand more from the modern military anesthesiologist.

The Battlefield in Your Backyard: Orthopaedic Anesthesia in the Age of Terrorism

Historically, with the notable exceptions of the Revolutionary War and the Civil War, American military medicine has been practiced by physicians and nurses who follow armies into battle in other countries around the globe. Although many civilian populations have experienced the terror and destruction of modern war, the American continent has been largely spared. Apart from academic interest, American civilian health care providers have therefore had little need to be versed in the complexities of military medicine. The disaster of September 11, 2001, and the War on Terror have, however, changed the American medical landscape for the foreseeable future. Unlike previous wars, where civilian casualties were an unwanted result of military action (collateral damage), in the present age of terrorism, civilians are the primary target and means to effect change in political structures. In his book *The Transformation of War*, Martin van Creveld[6] describes modern conflict as a series of highly violent, low-intensity (more traditional weapons) conflicts where distinctions between "civilian" and "soldier" break down. Future war will be information-based, designed to influence public opinion in the target state by using all available networks (print media, radio, television, Internet) to carry its message. This new type of war, or "netwar," as it has been termed, seems very plausible, with the daily bombardment of terror images inflicted on civilian populations and received by Americans through various news media.[7] Although these images are horrific, they strengthen the terrorists' agenda and recruitment activities. With netwar, targets are often civilian, and campaigns are designed to have the greatest impact on public opinion. The battlefield for netwar can, in fact, be in the civilian anesthesiologist's community. The characteristics of caring for battlefield wounded and orthopaedic injury, outlined in this chapter, are now important for all anesthesiologists.

Modern War Injury

An understanding of modern weapons and their effects on the human body is prerequisite to any discussion of anesthesia for battlefield orthopaedic injury. Apart from help in planning proper anesthesia, knowledge of weapons is important for the sake of safety, since live munitions may sometimes accompany the evacuated casualty.

Small arms, explosives/fragmentary devices, and incendiary munitions are the three major conventional weapons responsible for war wounds. Small arms are further classified into low-velocity (less than 2000 ft/s) and high-velocity weapons (greater than 2000 ft/s). The damage any projectile causes is related to its kinetic energy at impact (kinetic energy = 0.5 (mass) × velocity).[2] Military small arms doctrine favors low-mass, high-velocity weapons (the M-16 and AK-47 assault rifles are examples), which generally cause more tissue damage. The volume of devitalized tissue is significantly greater with high-velocity projectiles. The projectile velocity estimated to fracture bone is only 200 ft/s, which can significantly complicate high-velocity wounds when bone is struck by the projectile.[8] Modern assault rifles can cause orthopaedic injury requiring extensive bone stabilization, tissue debridement, and infection prophylaxis (Fig. 34-1).

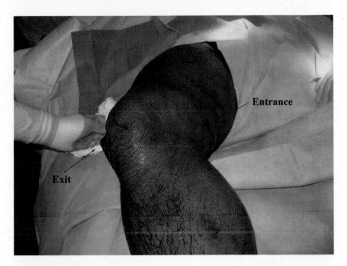

Figure 34-1. High-velocity gunshot injury to the knee.

Explosive/fragmentary weapons produce wounding by three mechanisms.[9] Primary blast injury is caused by the explosive pressure wave (shock wave) as it moves through air or water. Casualties with primary blast injuries are relatively rare, since these injuries are often lethal. In caring for a blast victim, the anesthesiologist should remain vigilant for signs of pulmonary and visceral injury from the blast, since external evidence of this injury is often lacking. Pulmonary contusion and pneumothorax caused by a blast is termed *blast lung* and is one example of the internal injuries that can develop from blast exposure. Secondary blast injury is caused by fragments of material propelled into the victim's body by the blast. This is the blast injury that most frequently requires orthopaedic intervention, as fragments damage soft tissue and bone. Home-made explosive devices or the unconventional use of conventional weapons (the roadside artillery shell remotely detonated) are termed *improvised explosive devices* (IED) and are a source of significant orthopaedic injury in Operation Iraqi Freedom. Fragments from exploding artillery shells can reach velocities up to 10,000 ft/s, resulting in massive soft tissue and bone injuries.[8] Tertiary blast injury results from the victim being thrown on other structures by the blast. This can also result in significant orthopaedic injury.

Incendiary munitions are designed to ignite a target, driving the enemy from a fortified or hidden position. Burn injuries can also result from explosive weapons as a secondary injury, particularly when vehicles are attacked with armor-defeating munitions. Although standard burn care applies to all these wounds, burn injury can greatly complicate orthopaedic injuries.

Injury Survival

As warfare has changed from the pitched battles of history involving large armies to the global ambush tactics of netwar waged on soldier and civilian alike, the types of casualties seen by the military anesthesiologist have changed. Munitions have become increasingly lethal. Paradoxically, this results in a preponderance of casualties with superficial soft tissue and/or extremity wounds, because wounds from these munitions to the head, thorax, or abdomen tend to be fatal.[10] During the Vietnam War, three-fourths of the surviving wounded soldiers had soft tissue wounds and extremity fractures during an 18-month period from 1967 to 1969.[11] Modern helmets and body armor, while reducing penetrating wounds to the head and thorax, have not reduced extremity injuries.[12] The preponderance of orthopaedic injury in modern war is indicated by figures from the current conflicts in Afghanistan[13] and Iraq. Data from the Army Office of the Surgeon General on the 651 soldiers wounded in action (WIA) from May 1 until December 31, 2003, revealed that 42 percent were orthopaedic cases (the next closest category was general surgery cases, at 29 percent). Of the 2549 non-battle-related injuries during that same time period, 70 percent were orthopaedic injuries! Clearly, anesthesia in support of orthopaedic surgeons will be the most common activity for battlefield anesthesiologists.

Nuclear, Biological, and Chemical Warfare

The threat of unconventional nuclear, biological, or chemical (NBC) war cannot be ignored in the modern era. Military anesthesiologists are usually focused on the physical trauma produced by projectiles and blasts in conventional warfare. The introduction of NBC war will produce casualties that complicate the anesthesiologist's management, since injury from these weapons may be ongoing and not readily apparent. Recent experiences with NBC terrorism (Halabja, Iraq gas attack in 1988, Tokyo subway sarin gas attack 1995, and anthrax mail attacks of 2001 are examples) suggest that NBC warfare is certainly not limited to the battlefield. All anesthesiologists should be familiar with these weapons and the clinical effects they produce. The ongoing threat of NBC war or NBC terrorism will likely continue. Medical providers should become thoroughly educated in the use of available NBC personal protective equipment, and opportunities to practice with this equipment should be aggressively sought. Although the management of NBC casualties is beyond the scope of this chapter, many excellent resources are available on the Internet, such as e-Medicine (*www.emedicinehealth.com/collections/CO1542.asp*) or the National Library of Medicine (*www.nlm.nih.gov*).

Environmental Issues

The tremendous infrastructure support and technology that assist anesthesiologists caring for civilian trauma patients in the industrialized world is hardly noticed and certainly underappreciated. Furthermore, the benefits of modern civilization begin to aid the patient from the moment of injury. Communications technology is ubiquitous and reliable in calling for help. Modern road infrastructure and medical air evacuation place most Americans within minutes of a major trauma hospital. In the hospital, the anesthesiologist is surrounded by all kinds of technology and utilities that assist in caring for the patient. Additionally, the anesthesiologist in this scenario is rarely confronted with large numbers of casualties at once and resources are seemingly limitless.

In contrast, the military anesthesiologist (or civilian anesthesiologist following a terrorist act) will often find the benefits of modern society lacking or nonexistent in the practice environment. Military anesthesiologists must learn to provide quality anesthesia in places where the most basic resources are absent. The local environmental effects of extreme temperature and weather, which have little impact on the anesthetic decisions of the anesthesiologist in a modern hospital environment, can greatly modify the choices of the modern battlefield anesthesiologist.

In civilian practice, care and transport of the patient beyond the postanesthesia care unit (PACU) is rarely a concern. Terrain, distances, and evacuation routes must be considered by the battlefield anesthesiologist. From a purely military viewpoint, it is far better to wound rather then kill an enemy soldier. A dead soldier, while reducing combat power, ceases to be a logistic or leadership burden. A wounded soldier, on the other hand, becomes a tremendous liability. Wounded soldiers reduce combat effectiveness and overall unit morale exponentially, since other soldiers are employed for evacuation duties rather then mission completion. Most significantly, wounded soldiers require the military organization to expend a massive logistic effort in the care and management of battlefield casualties. The U.S. Army Combat Support Hospital (Fig. 34-2) is an example of this logistic effort in the 2002 Iraq conflict, demonstrating both the enormous commitment and power projection the United States can bring to the modern field of battle. Because of the significant reduction in combat effectiveness and the logistic burden that casualties represent on the battlefield, current military doctrine in the United States emphasizes rapid evacuation of the wounded out of the theater of operations. The remarkable airlift capabilities of the Coalition forces in Iraq and Afghanistan make this possible. Evacuation of wounded from the war operations theater that was historically measured in days is now often measured in hours. Anesthetic choices made at the Combat Support Hospital (CSH) or by the forward surgical team (FST) must be made with this extremely fast evacuation in mind. Although anesthesiologists in future conflicts may not enjoy such a rapid evacuation capability, the current conflict demonstrates how the military anesthesiologist must adapt care decisions to changing environments.

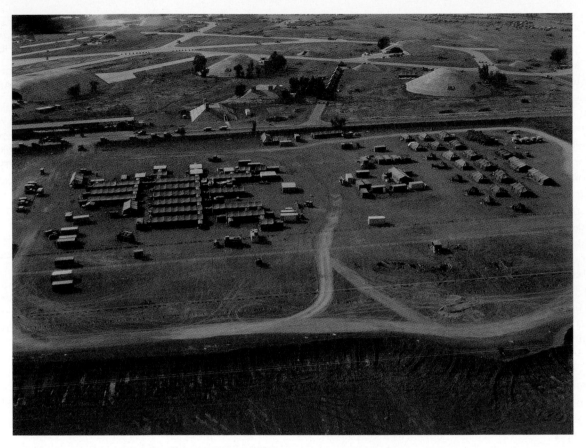

Figure 34-2. Combat Support Hospital (CSH) in Iraq.

Personal Safety

"It is well that war is so terrible—we shouldn't grow too fond of it."

General Robert E. Lee

The modern battlefield is a horrific and dangerous place. For those special individuals who place themselves at risk in order to ease the suffering of the battle wounded and care for them, attention to personal safety is paramount. Apart from self-preservation, medical personnel add directly to the overall fighting effectiveness of an army and are not readily replaced when lost. Anesthesiologists sent to war (or thrust into war from acts of terrorism) must develop situational awareness (SA). As defined by the Naval Aviation Schools Command in Pensacola, Florida, "SA refers to the degree of accuracy by which one's perception of his current environment mirrors reality." Although anesthesiologists are normally highly skilled at monitoring and evaluating the patient's reality, in the combat environment constant attention to the unpredictable battlefield is imperative if dangerous situations are to be avoided. Obviously not all personal risk can be eliminated in a war zone, but it can be reduced to a minimum through careful analysis of wartime threats and dangers (good SA). Once

enemy and environmental threats are identified, a proactive response to the dangers is possible. For example, enemy mortar or rocket attacks within a hospital compound should cause medical personnel to harden sleeping areas to these attacks (i.e., by using sand bags), know where bomb shelters are located within the compound, keep body armor nearby and serviceable, and recognize the times or patterns of the attacks. Although this example may seem simplistic or plain "common sense," it can be all too easy in the fatigue-ridden, harsh combat environment to lose SA and fail to employ commonsense protection strategies. The wartime anesthesiologist cannot depend on others for SA, and attention to these details can be lifesaving.

As noted previously, improved modern body armor and helmets have greatly reduced the severity and lethality of combat wounds. Anesthesiologists should strive to use them and integrate their use into battlefield medical practice. Although body armor may be unnecessary in a *secured* hospital compound, it should always be used in triage situations or when missions require the physician to leave secured areas. Physician bravado is a poor substitute for Kevlar when rounds are incoming.

Deployed medical personnel should be proficient and familiar with issued firearms. Weapons are an ever-present reality of war and will be encountered during the care of casualties. Anesthesiologists must be familiar with firearms in order to recognize and safely remove them from war victims. Although each physician must make a personal decision to use lethal force for self-defense or the defense of patients, this situation does occur and mental preparation for the event is prudent. Before any anesthetic or intervention is begun on any (regardless of nationality) patient, a thorough search for weapons (guns, knives, explosives) should be made and these items confiscated. The best policy is complete removal of all clothing and equipment when the casualty arrives at the medical facility. The realities of physical injury during war are readily apparent, but physicians and medical commanders can take precautions to reduce this risk.

War is also mentally stressful, and mental injury, though harder to detect, can be no less devastating than wounds. Prolonged separation from home and family, the constant threat of personal injury, and exposure to the aftermath of combat can cause significant stress leading to mental health problems. Unfortunately, war-related mental stress is not easy to categorize, hard to define, and difficult to protect against. However, physical health through proper diet and exercise, discussion about traumatic events with comrades, and frequent communication with loved ones (in the current conflicts, e-mail has had a profoundly positive impact) seem effective strategies to lessen stress.

Patients

"There was never a good war, or a bad peace."
Benjamin Franklin

As warfare on civilian targets has become increasingly common, the makeup of casualties requiring military care has also changed. Although injured soldiers continue to occupy most of the military anesthesiologist's operating room schedule, other casualties are becoming more common. Since the Vietnam War, the enemies of the United States and its allies have rarely had an organized military medical infrastructure. Many enemy wounded have therefore been cared for by U.S. military medical units. The U.S. military prides itself on providing the same standard of care for wounded enemy prisoners of war (EPW) as it does for its own personnel, but these people are not evacuated from the theater of war. Severely wounded EPW end up at the CSH (the highest level of care within a theater currently) and can remain there for weeks or months (Table 34-1). This puts a significant strain on the CSH, which is not designed for the prolonged management and rehabilitation of the wounded. The anesthesiologist is forced to provide repeated surgical anesthetics and chronic pain management services with limited resources for many EPW orthopaedic patients. Some innovative solutions used in the current Iraq war in managing EPW are discussed further on.

▶ **TABLE 34-1.** BASIC DESCRIPTION OF THE LEVELS OF MILITARY MEDICAL SUPPORT AND EVACUATION CHAIN FROM THE BATTLEFIELD

Basic Level	Immediate First Aid by Nearest Person or Medic ("Buddy Aid")
Level 1	First structured (usually a tent) aid post. Resuscitation and stabilization care. Battalion aid stations are an example.
Level 2	First stabilization surgical capability. The forward surgical team (FST), which provides trauma resuscitation, is an example.
Level 3	Multidisciplinary general hospital within or near the theater of war. The Combat Support Hospital (CSH) is an example and provides specialized surgical and medical services. Ancillary laboratory, radiology, and dental facilities exist at the CSH.
Level 4	Definitive medical care hospital within the United States or allied country.

SOURCE: *Seet,[30] with permission.*

The insurgent style of ambush that predominates in the current conflicts, often targeting civilians, has also resulted in large numbers of wounded adults and children. Though policy and resource availability discourages the acceptance of these civilian casualties in military medical facilities, they are often admitted because of politics, news media pressure, and compassion. In short, the modern battlefield anesthesiologist must be ready for anything.

Roles of the Anesthesiologist in Modern War

The anesthesiologist brings unique capabilities in support of the wartime medical mission beyond traditional operating room responsibilities. As resuscitation medicine specialists, anesthesiologists are eminently qualified to assist with the triage system in sorting casualties. In collaboration with surgeons, the anesthesiologist can plan the most efficient surgical schedule that will utilize operating room resources efficiently and provide the maximum benefit when large numbers of casualties arrive at the same time. Anesthesiologists are often called on to mediate surgeon subspecialty concerns about operating room case order in routine practice. This role is vitally important in wartime casualty scenarios.

The practice of anesthesiology is surgical critical care medicine. Resident training in anesthesiology usually provides extensive experience in surgical intensive care. The anesthesiologist can provide valuable consulting experience in the management of difficult intensive care patients.

The anesthesiologist is the pain medicine consultant on the battlefield, and the profound impact of effective pain control on wounded soldiers cannot be overstressed. In the 2002 Iraq war, Lieutenant Colonel Allen Hayes, while serving with the 21st CSH, used his skills as a pain specialist on approximately 30 soldiers with a variety of chronic pain complaints. Colonel Hayes reported that 80 percent of these patients were retained in the Iraq theater. In other circumstances they would have required evacuation and replacement.

The anesthesiologist plays a vital role in casualty stabilization and preparation for evacuation from the battlefield. Optimization of vital signs, respiratory status, fluid status, and pain management are more important now that casualties may be at the CSH for only hours before being evacuated from the war theater on long flights.

The anesthesiologist can also supervise several nurse anesthetists collaboratively managing several patients in the operating suites while also performing the perioperative roles previously mentioned. Anesthesiologists are medical force multipliers on the modern battlefield.

Anesthesia Logistics on the Battlefield

Anesthesia supply, and medical supply in general, is governed by the classic military slogan: "Beans, bullets, and Band-Aids." The first two necessities of war, food and ammunition, directly compete with medical supplies. Lessons learned from the Desert Shield/Desert Storm war of 1991 revealed that the army had essentially oversupplied medical assets in preparation for thousands of casualties that never materialized.[14] After September 11, medical planners envision a significantly smaller medical response (reduced medical logistics footprint) designed to support small numbers of high-technology war fighters against terrorists or rogue states.[15] Current conflicts appear to support this premise. The new goal for casualty care on the battlefield is "stabilization for evacuation." For the anesthesiologist, this means providing quality anesthesia services with the smallest logistic footprint possible. The marked increase in the speed of evacuation from battle will challenge military anesthesiologists to provide a better patient "product" to the PACU. The patient product goal following surgery should be a stable, alert, and pain-free patient who can be a proponent of his or her own evacuation. A sedated, possibly overnarcotized, nauseated and vomiting patient brought to a modern civilian PACU is not a difficult problem when nursing and monitoring facilities are abundant. However, the same patient in chaotic battlefield conditions can divert scarce nursing and other medical resources away from more critical patients and even delay evacuation. New anesthetic techniques and technology introduced into future battlefields should focus on improving the patient product for the new realities of fast battlefield evacuation.

On the battlefield, anesthesiologists must concern themselves with sparing anesthetic resources. Unlike the case in civilian medicine, where supplies are rarely a problem, medical supply in war is often variable or inadequate and subject to disruption by the enemy. The military anesthesiologist should know the medical unit's anesthetic supply situation at all times. Regardless of the state of medical supply, strict conservation of anesthetic resources should always be a priority. Simple mistakes that seem insignificant in civilian anesthesia, such as forgetting to turn off the oxygen at the end of a case, can damage a unit's medical readiness on the battlefield. Medical logistics are therefore important in anesthetic selection.

The storage of anesthetic equipment and consumables must also be among the military anesthesiologist's daily concerns. Environmental control is not always available in the field, and extremes of heat or cold can degrade medications and damage equipment. Supply personnel may not be aware of the environmental requirements for the storage of medical material. The anesthesiologist for the unit must be proactive in ensuring that anesthetic supplies are not lost due to improper handling and storage.

The prudent military anesthesiologist will deploy with a personal tool bag containing a complete set of airway instruments, stethoscope, reference handbook, calculator, and other items that facilitate anesthesia practice in austere environments. The military anesthesiologist should always be on the lookout for new technology that will improve anesthetic care in the stern battlefield environment while working to decrease the medical logistics burden. An excellent example of "off the shelf" technology that has tremendous potential in military anesthesia is the Onyx digital finger-pulse oximeter (Nonin Medical Inc., Plymouth, MN). This very compact, portable device ($5 \times 3 \times 3$ cm) allows spot or continuous checks of pulse and hemoglobin oxygen saturation at any time. In the author's experience, the device has proven itself as the sole patient monitor in extremely harsh anesthesia situations where typical monitoring equipment is unavailable or its use impractical. Research and development of this type of "field friendly" anesthesia equipment is the business of the military anesthesiologist.

General Anesthesia

General anesthesia (GA) is the standard technique to which all other anesthetic techniques for orthopaedic surgery are compared. The ability to perform a GA on the battlefield is vital, since it is often the safest option for the patient, particularly when wounds to the head, chest, or abdomen are involved. Much of the success of modern military medicine in treating battlefield wounded can be attributed to the use of GA on the battlefield. As practiced in the developed world, GA depends a lot on resources and technology. Unfortunately, the lack of resources (electricity, compressed gas, modern anesthesia machines, operating rooms, etc.) on the battlefield can severely limit the usefulness of this anesthetic. Currently, the U.S. Army is using the Dräger Narkomed M at the CSH level. This machine has most of the standard features of any modern anesthesia machine. As previously noted, military anesthesiologists are frequently faced with situations in which the resources needed to operate a machine as advanced as the Dräger Narkomed M are unavailable. In these situations, simple bag-valve-mask systems can be used with a draw-over vaporizer and room air to provide a GA (Fig. 34-3). The U.S. Army Medical Materiel Development Activity (USAMMDA) has established guidelines for a far-forward battlefield anesthesia machine (Table 34-2). The combination of the Ohmeda Portable Anesthesia Complete draw-over vaporizer with an Impact 754 Eagle ventilator has been suggested to meet many of the guidelines outlined by USAMMDA.[16]

Regardless of the indication for GA, the use of volatile anesthetics poses problems on the modern battlefield. Volatile anesthetics are triggers for malignant hyperthermia (this has been an issue in current conflicts), scavenging of waste gases can be difficult, and gas monitoring is rarely available, so that depth of anesthesia is more difficult to ascertain and wake-up times are unpredictable. Compared with other options, volatile anesthetics are affected by extremes of environmental temperature or pressure and require a larger logistics footprint because specialized equipment is needed to deliver them. Also, the increased incidence of nausea and vomiting associated with the use of volatile anesthetics has been well documented.[17,18] These factors

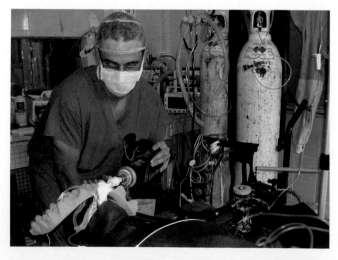

Figure 34-3. In the absence of sophisticated anesthetic equipment, a simple bag-valve-mask system can be used with a draw-over vaporizer and room air to provide general anesthesia.

► **TABLE 34-2.** U.S. ARMY MEDICAL MATERIEL DEVELOPMENT ACTIVITY GUIDELINES FOR A FAR-FORWARD FIELD ANESTHESIA MACHINE

Has a functional ventilator
Does not rely on compressed gases for operation
Compatible with low-flow/low-pressure oxygen from a concentrator
Electrical operation (for electronic pumps)
Operation for 3 h on battery backup
Compact
Digital ventilator display
FDA approval
Multiagent capability
Inspired and expired gas-monitoring capabilities

impede the successful management of a casualty in the chaos of a battlefield.

A viable alternative to volatile anesthetics is total intravenous anesthesia (TIVA). These anesthetics, such as propofol, can be delivered via computerized pumps that allow target-controlled infusion (TCI), permitting more precise control of anesthetic blood levels. TIVA with computerized pumps offers a means to the rapid induction of GA and to planning for emergence.[19] Compared with volatile anesthetics, the use of propofol is associated with fewer postoperative complications.[20,21] The same TCI pump can be used for postoperative sedation if required. Intravenous anesthesia also works synergistically with regional anesthesia for moderate sedation during orthopaedic procedures. The use of TIVA with pumps in the modern battlefield will reduce equipment needs and improve the condition of the patient to be evacuated. TIVA is an active area of research in military medicine by the Triservice Anesthesia Research Group Initiative (TARGET) based at Brooke Army Medical Center, Texas.

Modern weapons can produce overwhelming orthopaedic injury (Fig. 34-4). The anesthesiologist in these situations is primarily responsible for the lifesaving resuscitative anesthesia (airway, breathing, and circulation, or ABC) needed to manage severe hypovolemic shock (see Chap. 2). Significant hemorrhage into limbs following blunt trauma can be another source of hypovolemic shock; therefore both the anesthesiologist and the surgeon must be vigilant for occult fractures. Standard anesthesia-induction drugs (particularly with inhalational agents) for airway management and anesthesia can be fatal in the shock patient. Patients in severe hypovolemic shock usually require little or no sedative or analgesic medication for intubation. Excessive anesthetic use in these patients will cause further deterioration of blood pressure and possibly cardiac arrest. The clinical situation and the anesthesiologist's estimate of the severity of the patient's hypovolemia will determine anesthetic use. The main effort in these patients is to restore blood volume and maintain hemodynamic stability while surgeons rapidly manage sources of bleeding. As these goals are achieved and the patient's vital signs improve, anesthetic agents can be administered carefully. Essentially, the patient earns the anesthesia as bleeding is controlled, volume is restored, and vital signs improve.

One important aspect in managing the patient with hypovolemic shock is not to delay moving the patient to the operating room for definitive care. Some delay is unavoidable while the patient undergoes physical examination, diagnostic procedures, and the placement of intravenous lines. Occasionally, lifesaving surgery is postponed while medical personnel attempt to provide central venous access and begin aggressive restoration of volume. The anesthesiologist should discourage these activities until a surgeon is available to control hemorrhage.

Venous access in trauma patients is vital, but it is often difficult to obtain in the hypovolemic patient with collapsed veins. Central venous access or venous cut-down procedures can be time-consuming, especially in the chaos of combat situations. Intraosseous vascular access, a technique that is often used in children, may offer a time-saving alternative for emergencies when standard techniques fail. Manual placement of intraosseous needles in adults has usually been avoided because harder adult bone causes the needle to bend or slip off. New spring-driven, trigger-operated intraosseous needles overcome this problem. These devices have been successfully used by medical personnel in full chemical protective gear (a difficult situation for medical practice in the best of circumstances) and are easy to operate with minimal training.[22,23] They represent a simple, innovative solution to a common medical problem in the battlefield. While not a replacement for standard intravenous access methods, intraosseous needle systems provide an important emergency alternative and should become part of standard training for military anesthesia providers.

Rapid infusion systems are another example of technology that has been incorporated into battlefield use. Rapid infusion systems allow anesthesiologists to maintain organ perfusion despite massive hemorrhage. Currently, pressure infusion systems for army use are being replaced because of concerns over insufficient heating capacity, maintenance problems with water countercurrent baths, and the risk of air embolism. New semiocclusive, roller-head pump systems that heat fluid using magnetic induction, such as the FMS 2000 (Belmont Instrument Corp., Billerica, MA), obviate these problems and are quickly being added to the army's inventory. The benefit of rapid infusion systems for casualty survival is greatly amplified by the success of the Armed Services Blood Program (ASBP). This program, established in 1952, performs a tremendous service in providing blood and blood products to the military community worldwide and on the battlefield. The benefits that blood component therapy has had on the survival of casualties in past and current conflicts cannot be overestimated. Major Dennis Williams, working at the 31st CSH in Iraq, emphasized the importance of blood products in casualty care with his description of a 30-year-old Iraqi man who sustained multiple extremity injuries from a mortar attack. He was taken to the operating room for ligation of distal arteries as well as multiple open veins, debridement, fracture stabilization via external fixation, and four-compartment fasciotomies of both legs. Although the operation lasted only 85 min, blood loss was estimated at 4000 mL, and the patient received 10 units of packed red blood cells, 2 units of whole blood, 4 units of fresh frozen plasma, and recombinant factor VIIa.

Regional Anesthesia

"Those who cannot remember the past are condemned to repeat it."

George Santayana

Recognition of the advantages of RA in managing orthopaedic trauma on the modern battlefield is not unique to the current conflicts. Major Gale Thompson, writing about his experiences in Vietnam, noted that RA techniques were used whenever possible. In a series of 1000 battle casualties, RA was used 49 percent of the time (spinal and axillary blocks predominating).[24] Major Thompson reports, "Of course Vietnam was full of potential to produce extremity wounds because of the Punji sticks planted along trails. They would penetrate boots or legs or arms when the enemy would create some noise up ahead and at the alarm everyone would dive for cover, only to be impaled by those primitive, fecally contaminated sticks." The similarities in wounding patterns produced by primitive means in Vietnam and those seen in the insurgent conflicts today are striking.

Other innovators in battlefield anesthesia have also recognized the advantages of RA, as, for example, in the Angola Civil War in 1975 (personal communication, A. P. Boezaart). In that year, during his conscription to the South African Defense Force (SADF), Dr. Boezaart, then a young and inexperienced junior officer, was in charge of anesthesia for the number 1 Forward Surgical Unit (1FSU) under the command of Brigadier Tony Dippenaar. The unit was deployed just behind the front lines. In this conventional war, the SADF joined forces with the Unita movement of Dr. Jonas Savimbi and was supported by the United States against the MPLA forces supported by Cuba and the then Soviet Union. The 1FSU followed Alpha Brigade in their push northward toward Luanda from what was then Southwest Africa (now Namibia).

Before going to Angola, Dr. Boezaart worked as sole practitioner in a 250-bed mission hospital in northern South Africa with a nurse, the late Roelf Neuhoff, who introduced him to RA and presented him with a copy of the fourth edition of Daniel C. Moore's textbook *Regional Block*, with the words "Doc, you'd better take this book with you, otherwise you will kill more soldiers than the enemy will." This textbook saved many lives during this war. It was the philosophy of the surgical team to perform surgery as soon as possible after the injury occurred, and in many cases patients were on the operating table a few hours after injury. Land-mine injuries were very common in Angola (Angola to this day still has the highest concentration of land mines per square mile in the world), and all the operations following these injuries were done under single-injection epidural block performed with a 22-gauge spinal needle (Fig. 34-4). Except for surgery to the head, neck, and thorax, almost all other surgery was done with a regional technique. The facilities for general anesthesia were very basic, but with an old Manley ventilator and a basic Boyles machine, this was possible. With the aggressive use of RA, there was not one single operating room mortality out of a total of 113 major operations performed during a 2-month period. The most advanced monitoring device was a mercury baumanometer, while oxygen saturation, capnography, and electrocardiographic monitoring were unheard of in the battlefield in those years.

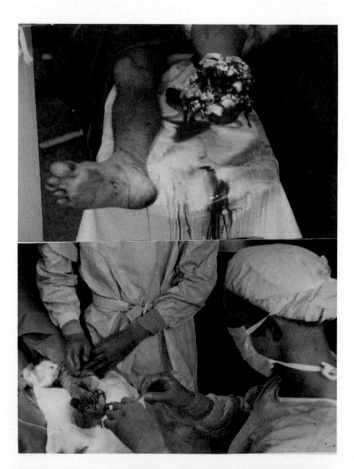

Figure 34-4. Injury from an antipersonnel land mine. Brigadier Tony Dippenaar performed the surgery with the patient under epidural anesthesia.

As far as can be established, Dr. Boezaart performed one of the early continuous peripheral nerve blocks for pain in 1975 during this war. The SADF captured a large number of recoilless mortar-launching guns, which produced a large "back blast," from the enemy forces, and the SA soldiers were not familiar with this equipment. The result was that a number of soldiers got their hands severely injured in the blasts. Toward the later days of the war, soldiers also discovered that a self-inflicted gunshot wound to the hand was a sure pass home. The debridement that followed was done under axillary block. Dr. Boezaart infiltrated the skin in the axillae of these patients with lidocaine and performed a 1-cm cut-down to expose the axillary artery. He then fed a central line catheter proximally next to the artery for approximately 10 cm, closed the small wound, and sutured the catheter to the skin. These catheters were left in place for weeks after the surgery—for long after the patients were evacuated back to South Africa. Patients were given a supply of 10-mL syringes filled with bupivacaine 0.5% and the patient or his comrade or "medic" would inject the agent through the catheter in the event of pain. These continuous blocks were also used for "topping up" of the block for repeated debridement surgery in the military hospital long after the patient had returned from the war zone.

Despite this encouraging early evidence of the utility of RA on the modern battlefield, RA use in the current conflicts is relatively rare. This is probably due to the availability of equipment to administer GA safely under field conditions. Anesthesiologists are also reluctant to use RA in orthopaedic patients partly from concerns voiced by orthopaedic surgeons. One such misgiving is the possible delay in the diagnosis of compartment syndrome following injury. Many orthopaedic surgeons rely on clinical indicators associated with developing compartment syndrome, including pain, paresthesia, pain with passive stretch, and paresis. Unfortunately, the predictive value of these clinical signs is unknown.[25] Effective pain management of orthopaedic injury using RA has been suggested as a possible contributing factor to delayed diagnosis of this complication. Although analgesia with RA certainly alters the patient's overall clinical presentation (usually for the better, with improved pain control), it does not necessarily preclude a timely diagnosis of compartment syndrome. In the presence of a regional block, both the orthopaedic surgeon and anesthesiologist must learn to adjust their interpretation of clinical signs suggesting compartment syndrome. A high index of suspicion should be maintained in managing patients at risk for compartment syndrome regardless of the pain management techniques used. The denial by surgeons of first-rate pain treatment out of fear that it may delay diagnosis of compartment syndrome should be carefully reconsidered.

Delay of postoperative neurologic examination has also been suggested as an indication to avoid RA. The delayed or temporarily changed postoperative neurologic examination in a patient whose orthopaedic injury is managed under RA cannot be contested. Whether this delay is clinically significant is debatable, since many surgeons often manage possible iatrogenic nerve injuries with observation. In most cases, discussion with the surgeon concerning anesthetic technique can facilitate timely postoperative neurologic examination if needed while still allowing the patient the benefits of RA. Before giving any anesthetic (particularly when RA is planned) for orthopaedic surgery, preoperative neurologic examination by the anesthesiologist is essential.

Another concern of orthopaedic surgeons with RA is case delay. Unwillingness to employ RA can be particularly valid in chaotic battlefield conditions. When casualty loads are high or patients are unstable, RA may not be the best initial choice for anesthesia. Nevertheless, depending on the casualty mix, RA can prove extremely useful. In the author's own experience in Iraq, after the most severely injured and unstable patients had been successfully managed and their operations started, time was available to prepare waiting cases for surgery, often with RA. This concept was employed at the 21st CSH many times; the following situation is illustrative. Six casualties arrived at the CSH (two were dead on arrival) requiring triage and operative management. The most critical cases were a patient with a shrapnel wound to the face, with significant soft tissue loss that threatened the patient's airway, and a patient with a massive wound from a high-velocity bullet to the buttock and femur that caused serious hemorrhage. After these patients had been stabilized and were under GA in the operating rooms, we (the author and Colonel Hayes) evaluated a coalition soldier wounded by an AK-47 bullet to the right knee (Fig. 34-1). This soldier was hemodynamically stable, neurologically intact, and in great pain. We decided to place catheters for lumbar plexus and sciatic nerve continuous peripheral nerve block (CPNB). After the block, the patient was very comfortable while waiting for surgery and required only light propofol sedation for his knee exploration. After the operation, the patient's pain was treated with local anesthetic infusions via the CPNB catheters. During this same period, a fourth patient with a shrapnel wound to the right anterior thigh was treated with a long-acting (ropivacaine) single-injection femoral nerve block. Both RA blocks were completed before operations on the previous cases had been concluded and both soldiers were alert and pain-free before and after their respective operations.

These actual case examples illustrate how RA can benefit battlefield orthopaedic patients by preemptively treating pain, facilitating casualty flow through the operating rooms, and providing effective analgesia postoperatively. In many casualty situations, the anesthesiologist trained in the use of RA can complete the anesthetic and have a comfortable patient waiting for the surgeon before the previous patient has left the operating room. More importantly, when RA techniques are used instead of GA with volatile anesthetics, the patient arriving in the recovery room tends to be alert and pain-free. Potential advantages of RA on the modern battlefield are listed in Table 34-3. In battlefield conditions, these advantages can be lifesaving, since alert and pain-free patients require fewer medical resources and can actively participate in their own evacuation.

Spinal and epidural anesthesia, though effective RA techniques, are currently underutilized on the modern battlefield. Concerns about cleanliness and possible increases in infection have caused many anesthesia personnel to avoid these methods. The successful use of these important techniques in austere environments and on the battlefield has been documented; however, shortcomings do exist.[10,24] A particular disadvantage of neuraxial block in hypovolemic trauma patients is hypotension. Other issues include unpredictable onset and regression, urinary retention, issues involving perioperative anticoagulation, and inclusion of the uninjured limb in the block. Despite these concerns, neuraxial RA can be a very useful technique for battlefield orthopaedic anesthesia.

Advances in peripheral nerve stimulation, stimulating needles, perineural catheter technology, and portable infusion pumps have renewed interest in peripheral nerve block (PNB) anesthesia. PNBs have the benefits of neuraxial RA while avoiding some of its limitations. The localized sympathectomy of PNB as opposed to the more generalized sympathectomy of neuraxial RA minimizes induced hypotension in trauma patients.

Recognizing an expanded role for RA on the modern battlefield, Colonel John Chiles, Anesthesiology Consultant to the Surgeon General, established RA as a training priority for army anesthesiology. In support of this mission, the Army Regional Anesthesia and Pain Management Initiative (ARAPMI) was established in 2000. The primary goal of the initiative is improved training in RA and acute pain treatment for military anesthesiology residents and to establish an expanded role of RA and CPNB for military patients at home and on the battlefield. Since the beginning of the wars in Afghanistan and Iraq, PNB and CPNB have played a major role in the care of many wounded soldiers returning to the United States with severe extremity injuries.

▶ **TABLE 34-3.** ADVANTAGES OF REGIONAL ANESTHESIA ON THE BATTLEFIELD

Small logistics footprint to support
Excellent operating conditions
Stable hemodynamics
Improved postoperative alertness
Minimal side effects
Profound perioperative analgesia
Reduced need for other analgesics (opioids)

In addition to the superior perioperative analgesia provided by CPNB between operative procedures, the catheters can be used repeatedly to reestablish a surgical block for the frequent trips to the operating room often required by these patients. At Walter Reed Army Medical Center (WRAMC) in Washington, D.C., where the ARAPMI is based, hundreds of wounded soldiers have been successfully managed with RA since the beginning of the Iraq War. Many soldiers have used CPNB catheters for weeks to provide analgesia and anesthesia for multiple operations and dressing changes. Considerable experience has also been gained in the use of peripheral nerve stimulation to place CPNB catheters for phantom limb stimulation in amputees.[26] These catheters have proven extremely useful for surgical intervention and the management of acute phantom limb and stump pain following traumatic amputation.

In the fall of 2003, the author was sent to Iraq to examine the feasibility of using PNB and CPNB on the modern battlefield. On October 7, 2003, lumbar plexus and sciatic CPNB catheters were placed in a soldier who had sustained an injury to his left calf caused by rocket-propelled grenade.[27] These catheters were used in the soldier's initial operation in Balad, Iraq, and were then connected to portable infusion pumps containing local anesthetic, which provided analgesia for the long flight to Landstuhl, Germany, and eventually WRAMC. This was the first use of CPNB catheters and portable peripheral nerve infusion pumps in a soldier's evacuation throughout the levels of care. He would use the catheters placed in Iraq for 16 days of analgesia, five operations, and multiple dressing changes. Since this initial success, the use of these nerve blocks in managing battlefield casualties has continued to expand, with many more soldiers receiving CPNB catheters in Iraq and using them throughout their evacuation. Continuous plexus block has been particularly useful at the CSH level in managing Iraqi wounded. These casualties are not evacuated and can be a significant strain on CSH resources because they may take weeks to recover. With CPNB, much of the routine wound care of these cases is handled at the bedside instead of in the operating room. This saves considerable time and resources.

Although these successes are encouraging, many questions remain about the use of CPNB in the battlefield. Considerable effort will be needed to establish the physical and educational infrastructure for RA in military anesthesia before this anesthetic technique can be fully implemented on the battlefield.

Conclusion

"If everyone is thinking alike, then somebody isn't thinking."
General George S. Patton

This chapter has outlined some of the many challenges military anesthesiologists face on the battlefield. As twenty-first-century warfare moves the battlefield ever closer to civilian population centers, concepts of care in military anesthesia will soon concern civilian anesthesiologists. To prepare for this new reality, the problems of battlefield anesthesia traditionally addressed by military anesthesiology training programs will need to be included in the curricula of all anesthesiology training programs. At WRAMC, an important program used to prepare our anesthesiology residents for the rigors of battlefield anesthesiology is our Operational Anesthesia Rotation (OAR).[10] Military staff and resident anesthesiologists participating in this rotation deploy to austere, medically underserved locations to provide anesthesia in a "field" environment (Fig. 34-3). The goals of this program are shown in Table 34-4.

Medical simulation is another training modality that military anesthesiology is actively pursuing. Through simulation, the anesthesiologist can be exposed to battlefield situations and stresses that otherwise could be experienced only on an actual battlefield. At WRAMC, efforts are under way to develop a "battle lab operating room" where field equipment and anesthetic techniques can be evaluated and tested in a controlled environment before they are actually used. This area will also serve as

▶ **TABLE 34-4.** OPERATIONAL ANESTHESIA ROTATION (OAR) PROGRAM GOALS

Preparation for working and living among patients and families with diverse cultural backgrounds while providing their health care

Preparation for deployment to areas with a high prevalence of endemic infectious diseases, including estimation of medical threat, collection of medical intelligence information, development of medical operational plans, and individual consultation on travel medicine

Public health aspects of humanitarian missions such as relevant infectious diseases and risk/benefit issues of prophylaxis options

Understanding of basic food and water sanitation

Effects of extreme environmental conditions on patients, staff, anesthetic equipment, and medications

Universal precautions in austere environments

Medical supply logistics with travel to and operations in harsh environments

Fatigue and stress management

Triage and medical resource allocation

Spontaneous ventilation: Its use in the field to avoid the need for ventilators, increase safety, and extend capabilities and its limitations in complex surgical procedures

Total IV anesthesia (TIVA): Its use in austere conditions and the risks/benefits of this anesthetic

Regional anesthesia: The appropriate use of RA to extend capabilities in a mass casualty situation, improve postoperative analgesia with limited patient monitoring, and minimize risk in austere environments

SOURCE: *From Buckenmaier et al.,[10] with permission.*

a location for simulated battlefield scenarios. Using modern simulation and telecommunications technology, any number of wartime or terrorist casualty situations can be explored, so that the anesthesiologist's first encounter with these difficult circumstances will not also represent their first casualty.

New techniques and devices are on the horizon that will greatly influence anesthetic care for battlefield wounded. The possibility of ultra-long-acting local anesthetics that provide analgesia for days rather than hours would enhance the application of RA on the battlefield, since single injections could replace sophisticated infusion pumps or catheters and provide analgesia for evacuation. Recently, there has been some success in increasing the duration of bupivacaine analgesia by using liposomal encapsulation as a slow-release delivery vehicle.[28,29] The Special Forces community within the military has called for innovative methods to manage pain that would, unlike opioid therapy, not significantly degrade mental acuity or combat performance after a painful but not incapacitating wound. Regional anesthesia, possibly with ultra-long-acting local anesthetics, might offer one solution. Additional research into a more comprehensive approach to managing pain on the battlefield pain is sorely needed. Military anesthesiologists should avoid practicing the anesthesia of the last war; soldiers deserve better. Advances in anesthesia practice and technology should not be prevented from being used on the battlefield merely because the operating room happens to be in a tent and functioning under less then ideal conditions.

Military anesthesiology is a challenging and constantly changing field of medicine. As a military anesthesiologist, I have had the honor of relieving pain and suffering in many of America's servicemen and women. Few experiences in my life have been as rewarding.

REFERENCES

1. Cozen LN. Military Orthopaedic surgery. *Clin Orthop* 50–53, 1985
2. Dougherty PJ. Wartime amputations. *Mil Med* 158:755–763, 1993.
3. Oreck SL. Orthopaedic surgery in the combat zone. *Mil Med* 161:458–461, 1996.
4. Condon-Rall ME. A brief history of military anesthesia, in Zajtchuk R, Grande CM (eds): *Anesthesia and Perioperative Care of the Combat Casualty*. Washington DC: Office of the Surgeon General at TMM Publications, Bordon Institute, 1995:855–896.
5. Hrutkay JM, Hirsch E, Hockenbury T. Orthopaedic surgery at a MASH deployed to the former Yugoslavia in support of the United Nations Protection Force. *Mil Med* 160:199–202, 1995.
6. Van Creveld ML. *The Transformation of War*. New York: Free Press, 1991.
7. Hammes, TX. The evolution of war: The fourth generation. *Marine Corps Gazette* 78:35, 1994.
8. Bartlett CS. Clinical update: Gunshot wound ballistics. *Clin Orthop* 28–57, 2003.
9. Phillips YY III, Richmond DR. *Primary blast injury and basic research*, in Zajtchuk R, Jenkins DP, Bellamy RF, Quick CM (eds): *A Brief History, Part I: Warfare, Weaponry, and the Casualty*. Washington DC: Office of the Surgeon General, 1991:221–240.
10. Buckenmaier CC III, Lee EH, Shields CH, et al. Regional anesthesia in austere environments. *Reg Anesth Pain Med* 28:321–327, 2003.
11. Bellamy RF. Combat trauma overview, in Zajtchuk R, Bellamy RF (eds): *Textbook of Military Medicine, Part IV: Anesthesia and Perioperative Care of the Combat Casualty*. Washington, DC: Office of the Surgeon General, 1995:11–13.
12. Mabry RL, Holcomb JB, Baker AM, et al. United States Army Rangers in Somalia: An analysis of combat casualties on an urban battlefield. *J Trauma* 49:515–528, 2000.
13. Bilski TR, Baker BC, Grove JR, et al. Battlefield casualties treated at Camp Rhino, Afghanistan: Lessons learned. *J Trauma* 54:814–821, 2003.
14. Gunby P. Another war ... and more lessons for medicine to ponder in aftermath. *JAMA* 266:619–621, 1991.
15. Mitka M. US military medicine moves to meet current challenge. *JAMA* 286;2532–2533, 2001.
16. Reynolds PC, Calkins M, Bentley T, et al. Improved anesthesia support of the forward surgical team: A proposed combination of drawover anesthesia and the life support for trauma and transport. *Mil Med* 167:889–892, 2002.
17. Chung F, Mezei G. Factors contributing to a prolonged stay after ambulatory surgery. *Anesth Analg* 89:1352–1359, 1999.
18. Pavlin DJ, Rapp SE, Polissar NL, et al. Factors affecting discharge time in adult outpatients. *Anesth Analg* 87:816–826, 1998.
19. Russell D, Wilkes MP, Hunter SC, et al. Manual compared with target-controlled infusion of propofol. *Br J Anaesth* 75:562–566, 1995.
20. Fombeur PO, Tilleul PR, Beaussier MJ, et al. Cost-effectiveness of propofol anesthesia using target-controlled infusion compared with a standard regimen using desflurane. *Am J Health Syst Pharm* 59:1344–1350, 2002.
21. Suttner S, Boldt J, Schmidt C, et al. Cost analysis of target-controlled infusion-based anesthesia compared with standard anesthesia regimens. *Anesth Analg* 88:77–82, 1999.
22. Calkins MD, Fitzgerald G, Bentley TB, et al. Intraosseous infusion devices: A comparison for potential use in special operations. *J Trauma* 48:1068–1074, 2000.
23. Vardi A, Berkenstadt H, Levin I, et al. Intraosseous vascular access in the treatment of chemical warfare casualties assessed by advanced simulation: Proposed alteration of treatment protocol. *Anesth Analg* 98:1753–1758, 2004.
24. Thompson GE. Anesthesia for battle casualties in Vietnam. *JAMA* 201:215–219, 1967.
25. Ulmer T. The clinical diagnosis of compartment syndrome of the lower leg: Are clinical findings predictive of the disorder? *J Orthop Trauma* 16:572–577, 2002.
26. Klein SM, Eck J, Nielsen K, et al. Anesthetizing the phantom: Peripheral nerve stimulation of a nonexistent extremity. *Anesthesiology* 100:736–737, 2004.

27. Buckenmaier CC III, Mcknight GM, Winkley JV, et al. Continuous peripheral nerve block for battlefield anesthesia and education. *Reg Anesth Pain Med* 30:202–205, 2005.

28. Grant GJ, Barenholz Y, Bolotin EM, et al. A novel liposomal bupivacaine formulation to produce ultra-long-acting analgesia. *Anesthesiology* 101:133–137, 2004.

29. Malinovsky JM, Benhamou D, Alafandy M, et al. Neurotoxicological assessment after intracisternal injection of liposomal bupivacaine in rabbits. *Anesth Analg* 85: 1331–1336, 1997.

30. Seet B. Levels of medical support for United Nations peacekeeping operations. *Mil Med* 164:451–456, 1999.

INDEX